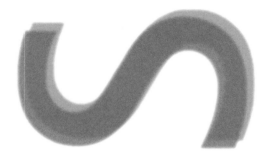
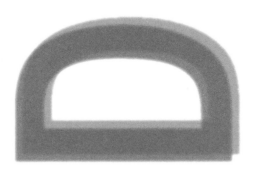
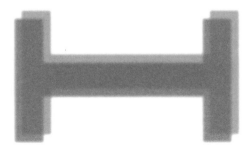
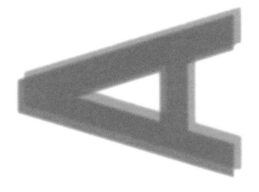

AIDS IN NIGERIA

A Nation on the Threshold

EDITORS

Olusoji Adeyi, MD, MPH, DrPH
Coordinator, Public Health Programs
World Bank
Washington, DC, USA

Phyllis J. Kanki, DVM, DSc
Director, AIDS Prevention
Initiative in Nigeria
Principal Investigator, APIN Plus/
Harvard PEPFAR
Professor of Immunology and Infectious
Diseases, Harvard School of Public Health
Boston, Massachusetts, USA

Oluwole Odutolu, MD, MBA
Senior Program Manager
AIDS Prevention Initiative
in Nigeria
Abuja, Nigeria

John A. Idoko, MD, FMCP
Professor of Medicine,
University of Jos
Director of APIN and APIN
Plus Programs
Jos University Teaching Hospital
Jos, Nigeria

Harvard Series on Population and International Health   *Distributed by Harvard University Press*

Published by:

Harvard Center for Population and Development Studies

9 Bow Street, Cambridge, MA 02138 USA

Sponsored by the AIDS Prevention Initiative in Nigeria
(www.apin.harvard.edu), through a generous grant
from the Bill & Melinda Gates Foundation

A copy of Cataloging-in-Publication data
is available from the Library of Congress.

ISBN 0-674-01868-0

The photograph on pages 2–3, by Dominic Chavez, was
provided courtesy of the *Boston Globe*.

The material contained in this volume was submitted as
previously unpublished material, except in the instance
in which some of the illustrative material was derived.

Great care has been taken to maintain the accuracy of
the information contained in the volume. However,
neither the publisher nor the editors can be held responsible
for errors or for any consequence arising from the use of the
information contained herein.

9 8 7 6 5 4 3 2 1

Photography by Dominic Chavez

Design by Laura McFadden

DEDICATION

*This book is dedicated to those battling the HIV epidemic in Nigeria—and
the millions of Nigerians living with the virus.*

ACKNOWLEDGMENTS

The editors are deeply grateful to the authors of *AIDS in Nigeria* for their contributions not only to this book but also to the fields of HIV/AIDS prevention, research, care, and treatment. We give thanks as well to those willing to share their lives with us through words and images.

We are indebted to the Bill & Melinda Gates Foundation, which awarded the Harvard School of Public Health with a $25 million grant in 2000 to create the AIDS Prevention Initiative in Nigeria (APIN). In partnership with government agencies, universities, and nongovernmental organizations in Nigeria, APIN strives to reduce the rate of growth of Nigeria's HIV epidemic and ultimately reverse its course. Without the support of the Gates Foundation, this book—and the work of APIN—would not have been possible. Luke Nkinsi and Helene Gayle played especially important roles in ensuring that the vision of APIN became a reality.

A number of other people deserve our gratitude. Managing editor Seyed Jalal Hosseini heroically coaxed chapters from harried authors. Before Jalal took on the role of shepherding the book, Hope Bryer and Sarai Walker played early roles in helping to shape it. Our consulting editor, Paula Brewer Byron, gave the book its humanistic touches—and provided us with invaluable publishing expertise. Our designer, Laura McFadden, contributed her visual talents and Matt Mayerchak his production prowess. Photographer Dominic Chavez helped translate the statistics of the epidemic through his powerful portraits of Nigerians affected by HIV.

The Advisory Council of APIN—Professor Adetokunbo Lucas, Professor Souleymane Mboup, Dr. Abdulsalami Nasidi, Professor Babatunde Osotimehin, and Professor Lateef Salako—provided outstanding guidance and inspiration. Professor Michael Reich contributed wise counsel to the book overall as well as to individual chapters. Dr. Jason Blackard spent long hours critiquing book chapters and requesting additional content. Our thanks also go to Professor Max Essex, Molly Pretorius Holme, Lendsey Melton, Guy Sciacca, Michael Simon, Connie Smith, Jean Weinshel, Anna Weiss, and Betsy Wise for their roles in ensuring the completion of this book.

PREFACE

Every minute a Nigerian man, woman, or child becomes infected with HIV. Soon Nigeria will be home to more people living with HIV than any other country in Africa. With 5 percent of its inhabitants already infected, Nigeria has reached the critical threshold that can catapult rates to nearly 40 percent of a country's population. The full magnitude of Nigeria's epidemic will be determined by its response now.

AIDS in Nigeria is intended to help guide that response. Written by dozens of the country's leading HIV experts, the book explores the dynamics of the epidemic, analyzes prevention efforts, identifies crucial gaps, and formulates effective strategies for controlling the epidemic. Complementing the experts' words are the dramatic portraits of people whose lives have been forever transformed by AIDS. Their stories reveal the human costs of the epidemic—and the courage required to overcome it.

We hope this book's reach will extend beyond Nigeria's borders, offering not only valuable lessons for other countries, but also inspiration, as it reveals a nation's determination to redirect what may seem like an inevitable, tragic course.

Olusoji Adeyi, MD, MPH, DrPH

Phyllis J. Kanki, DVM, DSc

Oluwole Odutolu, MD, MBA

John A. Idoko, MD, FMCP

FOREWORD

The HIV/AIDS pandemic has been the most serious natural disaster to hit the world in recent centuries. In the worst affected regions, notably sub-Saharan Africa, this steadily progressing catastrophe threatens to become a calamity of cataclysmic proportions.

The massive growth of literature on this subject reflects the extensive work that practitioners and scientists around the world are doing to confront the daunting challenge of HIV/AIDS. Writing mainly for specialist audiences, biomedical scientists have reported on the biology of the virus, the range of host responses to the infection, the clinical features of the disease, and innovations in treatment. For their part, social scientists have analyzed the cultural and behavioral aspects of the epidemic, as well as its impact on families, communities, and nations. This widening base of knowledge about the virus and its effects, accumulated over the past few decades, provides health practitioners and other stakeholders with critical information. This literature also tracks scientific discoveries and observations that we hope will generate improved technologies, including vaccines and new drugs.

Yet most of these publications offer research findings without providing a clear picture of their application to individual countries. Public health practitioners, policy makers, nongovernmental organization leaders, and other stakeholders face the difficult task of accessing this massive literature, identifying the best information to guide policies and strategies, and adapting the findings to the local situation. *AIDS in Nigeria: A Nation on the Threshold* provides a scholarly synthesis of the biological, social, behavioral, and economic features of HIV/AIDS as they apply to Nigeria. This country-based analysis provides a useful tool for all stakeholders involved in the control of Nigeria's epidemic.

In some respects, Nigeria has been granted several advantages over many other African nations. The epidemic reached the country at a relatively late stage, permitting health authorities to apply the valuable lessons other countries had already learned. Furthermore, the prevalence rates and patterns of progress of the epidemic show significant geographic variations within the country. The most recent sentinel survey, in 2003, showed that the HIV prevalence rate ranged from 1.2 percent in Osun State to 12.0 percent in Cross River State. This variation not only reflects the social and cultural diversity of a nation populated by hundreds of language groups, but it also may provide clues about the local determinants of the epidemic—information that can be translated into highly focused, effective interventions.

The dynamics of the epidemic in Nigeria—as in all countries—reflect the complex interaction of biological and social factors, as well as the effects of public health and medical interventions. The chapters in this book capture that complexity as they cover a range of relevant topics, from the evolution of the epidemic in Nigeria, to the biomedical and social dimensions of HIV/AIDS, to the national response to the crisis.

This volume had its genesis in the work of the AIDS Prevention Initiative in Nigeria, when people working on the frontlines—whether in laboratories or clinics or outreach sessions for sex workers—felt the need for a single, authoritative source on HIV/AIDS in Nigeria. For all its value, *AIDS in Nigeria* should be regarded as an interim report to be supplemented by later accounts as the epidemic continues to evolve. In the meantime, the information contained in this book will guide all stakeholders in making a more robust and effective response to the epidemic in Nigeria.

Adetokunbo O. Lucas, MD
Adjunct Professor
Harvard School of Public Health
Boston, Massachusetts, USA

CONTENTS

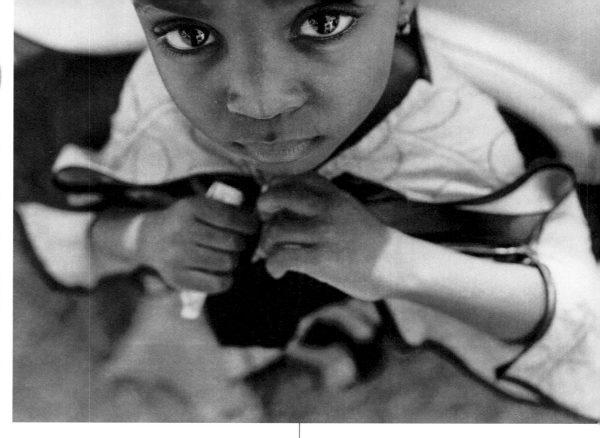

PART II: CONTROLLING HIV/AIDS IN NIGERIA

PART III: FUTURE POLICIES AND STRATEGIES

CONCLUSION

I

THE IMPACT OF THE EPIDEMIC IN NIGERIA

An Awakening to AIDS

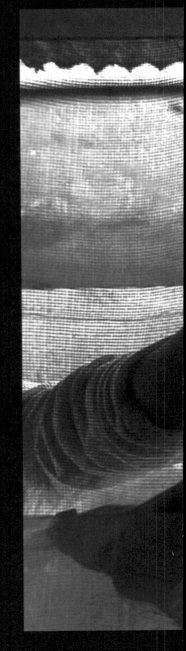

THE DAY SHE LEARNED SHE WAS INFECTED with HIV, Olayinka Jegede-Ekpe took to her bed and eventually fell into a troubled sleep, never expecting to awaken. The images she knew of AIDS had come from television and newspaper reports, which illustrated their stories with skeletons and skulls. The behavior of the doctors and nurses that day only confirmed her fears; they had stared at her as if she were a living corpse. When they broke the news,

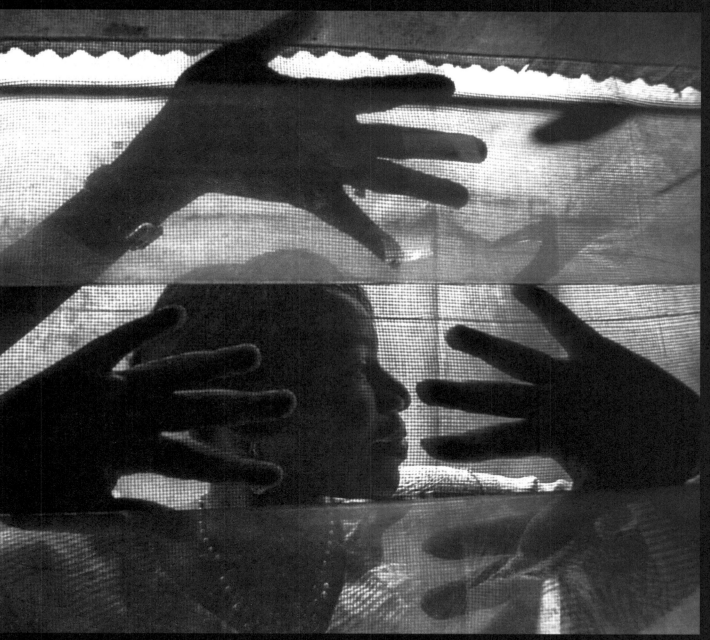

Olayinka Jegede-Ekpe is putting her energy into supporting other African women living with HIV/AIDS.

she expected death to be instantaneous. But the next morning she did wake up. "There, in the mirror," she says, "I looked just the same. I realized I wasn't dying immediately, so I thought, what should I do?"

It was 1997 and, like many of her fellow Nigerians, Jegede-Ekpe was ignorant of what it meant to be infected with HIV. Her country was still in denial about its growing epidemic, and the stigmatization of AIDS could sometimes be as deadly as the virus itself. One woman inadvertently betrayed her seropositive status on national television. Although the television producers had masked the woman's face, her clothes betrayed her identity. Her neighbors later stoned her to death.

Jegede-Ekpe feared similar retribution. Even more, though, she feared for the future of her country. So she decided to take her diagnosis public. "I was afraid," she says. "But I knew that Nigerian youth needed to hear about AIDS, that we were all vulnerable. I knew if I didn't speak out, millions of young people would soon be infected with HIV. And when I came forward, others would be willing to come forward."

The reactions were swift. Members of her church choir asked her to stop singing with them. The principal of her nursing school tried to expel her, and her fellow students shunned her. The administration installed a lock on the door to the women's bathroom in her dormitory and refused to give her a key. Yet Jegede-Ekpe fought for her rights, completed her training, and received her nursing degree.

The early stigmatization and discrimination she endured only fueled her determination to act on behalf of those infected. With a small group of activists, she helped establish the AIDS Alliance in Nigeria, the country's first organization for people living with HIV/AIDS. When she discovered she had been infected through the poor hygienic practices of her dentist, she demanded that he change those practices. As a prominent member of the National Action Committee on AIDS, she became active in helping to implement the country's HIV prevention policies. Her work with the Civil Society Consultative Group on HIV/AIDS in Nigeria and other organizations contributed to the adoption, by the federal government and several state governments, of the principle of "greater involvement of persons living with HIV/AIDS" in policy making and program development.

When Jegede-Ekpe realized that women's concerns were being neglected, she founded the Nigerian Community of Women Living with HIV/AIDS (NWC+). Now, as executive director of NWC+, she tries to empower women infected with HIV by teaching them their rights and providing them with gender-specific information about HIV/AIDS. Also through NWC+, she works to link together support groups of women living with HIV/AIDS across Nigeria and to empower others to become advocates for the human rights of women affected by AIDS.

Through this work, Jegede-Ekpe has lent a powerful voice to the large, growing, and often voiceless population of African women living with HIV/AIDS. Of the estimated 25 million HIV-infected people in sub-Saharan Africa, roughly 57 percent are women and girls.

"Many more African women than men are infected with HIV," she says. "Women have a biological vulnerability to HIV, as well as an economic one, and many cultural factors contribute to the high rates of infection among women in Africa. So I started focusing my attention on women, because we are the ones who will be dying at home or caring for people who are sick and dying of AIDS."

For her advocacy of people living with HIV/AIDS, Jegede-Ekpe was named a recipient of the prestigious Reebok Human Rights Award in 2004. She has used the grant that accompanies the award to bolster the work of NWC+. Her organization has since established an educational trust fund for orphans and a crisis fund for women. "Until women are seen as equal partners," she says, "all the science in the world will not solve the AIDS crisis."

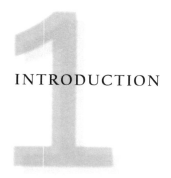

INTRODUCTION

Phyllis J. Kanki* and Olusoji Adeyi†

The HIV/AIDS epidemic has already devastated Nigeria, with nearly a million people dead and more than two million children orphaned. By 2003, the virus had infected approximately 5.0% of the adult population (1); within two years, an estimated four to six million Nigerians were carrying the virus.

In 2002, the National Intelligence Council identified the five countries expected to bear the heaviest burden of HIV infection in the expanding worldwide epidemic: India, China, Nigeria, Ethiopia, and Russia (2) (Figure 1-1). The council predicted that Nigeria and Ethiopia would be especially hard hit, with the number of people living with HIV/AIDS in Nigeria projected to balloon to ten to fifteen million by 2010, or as much as 26 percent of the adult population. Without effective prevention on a large scale, Nigeria will experience not only the tragedy of countless lives forever altered by the virus, but also untold adverse social and economic effects.

THE NATIONAL RESPONSE

Nigeria, like many countries around the world, initially responded to the epidemic with denial and little action (3,4). In 1987, the Nigerian government formed the National Expert Advisory

*AIDS Prevention Initiative in Nigeria, Harvard PEPFAR, and Harvard School of Public Health, Boston, Massachusetts, USA
†World Bank, Washington, DC, USA

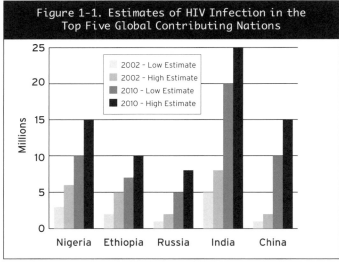

Figure 1-1. Estimates of HIV Infection in the Top Five Global Contributing Nations

Legend:
- 2002 - Low Estimate
- 2002 - High Estimate
- 2010 - Low Estimate
- 2010 - High Estimate

Y-axis: Millions (0 to 25)

X-axis: Nigeria, Ethiopia, Russia, India, China

Source: Eberstadt N. The future of AIDS. *Foreign Aff*, 2002;81(6).

Committee on AIDS. A year later, the National AIDS and STDs Control Program (NASCP), coordinated by the Federal Ministry of Health, replaced this advisory board. Yet the response remained tepid.

Nigeria's political leadership has since taken a more proactive approach to HIV/AIDS control (5), with an increase in local activities and external donor support. President Olusegun Obasanjo, elected in 1999, has been actively involved in HIV/AIDS prevention and control. In January 2000, the federal government, recognizing the need for a multisectoral approach, established a Presidential Committee on AIDS and a National Action Committee on AIDS (NACA). The government established the three-year HIV/AIDS Emergency Action Plan (HEAP) in 2001. That same year President Obasanjo created the Nigerian National ART Program with the purchase of anti-retrovirals (ARVs) for 10,000 adults and 5,000 children. He also hosted African heads of state for the first Organization of African Unity Summit on HIV/AIDS, Tuberculosis and Other Related Infectious Diseases, and he has continued to be a strong advocate and spokesperson for HIV prevention programs throughout Africa.

More recently, the government devised the National HIV/AIDS Strategic Framework, which is intended to guide the nation's response from 2005 to 2009. The partners implementing these plans include governmental institutions, nongovernmental organizations, community-based organizations, faith-based organizations, and people living with or affected by HIV/AIDS. NASCP, in the meantime, continues to take responsibility for the Nigerian health system's response to HIV/AIDS. It develops guidelines on key interventions and supports monitoring and surveillance of the epidemic.

Although data suggest that Nigeria's nationwide prevalence has not dramatically increased since 1999, the sheer magnitude of the population and the high prevalence rate together indicate a generalized epidemic. Since HEAP was written, all sectors—including advocacy, prevention, care, and treatment—have seen activity, yet the need remains great to scale these activities up significantly. For example, more than one million Nigerians would be considered eligible to receive antiretroviral therapy (ART), yet the fewer than 50,000 eligible patients treated by the end of 2005 represent only a fraction of those who need ART.

SPECIAL CHALLENGES FOR NIGERIA
IN TACKLING THE EPIDEMIC

Nigeria faces a number of important challenges in its efforts to control the HIV/AIDS epidemic, including widespread poverty, a large and youthful population, extensive variation in epidemic trends, and viral heterogeneity.

An Impoverished Population

With its annual income per capita below the average for other low-income countries, Nigeria is considered a "poor" nation (Table 1-1). The country's health status indicators also are worse than average; Nigeria spends less than average on health and has received less external aid than other low-income countries. The United Nations Development Programme has ranked Nigeria 152 out of 175 on the Human Development Index, a composite measure of income coupled with access to education and health services (6). By some estimates, two-thirds of Nigerians live on less than US$1 per day. Youth unemployment is a major problem, with estimates ranging between 40% and 60% (7).

Poverty—combined with economic vulnerability, institutional weaknesses, and sociocultural complexity—exacerbates the difficulties inherent in tackling the Nigerian epidemic. At the same time, an increased commitment by the government, local professionals, and civil society organizations and a growing international attention provide a basis for cautious optimism that the epidemic can be contained. The deciding factor may be the extent to which the country deploys local and international expertise to meet the challenge within the local context. The fact that the national HIV prevalence rate has been hovering in the 5% range suggests that such cautious optimism may be warranted. Increased efforts to demonstrate the efficacy of current programs will further support the view that the HIV prevalence has reached a plateau as a result of the national response.

A Youthful and Populous Nation

Nigeria's population has grown rapidly in recent decades. In 1991 the total population was 88.9 million, and projections by the National Population Commission of Nigeria estimated that by 2003 the population would rise to 133 million (8). The annual rate of growth of the Nigerian population is estimated at 2.8%. Nigeria has been undergoing a demographic transition from a high-fertility and high-mortality population to a low-fertility and declining-mortality population. The effect of this transition has brought about a population structure with a wide base of people younger than 15 years. While the median age of the population is 17 years, the 15-to-24-year age group constitutes about 20% of the population. Life expectancy rose from 45 years in 1963 to 51 years in 1991. More recently, however, the life expectancy has been falling, at least in part because of the HIV/AIDS epidemic. In 2002, life expectancy in Nigeria was estimated at 45 years. The infant mortality rate is 88.4 per thousand and the under-five mortality rate is 201 per 1,000.

Table 1-1. Selected Indicators of Development, Health Expenditures, and Outcomes		
Indicators	**Nigeria**	**Low-Income Countries (average)**
Population (millions, in 2002)	133	
Gross national income per capita in 2002 (US$)	300	430
Under-five mortality rate per 1,000 live births in 2002	201	121
Incidence of tuberculosis per 100,000 people in 2002	304	226
Average life expectancy at birth (years, in 2002) • Male • Female	 45 46	 58 60
Dependency ratio (young dependents as percent of working age population) in 2002	80	60
Health expenditure (in 2001, US$) • Total as % of gross domestic product • Public as % of gross domestic product • Health expenditure per capita	 3.4 0.8 15	 4.4 1.1 23
Aid dependency (as of 2002) • Aid as % of gross national income • Per capita (US$)	 0.8 2	 2.7 12

Source: World Development Indicators. Washington, DC: World Bank, 2004.

Note: Low-income countries are those with a gross national income per capita of $735 or less in 2002.

Wide Variations in Epidemic Trends

In just a few decades the HIV epidemic has reached global proportions, with approximately 40 million people infected worldwide. Since Nigeria's first AIDS case was reported in 1986, as many as six million Nigerians may have become infected with HIV. To estimate HIV prevalence rates in the country, beginning in 1991, the Federal Ministry of Health began conducting a countrywide survey of HIV infection in pregnant women, a representative population. These surveys show that the adult HIV prevalence increased from 1.8% in 1991 to 4.5% in 1996 and to 5.8% in 2001.

In 2001, the survey was expanded nationwide and readily demonstrated the incredible capacity of the country in its implementation. Conducted over a three-month period, the survey included approximately 300 pregnant women from each of 85 sites, which represented all 36 states and the Federal Capital Territory (FCT). More than 24,200 samples were collected and tested for HIV. A nationwide median prevalence rate of 5.8% was reported, ranging from 0.8% to 16.4% by state (9). In 2003, the nationwide survey was repeated, with a countrywide prevalence of 5.0% (10). All states and the FCT reported HIV infection, which in all cases exceeded 1%. Thus, Nigeria is experiencing a "generalized" epidemic, in which transmission within low-risk populations not only is occurring, but also is independently fueled by transmission from higher risk and "bridge" groups. In a country with such as sizable population, this represents a significant fraction of the worldwide pandemic.

A review of the prevalence figures from each of the states and the FCT demonstrates tremendous diversity in the rates of HIV infection, ranging from 1% to 16.4%. Although subject to continued discussion and speculation, it seems clear that multiple determinants must be considered to explain this tremendous heterogeneity in infection rates. HIV is thought to have entered the Nigerian population in the mid-1980s, just as it did with Nigeria's West African neighbors; however, the origin of the infection and the factors responsible for its early spread in the country remain unknown. Geopolitical zones and differences in ethnic, religious, and sexual networking are but a few of the many possible factors that contributed to the differences in HIV infection that we now appreciate decades later. As HIV continues to spread, it has become increasingly apparent that the epidemic does not follow the same course in different locales or among various subpopulation groups. This variation has complicated the task of monitoring the epidemic's course, planning intervention measures, and projecting needs for the care and support of infected people. Therefore, a thorough understanding of the nature of the epidemic, especially the factors enhancing the spread of the virus among different subpopulations, is still needed.

Until 2002, the federal government had monitored the epidemic primarily using cross-sectional sero-surveys of HIV infection. While this method has its merits, its inability to provide specific behavioral information on at-risk subpopulations or to explain changes in levels of infection in mature epidemics creates serious limitations. According to UNAIDS, such an understanding can only be achieved with more information on the most-at-risk subpopulations and on the behaviors that place them at risk (1). The second generation of HIV surveillance provides warning signals for the spread of HIV along with some important biological markers of spread. It also allows the identification of relevant high-risk and bridge populations. These data then provide the basis for development of targeted interventions. Because Nigeria demonstrates such cultural and ethnic diversity, obtaining up-to-date surveillance data with the best available methods is a critical first step in developing targeted interventions. To accomplish this step, it is crucial to have continued high-quality surveillance and monitoring systems as well as expanded scientific research.

Viral Heterogeneity

HIV, the first human lentivirus from the retrovirus family, was first described in the early 1980s coincident with the description of AIDS in the developed world. HIV integrates its genetic material into the infected host's DNA; therefore, infection is lifelong, even with currently available treatment. Although mortality is high without treatment, the incubation time from infection to AIDS can range from eight to ten years in the developed world.

Perhaps the most striking feature of HIV is its tremendous genetic diversity. Viral dynamics studies have indicated that 10^{12} virus particles are generated each day, with mutation occurring at every round of replication, suggesting that the high replication rate also contributes to viral genetic diversity (11).

This high degree of diversity has a number of important implications. First, there are two HIV types—HIV-1 and HIV-2—with a number of related viruses in non-human primates. Both HIV-1 and HIV-2 have been described in Nigeria and other parts of West Africa. Second, HIV-1 has multiple subtypes

(A–D, F–H, J, and K) and a number of circulating recombinant forms (CRFs), which are associated with significant transmission and disease in various populations worldwide (12). Molecular surveillance studies have made use of polymerase chain reaction (PCR) and molecular sequencing techniques to characterize the viral subtypes and describe their prevalence and geographic distribution worldwide. Subtype B, for example, accounts for an estimated 12.3% of cases worldwide, but infections with this subtype are primarily seen in the Americas, Western Europe, and Australia. Conversely, subtype C is estimated to have caused more than 47% of the worldwide infections, with highest incidence in southern African countries, Ethiopia, and India.

Areas of the world with a significant circulation of multiple viral subtypes also appear to have a unique and heterogeneous distribution of CRFs. CRF_02 A/G, originally described by David Olaleye from the University of Ibadan, has been considered the prototype West African HIV-1 subtype; the "IbNG" strain name designates Ibadan, Nigeria, as the source. CRF_02 A/G is responsible for a significant proportion of the new infections in Nigeria, as it is in other West African countries (12).

The status of HIV genetic diversity appears to be ever changing, with the possibility of additional new recombinant forms ever present. The potential for this event is highest in Africa, where multiple subtypes are actively circulating. The underlying causes of the varied geographic distributions are unknown and could conceivably represent founder effects, whereby viruses present in a given locale would predominate over time. This heterogeneity may also represent a complex interaction between viral parameters, however, such as infectivity, transmissibility, and immunogenicity, as well as host characteristics, such as genetic background and immune system competence.

Research continues into the mechanisms and impact of viral diversity, which represents a major obstacle to vaccine development. Current vaccine development approaches are often subtype specific, with most developed for the prototype subtype B, which is found predominantly in the United States and Europe. In recent years, some vaccine candidates have been developed for trials with non-B subtypes. A vaccine candidate for West African CRF_02 A/G has yet to reach human trials.

Triple-drug regimens have been shown to significantly prolong life in the developed world, yet HIV/AIDS treatment is complex and expensive. When Nigeria embarked on its national ART program in 2001, initial data indicated early efficacy in the first 50 patients treated with generic ARVs (13). It is well recognized, however, that the ultimate success and longevity of ART depend heavily on patient adherence. In addition, toxicity to different drugs in the multiple-drug regimens will be responsible for a significant proportion of patients who fail to benefit from ART over time. The Nigerian experience with these drugs is limited and based on clinical trials data conducted in the United States and Europe. The circulating HIV subtypes in Nigeria are distinct from subtype B; thus, it remains to be seen whether this distinction will alter the efficacy of these drugs or the rate at which drug resistance develops. Early data suggest a 10% to 17% baseline resistance to major classes of ARVs in viruses from Nigerians not undergoing ART (14,15). Therefore, the genetic diversity of Nigerian HIV-1 subtypes would seem to suggest that drug-resistance mutations might lower the overall efficacy of ART in Nigeria.

HIV/AIDS has created new challenges for physicians, other health care providers, and laboratory investigators. New methods to detect antibodies to HIV were needed for diagnosis, and although the simple rapid test and the enzyme-linked immunosorbent assay formats have been improved, they remain expensive for Nigerian patients. Furthermore, voluntary counseling and testing (VCT) programs are still based in urban centers, where they remain inaccessible to many Nigerians. Clinical management of HIV infection requires the regular measurement of CD4+ lymphocytes in the blood; these laser-based flow techniques are expensive and require a significant infrastructure to perform. In addition, the measurement of quantities of virus in the blood—known as viral load—is an important clinical parameter to evaluate the severity of disease and to monitor the efficacy of therapy. These expensive laboratory tests require complex technologies not previously used in much of the developing world. Scientists are devising new methodologies that they hope will be as sensitive as existing methodologies yet more cost effective. To accommodate these new and critical diagnostic clinical tools, Nigerian institutions will need ongoing training, capacity building, and infrastructure development. These requisites will grow even more acute as the country scales up its ART program.

THE POWER OF TARGETED INTERVENTIONS

Despite the rising toll of the global HIV/AIDS epidemic, compelling evidence—based on work in Senegal, Uganda, and Thailand—has emerged that early interventions can make a significant difference in reducing HIV infection rates and preventing explosive increases in AIDS (1). The most effective interventions have been multisectoral, with a high-level government commitment to tackle the problem, policy changes resulting from an awareness of the impact of HIV/AIDS on society, and the development of communications and media efforts, health interventions targeting high-risk populations, laboratory and field research, and scientific training.

HIV prevention initiatives include an array of education, behavioral change, and condom promotion programs. Through second-generation surveillance, the epidemiologic and behavioral characterization of high-risk and bridge populations provides the necessary data to design such interventions for maximum efficacy. The promotion of VCT centers provides a venue for community education and risk reduction messages, as well as the identification of HIV-infected individuals for intervention and treatment.

Programs that prevent sexually transmitted infections (STIs) through education, early diagnosis, and treatment are considered critical components to HIV prevention and intervention, as STIs are significant cofactors for HIV transmission. Population groups at high risk for HIV are similarly at high risk for STIs; therefore, HIV and STI prevention are often integrated. The monitoring of the efficacy of HIV prevention programs may include lowering of HIV incidence rates, while STI rates may serve as important proxy indicators of the success of HIV prevention programs.

In much of the developing world, HIV infection in pregnant women contributes to the spread of the epidemic through mother-to-child transmission. In 2004, more than 640,000 children under the age of 15 were infected with HIV, the vast majority in Africa. In that year alone, more than 75,000 infants were born with

HIV in Nigeria (16). Prevention-of-mother-to-child-transmission (PMTCT) programs that provide ARVs such as zidovudine and nevirapine to infected pregnant women and their exposed babies can significantly reduce HIV transmission rates. The use of triple-drug regimens to HIV-infected pregnant women can further reduce transmission to negligible rates; however, this has yet to be implemented in most of Africa.

PMTCT trials have demonstrated disturbing levels of nevirapine resistance (12% to 40%) in the HIV virus sequences from mothers receiving a single dose of nevirapine as part of typical developing country PMTCT programs (17). The nevirapine resistance in these mothers may diminish the efficacy of ARV regimens that include nevirapine, which becomes problematic because nevirapine is often used in the first-line drug regimens in most developing country ART programs.

Sentinel surveillance in Nigeria conducted on pregnant women throughout the country can help predict the magnitude of the impact of mother-to-child transmission on the epidemic. Nigeria has one of the world's highest numbers of children orphaned by AIDS, and already an estimated 290,000 Nigerian children are infected with HIV (1). PMTCT programs have been an important part of the Nigerian national response to the epidemic since 2001. Federal PMTCT centers were first established in seven target states providing HIV testing to pregnant women and single-dose nevirapine to thousands of HIV-infected women and their babies. Expansion and refinement of the Nigerian PMTCT program is under way, with different and more effective ARV combinations administered to both mothers and infants. Nonetheless, there is a critical need to provide broader coverage of these programs across the country. This will no doubt constitute a major challenge to the Nigerian PMTCT program in the short term. The infrastructure and capacity building needed for such a scale-up is substantial, as the PMTCT program is both expensive and medically complex.

Effective treatment is available to HIV-infected populations in most of the developed world. However, the costs and complexities of these treatment programs have prevented these lifesaving therapies from reaching the developing world. In recent years, international donor organizations have committed tremendous funds to provide treatment and care programs to African nations. In addition, many African governments, including that of Nigeria, have committed substantial resources to initiate and scale up national treatment and care programs. ART programs require enormous resources, training, capacity building, and infrastructure development. Training of physicians in HIV care and treatment is required, accompanied by significant bolstering of health care systems that are already constrained in most African nations. Thus, ensuring the sustainability of such programs needs to be considered in their design.

In 2004, more than 16,000 people living with HIV/AIDS were treated under the national ART program. The U.S. President's Emergency Plan for AIDS Relief (PEPFAR) program has since augmented the national program, providing treatment to 25,000 people and care to tens of thousands more by the end of 2005. Yet these treated individuals still represent only a fraction of the millions of Nigerians living with HIV/AIDS who will eventually require treatment. It is hoped that the increased access to treatment and care will augment prevention efforts, by decreasing societal stigma and lowering the transmission potential of treated patients.

CONCLUSION

Nigeria faces many challenges in dealing with its HIV/AIDS epidemic. Public education must play a key role in the success of prevention programs and increase the uptake of HIV testing. Behavioral change programs must encourage individuals to reduce their risk of HIV acquisition. The stigmatization and discrimination that have typified societal responses must be dealt with promptly, as they compromise the effectiveness of prevention programs. The early involvement and support of the government in the HIV/AIDS campaign set the necessary groundwork for a continuing strong leadership that will be critical for initiating and sustaining an effective nationwide prevention program. As Nigeria and much of Africa await more effective and affordable ARV interventions, additional scientific research will be necessary to monitor the epidemic, to consider unique aspects of the viruses required for therapeutic intervention, and to develop an appropriate HIV vaccine. Nigeria's remarkable progress in the past several years demonstrates the country's capacity and resolve to combat the epidemic. We remain optimistic that the country will rise to the occasion and meet its many challenges.

REFERENCES

1. UNAIDS/WHO. *AIDS Epidemic Update: December 2005.* Geneva: UNAIDS, 2005.

2. Eberstadt N. The future of AIDS. *Foreign Aff,* 2002;81(6).

3. Barnett T, Whiteside A. *AIDS in the Twenty-First Century: Disease and Globalization.* New York: Palgrave Macmillan, 2002:3–23.

4. Caldwell J. Rethinking the African AIDS epidemic. *Popul Dev Rev,* 2002;26(1):117–135.

5. Ajakaiye D. *Socio-economic Burden of HIV/AIDS Epidemic in Nigeria.* Ibadan: Nigerian Institute of Social and Economic Research, 2002:23–25.

6. United Nations Development Programme. *Human Development Report.* New York: United Nations Development Programme, 2004:141.

7. World Bank. *Memorandum of the President of the International Development Association and the International Finance Corporation to the Executive Directors on a World Bank Group Second Joint Interim Strategy Progress Report for the Federal Republic of Nigeria.* Washington, DC: World Bank, 2004.

8. National Population Commission of Nigeria. *Population Census of the Federal Republic of Nigeria: Analytic Report at the National Level.* Abuja: National Population Commission of Nigeria, 1991.

9. Federal Ministry of Health. *HIV/Syphilis Seroprevalence and STD Syndromes Sentinel Survey among PTB and STD Patients in Nigeria.* Abuja: Federal Ministry of Health, 2001.

10. Federal Ministry of Health. *HIV/Syphilis Seroprevalence and STD Syndromes Sentinel Survey among PTB and STD Patients in Nigeria.* Abuja: Federal Ministry of Health, 2003.

11. Wei X, Ghosh SK, Taylor ME, et al. Viral dynamics in human immunodeficiency virus type 1 infection. *Nature,* 1995;373(6510):117–122.

12. Kanki P. Viral determinants of the HIV/AIDS epidemic in West Africa. *BMJ, West Africa Edition,* 2004;7(2):69–71.

13. Idigbe E, Adewole T, Eisen G, et al. Management of HIV-1 infection with a combination of nevirapine + stavudine + lamivudine: a preliminary report on the Nigerian ARV program. *J Acquir Immune Defic Syndr,* 2005;40(1):65–69.

14. Agwale S, Zeh C, Robbins K, et al. Molecular surveillance of HIV-1 field strains in Nigeria in preparation for vaccine trials. *Vaccine,* 2002;20(16):2131–2139.

15. Ojesina A, Sankalé J, Odaibo G, et al. Subtype-specific patterns in HIV-1 reverse transcriptase and protease in Oyo State, Nigeria: implications for drug resistance and host response. *AIDS Res Hum Retroviruses,* 2006;in press.

16. Federal Ministry of Health. *HIV/Syphilis Seroprevalence in Antenatal Patients.* Abuja: Federal Ministry of Health, 2004.

17. Mofenson L. Advances in the prevention of vertical transmission of human immunodeficiency virus. *Semin Pediatr Infect Dis,* 2003:14(4):295–308.

2

THE EPIDEMIOLOGY OF HIV/AIDS IN NIGERIA

Abdulsalami Nasidi* and Tekena O. Harry†

During the past two decades, researchers have made significant progress in understanding the epidemiology of HIV/AIDS worldwide. Despite this improved understanding, the epidemic in Africa has continued to grow, with disastrous consequences. AIDS has begun to erase decades of health, economic, and social progress as it has reduced life expectancy, deepened poverty, exacerbated gender inequalities, lessened labor productivity, and eroded the capacity of governments to provide essential services.

Africa, with just over 10% of the world's population, carries well above 75% of the burden of this epidemic (1). While African nations are facing a virulent epidemic, there is no such thing as "the African epidemic." The continent shows tremendous diversity in the levels and trends of HIV infection. Prevalence rates in East Africa and southern Africa include some of the highest in the world, with prevalence rates exceeding 35% in Botswana and Swaziland. Rates have remained lower in West Africa, with no country having a rate above 10% and most having a rate between 1% and 5%. Across the continent, an increasing number of children are now either infected with the virus, through mother-to-child-transmission, or have lost one or both parents to AIDS. By all indications, HIV has continued to spread largely through unprotected sexual relationships between men and

*Federal Ministry of Health, Abuja, Nigeria
†Department of Immunology and Microbiology, University of Maiduguri Teaching Hospital, Maiduguri, Nigeria

women and through mother-to-child transmission. With the traditional support systems in these countries already under severe pressure, many extended families are—or soon will be—overwhelmed and in great need of external support and protective safety nets.

BACKGROUND

For many years now the devastating effects of HIV/AIDS on the world's population, particularly people in sub-Saharan Africa, have ceased to be in doubt. Unfortunately, realization of these effects came relatively recently to Nigeria, the continent's most populous country. For a long time many Nigerians viewed AIDS as a scourge of distant lands, or even a product of the imaginations of some scientists. The country has since become among the most affected countries in the world, however, and it now ranks second among sub-Saharan African nations in the number of HIV-infected adults (2).

History and Government Response
Nigeria's first two AIDS cases were diagnosed in 1985 in Lagos, the largest city in the country, and reported at the international AIDS conference that took place the following year (3). The reporting of those findings to the Federal Ministry of Health (FMOH) created panic in government circles. That same year the FMOH set up the National Expert Advisory Committee on AIDS (NEACA) and requested the assistance of the World Health Organization (WHO). In 1987, with this assistance, the government established the first of nine HIV testing centers in the country. As work continued, additional AIDS cases were diagnosed, and a small number of apparently healthy blood donors were found to be HIV antibody-positive through routine pre-transfusion screening.

Following the increasing detection of HIV-infected individuals in the country, NEACA recommended the development of a short-term plan to combat the spread of the virus. With the assistance of the WHO and under the guidance of NEACA, the FMOH implemented the comprehensive Medium-Term Plan for the nation's battle against HIV/AIDS. NEACA also played a key role in providing the initial epidemiologic information that was used for charting Nigeria's prevention and control strategies.

In 1988, the National AIDS Control Program replaced NEACA, still under the auspices of the FMOH. The program was expanded in 1991 to include sexually transmitted infections (STIs) and renamed the National AIDS and STDs Control Program (NASCP). Unfortunately, those changes altered the multisectoral approach of NEACA, as NASCP began to focus primarily on the health sector responses to HIV and other STIs. It developed guidelines on key interventions, which included syndromic management of STIs, voluntary counseling and testing (VCT), prevention of mother-to-child transmission of HIV (PMTCT), and management of HIV/AIDS, including treatment of opportunistic infections, administration of antiretrovirals (ARVs), and home-based care. It also supported monitoring and surveillance of the epidemic.

Despite these actions, it wasn't until the restoration of democracy in 1999 that the nation launched a serious effort to tackle the epidemic. President Olusegun Obasanjo has since placed high priority on HIV prevention, treatment, care, and support activities both in Nigeria and in the international community. In 2001, for example, he hosted the Organization of African Unity's first African Summit on HIV/AIDS, Tuberculosis, and Other Related Infectious Diseases.

President Obasanjo also replaced NASCP with a broader AIDS control program, which included the Presidential Committee on AIDS and the multisectoral National Action Committee on AIDS (NACA). This initiative further extended to all states through the state action committees on AIDS (SACAs) and to the district level through the local action committees on AIDS (LACAs). NACA was charged with developing policies for the prevention and control of HIV/AIDS, and its mandate included developing effective multisectoral response strategies nationwide (4). NACA developed the first multisectoral medium-term plan of action, the HIV/AIDS Emergency Action Plan (HEAP).

NACA's main responsibility then became the execution and implementation of activities under HEAP. The action plan had two main components: to break down barriers to HIV prevention at the community level and support community-based responses, and to provide prevention, care, and support interventions directly. Despite progress toward achieving these goals, huge gaps remained in HIV prevention, treatment, and care services, particularly at the community level. In 2004, the National HIV/AIDS Strategic Framework (2005–2009) was developed to succeed HEAP (4,5).

Civil Society and Uniformed Services

As soon as the government initiated its HIV/AIDS prevention and control program, several nongovernmental organizations, community-based organizations, and faith-based organizations established similar programs. A coalition—the Civil Society Consultative Group on HIV/AIDS in Nigeria, or CISCGHAN—was subsequently formed to help coordinate and advocate for this sector. Immediately after the group's establishment, the Global Fund to Fight AIDS, Tuberculosis and Malaria provided funds to help strengthen its work. In addition, the National Network of People Living with HIV/AIDS in Nigeria (NEPWHAN) organized, leading advocacy efforts for the human rights and greater involvement of people living with HIV/AIDS (PLWHAs) in all sectors. These associations—together with the military, police, and other uniformed services, which occupy critical positions within Nigerian society—contributed immensely toward HIV prevention and control. The Armed Forces Program on AIDS Control, apart from developing a military HIV/AIDS policy, also runs its own treatment, care, support, prevention, and laboratory service activities.

Demographic Profile

Nigeria, which is in West Africa, borders the Gulf of Guinea to the south, Benin to the west, Cameroon to the east, and Niger and Chad to the north. It is primarily rural, with a land area of 923,768 square kilometers and a population density of about 96.3 people per square kilometer. The most populous country in sub-Saharan Africa, Nigeria is also the tenth most populous country in the world. It has an estimated population of more than 130 million with 36 states and a Federal Capital Territory (FCT). Nigeria is subdivided into six geopolitical zones: North-West, North-East, North-Central, South-West, South-East, and South-South. Nigeria has more than 350 ethnic and linguistic groups, and its citizens have diverse religious and cultural backgrounds. Development is complicated by the poor economic status of the country, which has a human development index of 152 out of 175, placing Nigeria among the 25 poorest countries in the world (6).

Nigeria has been undergoing a demographic transition from a high-fertility, high-mortality population to a low-fertility, declining-mortality one. The base of the population pyramid is wide because of the large number of people younger than 15. The median age of the population is 17 years, and the 15-to-24-year age group constitutes about 20% of the population, with a 1:1 male-to-female ratio.

National Sentinel Surveillance

For strategies for the control of HIV/AIDS to succeed, the rates of HIV infection must be determined and the emerging trends in infection rates and risk-taking behaviors must be identified. One of the most efficient means of determining these rates and trends is to conduct sentinel surveillance surveys among specific groups of at-risk people within a specified time period. Thus, in 1991, the Federal Ministry of Health established the first HIV sentinel surveillance as a means of monitoring HIV/AIDS in the country. Subsequent surveys were conducted in 1993, 1995, 1999, 2001, and 2003 for a total of six national sentinel surveillance surveys between 1991 and 2003 (Figure 2-1) (7–10). These studies have shown that all 36 states now report HIV/AIDS, though the rates vary significantly from state to state and from zone to zone.

In Nigeria, HIV prevalence increased from 0.9% in 1986–1989, to 1.8% in 1991, to 4.5% in 1996. By 1999, 5.4% of people aged 15 to 49 were infected. In 2003, the prevalence was found to be 5.0% (Figure 2-2). The wide variation in HIV prevalence rates illustrates the importance of constant surveillance at several levels in a country as large and heterogeneous as Nigeria. In 2003, the states with the highest prevalence rates were Cross River (12.0%), Benue (9.3%), Adamawa (7.5%), and Akwa Ibom (7.2%); the FCT had a rate of 8.5%. The states with the lowest prevalence rates were Osun (1.2%), Ogun (1.5%), Ekiti (1.95%), Jigawa (1.95%), Ondo (2.2%), and Kebbi (2.6%) (Figure 2-2).

MODES OF TRANSMISSION

HIV is spread by sexual contact with an infected person and by blood or body fluid exchange through sharing of contaminated needles or transfusions of infected blood or blood clotting factors. Infants born to HIV-infected women may become infected in gestation, during birth, or through breastfeeding. Heterosexual transmission accounts for up to 80% of all HIV infection in Africa. Other transmission routes in Africa include injection drug use (2.8%), mother-to-child (2.6%), and blood products and transfusion (2.5%). Unknown modes of transmission result in 7% of HIV infections (11). In Nigeria, the heterosexual route of infection accounts for 82 percent of all transmissions and together with bloodborne and mother-to-child transmission account for the vast majority of different routes of HIV transmissions (12).

Sexual Route of Transmission

During heterosexual transmission, HIV can enter the body through the lining of the vagina, vulva, penis, rectum, or mouth, through vaginal, anal, or oral sexual intercourse (13–17). Based on gender-spe-

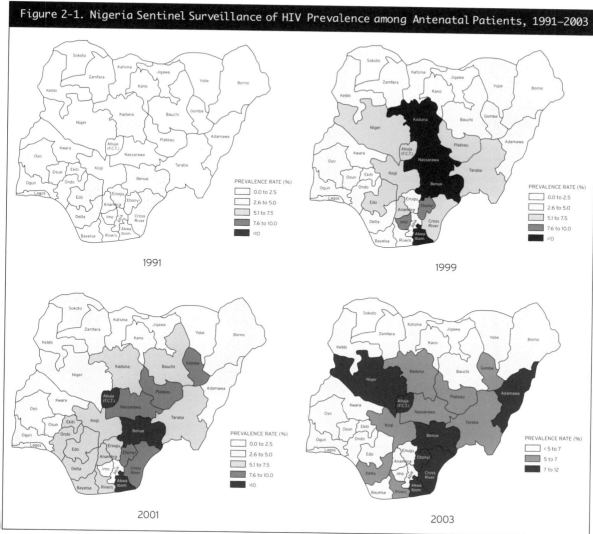

Figure 2-1. Nigeria Sentinel Surveillance of HIV Prevalence among Antenatal Patients, 1991–2003

1991

1999

2001

2003

PREVALENCE RATE (%)
0.0 to 2.5
2.6 to 5.0
5.1 to 7.5
7.6 to 10.0
>10

PREVALENCE RATE (%)
< 5 to 7
5 to 7
7 to 12

Source: Federal Ministry of Health. National HIV Seroprevalence Sentinel Surveys for 1991, 1999, 2001, and 2003.

cific anatomical and physiologic characteristics, it has been generally believed that male-to-female transmission is higher than female-to-male transmission. In addition, men tend to be more likely to have multiple sexual partners than women, which might contribute to HIV infection dynamics in heterosexual populations. Homosexual intercourse does not appear to contribute significantly to the HIV epidemic in Nigeria.

It has been well recognized that STI prevalence rates are generally high in Africa (13,14); this fact may reflect both casual attitudes toward sex and tendencies toward multiple sex partners in some African communities, as well as the lack of easily available treatment for STIs. Sex workers are considered important in the transmission of HIV and other STIs in Africa (14–20). Figure 2-3 depicts the increase in

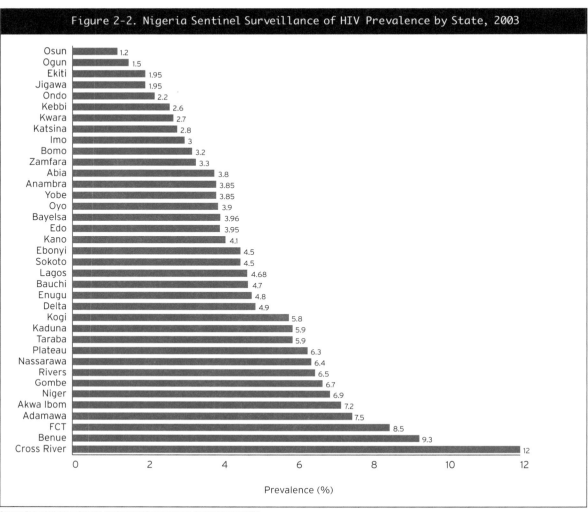

Figure 2-2. Nigeria Sentinel Surveillance of HIV Prevalence by State, 2003

State	Prevalence (%)
Osun	1.2
Ogun	1.5
Ekiti	1.95
Jigawa	1.95
Ondo	2.2
Kebbi	2.6
Kwara	2.7
Katsina	2.8
Imo	3
Bomo	3.2
Zamfara	3.3
Abia	3.8
Anambra	3.85
Yobe	3.85
Oyo	3.9
Bayelsa	3.96
Edo	3.95
Kano	4.1
Ebonyi	4.5
Sokoto	4.5
Lagos	4.68
Bauchi	4.7
Enugu	4.8
Delta	4.9
Kogi	5.8
Kaduna	5.9
Taraba	5.9
Plateau	6.3
Nassarawa	6.4
Rivers	6.5
Gombe	6.7
Niger	6.9
Akwa Ibom	7.2
Adamawa	7.5
FCT	8.5
Benue	9.3
Cross River	12

Prevalence (%)

Source: Federal Ministry of Health. National HIV Seroprevalence Sentinel Survey, 2003.
Abbreviation: FCT: Federal Capital Territory

HIV prevalence rates by risk group population surveyed over time, demonstrating higher rates of HIV prevalence among sex workers and STI patients than among antenatal populations (20,21).

The 2003 National HIV/AIDS and Reproductive Health Survey (NARHS) found that many Nigerians contract STIs during their sexually active years and engage in multiple-partner sex (22). Therefore, understanding the patterns of sexual behavior and partner exchange is important to gauge the forces driving the spread of HIV and other STIs in communities. This information can then be used to determine how intervention strategies may be adopted to curb further spread of HIV and other STIs and to minimize the impact of the HIV epidemic on the individual, the community, and society as a whole.

Mother-to-Child Transmission of HIV

Women can transmit HIV to their babies in utero, during birth, and through breast-feeding. Most infection is thought to occur at the moment of delivery (60% to 70%), followed by transmission through breast-feeding (20% to 30%), and then transmission in utero (less than 10%) (23). Without preventive interventions, approximately 25% to 40% of infants born to HIV-positive mothers will contract the virus. In the developed world with lower HIV prevalence rates, mother-to-child transmission has dropped to less than 2% with the implementation of universal VCT, ARV prophylaxis, elective Caesarean section, and the avoidance of breastfeeding (23). Unfortunately, in Nigeria and other countries with poor health systems, particularly poor maternal and child health programs, this transmission route continues to cause great concern.

Figure 2-3. Nigeria Sentinel Surveillance of HIV Prevalence in Sentinel Groups, 1991–2001

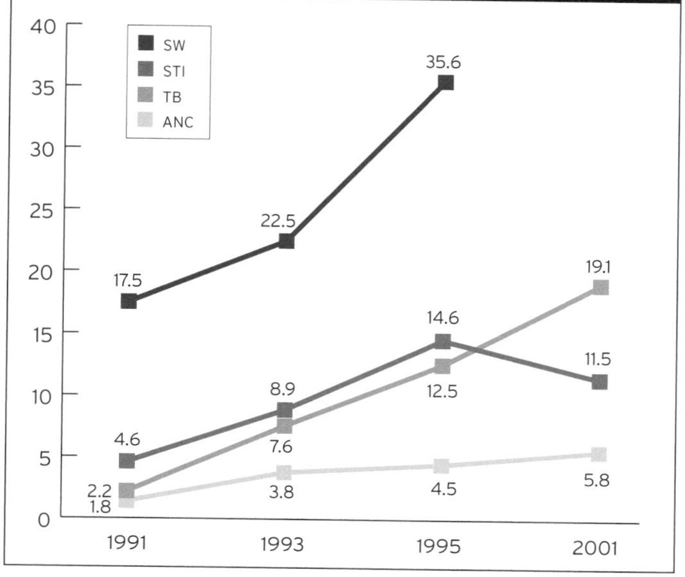

Source: Federal Ministry of Health. National HIV Seroprevalence Sentinel Surveys for 1991, 1993, 1995, and 2001.
Abbreviations: ANC: antenatal clinic attendees; TB: people with tuberculosis; STI: people with sexually transmitted infections; SW: sex workers

The key entry point to PMTCT programs is the VCT offered to pregnant women. The experiences of PMTCT programs in Nigeria and other African nations demonstrate that much of their success is determined by the proportion of women who agree to be tested for HIV, return to obtain their test results, and accept the ARV prophylaxis, which is often a single dose of nevirapine. The infrastructure, capacity building, and training are required to maximize the "uptake" of VCT, as well as the development of clinically proven ARV prophylaxis protocols.

ARV prophylaxis significantly reduces the rate of mother-to-child transmission of HIV. This consists of single or double ARVs during the last trimester of pregnancy or at delivery with a goal of lowering viral load to decrease the risk of transmission. Trials of various PMTCT protocols have been conducted in the developing world, yet viral drug resistance remains a problem (23,24). Although the current use of single-dose nevirapine to HIV-infected pregnant women does significantly reduce mother-to-child transmission, it also leads to the development of nevirapine resistance in 12% to 40% of women (23–25). The development of drug resistance in either the mother or infant compromises ARV provision since nevirapine is often used in first-line regimens for adults and infants in developing country programs (26).

To date, the use of various short courses of ARVs given during the last trimester of pregnancy reduce levels of viral load and significantly lower the risk of in utero and intrapartum infection. HIV transmission through breast milk, however, continues to be a major obstacle for PMTCT efforts, particularly in

Africa, where strong cultural and economic factors favor breast milk feeding rather than expensive breast milk substitutes. Furthermore, employment of safe breast milk substitutes is complicated by the fact that many HIV-infected women lack access to clean water and sanitation. Given these constraints, the development of successful HIV vaccines for pediatric use may prove invaluable for overcoming mother-to-child HIV transmission.

To understand the critical role mother-to-child transmission of HIV plays in Nigeria, it will be necessary to relate the poor reproductive health status in the country with the HIV prevalence among women of reproductive age. The 2003 NARHS found that Nigeria still has a high maternal mortality rate of 704 per 100,000 live births; this means that with about 2.4 million live births occurring annually, some 170,000 Nigerian women die as a result of complications associated with pregnancy or childbirth (22). The maternal mortality rate in Nigeria is about 100 times higher than those in industrialized countries. Moreover, only one-third of Nigerian women who gave birth in the last five years reported being attended to during their last delivery by skilled health care professionals. Thus, unless health care systems undergo a dramatic overall improvement, significant progress with widespread implementation of PMTCT programs will be difficult to achieve.

Nigeria initiated its PMTCT program in 2003 with a goal of reducing mother-to-child transmission of HIV by 50% in 2010. During 2003 and 2004, the AIDS Prevention Initiative in Nigeria supported 5 of the 11 federal PMTCT sites established.

Transmission Through Contact with Blood and Blood Products

Contact with infected blood is responsible for HIV transmission in many communities, particularly in those where screening of blood and blood products is not performed routinely, as is the case in much of Nigeria. Although blood bank centers exist at most tertiary care institutions, the support for a robust HIV blood bank screening program has been sorely lacking. In communities where blood bank screening and inactivation of blood products are routine, the risk of acquiring HIV infection from blood transfusion is extremely small. Nonetheless, as the HIV epidemic becomes more generalized in Nigeria, capacity building and support for a national blood bank screening program should be prioritized in the National AIDS Control and Prevention Plan (4).

The FMOH has developed a national protocol for proper blood bank screening of HIV. However, a number of gaps exist in enforcing adherence to the protocol, including pre- and post-test counseling of all donors, testing of donated blood using ELISA or rapid test before transfusion, and discarding blood that is reactive on the first ELISA or rapid test.

Transmission Through Needles and Other Skin-Piercing Procedures

The sharing of needles and syringes is considered the main route of HIV transmission among injection drug users. Injection drug use is uncommon in Nigeria, as it is in other parts of sub-Saharan Africa, and it is not considered a major mode of transmission in the Nigerian epidemic. Other modes of transmission may include the sharing of HIV-contaminated skin-piercing objects, such as blades, clippers, and injection needles. Skin-piercing instruments may be shared during tattooing, manicures, pedicures, and even barbering and shaving. Although these practices are widespread, there is a general lack of studies that verify or quantify their role in transmitting HIV infection. Nonetheless, we describe some of them below, as they play a role in Nigerian society's perceptions of HIV risk.

Tribal and medicinal scarification, group circumcision, and genital tattooing are common in Nigeria (27–29), particularly in the west among the Yoruba and the middle-belt region among the Tiv. Among these and some other Nigerian tribes, cuts are made for identification, beautification, and other ritual purposes. A proportion of the Hausa, an ethnic group in northern Nigeria, and some other northern tribes also engage in the practice of scarification for medical purposes. Another important traditional practice that may play a role in the transmission of HIV in Nigeria is an obstetric incision procedure performed at delivery termed a "gishiri cut." In this traditional Hausa practice, the wanzami, who are generally accepted as local surgeons by the Hausa community, use non-sterilized instruments.

The true risk of HIV transmission attributed to these practices has not been rigorously studied, yet these ethnically linked practices have been prominently included in HIV education and prevention messages throughout the country. This does not, however, exclude the possibility that HIV could be transmitted if instruments contaminated with infected blood are not sterilized or disinfected between clients.

In 1985, the U.S. Centers for Diseases Control and Prevention (CDC) and the WHO recommended standards and practices of good personal hygiene, food sanitation, and routine precautions that all personal-service workers — such as hairdressers, barbers, and massage therapists — should follow, even though there has been no evidence of transmission from a personal-service worker to a client or vice versa (11). It has been recommended that instruments intended to penetrate the skin — such as tattooing and acupuncture needles and ear-piercing devices — should be used once and disposed of or thoroughly cleaned and sterilized. Personal-service workers can use the same cleaning procedures as those recommended for health care institutions (11).

Transmission in Health Care Settings

HIV transmission in health care settings occurs when workers are stuck with needles or sharp instruments contaminated with HIV-infected blood or, less frequently, when workers are exposed to infected blood through an open cut or a mucous membrane, such as the eyes or nasal passages (30,31). Patients in African settings may be more likely to be infected with HIV, increasing the risk to health care workers if proper universal precautions are not well established. In developed countries, post-exposure prophylaxis is part of most health care policies. Post-exposure prophylaxis — a short course of triple-drug ART provided to prevent possible HIV infection (31) — has yet to be broadly institutionalized in Nigeria's health care facilities, though increased availability of ARVs should improve this situation in the near future.

Other Modes of Transmission

Although HIV is found in varying concentrations or amounts in blood, semen, vaginal fluid, breast milk, saliva, and tears, scientists agree that HIV does not survive long outside of the human body, making the possibility of environmental transmission extremely remote. Several studies have found HIV in very low quantities in the saliva and tears of some PLWHAs, yet the risk of exposure and infection via these fluids is considered minimal. Some people fear that, despite the lack of scientific evidence, HIV may be transmitted through air, water, and or insects. Even in Africa, where the fear of mosquitoes transmitting HIV is highest, mosquito transmission of HIV has never been reported. Studies conducted by researchers at the CDC and elsewhere have shown no evidence of HIV transmission through insects, even in areas where there are many AIDS cases and large insect populations (32,33).

Transmission of HIV During Wars and Civil Conflicts

In sub-Saharan Africa, the number of states at war or involved in significant lethal conflicts increased from 11 in 1989 to 22 in 2000 (34,35). In a survey conducted in Sierra Leone recently, Physicians for Human Rights estimated that 215,000 to 257,000 internally displaced women and girls experienced rape or other forms of sexual violence in war, as well as non-combat situations. This demonstrates the potential for women to be exposed to HIV during conflicts (36). Although Nigeria has not experienced a national war in the past 37 years, limited internal, inter-ethnic, and religious skirmishes have occurred in several regions. Moreover, women and children have become victims of forced sex and other human rights abuses. As no specific epidemiologic data exist to prove increased HIV transmission in those regions, additional research is needed.

Several studies have shown that HIV prevalence among soldiers in Africa is elevated, with prevalence rates as high as 60% in the militaries of Angola and the Democratic Republic of Congo (37). Many African military forces have infection rates as high as five times those of civilian populations (34–39). It is important to remember that HIV transmission does not end when conflict ceases; when infected soldiers return to their communities, they continue to spread the virus. In Nigeria, this trend was confirmed by the increased HIV seroprevalence among soldiers returning home from a peacekeeping mission (36).

TUBERCULOSIS AND HIV IN NIGERIA

Nigeria, with an estimated 259,000 cases, has the sixth largest population of people with tuberculosis (TB) in the world. The arrival of HIV/AIDS has caused a secondary tuberculosis epidemic in many African countries. Before the HIV epidemic, the incidence rate of new cases of tuberculosis had been estimated at 2 per 1,000 (40). This led to the estimation of 100,000 cases of tuberculosis occurring every year in Nigeria. The WHO now estimates that the incidence is 3.05 per 1,000, implying a 50% increase in the incidence rate (41). These dramatic increases in TB are thought to be because of the expanding HIV epidemic and the strong biological association between HIV and *Mycobacterium tuberculosis*. It is estimated that at least 50% of sub-Saharan Africans are living with latent tuberculosis infection, which can be reactivated during periods of diminished immunity, as seen following HIV infection.

Nigeria's National Tuberculosis and Leprosy Control Program was formally launched in 1991 to address tuberculosis and leprosy infections in a comprehensive manner. The overall objective of the program is to reduce the prevalence and incidence of the disease to a level at which it no longer constitutes a public health problem in the country. In some states, the tuberculosis problem has not been addressed adequately due to a lack of funds for anti-TB drugs, weak laboratory services, and inadequate training of health personnel in the current protocol for TB management and control. As of 2002, functional TB control services were available in 22 of the 36 states and the FCT.

HIV seroprevalence studies that have been carried out regularly among TB patients in Nigeria have demonstrated a rapid increase in prevalence of HIV infection among TB patients (Figure 2-3). In 1991, the seroprevalence of HIV in tuberculosis patients was 2.2%; it has risen rapidly and was found by 2003 to be 19.1% (9,10,40). Conservative estimates suggest that at least 1 million adults in Nigeria are coinfected with HIV and TB.

Although the number of TB cases detected has been increasing over the years, the number falls well below the estimated incidence for the country as a result of the relatively limited coverage. To manage the increasing burden of tuberculosis, the directly observed therapy, short course (DOTS) expansion plan has been developed as the National DOTS Expansion Strategic Plan, 2002–2005. This will ensure ongoing training of DOTS providers and social mobilization for TB control. Quality control of TB diagnostic and treatment services will be ensured through supervision and monitoring. Furthermore, to foster the collaborative effort of TB and HIV/STI control programs, a TB/HIV working group was established in February 2002. In this regard, the 25 recently established ARV centers in the country will also implement DOTS, while HIV counseling programs will be made available in TB centers implementing DOTS.

THE NIGERIAN HIV/AIDS EPIDEMIC

A 2004 report from UNAIDS the United Nations projected that more than 80 million Africans could die from AIDS by 2025, and infections could soar to 90 million—or more than 10 percent of the continent's population (1). Sub-Saharan Africa carries the largest burden of the global pandemic; more than 25 million Africans have been infected with HIV (1). The HIV prevalence in many other African countries, especially those in East Africa and southern Africa, is much higher than that of Nigeria. For example, Kenya's prevalence rate is 15%, South Africa's is 20%, Zambia's is 21.5%, and Zimbabwe's is nearly 34% (Figure 2-4). The higher infection rates in these countries may be attributed to an earlier start of the epidemic, different behavior patterns and risk factors, more pathogenic and/or transmissible strains of HIV, a variation in susceptibility to HIV, or a combination of these factors.

For many years, Nigeria was considered to be at a relatively early stage of the HIV/AIDS pandemic compared to the more heavily affected nations of East Africa and southern Africa and even some countries of the West Africa, such as Côte d'Ivoire and Ghana. Although Nigeria's prevalence rate is lower than those of neighboring countries, because of its large population size, it has the second highest number of HIV-positive adults in sub-Saharan Africa. It ranks third in the world in terms of the total number of people infected, behind India and South Africa (1,2).

One commonly used measure of the extent of HIV infection in a population is adult prevalence, or the proportion of adults infected with HIV in a given population. Studies in a number of African countries have shown

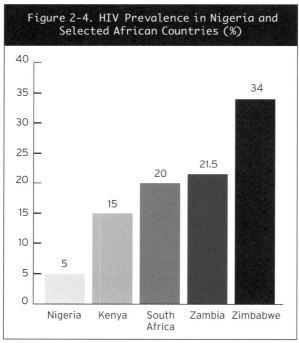

Figure 2-4. HIV Prevalence in Nigeria and Selected African Countries (%)

Source: UNAIDS. *2004 Report on the Global AIDS Epidemic.* Geneva: UNAIDS, 2004.

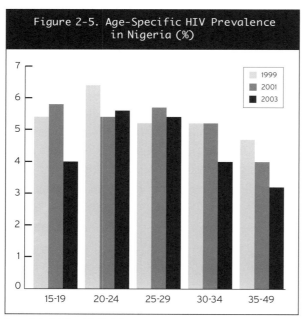

Figure 2-5. Age-Specific HIV Prevalence in Nigeria (%)

Source: Federal Ministry of Health. National HIV Seroprevalence Sentinel Surveys for 1999, 2001, and 2003.

that HIV prevalence among pregnant women is a good estimate of prevalence among all adults between the ages of 15 and 49 (7–10). These surveys—coupled with high-quality behavioral data collection—can provide important information on the status of the epidemic. Nigeria's most recent national sentinel surveillance study, in 2003, tested more than 85,000 women from 86 sites throughout the federation (10). The survey estimated that of the millions of Nigerians living with HIV/AIDS, 48% are women and 7.7% are children. More than 25,000 deaths occur from AIDS annually and close to 2 million AIDS orphans now live in Nigeria (2).

Patterns of Infection by Age

When the cases of HIV infection identified in the surveys were broken down by age and sex, the distribution showed that most infections were in men and women between the ages of 20 and 39 years (Figure 2-5) (10). The survey also showed that more males were infected than females. This higher ratio of males to females has been previously described in other African countries and is usually seen in the early phases of the epidemic. As the HIV epidemic matures, the ratio reverses and women are more affected. To more adequately address age- and gender-specific trends, a population-based survey of HIV prevalence is necessary but has yet to be done.

Although the prevalence rate decreased slightly from 5.8% in 2001 to 5.0% in 2003, it is not known whether that drop is statistically significant (Figure 2-6) (7–10). It may also be due to differences in study design between the two surveys. As always, it is not clear whether the antenatal population studied in the national sentinel surveillance is representative of the country. Nonetheless, it would be encouraging to believe that this slight decline is attributable to Nigeria's nationwide prevention campaigns. In the recent past, other African countries such as Uganda and Zambia have experienced similar slight declines in HIV prevalence during enhanced government efforts to increase support for prevention and control activities. Regardless, the statistical trend would still suggest caution in interpreting small differences in the national HIV prevalence (Figure 2-6).

Forces Driving the Spread of HIV in Nigeria

Among the most important factors driving the HIV epidemic in Nigeria are sexual behavior, the presence of other STIs, stigmatization and discrimination, cultural factors, and the inadequacy of health care systems.

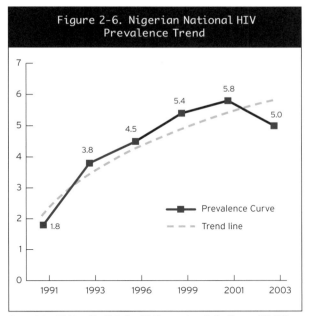

Figure 2-6. Nigerian National HIV Prevalence Trend

Source: Federal Ministry of Health. National HIV Seroprevalence Sentinel Surveys, 1991-2003.

Sexual Behavior

The sexual behavior determinants of HIV transmission are often difficult to study and identify. For cultural and religious reasons, sex is traditionally a very private subject in Nigeria, as in many other African nations. Discussions about sex with adolescents, particularly girls, are not considered culturally acceptable. Until recently, young people received little or no sexual health education, which has proved a major barrier to behavioral interventions aimed at reducing rates of HIV and other STIs. The lack of accurate information about sexual health has fostered myths and misconceptions, contributed to rising transmission rates, and helped fuel the stigmatization and discrimination of PLWHAs.

The 2003 NARHS confirmed that virtually all respondents surveyed over the age of 30 had had sexual intercourse (22). Among the respondents who had never married, about 39% of females and 48% of males reported that they had had sexual intercourse in the past year. The same survey showed that the median age at first sex was 16.9 years for females and 19.8 years for males. Females in the North-West and North-East zones reported the lowest median age at first sexual intercourse. The median age of first sex for both females and males was lower in rural areas than in urban areas.

An important behavioral determinant of HIV sexual transmission is the level of multiple partnering within a community. Of all respondents who have ever had sex, only 3% women reported having multiple partners, compared to 26% of men. Different zones, age groups, and levels of education showed substantial differences (22). For women, the lowest levels of multiple partnering were reported in the North-West (1%) and the North-East (2%) zones, while the highest for males was from the North-Central zone (33%), which may explain the extensive HIV transmission observed within this zone. Interestingly, females with higher levels of education were more likely to report having multiple partners.

Other Sexually Transmitted Infections

STIs pose a major public health problem as they affect hundreds of millions of people globally with far-reaching health, social, and economic consequences. Although the probability of transmitting HIV during a single sexual act can be low, such factors as frequency of intercourse and a multiplicity of partners can increase the risk of infection dramatically. Among those factors is the presence in either partner of an STI, the practice of multiple partner sex, and a high prevalence of STIs among men who have sex with men. Some cultural practices—including female circumcision and infibulation—may influence sexual transmission in Africa (28,29).

The level of awareness of STIs and their symptoms in Nigeria is generally high, though it is generally lower among women (22,42). The NARHS showed that STI symptoms were most commonly seen in South South at 10%, while the lowest (2%) was seen in the North-East zone (22). Generally, women were more likely to report having experienced STI symptoms in the last year. For both sexes, genital ulcers were the least reported symptom (1%), while itching was the most commonly reported symptom (4%). Sexually active adults with higher levels of education were more likely to report genital discharge or genital itching. Among sexually active individuals, 8% and 4% of females and males respectively had at least one of these symptoms in the preceding 12 months.

The most commonly used sources for STI treatment included government health institutions (24%), traditional healers (17%), and private health institutions (14%). Urban dwellers reported higher use of government health institutions and private health facilities, while a higher proportion of people living in rural areas received treatment from traditional healers. Some traditional healers in Nigeria have continued to claim having new treatments for HIV/AIDS and have even challenged orthodox medical centers with their claims.

Stigmatization and Discrimination

Stigmatization and discrimination against PLWHAs are common in Nigeria. Often both Christian and Muslim religious leaders view immoral behavior as the cause of the HIV/AIDS epidemic. PLWHAs often lose their jobs or are denied health care services because of the ignorance and fear surrounding the disease. Moreover, early surveys showed that 60% of health care workers believed HIV-infected patients should be isolated from other patients. Nevertheless, some progress has been made more recently because of increased national campaigns and more visible and vocal societies and support groups for people infected with or affected by HIV. Their efforts have helped educate the public about HIV/AIDS, dispelling myths and giving the disease a human face.

Cultural Factors

Nigeria is a male-dominated society and women are viewed as inferior to men. Women's traditional role is to have children and be responsible for the home. Their low status, their lack of access to education, and certain social and cultural practices increase their vulnerability to HIV infection. Many marriage practices violate women's human rights and contribute to increasing HIV rates among women and girls. Nigeria has no legal minimum age for marriage, and in some areas early marriage is still the norm, as parents consider it a way to protect their young daughters from the outside world and maintain their chastity. Girls may get married between the ages of 12 and 13, and a large age gap usually exists between husbands and wives. Young married girls are at risk of contracting HIV from their husbands because it is considered acceptable for men to have sexual partners outside of marriage and even for some men to have more than one wife. Because of their age, lack of education, and low status, young married girls cannot negotiate condom use to protect themselves against HIV and other STIs.

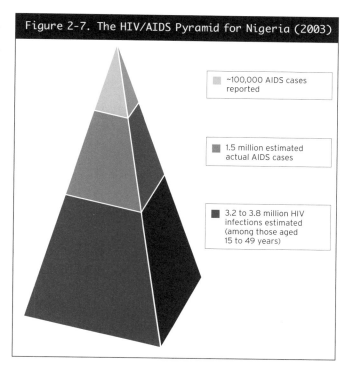

Figure 2-7. The HIV/AIDS Pyramid for Nigeria (2003)

~100,000 AIDS cases reported

1.5 million estimated actual AIDS cases

3.2 to 3.8 million HIV infections estimated (among those aged 15 to 49 years)

Inadequate Health Care Systems

Until democracy was reestablished in 1999, Nigeria's health care system had deteriorated significantly because of political instability, corruption, and a mismanaged economy under military rule. Large parts of the country still lack even basic health care provision, making it difficult to establish HIV testing and prevention services such as those for PMTCT and HIV/AIDS treatment and care. Sexual health clinics provide contraception, but testing and treatment for STIs are frequently absent.

Projections for the Epidemic

The HIV/AIDS Pyramid

By the end of 2003, an estimated 100,000 AIDS cases had been officially reported in Nigeria. Since then, all states have reported cases. The number of AIDS cases, however, represents only the clinically visible portion of the epidemic, as many more people are HIV infected than have received a clinical AIDS diagnosis (Figure 2-7). In addition, official reporting of AIDS is thought to represent only a fraction of actual cases, with estimates for 2003 of 1.5 million (1,2). Because of the long incubation period of HIV infection and the time to disease, it is generally believed that the number of AIDS cases represents less than half of all those infected with HIV. Thus, the 1.5 million AIDS cases would correspond to 3.2 to 3.8 million people infected with the virus. The number of new cases occurring in future years is a reflection of the number of individuals already infected with HIV but who have not yet developed the disease. New infections would increase the pyramid base and contribute to larger numbers of AIDS cases in the future. Even if new infection rates were to drop to zero, AIDS cases would still be detected for years to come.

Using these data, UNAIDS has predicted that the number of Nigerians infected will continue to rise through 2010 (42). Under the lower-prevalence scenario, the number would rise steadily, reaching a plateau of 5.5 million in 2010. In the higher-prevalence scenario, the number of infected people would continue to climb, reaching 8.4 million by 2015.

HIV/AIDS Underreporting in Nigeria

AIDS projection models are based on a number of important assumptions specific to the model and the validity of the data used. As epidemics mature, models and their projections tend to become more useful. At least one reason for this is the increased accuracy of the data used. HIV infection rates and the number of reported AIDS cases heavily depend on well-designed studies or systems to accurately reflect these important statistics. It is therefore not surprising that we have repeatedly seen underreporting of both HIV infection and AIDS cases, particularly early in a country's epidemic. The following reasons may have contributed to the underreporting of AIDS in Nigeria:

- The stigma of AIDS may discourage PLWHAs from seeking medical care;
- Health care workers may not want to record an AIDS diagnosis because of the stigma attached to the disease;
- Some people with HIV infection may die of other diseases before they are diagnosed with AIDS;
- Some rural hospitals and district heath care facilities may not have the capability to test for HIV infection, or may not be able to recognize the disease;
- Most private clinics and laboratories do not report their HIV/AIDS statistics; and
- Misdiagnosis, attributing HIV disease to other ailments.

Life Expectancy and Mortality

One dramatic impact of AIDS deaths is the decline in life expectancy. The impact of HIV/AIDS on life expectancy at birth is felt through the various age groups most affected by HIV/AIDS. Infants who are born HIV infected, or who develop HIV through transmission from their mothers, have a shortened lifespan, as discussed earlier. Most HIV infections occur, however, among those in their early to mid-20s in Nigeria, which means, with an incubation period of 5 to 8 years, they may die in their early 30s.

The United Nations projection model estimates the effect of HIV/AIDS on a country's life expectancy (42). It shows that life expectancy had already fallen to about 45.5 years in 2002, from 53.0 years in 1990. If the epidemic did not exist, the current life expectancy rate would have been about 57 years. Again, without the epidemic, life expectancy should gradually improve, reaching nearly 62 years by 2015. However, the significant mortality associated with HIV/AIDS will diminish any positive effects that might have occurred as a result of other improvements in life standards and health care. Fortunately, the effects of the epidemic are reversible in the long-term if the epidemic is brought under control by effective prevention and therapeutic programs. This is forecast by the fact that life expectancy is expected to begin to rise after 2012, the time at which the prevalence is expected to level off (42).

The epidemic will increase the death rate in all age groups (Figure 2-8). The impact will be most severe among adults in their prime working years and among children under the age of five. Without AIDS, we would have expected a slight increase in the number of deaths per year, mainly due to the increase in the size of the population. The crude death rate in Nigeria is 14 per 1,000, which implies approximately 1.65 million deaths annually. However, the number of deaths among people in the 15- to 49-year age group is usually small because that group typically represents the healthiest fraction of the population. The HIV/AIDS epidemic has reversed this trend. In 2000, more than 100,000 Nigerians died of AIDS. This rapid increase in deaths in this productive age group will have serious consequences for the economic and social development of the country.

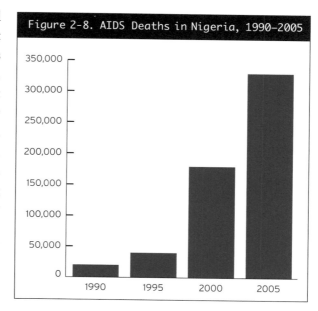

Figure 2-8. AIDS Deaths in Nigeria, 1990–2005

From the beginning of the epidemic through 2000, the cumulative number of AIDS deaths has been estimated at 800,000 — and the worst is yet to come. By 2010, an additional 4.3 to 4.7 million people in Nigeria could die from the disease (42). Under the high-prevalence scenario, by the year 2015, the cumulative number of AIDS deaths could reach a staggering 9.4 million.

Demographic and Sociocultural Impact

Generally, because of the severity of the HIV/AIDS epidemic on the African continent and the speed of its spread and impact on mortality, AIDS is now the leading cause of death in Nigeria. In its report *AIDS in Africa*, UNAIDS examines three potential scenarios for the continent in the next 20 years depending on the international community's response (43). Researchers determined that even with massive funding and better treatment, the number of Africans who will die from AIDS is likely to top 67 million in the next two decades. This is the total population of more than ten countries on the continent and may constitute 20% of the total population of the entire continent by that period.

From this interpretation and the projection for the epidemic and its impact on the African continent, it is obvious that the global AIDS epidemic is one of the greatest challenges facing Nigeria and, in fact, the most serious public health and international development problem. The epidemic has such far-reaching social and economic dimensions that it requires a multisectoral approach, one that addresses gender inequities and homelessness among AIDS-affected families, improves farm productivity to shore up agrarian incomes against hard times, provides shelter and education for orphans, enlists the help of traditional healers in education campaigns, and pursues dozens of other promising interventions.

PREVENTION OF HIV TRANSMISSION

The main thrust of HIV prevention strategies in Nigeria is based on the following: information, education, and communication; condom promotion; behavior change; and vaccine development. Since 2000, the government of Nigeria, with outside support and the help of nongovernmental organizations in the country, has been conducting public education campaigns about HIV/AIDS. Interventions currently being used to limit transmission include promoting abstinence before marriage; encouraging, through a combination of mass media campaigns and counseling, faithfulness to one partner; and various HIV education programs. Although some of these efforts are likely to bear fruit if they are sustained and spread across the entire country, prevention efforts are at risk of being eclipsed by official, popular, and international emphasis on ARV therapy. Again, poverty, enormous cultural and religious diversity, and an increased allocation of funds to AIDS treatment threaten the maintenance of effective prevention and control strategies.

Overall, there are several important lessons to be learned about prevention. Pilot tests have shown that interventions can be successful in significantly reducing the spread of HIV. It is important to intervene as early as possible with a mix of interventions that have proved effective in reaching the largest possible number of people and that can achieve maximum impact. The most effective interventions are those that focus on population groups with the highest transmission rates. Prevention through behavior change, condom promotion, and STI treatment is thought to be the most cost effective approach.

Applying interventions on a large scale is costly, and success is difficult to measure. Yet there is now evidence from Senegal, Uganda, and Thailand that significant reductions in HIV incidence and prevalence can occur at a national level. Those countries recognized the seriousness of the epidemic early and implemented strong national programs to reduce the spread of HIV and to support PLWHAs and their families.

CONCLUSION

By the time the first two AIDS cases in Nigeria were reported in 1986, much had been learned about the character of the epidemic from other African countries and beyond. From 1986 to 1990, only a few AIDS cases were reported in Nigeria, even in major hospitals where conscious efforts were made to find cases. In the hospitals that screened blood routinely, the percentage of HIV antibody-positive blood units remained below 1% during the same period. Nigeria had the opportunity to limit the spread of HIV by instituting elaborate measures across the country. Unfortunately, this did not happen. Now the country appears to be paying the price for a less than vigorous response to the HIV/AIDS problem at the early stage of the epidemic.

There is an increasing volume of data on the spread of HIV generated now in Nigeria and most of these are based on the population-based surveys with HIV testing. Since 1999 serological surveys have shown evidence of HIV infection in all geographic locales sampled. Since 1991 surveys, pregnant women have consistently shown the lowest HIV prevalence rates, and increased HIV infections have been identified in sex workers and TB patients. Nigeria now has a significant HIV/AIDS problem, and it needs to commit attention and resources to prevent further deterioration of the situation.

Improvement of the health system and medical care services especially at the level of primary health care could help reduce HIV transmission and strengthen case management. Increasing levels of poverty could indirectly affect the increase in the prevalence of HIV in Nigeria. Moreover, the poor level of maternal health system in the country may enable further transmission of HIV.

Most prevention programs have failed, in part because they were not evidence based on the appropriate specific population group, the behavioral and cultural factors involved, and the mechanism of transmission. To develop effective prevention and control strategies, therefore, it is important that we understand the multiple cultural characteristics of the population and address issues of worsening poverty and the negative impact of frequent conflicts and wars on our efforts. Ultimately, HIV/AIDS will not diminish in Africa until sociocultural, gender, and economic inequities are addressed in a meaningful manner.

ACKNOWLEDGMENTS

We wish to acknowledge the immense contributions of the following in the preparation of this chapter: Dr. Sani Gwarzo, Dr. Mohammed Muktar, Dr. Levi Uzono, and Dr. Johnson Onoja. The efforts of the Federal Ministry of Health secretariat — Dr. Aliyu Gumel and Ms. Lola Adeniji — and the support of Dr. Nasidi's deputy, Dr. Razaq Gbadamosi, are highly appreciated.

REFERENCES

1. UNAIDS. *2004 Report on the Global AIDS Epidemic.* Geneva: UNAIDS, 2004.

2. UNAIDS. *Epidemiological Fact Sheet Nigeria, Update 2004.* Geneva: UNAIDS, 2004.

3. Nasidi A, Harry TO, Ajose-Coker OO, et al. Evidence of LAV/HTLV III infection and AIDS-related complex in Lagos, Nigeria. *II International Conference on AIDS*, Paris, France, June 23–25, 1986 (abstract FR86-3).

4. Federal Ministry of Health. *HIV/AIDS Emergency Action Plan.* Abuja: Federal Ministry of Health, 2001.

5. National Action Committee on AIDS. *HIV/AIDS National Strategic Framework: 2005 to 2009.* Abuja: National Action Committee on AIDS, 2005.

6. United Nations Development Program. *Human Development Report.* New York: United Nations Development Program, 2004:141.

7. Federal Ministry of Health. *1991 National HIV Seroprevalence Sentinel Survey.* Abuja: Federal Ministry of Health, 1991.

8. Federal Ministry of Health. *1999 National HIV Seroprevalence Sentinel Survey.* Abuja: Federal Ministry of Health, 1999.

9. Federal Ministry of Health. *2001 National HIV Seroprevalence Sentinel Survey.* Abuja: Federal Ministry of Health, 2001.

10. Federal Ministry of Health. *2003 National HIV Seroprevalence Sentinel Survey.* Abuja: Federal Ministry of Health, 2003

11. Federal Ministry of Health. *Handbook on HIV/AIDS Management for Healthcare Workers.* Abuja: Federal Ministry of Health, 1992.

12. UNAIDS Reference Group on Estimates, Modelling and Projections. Improved methods and assumptions for estimation of the HIV/AIDS epidemic and its impact: recommendations of the UNAIDS Reference Group on Estimates, Modelling and Projections. *AIDS*, 2002;16:W1–W14.

13. Piot P, Quinn TC, Taelman H, et al. Acquired immunodeficiency syndrome in a heterosexual population in Zaire. *Lancet*, 1984;2:527–529.

14. Kreiss JK, Koech D, Plummer FA, et al. AIDS virus infection in Nairobi prostitutes: spread of the epidemic in East Africa. *N Engl J Med*, 1986;314:414–418.

15. Melbye M, Njelesani EK, Bayley A, et al. Evidence for heterosexual transmission and clinical manifestations of human immunodeficiency virus infection and related conditions in Lusaka, Zambia. *Lancet*, 1986;2:1113–1115.

16. Harry TO, Bubbuk DN, Idrisa A, Akoma MB. HIV infection among pregnant women: a worsening situation in Maiduguri, Nigeria. *Trop Geogr Med*, 1994; 46:46–47.

17. Mohammed I, Nasidi A, Chikwem JO, et al. AIDS in Nigeria. *AIDS*, 1988;2:61–64.

18. D'Costa LJ, Plummer FA, Bowner I, et al. Prostitutes are a major reservoir of sexually transmitted disease in Nairobi, Kenya. *Sex Trans Dis*, 1985;12:64–67.

19. Vandeperre P, Clumeck N, Carael M, et al. Female prostitutes: a risk factor for infection with human T-cell lymphotropic virus type III. *Lancet*, 1985;2: 524–526.

20. Obi CL, Ogbonna BA, Igumbor EO, et al. HIV seropositivity among female prostitutes and non-prostitutes: obstetrics and perinatal implications. *Viral Immunol*, 1993;6:171–174.

21. Harry TO, Kabeya, Claire M, Okpudo-Itata E, et al. Rapid increase in prevalence of HIV infection among prostitutes in Maiduguri, Nigeria. *Afr J Med Pract*, 1997;4:182–186.

22. Federal Ministry of Health. *National HIV/AIDS and Reproductive Health Survey (NARHS)*. Abuja, Federal Ministry of Health, 2003.

23. Mofenson, LM. Advances in the prevention of vertical transmission of human immunodeficiency virus. *Semin Pediatr Infect Dis*, 2003;4(4):295–308.

24. Mofenson LM, Lambert JS, Stiehm ER, et al. Risk factors for perinatal transmission of human immunodeficiency virus type 1 in women treated with zidovudine. *N Engl J Med*, 1999;341:385–393.

25. Eshleman SH, Mracna M, Guay L, et al. Selection and fading of resistance mutations in women and infants receiving nevirapine to prevent HIV-1 vertical transmission (HIVNET 012). *AIDS*, 2001;15: 1951–1957.

26. Lallement M. Response to the therapy after prior exposure to nevirapine. *3rd IAS Conference on HIV Pathogenesis and Treatment*, Rio de Janeiro, Brazil, July 24–27, 2005 (abstract TuFo0205).

27. Morfeldt-Manson L, Lindquist L. Blood brotherhood: a risk factor for AIDS? *Lancet*, 1984;2:1346.

28. Adesoji FA, Moronkola OA. Changing social and cultural practices in the face of HIV/AIDS in Nigeria. *Afr Q*, 2003;43(3):55–60.

29. Futuh-Shandall AA. Circumcision and infibulations of females. *Sudan Med J*, 1967;5:178–211.

30. Hirsch MS, Wormser GP, Schooley RT, et al. Risk of nosocomial infection with human T-cell lymphotrophic virus III (HTLV-III). *N Engl J Med*, 1985; 312:1–4.

31. Campbell S. Management of HIV/AIDS transmission in health care. *Nurs Stand*, 2004;18(27):33–35.

32. Iqbal MM. Can we get AIDS from mosquito bites? *J La State Med Soc*, 1999;151(8):429–433.

33. Bockarie MJ, Paru R. Can mosquitoes transmit AIDS? *P N G Med J*, 1996;39(3):205–207.

34. United States Institute of Peace. *AIDS and Violent Conflict in Africa*. Special Report. Washington, DC: United States Institute of Peace, 2001.

35. UNAIDS. *AIDS and the Military*. Best Practice Collection. Geneva: UNAIDS, 1998.

36. Lovgren S. African Army hastening HIV/AIDS Spread. *Jenda: A Journal of Culture and African Women Studies*, 2001;1:2.

37. Fleming AF. Seroepidemiology of human immunodeficiency viruses in Africa. *Biomed Pharmacother*, 1988;42(5):309–320.

38. Nwokoji UA, Ajuwon AJ. Knowledge of AIDS and HIV risk-related sexual behavior among Nigerian naval personnel. *BMC Public Health*, 2004;4:24.

39. Bakhireva LN, Abebe Y, Brodine SK, et al. Human immunodeficiency virus/acquired immunodeficiency syndrome knowledge and risk factors in Ethiopian military personnel. *Mil Med*, 2004;169(3): 221–226.

40. Federal Ministry of Health. *2004 National HIV Seroprevalence Sentinel Survey among PTB and STD patients*. Abuja: Federal Ministry of Health, 2004.

41. World Health Organization. *Global TB Control, Nigeria Country Report*. Geneva: World Health Organization, 2005.

42. UNAIDS. *AIDS in Africa: Three Scenarios to 2025*. Geneva: UNAIDS, 2005.

THE VIROLOGY AND DYNAMICS OF THE EPIDEMIC

David O. Olaleye,* Tekena O. Harry,† and Georgina N. Odaibo*

Viruses are submicroscopic, obligate intracellular parasites that can neither grow nor reproduce outside a living cell. Their survival therefore depends completely on the continued survival of their hosts. They are unique among all other living organisms, with the following main features:

- The genome of a complete virion—or an infective virus particle—is either RNA or DNA;
- Virus particles are produced from the assembly of preformed components, whereas other agents "grow" from an increase in the integrated sum of their components and reproduce by division;
- Matured virus particles themselves do not "grow" in size or undergo division, but multiply by a process called replication (of their genetic material);
- Viruses lack the genetic information that encodes the apparatus (mitochondria) necessary for the generation of metabolic energy or for protein synthesis (ribosomes); they therefore depend on the host machinery for these functions; and
- They are composed mainly of nucleic acid and proteins (that is, products of the various genes).

*Department of Virology, College of Medicine, University of Ibadan, University College Hospital, Ibadan, Nigeria
†Department of Immunology and Microbiology, University of Maiduguri Teaching Hospital, Maiduguri, Nigeria

Table 3-1. Host Range and Associated Diseases of Lentiviruses		
Virus	**Natural Host Species**	**Clinical Presentation**
Equine infectious anemia virus	Horse	Cyclical infection in the first year, autoimmune hemolytic anemia, occasional encephalopathy, arthritis
Visna maedi virus	Sheep	Encephalopathy, pneumonitis, arthritis, wasting
Caprine arthritis-encephalitis virus	Goat	Lymphadenopathy, lymphocytosis, anemia, wasting, arthritis, encephalitis
Bovine immune deficiency virus	Cow	Lymphadenopathy, lymphocytosis, possible central nervous system disease
Feline immunodeficiency virus	Cat	Immune deficiency, wasting, encephalitis
Simian immunodeficiency virus	Primates	Immune deficiency and encephalopathy
Human immunodeficiency virus	Human	Immune deficiency and encephalopathy
	Chimpanzee	None

Source: Adapted from the International Committee on Taxonomy of Viruses database (http://phene.cpmc.columbia.edu/index.htm)

The morphology of viruses may be circular, oval, cylindrical, spiral, filamentous, hexagonal, or helical. The shape of the viral capsid usually determines its morphology. The smallest viruses are approximately 20 nm in diameter and the largest around 250 nm. The nucleic acid polymer may either be double-stranded or single-stranded DNA or RNA. This viral nucleic acid polymer may contain as few as 4 to 7 genes for the tiniest viruses to as many as 150 to 200 genes for the largest viruses. In some viruses, the nucleic acid may occur as more than one molecule or as intermediate forms during the process of replication.

Furthermore, some viruses contain a few enzymes while others contain none. All viruses are covered with a protein coat called the capsid. If a virus has only a protein capsid covering it, it is termed a naked capsid virus or a naked virus. Some viruses acquire a lipid membrane from the host cell during the process of release. This lipid membrane surrounds the virus capsid and is called the virus envelope; such viruses are termed enveloped viruses. In addition, virus particles may contain small quantities of carbohydrate moieties on the envelope, called glycoproteins.

Virus infection of higher organisms is the cumulative result of infection, replication, and expression of the viral genome. Virus infections range in complexity and duration from a brief, superficial interaction between the virus and its host, to chronic or persistent infection, which may encompass the entire life of the host organism. A common misconception is that virus infection invariably results in disease; instead, only a small proportion of viral infections give rise to any disease symptoms. The course of virus infections may be abortive, acute, chronic, latent, persistent, or steady state.

CHARACTERISTICS OF RETROVIRUSES

The virus family Retroviridae includes three sub-families: Oncovirinae, Lentivirinae, and Spumavirinae. Each member contains an enzyme called reverse transcriptase, which generates proviral DNA from the infecting viral RNA genome. The provirus (also called the complementary or cDNA) integrates itself into the chromosome of the host cell with the aid of additional enzymes encoded by the viral *pol* gene. The integration of the viral cDNA into the host cell genome permits the continuous viral replication that characterizes retroviruses (1) as well as the unconventional method of "reverse" transcription used by this group of viruses (2).

Table 3-2. Summary of Properties of Lentiviruses	
Family	**Retroviridae**
Major human viruses	HIV-1, HIV-2
Size of virion	80-130 nm
Capsid symmetry	Icosahedral
Envelope	Yes
Genome	Diploid linear + sense single-stranded RNA; 10kb
Genome replication site	Nucleus
Virus assembly	Cytoplasm
Characteristic feature	Slow disease
Associated diseases	AIDS; neurologic; arthritis; pneumonia

Source: Adapted from the International Committee on Taxonomy of Viruses database (http://phene.cpmc.columbia.edu/index.htm)

The subfamily Lentivirinae, to which HIV belongs, includes multiple viruses that infect a diverse group of animals (Table 3-1). Interestingly, one of the first viruses identified in nature was a lentivirus, the equine infectious anemia virus, discovered in 1904 (3,4). Lentiviruses typically cause a slowly progressive disease with prolonged subclinical infection (1). Additional characteristics include a long incubation period, suppression of the immune system, tropism for cells of the hematopoietic system, involvement of the nervous system, malignancies, wasting disease, association with autoimmunity and arthritis, and sustained viremia in the absence of any obvious clinical disease. Lentiviruses are host specific and non-oncogenic. They induce syncytia, a phenomenon that occurs when viral fusion proteins that are normally used by the virus to enter host cells are transported to the cell surface, cause the host cell membrane to fuse with neighboring uninfected cells, and cause noncytopathic infection of macrophages. Formation of syncytia, which is caused by the fusion of HIV-infected cells to form large cells with many nuclei, has also been suggested as a possible cause of CD4+ cell depletion in HIV-infected people (5).

The viral cDNA, typically 9 to 10 kb in length, integrates into the host genome. In addition to the structural genes (*gag* and *env*) and enzyme genes (*pol*) that are found in other retroviruses, lentiviruses also encode regulatory proteins such as Tat and Rev, which have been shown to regulate viral transcription and viral RNA transport, respectively (6). Unlike oncoretroviruses, lentiviruses can efficiently infect terminally differentiated, non-dividing cells, such as macrophages and microglia. Table 3-2 shows additional properties of lentiviruses.

Lentiviruses were initially thought to have a latent stage due to their prolonged subclinical infection. It has been shown, however, that these viruses continue to replicate throughout the infection, regardless of the observation or diagnosis of clinical disease (3,4). The first cases of lentivirus-associated disease were reported in Iceland where a virus caused slow demyelinating brain disease (visna) and a progressive lung disease (maedi) in sheep (1). To date, at least six additional lentiviruses have been identified.

Human immunodeficiency virus types 1 and 2 (HIV-1 and HIV-2) and related viruses in non-human primates, such as simian immunodeficiency virus (SIV), cause a severe immunodeficiency disorder in their primary hosts (7). HIV-1 is closely related to a naturally occurring virus of certain sub-species of chimpanzees called SIVcpz, while HIV-2 has been shown to be closely related to SIVsm, a virus that naturally infects sooty mangabey monkeys (8). Other members of the genus lentivirus include the feline immunodeficiency virus, the equine infectious anemia virus (3,4,6,7), the caprine arthritis-encephalitis virus, and the bovine immune deficiency virus.

HUMAN IMMUNODEFICIENCY VIRUSES

Retroviruses were initially believed to cause disease only in animals, as no retroviruses were isolated from humans for some time (9). In 1978, however, Poiesz et al. reported the isolation of a retrovirus called human T-cell lymphotropic virus (HTLV) from a patient with mycosis fungoids (10). Since the initial discovery of HTLV, many other retroviruses, including HIV-1 and HIV-2, have been isolated from humans.

Human immunodeficiency viruses, like other retroviruses, have a positive-sense, single-stranded RNA genome (11). In the mature virus, the genome is diploid, with a 60-70s complex of the two identical RNA copies. Electron-microscopy studies have showed that HIV has a dense, cylindrical core encoded by the Gag protein that surrounds the RNA genome. The central core is enclosed by a highly glycosylated protein envelope that is partially acquired from the surface of the host cell as mature virions are released (Figure 3-1A) (12).

HIV Genes and Proteins

The HIV proviral genome is approximately 10 kb in length with an open reading frame that codes for several viral proteins (3). The genome is flanked at both ends by long terminal repeat sequences that contain regulatory elements required for HIV replication (11). The genome includes the *gag, pol,* and *env* structural genes that code for the capsid proteins, the viral enzymes, and the internal and external envelope proteins, respectively. In addition to these major genes, the HIV genome has at least five other regulatory or accessory genes: *tat, rev, nef, vif,* and *vpu/vpx. Vpu* is present in HIV-1, while *vpx* is present in HIV-2 (3) (Figure 3-1B). At least four of these minor genes are involved in regulating HIV expression (11). Although much remains to be elucidated about the pathways for controlling HIV expression in infected cells, these genes have been characterized and their functions are now fairly well understood.

The *env* gene encodes the envelope precursor, gp160, which is split into two smaller glycoproteins, gp120 and gp41, via cellular enzymes in the Golgi apparatus (4). These glycoproteins have molecular weights of 120,000 and 41,000 (gp120 and gp41, respectively) for HIV-1 and 105,000 and 36,000 (gp105 and gp36, respectively) for HIV-2 (12). The gp120 forms the external surface envelope protein and contains the binding site for cellular entry receptors, as well as major immunodominant domains, while gp41 forms the transmembrane protein (Figure 3-1A; Table 3-3) (4). The structures of these small pro-

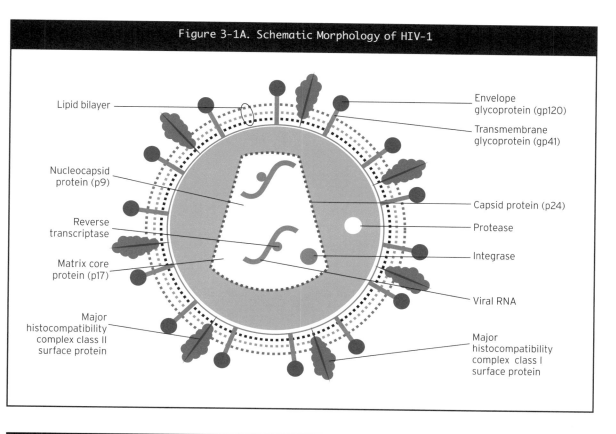

Figure 3-1A. Schematic Morphology of HIV-1

Lipid bilayer

Envelope glycoprotein (gp120)

Transmembrane glycoprotein (gp41)

Nucleocapsid protein (p9)

Capsid protein (p24)

Reverse transcriptase

Protease

Matrix core protein (p17)

Integrase

Viral RNA

Major histocompatibility complex class II surface protein

Major histocompatibility complex class I surface protein

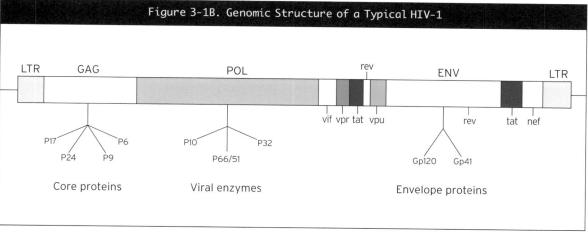

Figure 3-1B. Genomic Structure of a Typical HIV-1

LTR   GAG   POL   rev   ENV   LTR

vif vpr tat vpu   rev   tat nef

P17   P6   P10   P32

P24   P9   P66/51

Core proteins   Viral enzymes   Envelope proteins

Gp120   Gp41

Gene	HIV-1	HIV-2	Protein/Function
			Table 3-3. Structural Genes of Human Immunodeficiency Viruses
Gag	P24 P17 P9 P6	P26	Capsid (CA) structural protein Matrix (MA) protein-myristoylated RNA binding protein RNA binding protein
Pol	P66 P10 P32	P51 P14	Reverse transcriptase (RT) Post-translational processing of viral proteins (PR) Integration of viral DNA (IN)
Env	Gp120 Gp41	Gp105 Gp36	Envelope surface protein Envelope transmembrane protein
Tat	P14		Transactivation
Rev	P9		Regulation of viral mRNA expression
Nef	P27		Pleitropic, including virus suppression; myristoylated
Vif	P23		Increases virus infectivity and cell-cell transmission; helps in proviral DNA synthesis and/or in virion assembly
Vpr	P15		Necessary in virus replication; transactivation
Vpu	P16		Helps in virus release; disrupts gp160-CD4+ complexes
Vpx		P15	Associated with infectivity

jections appear to be one of the major differences between HIV-1 and HIV-2 (12); antibodies to these two sets of proteins do not usually cross-react and thus differentiate the serologic response to the two distinct human immunodeficiency viruses (12–14).

The envelope surrounds the core proteins that enclose the viral RNA genome and enzymes. The core proteins are encoded by the *gag* gene, whose precursor, p55, gives rise to four smaller proteins (p24, p17, p9, and p6) by proteolytic cleavage (4). The core itself is made up of two proteins of approximately 18,000 and 24,000 daltons in size (p18 and p24). The Pol precursor protein is cleaved into products consisting of the reverse transcriptase (RT), the protease (PR), and the integrase (IN) proteins by protease enzyme. The RT, IN, and PR enzymes have molecular weights of 66,000/51,000 (p66/p51), 32,000 (p32) and 12,000 (p12), respectively (11).

Cellular Receptors

The primary receptor for HIV is the CD4+ molecule located on T-helper cells; a number of other cell types — including macrophages, microglial cells, dendritic cells, and Langerhans cells — also bear these CD4+ receptors (15). Studies on the genetics of infectious diseases have shown that human genetic variation might influence susceptibility to pathogenic organisms, including HIV (16,17). Variation in the number of CD4+ molecules on the T-cell surface may influence the ability of HIV to bind and eventually penetrate the target cell (18). In addition, attachment to and fusion with target cells are determined not only by binding with CD4+ molecules, but also with secondary chemokine co-receptors (19–21).

The chemokine receptor family members have seven transmembrane helices and interact with G proteins. This family includes receptors for IL-8, MIP-1, and RANTES. The chemokine receptors CCR5 and CXCR4 are commonly used by HIV to preferentially enter either macrophages or T cells, respectively (16). CCR5 is the major co-receptor used for entry of macrophage (M-tropic or R5) isolates of HIV-1, while CXCR4 facilitates entry of T-tropic (or X4) HIV-1 strains. Cells of the myeloid lineage may be infected predominantly with R5 strains, although infection with dual-tropic isolates of HIV-1 or some strains of X4 isolates is possible. Several studies have found that individuals who are homozygous for a deletion in the CCR5 gene are less frequently infected with HIV, while those who are heterozygous for the same mutation still become infected but can be better protected against rapid progression than individuals who are homozygous for the wild-type CCR5 receptor gene (16,17,22).

Replication

Replication of the virus particle begins with attachment of gp120 to the CD4+ on the surface of a target cell. Following the gp120-CD4+ binding, a structural change allows for the interaction of the V3 loop region in the gp120 with a chemokine receptor, including CCR5 and CXCR4. The reaction with the co-receptor results in another conformational change in the viral surface glycoprotein, which exposes a fusion domain contained within the envelope transmembrane glycoprotein. Exposure of the fusion domain results in the insertion of the gp41 into the cellular membrane. Subsequent to the fusion event, the viral core is released into the cytoplasm of the host cell (1,7).

Once in the cytoplasm, the viral RNA genome is uncoated and reverse transcribed by the virally encoded RT enzyme to generate a double-stranded viral DNA preintegration complex. The double-stranded DNA is then transported into the host cell nucleus and, via catalysis by IN, becomes integrated into the host cell chromosome, where it resides as provirus. Once the viral genome has been integrated into the host cell genome, it can remain in a latent state for many years or can begin the production of new viral RNA. If the host cell is activated, the host cell enzyme RNA polymerase II will transcribe the proviral DNA into messenger RNA (mRNA). The mRNA is then translated into viral proteins that undergo extensive post-translational modifications. The viral RNA becomes the genetic material for the next generation of viruses. Viral RNA and viral proteins assemble at the cell membrane. After proper assembly and processing, new infectious virus particles are released by budding from the cell membrane.

GENETIC VARIABILITY OF HIV ISOLATES

An interesting feature of HIV is the marked genetic diversity among its different isolates. The viral reverse transcriptase is error-prone, with a mutation rate of approximately 7×10^6 to 1.4×10^4 base pair substitutions; thus, RT can quickly and efficiently give rise to mutations throughout the HIV genome (23). The average rate of base substitution would suggest that HIV-1, with a genome size of about 10 kb, mutates approximately one nucleotide per genome per replication cycle (24). Therefore, within an individual or a population, HIV-1 will contain few, if any, identical genomes. HIV within any individual actually exists as a population of related, yet distinct, viral variants termed the viral *quasispecies*. This variation may have profound effects on the development of immunologic escape, drug resistance, and vaccine-induced immunity. The molecular epidemiology of HIV and the possible implications of this genetic heterogeneity will be discussed in greater detail in Chapter 4, *this volume*.

THE PATHOGENESIS OF HIV INFECTION

Cellular Targets of HIV

The name "human immunodeficiency virus" suggests that this virus ultimately brings about deficiencies in the immune system of infected individuals. To exert such effects, the virus attacks and destroys the very cells that form the immune defense mechanisms of humans. The most important of these cells and their functions are T-lymphocytes, B-lymphocytes, plasma cells, macrophages, and natural killer cells.

T-Lymphocytes

These cells, consisting of several subpopulations, play a vital role in cell-mediated immune responses and help B lymphocytes in humoral antibody production. The most important T-lymphocyte subpopulations are CD4+ T cells (or T4 cells) and CD8+ T cells (or T8 cells). CD4+ T cells help or induce other cells of the immune system to carry out their various functions; hence, they are called helper/inducer cells. CD4+ cells carry out these functions either by direct contact with these or other cells of the immune system or by secreting soluble substances, called cytokines, that serve as chemical messengers and/or chemoattractants that direct cells to the appropriate sites of infection throughout the body. The activities of T4 cells also result in the maturation, activation, and proliferation of other cells of the immune system. T8 cells either suppress the activities of other cells (T4 and B cells), or function as cytotoxic cells, killing virus-infected and tumor cells. They directly bind to cells carrying a foreign antigen and lyse such cells, thus eliminating them from the body. T8 cells have been proposed to play a key role in the immunologic defense against HIV by controlling viral replication through at least two mechanisms: direct antigen-specific cytolysis, which appears to be required for optimal suppression, and release of soluble antiviral factors (24,25). The antiviral activity of T8 cells was first described when investigators observed a depletion in CD8+ cells from the peripheral blood mononuclear cells of HIV-infected people and a corresponding increase in viral replication in the remaining CD4+ cells (26,27). On the other hand, replacement of the CD8+ cells caused a dose-dependent suppression of viral replication.

B-Lymphocytes and Plasma Cells

B-lymphocytes, on maturation, lead to the production of plasma cells, which, in turn, produce antibodies that clear infecting organisms. For the efficient performance of their functions, B-lymphocytes require the assistance of T4 lymphocytes. Plasma cells are small cells produced from the maturation of B cells and in turn produce antibodies against a variety of foreign agents.

Macrophages

Macrophages are large cells that engulf and kill pathogens. These pathogens are digested by macrophages into multiple antigens that are then presented on the surface of macrophages for recognition and processing by other cells of the immune system. Monocytes constitutively migrate out of the bloodstream into the tissues to replenish the tissue macrophage pool and scout for infection. This physiologic tissue migration of macrophages also provides a means by which HIV-1 can infect the brain, lungs, and many other organs.

Natural Killer Cells

Natural killer cells, otherwise known as NK cells, kill malignant, altered, or deformed cells. Morphologically, NK cells resemble T-lymphocytes. Like the B- and T-lymphocytes, they exist in resting form in normal individuals who have not previously encountered the particular infectious agent or cancerous cells. Unlike T and B cells, NK cells are not specific for the cells they attack.

Effects of HIV on the Immune System

As the principal cellular target of HIV infection is the CD4+ T helper lymphocyte, the depletion of T lymphocytes is a central factor in the progression of HIV/AIDS. Because these cells play a vital role in regulating and amplifying the immune response, any decline in their number results in deficits in both humoral and cell-mediated immunity, resulting in the immune dysfunction that is a hallmark of HIV infection (28). The mechanisms by which HIV induce CD4+ T-cell death are not yet fully understood, however. At least three major mechanisms have been proposed (29):

- the killing of productively infected CD4+ T-cells is caused either by direct viral cytopathic effects or by antiviral cytotoxic CD8+ T lymphocytes;
- viral-mediated killing of bystander uninfected CD4+ T-cells is induced by viral proteins that are released from infected cells; or
- excessive, ongoing immune activation caused by a high, persistent viral antigen load leads to the activation-induced death of various uninfected immune cells, including CD4+ T-cells.

The normal function of CD4+ cells in maintaining an efficient immune response to infection is thus progressively reduced by the cytopathic effects of HIV. Macrophages and CD8+ cells become less efficient at clearing virally infected cells, because CD4+ helper cells are no longer functioning properly. Subsequently, production of specific antibodies is also reduced. Collectively, this severe immunosuppression allows opportunistic pathogens to replicate unchecked within an individual. Thus, as HIV infection progresses, the victim develops immune abnormalities as the virus interferes with the normal interactions and regulation of cells in the immune system.

Viral Load and CD4+ Natural History

Before the widespread use of viral load assays, the CD4+ cell count has been used extensively as a surrogate marker for HIV disease progression. In Nigeria, CD4+ cell counts in healthy individuals have been found to range from 636/mm^3 to 977/mm^3 of blood (unpublished data). In Western countries, the mean value has been reported to be 1,000/mm^3 to 1,100/mm^3 (30,31). Thus, constant exposure to a number of other pathogens in sub-Saharan Africa may result in an overall less healthy immune system with which to fight HIV infection.

The course of HIV infection varies within a population. Nonetheless, a typical infection can be divided into three stages: primary infection, asymptomatic infection, and symptomatic infection, or AIDS. Following primary HIV infection, the CD4+ cell count decreases, while HIV RNA rises to high levels. With sufficient exposure to viral antigens, cytotoxic T-lymphocyte responses are generated and the HIV viral load typically declines to an equilibrium known as a virologic "setpoint," which occurs within 6 to 12 months of initial infection. Once this viral setpoint is reached, the CD4+ cell count may rebound again marginally, although it does not often return to baseline values (32). Concurrent with these events are clinical manifestations of acute HIV infection in 30% to 60% of people (Figure 3-2). About half of newly infected people experience flu-like symptoms; the remainder are asymptomatic.

Once infected, humans experience an asymptomatic clinical latency that lasts 2 to 10 years, during which HIV is produced and removed by the immune system, and CD4+ T cells are killed and replaced. During this asymptomatic period, the number of infected circulating CD4+ cells and free virions is relatively low. Moreover, the hematopoietic system is able to replace most T cells that are destroyed, thus keeping the CD4+ cell counts in the normal range (800 to 1200/mm^3 of blood). Later in infection, replicating virus disrupts the follicular dendritic cells' architecture, and more infected T cells appear in the circulation. Viruses are no longer retained in the lymph nodes; thus, the circulating levels of free virus increase. Eventually, the circulating CD4+ T cell levels fall to less than 500/mm^3 and opportunistic infections may occasionally occur. During the later stage of infection, the CD4+ cell count declines below 200/mm^3, a level at which the infected individual is said to have developed AIDS. A number of opportunistic infections — including oral candidiasis and recurrent tuberculosis — are common during the early symptomatic phase of AIDS. As the CD4+ cell count declines to an even lower level, additional life-threatening opportunistic infections — such as herpes zoster, amoebiasis, and dermatomycoses — may occur with increasing frequency.

In the later stages of symptomatic HIV infection, the viral load levels rise again. Reports involving accurate quantification of virus in infected patients have revealed that much more virus is present than originally thought (33). Quantitative PCR methods, the so-called viral load assays, have shown that:

- Continuous replication of HIV occurs in nearly all infected individuals, although the rates of virus production vary by as much as 70-fold in different individuals;
- The average half-life of an HIV particle/infected cell in vivo is 2.1 days. Recent reports have suggested an even faster turnover of plasma virus of 28 to 110 per minute;
- Up to 10^9–10^{10} HIV particles are produced each day; and
- An average of 2×10^9 CD4+ cells are produced each day.

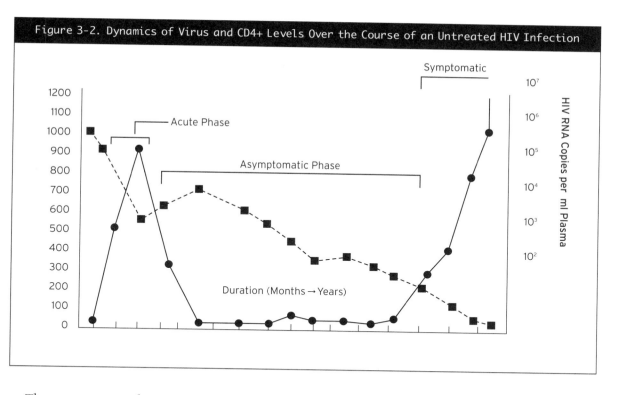

Figure 3-2. Dynamics of Virus and CD4+ Levels Over the Course of an Untreated HIV Infection

Thus, contrary to what scientists initially believed, there is a very dynamic situation in HIV-infected people involving continuous viral replication and destruction and replacement of CD4+ cells.

While the CD4+ cell count is a less expensive and less technical measure of HIV disease progression, quantifying the viral load is currently the most direct measurement of the HIV disease process. It has also been used to assess the risk of disease progression and the response to antiretroviral therapy (ART) (33). As the disease progresses, CD4+ cell count declines but may rebound if therapy is efficacious; however, this parameter alone is an incomplete marker for clinical assessment of a patient. Nevertheless, in resource-poor settings (which include a large proportion of the most affected countries), the CD4+ cell count is a more affordable and hence more practical yardstick for monitoring disease progression and ART efficacy. The following CD4+ cell counts are useful in staging a person's disease progression:

- Acute seroconversion syndrome: > 1000/mm³
- Early disease: > 500/mm³
- Middle-stage disease: 200–500/mm³
- Late disease: 50–200/mm³
- Advanced disease: < 50/mm³

Clinical Latency (Asymptomatic Infection)

Studies in industrialized countries have shown that the median time from initial HIV-1 infection to the development of AIDS ranges from 9 to 11 years (32). In Nigeria, such figures are not available. The course of infection with HIV-1 varies dramatically, even when the primary infections arose from the same source. In some individuals with a long-term non-progressive HIV-1 infection — that is, a lack of decline in CD4+ cell counts, or chronic infection for at least seven years without the development of AIDS — defective viruses have been identified (34–37). Thus, infection with a defective virus, or one with a poor capacity to replicate, may prolong the clinical course of HIV-1 infection.

As a result of immune activation and other factors, CD4+ cells in the lymph nodes produce virus more rapidly than latently infected cells. As these infected cells are ruptured, they release progeny virions that infect other susceptible cells. After acute HIV infection, a long clinical latency period occurs prior to the onset of symptomatic disease, or AIDS. Although the period is often called the latency period, the virus is not actually dormant. It continues to replicate, mostly in lymph nodes, leading to swollen lymph nodes or lymphadenopathy.

AIDS

Acquired immune deficiency syndrome, or AIDS, is a clinical diagnosis that represents the late stages of HIV disease progression. People classified as having progressed to AIDS either have CD4+ cell counts lower than 200/mm³ or one or more AIDS-defining conditions. The most common AIDS-defining conditions in Nigeria are severe weight loss; pulmonary tuberculosis; candidiasis (of the esophagus, trachea, bronchi, and lungs); herpes zoster infection; recurrent bacterial pneumonia; and Kaposi's sarcoma (38,39). In industrialized countries, the most prominent AIDS-defining diagnosis is *Pneumocystis carinii* pneumonia, which has been rare among AIDS patients seen in Nigeria (4,7,38,39).

Upon diagnosis of AIDS or symptomatic disease, the median survival time ranges from 12 to 18 months. Nearly all patients who die of HIV-related complications are in this CD4+ cell count category. With the recent introduction of highly active antiretroviral therapy, or HAART, as well as better education and management of people living with HIV/AIDS in Nigeria, people infected with HIV live longer and are healthier even with CD4+ cell counts of less than 200/mm³ (40–43).

TRANSMISSION OF HUMAN IMMUNODEFICIENCY VIRUS

After the first AIDS cases were reported in the United States, several risk groups were identified — homosexual men, hemophiliacs, and injection drug users — which suggested several possible modes of HIV transmission even before the isolation of the causative agent. Today, we know that both HIV-1 and HIV-2 are transmitted through three principal routes: sexual transmission; transfusion of blood and blood products; and mother-to-child transmission. These routes include the four bodily fluids responsible for all HIV transmission: semen, vaginal fluids, blood, and breast milk.

Sexual Transmission
HIV can be transmitted by vaginal, anal, or oral sexual intercourse. Like other sexually transmitted infections (STIs), the likelihood of infection with HIV is related to the number of sexual partners; the

infectiousness of infected individuals (for example, people with higher viral loads may be more likely to transmit HIV than people with lower viral loads); and the duration of infection. Globally, about 90% of HIV infection is acquired sexually (44).

In North America and Western Europe, homosexual anal intercourse was initially the major mode of HIV transmission (45). However, heterosexual transmission has since become the major mode of transmission in nearly all countries (46). In addition, heterosexual transmission of HIV-1 is more frequent than for HIV-2 (47). In Africa, the male-to-female ratio of HIV infection remains approximately 1:1 (48–51), suggesting that the main mode of transmission is heterosexual. It has been postulated, however, that the efficiency of male-to-female transmission is higher than female-to-male transmission (52). It also has been observed that some people became infected after a single exposure, while others escape infection even after prolonged, unprotected intercourse with HIV-infected people (53,54).

Moreover, the existence of highly exposed but uninfected individuals suggests that additional factors can influence the sexual transmission of the virus (53,54). Certain factors — such as duration of infection, genetic susceptibility of the host, infecting virus load, virulence of the particular HIV strain, and the status of the immune system — may also affect the rate of heterosexual transmission (52,55). Among the key factors are host infectiousness, viral infectivity and virulence, and host susceptibility.

Host Infectiousness

Some of the factors that influence the host infectiousness include:

- State of infection. Holmberg et al. suggested that HIV-infected people may be more infectious in later stages of infection (18). A study by Hirsch and Curran, however, found no association between stages of HIV infection and amount of virus in the semen (7).
- Severity of the disease and the presence of p24 antigenemia in the infecting person (56).
- CD4+ cell count. It has been shown that transmitting partners have significantly few T-helper cells than non-transmitters (57,58).
- Mode by which a person acquired infection. It has been shown that partners of infected injection drug users are much more likely to be HIV seropositive than partners of HIV-infected transfusion recipients (54).
- Vaginal sex during menstruation. Menstruation might increase the likelihood of HIV transmission to male sex partners (59).

Viral Infectivity and Virulence

Viral infectivity and virulence tend to relate directly to transmissibility. HIV manifests a high degree of genetic variability in vitro, and genetically distinct isolates can often be recovered from the same patient at different times. Nelson and Perelson observed fast replicating strains during early and late infection, and, in the same individual, slow replicating strains during the intermediate latent stage (60). Increased virulence might lead to an increase in transmission rates by augmenting the number of viruses present in host secretions (61). Therefore, people infected with HIV variants of higher virulence could be expected to infect a higher proportion of their susceptible contacts than people with less virulent variants.

Host Susceptibility

It has been shown that a break in integrity of the vaginal or rectal mucosa also facilitates HIV infection (7). Herpes simplex virus infection and syphilis, which cause ulcerative diseases, are known risk factors for HIV transmission (4). Sources of abrasion for the rectum or vagina—such as rectal douching, perianal bleeding, and tampon use—may also facilitate HIV transmission (62–64).

Estrogen-containing contraceptives and sexual intercourse during menstruation have been associated with higher risk of HIV infection in women (18,59). Although estrogen thickens the cervical mucosa and might be expected to reduce HIV infection, it is associated with a change in the cervical ectopion and predisposes it to chlamydial infection, cervicitis, and cervical changes that may facilitate HIV infection. In men, a lack of circumcision has been associated with a higher risk of HIV infection (65).

Transfusion of Blood and Blood Products

Whole blood, cellular components, plasma, and clotting factors have all been implicated in HIV transmission. Most people infected with HIV through blood transfusions had an exposure to a single yet large inoculum and often had underlying medical conditions that influenced the rapid development of HIV-related illnesses (66).

Heat treatment of concentrated clotting factor, coupled with donor screening, has reduced the transmission risk associated with transfusion of blood and blood products in developed countries to fewer than one HIV infection per 500,000 transfusions. In developing countries, though, where HIV screening facilities for blood transfusion safety are inadequate, this mode of transmission remains a significant source of new HIV infections.

Parenteral exposure to HIV also results in a small but definite occupational risk of HIV infection for health care workers (67). For this transmission mode, the size of the inoculum is the most important factor determining the risk of HIV infection. Among adults and children in Africa, especially in rural areas, there is a relationship between AIDS and needle injection. These injections, administered primarily for medical purposes, are often by untrained practitioners who usually use a single needle for more than one person (68). In Africa, some practices such as facial scarification and group male and female circumcision may also promote transmission of HIV (48).

Injection drug use plays an important role in transmission of HIV in the developed world. In addition to sharing contaminated needles, injection drug users may also engage in high-risk sexual intercourse (69). It has been shown that female injection drug users and partners of male injection drug users represent the largest number of HIV-infected women of childbearing age in developed countries (70); thus, the association between perinatal transmission of HIV and injection drug use is strong in the developed world.

Mother-to-Child Transmission

Nearly all cases of HIV infection in infants in both developed and developing countries occur as a result of mother-to-child transmission through three potential routes: across the placenta (in utero); during delivery, through exposure to infected genital tract secretions (intrapartum); and, postnatally, through breastfeeding.

Studies have shown that breastfeeding accounts for most mother-to-child transmission of HIV (71–74). Profound stomatitis in children and cracks on mothers' nipples are additional factors leading to HIV transmission. Additional maternal factors that may influence perinatal transmission of HIV include a low CD4+ cell count, viral load, rupture of membrane more than 48 hours before delivery, and a low level or lack of anti-V3 loop antibodies (75,76). Recent reports also show that the absence of ART in the mother and/or child is an additional factor in transmission.

LABORATORY DIAGNOSIS AND MONITORING

The effectiveness of HIV control measures and the success of treatment of infected people in any country largely depend on the establishment and provision of accurate and reliable diagnoses. Testing techniques must be reliable for results to be unambiguous.

HIV testing programs tend to have the following objectives:

- To monitor the trends of HIV infection in a population or subgroup for planning interventions, such as surveillance or unlinked anonymous sentinel surveys;
- To ensure the safety of recipients by testing donated blood or donors of organs or tissues;
- To identify individuals with HIV infection for diagnosis of AIDS-related diseases or voluntary testing purposes in asymptomatic or AIDS cases; and,
- To enable research on various aspects of HIV infection and AIDS-related diseases.

HIV testing has generated interest not only in the scientific community, but also among the general public. Several factors—including HIV variability, type of laboratory facilities, and the competence of personnel handling the tests—are known to affect the accuracy and reliability of HIV testing in Africa (77). While some of these factors can be managed to a great extent in laboratory settings in some developing countries, the problem of genetic variability is a serious one in most parts of Africa, where multiple HIV-1 subtypes and/or HIV-2 may circulate.

The various technical, ethical, and legal issues that invariably accompany HIV testing have led many countries to develop their own HIV testing policies and guidelines. The development of tests to detect infection with HIV has made it possible to determine the prevalence of HIV and to monitor trends within various populations. While this information is of great value in designing, implementing, and monitoring public health programs for prevention and control, testing of any population for HIV requires careful consideration of a number of issues relating to logistics, laboratory operations, legal ramifications, and ethics.

Serologic Techniques

Detection of HIV-specific antibodies in the blood or other body fluids is the main method of testing for HIV and the standard procedure for diagnosis of HIV infection. The most commonly used serologic assay for diagnosing HIV infection is the enzyme-linked immunosorbent assay (ELISA) (7,78–80). In general, the assays used to detect specific HIV antibodies can be classified into two categories: screening tests, including ELISA/EIA, rapid, and simple; and supplemental or confirmatory tests, including Western blot, culture, antigen detection, and immunofluorescence assays.

Screening Tests

Screening assays are performed to test blood samples or blood products and for surveillance. These include different forms of ELISAs, which typically take two to three hours to complete. Rapid screening tests can provide results within a few minutes and, in most cases, include visual assays like dot-blot tests; particle (gelatin, latex, microbeads) agglutination; HIV spot and comb tests; and fluorometric microparticle technologies. Most of the simple screening tests are based on ELISA principles, but take about half an hour to conclude.

The indirect ELISA screening technique uses inactivated virus, synthetic peptides, or recombinant proteins as antigens to detect the presence or absence of HIV-specific antibodies in serum or plasma. While there may be some degree of cross-reactivity between HIV-1 and HIV-2, ELISAs that can specifically detect HIV-2 have also been developed. Thus, discrimination between HIV-specific antibodies against the two types of HIV can be ensured in the assay protocol.

A well-developed ELISA kit should have a specificity and sensitivity that exceed 98% to 99% (7). A sample reactive in an ELISA is usually retested using an ELISA with another antigen source. If the ELISA is found to be reactive a second time, it is considered to be repeatedly reactive and then a confirmatory test (Western blot) is performed. Cases of false positivity and false negativity have been reported, however (7). False positivity may reflect the presence of other retroviruses (48) or immunologic abnormalities. False negative reactions, on the other hand, may occur at the early stage of infection before HIV-specific antibodies have fully developed at sufficient quantities for detection (that is, during the "window period" of primary infection) (48). Several techniques — including PCR, p24 antigen detection assay, or viral culture — can detect HIV infection during the window period.

The first generation of ELISAs were sensitive yet not specific because whole viral lysates were used as antigens. These lysates usually contained small amounts of host cell components, which gave rise to false positive reactions. The ELISA technologies improved, and second- and third-generation kits were developed using recombinant and synthetic peptides as antigens. Thus, ELISA assays available in the market may be:

- **First generation:** Use antigens derived from detergent disruption of viruses grown in human lymphocytes.
- **Second generation:** Use artificially derived recombinant antigens expressed from bacteria.

- **Third generation:** Use chemically synthesized oligopeptides of 15 to 40 amino acids.
- **Fourth generation:** Detect both antibody and antigen in the same well of an ELISA plate.

First-generation ELISAs are no longer used for HIV testing, however, because of the high level of false positivity.

Rapid assays. A number of rapid assays based on the principles of agglutination and ELISA have been developed for ease of performance and quick results. These assays generally require less than 30 minutes to perform and do not require special equipment.

Agglutination assays. Agglutination assays incorporate various antigen-coated carriers, such as red cells, latex particles, gelatin particles, and microbeads. These particles are used to support or carry HIV antigens by non-specific attachment.

Agglutination assays have good sensitivity, do not require sophisticated equipment, are easy to perform and cost-effective, and require no wash procedures. Specificity is somewhat compromised, however, and a prozone reaction may occur. To overcome the prozone reaction, diluted specimens should be tested. During the agglutination reaction, HIV antibodies interact with HIV antigens on the carrier particles. Since all antibodies are multivalent, a lattice network between antibodies and antigens is formed that can be visualized macroscopically or microscopically.

Dot-blot assays/comb tests. These assays are rapid and easy to perform, can usually discriminate between HIV-1 and HIV-2, and do not require sophisticated equipment. The results are read by development of color. Sensitivity and specificity of most of these assays compare with ELISAs (81–84).

The assays use recombinant or synthetic peptides spotted onto nitrocellulose paper or micro particles. The antigen-containing matrix is housed in a plastic device containing absorbent pads to collect reactants or made as a comb and the antigens are spotted onto the tooth of the comb card. Each assay contains an immunoglobulin capture control to validate the result. These assays are good for single-test applications, such as in an emergency, during an autopsy, or in labor rooms or peripheral blood banks.

HIV Antibodies Detected in Other Fluids

As stated earlier, the standard specimens for detection of HIV antibodies are serum, plasma, or whole blood. Detection of HIV antibodies in other fluids is also possible, however. HIV antibodies can be detected in oral fluids, such as saliva and oral mucosal transudates. However, the level of HIV antibodies in these fluids is usually less than 1% of the level in serum (85–87). These tests may find better use if issues of confidentiality, counseling, and follow-up can be resolved. HIV antibodies can also be detected in urine using appropriate ELISA kits (88,89). Guidelines for using these tests need to be developed, however, as do adequate strategies for follow-up.

Choice of HIV Screening Assay

The following factors should be considered when choosing a particular protocol, kit, or strategy for HIV detection:

- The objectives of testing for HIV infection;
- The sensitivity and specificity of the test kit in a particular locality or country;
- The prevalence of HIV in the population;
- The cost-effectiveness of the choice;
- The appropriateness to the strategy and national guidelines of testing; and
- The infrastructure, facilities, and trained personnel available.

Sensitivity is the accuracy with which a test can establish the presence of an infection — that is, HIV antibodies in an appropriate specimen — and is determined as follows:

$$\text{Sensitivity} = \frac{\text{True positive (TP)}}{\text{TP + False negative (FN)}} \times 100$$

Specificity is the accuracy with which a test can confirm the absence of an infection — that is, truly negative specimens test negative. Tests with high specificity show few false positives; therefore, they are preferred for diagnosing HIV infection and/or are used as the second assay in screening. Specificity is defined as follows:

$$\text{Specificity} = \frac{\text{True negative (TN)}}{\text{TN + False positive (FP)}} \times 100$$

Confirmatory Tests

Studies have shown that the probability that a test will accurately determine the true infection status of a person being tested varies with the prevalence of HIV infection in the population (90–92); the higher the HIV prevalence, the greater the probability that a person testing positive is truly infected. This is referred to as the positive predictive value (PPV) of the test.

In contrast, the likelihood that a person showing a negative result is truly uninfected is termed the negative predictive value (NPV). NPV decreases as the prevalence of HIV among the general population increases (92).

Supplemental tests are performed on blood samples that are previously reactive in a screening test. When a blood specimen is reactive by any one of the screening tests, it is tested again by a different assay system to confirm the diagnosis. If a specimen is reactive in two different screening systems, it is tested again using a supplemental test, such as the Western blot or immunofluorescence assay.

HIV infection is confirmed by the detection of antibodies to specific HIV proteins using the Western blot — or immunoblotting — technique (93,94). This assay has certain drawbacks that limit its use, especially in developing countries. It is costly and technically demanding. Furthermore, indeterminate Western blot reactions are common, especially with African blood samples (95). Thus, alternatives to

Western blotting for developing countries have been proposed (96) and are currently being used in some laboratories.

These supplemental tests are used to resolve discordant results of ELISAs in voluntary counseling and testing or to establish diagnosis of HIV infection for the purpose of therapy. It is important to ensure that any commercial kit selected for this purpose is capable of detecting both HIV-1– and HIV-2–specific antibodies, as well as their respective subtypes.

Molecular Methods

Polymerase Chain Reaction
PCR is a molecular technique that rapidly amplifies specific nucleotide sequences (96). The usefulness of PCR for the direct detection of HIV genetic material was recognized immediately. Today, PCR has been widely applied to the detection and study of HIV infection in both clinical and basic research settings for detecting HIV during early or acute infection; subtyping HIV variants and identifying HIV strains; sequencing of the *pol* gene relevant to monitoring drug resistance and therapeutic efficacy; and detecting HIV in newborn babies of infected mothers.

Virus Isolation
HIV infection can also be detected by isolation of the virus from peripheral blood mononuclear cells, genital secretion, plasma, brain, bone marrow, or a variety of other tissues (97–99). Co-cultivation of the test specimen with uninfected mitogen-stimulated PBMCs is the technique most commonly used (7). After several days, the supernatant of the co-culture is evaluated for reverse transcriptase activity, the presence of HIV p24 antigen, or HIV RNA. In general, virus is present in PBMCs in high concentrations very early and very late in the course of HIV infection; thus, this approach is particularly important for the accurate detection of HIV infection during the window period before HIV-specific antibodies have fully developed. However, because virus isolation is quite slow and generates a large number of infectious particles, it must be conducted under conditions of strict biocontainment. Thus, it is not routinely attempted in most developing countries; in the developed world, it is primarily a research method.

Diagnosis of HIV Infection in Newborns
Transplacental transmission of HIV can occur from an infected pregnant mother to her fetus as early as eight weeks of gestation (100,101). Diagnosis of HIV infection in infants born to seropositive mothers is difficult because maternal antibody (IgG) to HIV-1 crosses the placenta and can persist for up to 15 months, making the distinction between maternal and neonatal IgG difficult. The various tests available to diagnose HIV infection in neonates under the age of 15 months include detection of IgA and/or IgM anti-HIV antibodies, detection of p24 antigen, PCR amplification of viral DNA or RNA, and virus isolation.

Monitoring Progression of HIV Infection and Therapy

Infection with HIV progresses to AIDS at different rates in different individuals, with a wide spectrum varying from rapid progression to long-term non-progression. This variability makes it essential to have tests that can accurately assess the stage of infection in an individual, as well as monitor the progression of disease. The response of individuals to ART is similarly monitored. The increased rate of HIV replication is reflected in an increase in plasma viral RNA load, which is considered the most representative and sensitive laboratory test for monitoring progression of HIV infection. Over time, increased HIV replication leads to a depletion of CD4+ cells. The CD4+ cell count, a useful surrogate marker for viral replication, was the first method described for monitoring HIV disease progression and is still used for staging infection and monitoring progression in many parts of the world.

The laboratory tests used for monitoring the progression of HIV disease can be classified into viral markers and surrogate markers.

Viral Markers

Plasma HIV RNA load. Plasma viral load (HIV RNA) quantification is considered the best method for monitoring progression and response to ART. Active replication of virus occurs during all clinical stages of infection; thus, it is possible to detect and quantify virus throughout the course of infection. The techniques available for quantifying viral RNA are: quantitative RNA-PCR; branched DNA assay (bDNA); and nucleic acid sequence based amplification (NASBA) (14).

P24 antigenemia. The *gag*-gene–encoded core protein antigen, p24, is one of the earliest viral antigens detectable in the blood after infection. It is useful for diagnosis during the "window period" of early infection and in the newborn. An increase in free p24 levels is an important predictor of increased virus replication (102–104). Until the development of HIV RNA load assays, the p24 assay was the major assay used to measure viral replication directly. The p24 antigen is poorly quantifiable, however, and may not be detectable in many individuals. In addition, p24 concentrations in the blood do not correlate well with ART efficacy.

Surrogate Markers

Virus-specific markers. A viral characteristic associated with progression of HIV infection is the conversion of the virus from a non-syncytium-inducing (NSI) phenotype to a syncytium-inducing (SI) phenotype (105–108).

Non-HIV–specific markers. A number of non HIV-specific cellular markers have been used for monitoring progression of HIV infection and assessing response to therapy. One of the most useful and commonly used cellular markers is the absolute count (or percentage) of CD4+ lymphocytes in the blood. Other lymphocyte phenotypic markers associated with progression include an increase in indicators of immune activation on T lymphocytes like CD38 (especially on CD8+ lymphocytes), HLA-DR, IL-2R, CD45RO, and markers of apoptosis, such as Fas. Flow cytometry is the most accurate method for determining these markers and CD4+ cell counts, though it is technically demanding and comparatively expensive both in terms of equipment and reagents.

CD4+ cell counts. The most commonly used cellular marker is the CD4+ lymphocyte count. Its decline is the hallmark of HIV infection, and the rate of CD4+ cell loss in each person is unique. CD4+ cell number changes during HIV infection in the following stages:

- A rapid decline for 6 to 18 months at the time of seroconversion;
- A plateau or gradual decline that can last several years during the asymptomatic period;
- A steeper decline for several months before AIDS develops; and
- A continued CD4+ cell decline and pronounced immunosuppression until the death of the infected individual.

The CD4+ cell count is extremely important in the staging of HIV infection. A revised classification of the U.S. Centers for Disease Control and Prevention stratifies HIV positive people into three CD4+ count categories: > 500/mm^3; 200–499/mm^3; and < 200/mm^3 (along with three parallel clinical stages: A, B, and C). It is known that a low CD4+ count (less than 10% or < 100/mm^3) and a low CD4+/CD8+ ratio (< 0.2) are highly predictive of death from AIDS-related complications (109–114). In developed countries, a combination of the CD4+ cell count and HIV viral load assays are used as markers of progression. A persistently high viral load is predictive of a poor prognosis, especially when accompanied by a very low CD4+ cell count. Viral load is considered a superior prognostic marker compared with CD4+ cell counts when monitoring patients on ART.

Soluble markers: A large number of soluble markers of immune activation have been evaluated as prognostic indicators in HIV infection. These include serum/plasma levels of neopterin, β2-microglobulin, tumor necrosis factor alpha (TNF-α), soluble CD8+, and soluble cytokine receptors (sIL-2R for IL-2 and sTNF-α RII for TNF-α) (115–117).

HIV INFECTION IN NIGERIA

Initial concern about HIV infection in Nigeria was first raised between 1984 and 1986 by a number of medical scientists, including C. K. O. Williams and A. F. Fagbami, then of the Departments of Hematology and Virology, respectively, at the University College Hospital in Ibadan; Abdulsalami Nasidi and Tekena Harry at the National Institute for Medical Research in Yaba, Lagos; and Idris Mohammed of the University of Maiduguri Teaching Hospital. Their persistent call for action resulted in the establishment of the National Experts Advisory Committee on AIDS in 1987 by the minister of health at the time, the late Olikoye Ransome-Kuti. Also in 1986, the Nigerian government officially publicly recognized the first HIV/AIDS infection in the country (69). Subsequent work by individual researchers or groups led to the identification of more cases of HIV/AIDS in different parts of the country. It should be noted, however, that investigations at that period were limited to institutions or individual scientists who had access to the appropriate diagnostic assays through collaborations with scientists in institutions in the United States, France, the United Kingdom, and Germany.

In late 1987, the Federal Ministry of Health, with technical assistance from the Overseas Development Agency of the British Council and the World Health Organization, established HIV screening facilities in 13 teaching hospitals in the country with the sole objective of ensuring transfusion safety. Hence, the facilities were usually located in the departments of hematology or the blood banks of these centers. The number of such HIV screening centers was later increased to cover more hospitals in the country. Results of the first 2,000 blood units tested at the various centers were negative for HIV antibodies. In addition, none of 586 archival sera from blood samples collected from 1983, when the first evidence of HIV infection in Africa was reported, to 1986 was positive for HIV (59). Unfortunately, the announcement of these initial negative results led to complacency on the part of health authorities in Nigeria and consequently the general population.

Seroepidemiology

Data from screening of blood donors and limited seroepidemiologic studies of the general population indicated that the rate of HIV infection was less than 1% in Nigeria until the late 1980s (118–121). However, a study using 3,854 serum samples collected from 1985 to 1990 showed a 10-fold rise in the rate of HIV infection in the country within the five-year period (49). This observation was corroborated by other workers from different parts of the country, indicating increased HIV infections in Nigeria during the early 1990s (119,122). Thus, contrary to initial beliefs, the virus may have been introduced into the Nigerian population in the late 1970s, like many other African countries, but it remained at low levels within the population until its explosion in the late 1980s. In retrospect, blood samples from a woman who presented with severe loss of weight in the early 1980s, then called "slim disease," was found to be positive for HIV antibodies (unpublished data). The highly celebrated story of the "strange disease" was published on several occasions by a local newspaper, *Sketch*, in the early 1980s.

The first national surveillance of HIV infection among pregnant women attending antenatal clinics (ANC), as well as patients attending sexually transmitted infection clinics, was conducted in 1991 (123–125). In addition, groups of long-distance truck drivers and sex workers were tested. Surveys among the ANC attendees and people with high-risk behaviors have been repeated at various intervals since then (123–126). These studies have shown that HIV has spread extensively in urban and rural areas of Nigeria. The rate of infection also varies significantly from one location to another. The median rate of infection among the general population represented by ANC attendees in different parts of the country increased from 1.8% in 1991 to 4.5% in 1995, 5.4% in 1999, and 5.8% in 2001; a small decline to 5.0% was noted in 2003 (123–126). Similarly, a 2000 survey found high HIV infection rates of 11.0% (ranging from 5.2% to 23.0%) and 17.0% (ranging from 4.2% to 33.0%) among patients presenting with other sexually transmitted infections and pulmonary tuberculosis, respectively (123).

As HIV continues to spread in Nigeria, it is apparent that the epidemic manifests different patterns among various subpopulations and in different parts of the country. Initially, the age of highest infection was among people in their late twenties. More recent surveys, however, have shown high rates of HIV infection among people aged 15 to 24 years. The rate of HIV infection among pregnant women 15 to 24

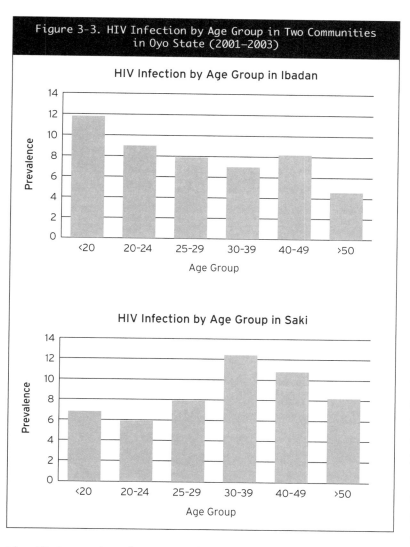

Figure 3-3. HIV Infection by Age Group in Two Communities in Oyo State (2001–2003)

years was 5.7% in 1999, 5.8% in 2001, and 5.4% in 2003 (125).

Apart from the periodic national surveys, testing of people with high-risk sexual behaviors, such as sex workers and long-distance truck drivers, also began in the late 1980s. The data showed a gradual increase in HIV infections among sex workers from about 2% in 1988–1989, to 15% in 1993, 24% in 1994, and greater than 50% in 1995 (126). By 2004, the rate of HIV infection among sex workers ranged from 35% to more than 80% in most parts of the country (126). Similar studies among long-distance truck drivers also demonstrated increased HIV infection rates from about 4% in the early 1990s to more than 20% in 2000 (126).

In a situation analysis report on HIV and other STIs in Nigeria in 2000, a ministerial committee of the Federal Ministry of Health identified several weaknesses in the national HIV data. With the rate based on the HIV seroprevalence among pregnant women attending government health facilities, little is known about HIV infections among pediatric populations or among men (124). The review also indicated a lack of information on incidence rates of HIV infection among various at-risk populations, few voluntary counseling and testing centers, and insufficient linkage of HIV with other STI prevention and control programs (124).

While several of these issues remain unresolved, surveillance has been the subject of the evidence-based prevention approach of the AIDS Prevention Initiative in Nigeria (APIN) of the Harvard School of Public Health. The goal of HIV surveillance is to determine the rate and incidence of the virus transmission among diverse subpopulations at the community level. Available baseline data from APIN-supported HIV surveillance projects in two occupational groups communities—Ibadan and Saki in Oyo State—showed that the actual HIV infection rate may be higher than previously suggested by the periodic national testing of ANC attendees. For instance, while the 2003 national HIV survey estimated a 4% prevalence in Oyo State, the results of a population-based study by APIN and the Department of Virology at the University College Hospital in Ibadan involving approximately 10,000 apparently healthy volunteers found HIV infection rates of 7% and 8% in Ibadan and Saki, respectively (Figure 3.3). The rates varied widely between occupational groups from 5.4% to 13.6% in Ibadan and 3.2% to 16.9% in Saki. The rate of HIV infection was significantly higher among males than females in the same geographic area.

In Nigeria, HIV transmission remains predominantly due to heterosexual sex. Males have been shown to be the main bridging route between people who engage in high-risk sexual behavior, such as female sex workers, and the general population (Olaleye et al., *unpublished data*). In addition, use of unscreened or improperly screened blood units for transfusion constitutes a major source of transmission. It is also pertinent to note that fewer than 1% of pregnant women in Nigeria have access to free HIV testing and prevention-of-mother-to-child-transmission counseling. Hence, mother-to-child transmission of HIV remains a significant problem in Nigeria.

Reported AIDS Cases

As part of the global strategy to monitor the HIV pandemic, all countries are expected to report new AIDS cases to UNAIDS. Although the value of AIDS case reporting is limited, as it only provides information on transmission patterns during the previous five to ten years, the data remain useful for advocacy and estimating the burden of HIV-related morbidity, as well as planning of AIDS-related health care services. The data also provide information on the demographic and geographic characteristics of the infected and affected population groups, including their risk factors for HIV infection.

In Nigeria, several attempts have been made to organize a proper AIDS case reporting system. Like many other public sector agencies seeking to collect data, the Federal Ministry of Health has had difficulty obtaining accurate data on AIDS cases from the local and state levels. In 2000 the ministry reactivated the AIDS reporting program in collaboration with several international developmental partners. The process of active data collection at the hospital level started in 2002–2003.

Although the government of Nigeria has been reporting AIDS cases to the World Health Organization since 1998, the data do not correspond with the reality of the problem in the country. As an alternative, the Federal Ministry of Health has adopted the UNAIDS projection method of estimating AIDS cases from HIV infection rates emanating from sentinel survey data. Based on the 2001 and 2003 HIV sentinel surveys, it has been estimated that at least four million adults between 15 and 49 years of age are infected with HIV in Nigeria, with another 350,000 already diagnosed or living with AIDS (125).

CONCLUSION

Our understanding of the biology, diversity, and pathogenesis of HIV has increased tremendously in the two decades since its discovery. These advances have enabled newer methods for epidemiologic surveillance, more rapid diagnoses, and more effective drugs to treat infection. Nigeria, already home to a large diversity of HIV viruses, may indicate that subtype-specific vaccine development will be difficult. The use of antiretrovirals in populations with limited resources may also suggest that drug-resistant virus is prevalent, creating obstacles for future ART programs if those strains begin to circulate widely. We remain hopeful, however, that continued research will advance the development of an effective vaccine that will prove a critical component in our efforts to stem the HIV/AIDS epidemic.

ACKNOWLEDGMENTS

We are very grateful for the kind opportunity given to us by the APIN director, Professor Phyllis Kanki, to contribute to this laudable initiative of the first book on AIDS in Nigeria. We would also like to thank APIN's senior program manager, Dr. Wole Odutolu, and project manager, Dr. Prosper Okonkwo, for their words of encouragement. The extensive and meticulous review work, advice, and constructive criticism by Dr. Jason Blackard is sincerely acknowledged, as is the deft editorial hand of Dr. Seema Thakore Meloni. The result of our collaboration with Dr. Jean-Louis Sankalé on the APIN surveillance project in Oyo State is evident in the data used on the molecular epidemiology of HIV in Nigeria. We are most grateful for this support. The tireless effort of Jalal Hosseini to get work done is appreciated. Many thanks are also due to M. O. Adewumi, A. S. Bakarey, and E. Donbraye, our graduate students in the Department of Virology at the University of Ibadan for their assistance. The versatility of Funke Adeniyi for the careful and faithful work of the illustrations and the typing of the manuscripts reaffirms her as a great asset to the group.

REFERENCES

1. Coffin M. Retroviridae and their replication. In: Fields BN, Knipe DM, Chanock RM, Hirsch MS, Melnick JL, Monath TP, Roizman B, eds. *Virology.* 2nd ed. Raven Press, 1990:1437–1488.

2. Gallo R, Salahuddin S, Popovic M. Frequent detection and isolation of cytopathic retroviruses (HTLV-III) from patients with AIDS. *Science,* 1984; 224:497–500.

3. Essex M, Mboup S. The etiology of AIDS. In: Essex M, Mboup S, Kanki PJ, Marlink RG, Tlou SD, eds. *AIDS in Africa.* 2nd ed. New York: Kluwer Academic/Plenum Publishers, 2002:1–10.

4. Levy J. *HIV and the Pathogenesis of AIDS.* Washington, DC: ASM Press, 1994.

5. Zijenah L, Katzenstein D. Immunopathogenesis of AIDS. In: Essex M, Mboup S, Kanki PJ, Marlink RG, Tlou SD, eds. *AIDS in Africa.* 2nd ed. New York: Kluwer Academic/Plenum Publishers, 2002:34–52.

6. Yu X, Lichterfeld M, Addo M, et al. Regulatory and accessory HIV-1 proteins: potential targets for HIV-1 vaccines? *Curr Med Chem,* 2005;12:741–747.

7. Hirsch M, Curran J. Human immunodeficiency viruses: biology and medical aspect. In: Fields BN, Knipe DM, Chanock RM, Hirsch MS, Melnick JL, Monath TP, Roizman B, eds. *Virology.* 2nd ed. New York: Raven Press, 1990:1545–1570.

8. Diop O, Gueye A, Ayouba A, et al. Simian immunodeficiency viruses and the origin of HIVs. In: Essex M, Mboup S, Kanki PJ, Marlink RG, Tlou SD, eds. *AIDS in Africa.* 2nd ed. New York: Kluwer Academic/Plenum Publishers, 2002:104–120.

9. Gallo R, Mann D, Broder S, et al. Human T-cell leukemia lymphoma virus (HTLV) is in T but not B lymphocytes from a patient with cutaneous T-cell lymphoma. *Proc Natl Acad Sci USA,* 1982;79:5680.

10. Poiesz B, Ruscetti F, Gazdar A, et al. Detection and isolation of type C retrovirus particles from fresh and cultured lymphocytes of a patient with cutaneous T cell lymphoma. *Proc Natl Acad Sci USA*, 1980; 77:7415–7418.

11. Wong-Staal F. Human immunodeficiency viruses and their replication. In: Fields BN, Knipe DM, Chanock RM, et al., eds. *Virology*. 2nd ed. New York: Raven Press, 1990:1529–1544.

12. Piot P, Plummer F, Mhalu F, et al. AIDS: An International Perspective. *Science*, 1998;239:573–579.

13. Clavel F, Guetard D, Brun-Vezinet F. Isolation of a new human retrovirus from West African patients with AIDS. *Science*, 1986;237:343–346.

14. Kanki P, Mani I. Monitoring viral load. In: Essex M, Mboup S, Kanki PJ, Marlink RG, Tlou SD, eds. *AIDS in Africa*. 2nd ed. New York: Kluwer Academic/Plenum Publishers, 2002:173–185.

15. Alimonti J, Ball T, Fowke K. Mechanisms of CD4+ T lymphocyte cell death in human immunodeficiency virus infection and AIDS. *J Gen Virol*, 2003; 84:1649–1661.

16. Connor R, Sheridan K, Ceradini D, et al. Change in coreceptor use correlates with disease progression in HIV-1 infected individuals. *J Exp Med*, 1997;185: 621–628.

17. McDermott D, Zimmerman P, Guignard F, et al. CCR5 promoter polymorphism and HIV-1 disease progression. Multicenter AIDS Cohort Study (MACS). *Lancet*, 1998;352:866–870.

18. Holmberg SD, Horsburgh CR Jr, Ward JW, et al. Biologic factors in the sexual transmission of human immunodeficiency virus. *J Infect Dis*, 1989;3: 361–366.

19. Dean M, Carrington M, Winkler C. Genetic restriction of HIV-1 infection and progression to AIDS by a deletion allele of the CKRS structural gene. *Science*, 1996;273:1856–1862.

20. Wells T, Proudfoot A, Power C, et al. Chemokine receptors: the new frontier for AIDS research. *Chemica Biologica*, 1996;3:603–609.

21. Zhang L, Huang Y, He T, et al. HIV-1 subtype and second receptor use. *Nature*, 1996;383:768.

22. McDermott D, Beecroft M, Kleeberger C, et al. Chemokine RANTES promoter polymorphism affects risk of both HIV infection and disease progression in the Multicenter AIDS Cohort Study. *AIDS*, 2000;14:2671–2678.

23. Pathak V, Temin H. Broad spectrum of in-vivo forward mutations, hypermutations and mutational hot spots in a retroviral shuttle vector after a single replication cycle: substitutions, frame shifts, and hypermutations. *Proc Natl Acad Sci USA*, 1990;87: 6019–6023.

24. Oxenius A, Price D, Trkola A, et al. Loss of viral control in early HIV-1 infection is temporarily associated with sequential escape from CD8+ T cell responses and decrease in HIV-1-specific CD4+ and CD8+ T cell frequencies. *J Infect Dis*, 2004;190: 713–721.

25. Yang O, Walker B. CD8+ cells in human immunodeficiency virus type 1 pathogenesis: cytolytic and noncytolytic inhibition of viral replication. *Adv Immunol*, 1997;66:273.

26. Flamand L, Crowley R, Lusso P, et al. Activation of CD8+ T lymphocytes through the T cell receptor turns on CD4 gene expression: implications of HIV pathogenesis. *Proc Natl Acad Sci USA*, 1998;96:3111.

27. Livingstone W, Moore M, Innes D, et al. Frequent infection of peripheral blood CD8-positive T-lymphocytes with HIV-1. *Lancet*, 1996;348:649.

28. Douek D, Brenchley J, Betts M, et al. HIV preferentially infects HIV-specific CD4+ T cells. *Nature*, 2002;417:95–98.

29. Lelievre J, Mammona F, Arnoult D, et al. A novel mechanism for HIV-1-mediated bystander CD4+ T-cell death: neighboring dying cells drive the capacity of HIV-1 to kill noncycling primary CD4+ T cells. *Nature*, 2004;11:1017–1027.

30. Wood E, Hogg R, Yip B, et al. Using baseline CD4 cell count and plasma HIV RNA to guide the initiation of highly active antiretroviral therapy. *Rev Invest Clin*, 2004;56:232–236.

31. Yaman A, Cetiner S, Kibar F, et al. Reference ranges of lymphocyte subsets of healthy adults in Turkey. *Med Princ Pract*, 2005;14:189–193.

32. Fauci A. The human immunodeficiency virus infectivity and mechanism of pathogenesis. *Science*, 1988; 275:617–622.

33. Plantier J, Gueudin M, Damond F, et al. Plasma RNA quantification and HIV-1 divergent strains. *J Acquir Immune Defic Syndr*, 2003;33:1–7.

34. Barbour J, Grant R. The role of viral fitness in HIV pathogenesis. *Curr HIV/AIDS Rep*, 2005;2:29–34.

35. Bernier R, Tremblay M. Homologous interference resulting from the presence of defective particles of human immunodeficiency virus type 1. *J Virol*, 1995; 69:291–300.

36. Sanchez G, Xu X, Chermann J, et al. Accumulation of defective viral genomes in peripheral blood mononuclear cells of human immunodeficiency virus type 1-infected individuals. *J Virol*, 1997;71: 2233–2240.

37. Zaunders J, Geczy A, Dyer W, et al. Effect of long-term infection with *nef*-defective attenuated HIV type 1 on CD4+ and CD8+ T lymphocytes: increased CD45RO+CD4+ T lymphocytes and limited activation of CD8+ T lymphocytes. *AIDS Res Hum Retroviruses*, 1999;15:1519–1527.

38. Akinsete I, Akanmu A, Okany C. Spectrum of clinical diseases in HIV-infected adults at the Lagos University Teaching Hospital: a five-year experience (1992–1996). *Afr J Med Med Sci*, 1998;27:147–151.

39. Anteyi E, Idoko J, Ukoli C, et al. Clinical pattern of human immunodeficiency virus infection (HIV) in pulmonary tuberculosis patients in Jos, Nigeria. *Afr J Med Med Sci*, 1996;25:317–321.

40. Laurent C, Ngom Gueye N, Ndour C, et al. Long-term benefits of highly active antiretroviral therapy in Senegalese HIV-1–infected adults. *J Acquir Immune Defic Syndr*, 2005;38:14–17.

41. Moore R, Keruly J, Gebo K, et al. An improvement in virologic response to highly active antiretroviral therapy in clinical practice from 1996 through 2002. *J Acquir Immune Defic Syndr*, 2005;39:195–198.

42. Resino S, Bellon J, Ramos J, et al. Impact of highly active antiretroviral therapy on CD4+ T cells and viral load of children with AIDS: a population-based study. *AIDS Res Hum Retroviruses*, 2004;20: 927–931.

43. Sungkanuparph S, Kiertiburanakul S, Manosuthi W, et al. Initiation of highly active antiretroviral therapy in advanced AIDS with CD4 < 50 cells/mm^3 in a resource-limited setting: efficacy and tolerability. *Int J STD AIDS*, 2005;16:243–246.

44. World Health Organization. State from consultation on HIV and routine childhood immunization. *Wkly Epidemiol Rec*, 1987;62:297.

45. Padian N, Shiboski SC, Jewell NP. Female-to-male transmission of human immunodeficiency virus. *JAMA*, 1991;266:1664–1667.

46. World Health Organization. Global AIDS surveillance Part II. *Wkly Epidemiol Rec*, 1998;73:373–380.

47. Gilbert P, McKeague I, Eisen G, et al. Comparison of HIV-1 and HIV-2 infectivity from a prospective cohort study in Senegal. *Stat Med*, 2003;22:573–593.

48. Williams AO. *AIDS: An African Perspective*. Ann Arbor, Michigan: CRC Press, 1991.

49. Olaleye D, Bernstein L, Ekwezor C, et al. Prevalence of human immunodeficiency virus type 1 and 2 infections in Nigeria. *J Infect Dis*, 1993;167: 710–714.

50. WHO Global AIDS News: Newsletter of the World Health Organization. *Global Programme on AIDS*, 1994;1020:1–5.

51. Subbarao S, Schochetman G. Genetic variability of HIV-1. *AIDS*, 1996;10(Suppl A):S513–S523.

52. O'Brien W, Namazi A, Kalhor H, Mao SH, Zach JA, Chen IS. Kinetics of human immunodeficiency virus type-1 reverse transcriptase in blood mononuclear phagocytes are slowed by limitations of nucleotide precursors. *J Virol*, 1994;68:1258–1263.

53. Georgi C, Chou J, Gudeman C, et al. Cell-mediated immune response to human immunodeficiency virus (HIV) type-1 in seronegative homosexual men with recent sexual exposure to HIV-1. *J Infect Dis*, 1992;165:1012–1019.

54. Peterman T, Stonenburner R, Allen J, et al. Risk of human immunodeficiency virus transmission from heterosexual adults with transfusion associated infection. *JAMA*, 1988;259:55–58.

55. Aaby P, Airyoshi K, Bucker M, et al. Age of wife as a major determinant of male-female transmission of HIV-2 infection: a community study from rural West Africa. *AIDS*, 1996;10:1585–1590.

56. Fischl M, Dickinson G, Scott G, et al. Evaluation of heterosexual partners, children and household contacts of adults with AIDS. *JAMA*, 1987;257.

57. Rate of vertical transmission of HIV high in black South Africans. *AIDS Wkly Plus*, Aug 12, 1996:17–18.

58. Gray C, Williamson C, Bredell H, et al. Viral dynamics and CD4+ T cell counts in subtype C human immunodeficiency virus type 1-infected individuals from southern Africa. *AIDS Res Hum Retroviruses*, 2005;21:285–291.

59. Hill JA, Anderson DJ. Human vaginal leukocytes and the effects of vaginal fluid on lymphocyte and macrophage defense functions. *Am J Obstet Gynecol*, 1992;166:720-6.

60. Nelson G, Perelson A. A mechanism of immune escape by slow replicating HIV strains. *AIDS*, 1992; 5:82–93.

61. Sheppard H, Lang W, Ascher M, et al. The characterization of non-progressors: long-term HIV infection with stable CD4+ T-cell level. *AIDS*, 1993; 7:1159–1166.

62. Coates R, Read S, Fanning M, et al. Transmission of HIV in the male sexual contacts of men with ARC or AIDS. *IV International Conference on AIDS*, Stockholm, Sweden, 1988.

63. Goedert J, Eyster M, Biggarm R, et al. Heterosexual transmission of human immunodeficiency virus: association with severe depletion of T-helper lymphocytes in men with hemophilia. *AIDS Res Hum Retroviruses*, 1988;3:355–361.

64. Guinan JJ, Kronenberg C, Gold J, Morlet A, Cooper DA. Sexual behavioural change in partners of homosexual men infected with human immunodeficiency virus. *Med J Aust*, 1988,149:162.

65. Simonsen J, Cameron W, Gakinya M, et al. Human immunodeficiency virus among men with sexually transmitted diseases. Experience from a center in Africa. *New Engl J Med*, 1988;319:274–278.

66. Ward J, Bush J, Perkins M, et al. The natural history of transfusion associated infection with human immunodeficiency virus. *New Engl J Med*, 1989;321:947–952.

67. Friedland G, Klein R. Transmission of the human immunodeficiency virus. *New Engl J Med*, 1987;317:1125–1130.

68. Guay L, Horn D, Kabengera S, et al. HIV-1 ICD p24 antigen detection in Ugandan infants: use in early diagnosis of infection and as a marker of disease progression. *J Med Virol*, 2000;62:426–434.

69. Focus on AIDS. *Nig Bull Epidemiol*, 1992;2:1–23.

70. U.S. Centers for Disease Control and Prevention. *Drug-Associated HIV Transmission Continues in the United States*. Accessed at www.cdc.gov/hiv/pubs/facts/idu.htm on March 1, 2006.

71. Coutsoudis A. Influence of infant feeding patterns on early mother-to-child transmission of HIV-1 in Durban, South Africa. *Ann NY Acad Sci*, 2000;918:136–144.

72. Ogundele M, Coulter J. HIV transmission through breastfeeding: problems and prevention. *Ann Trop Paediatr*, 2003;23:91–106.

73. Richardson B, John-Stewart G, Hughes J, et al. Breast-milk infectivity in human immunodeficiency virus type 1-infected mothers. *J Infect Dis*, 2003;187:736–740.

74. Rouet F, Elenga N, Msellati P, et al. Primary HIV-1 infection in African children infected through breastfeeding. *AIDS*, 2002;16:2303–2309.

75. McCarthy M. No-needle, HIV test approved by FDA. *Lancet*, 1996;347:1683.

76. Ryder RW, Manzila T, Baende E, et al. Evidence from Zaire that breast-feeding by HIV-1-seropositive mothers is not a major route for perinatal HIV-1 transmission but does decrease morbidity. *AIDS*, 1991;5(6):709–714.

77. Odaibo G, Ibeh M, Olaleye D. Reliability of HIV testing in Africa. *2nd IAS Conference on HIV Pathogenesis and Treatment*, Paris, France, 2003.

78. Beelaert G, Vercauteren G, Fransen K, et al. Comparative evaluation of eight commercial enzyme linked immunosorbent assays and 14 simple assays for detection of antibodies to HIV. *J Virol Methods*, 2002;105:197–206.

79. Menard D, Mavolomade E, Mandeng M, et al. Advantages of an alternative strategy based on consecutive HIV serological tests for detection of HIV antibodies in Central African Republic. *J Virol Methods*, 2003;111:129–134.

80. Rouet F, Ekouevi D, Inwoley A, et al. Field evaluation of a rapid human immunodeficiency virus (HIV) serial serologic testing algorithm for diagnosis and differentiation of HIV type 1 (HIV-1), HIV-2, and dual HIV-1-HIV-2 infections in West African pregnant women. *J Clin Microbiol*, 2004;42:4147–4153.

81. Foglia G, Royster G, Wasunna K, et al. Use of rapid and conventional testing technologies for human immunodeficiency virus type 1 serologic screening in a rural Kenyan reference laboratory. *J Clin Microbiol*, 2004;42:3850–3852.

82. Meless H, Tegbaru B, Messele T, et al. Evaluation of rapid assays for screening and confirming HIV-1 infection in Ethiopia. *Ethiop Med J*, 2002;40(Suppl 1):S27–S36.

83. Menard D, Mairo A, Mandeng M, et al. Evaluation of rapid HIV testing strategies in under equipped laboratories in the Central African Republic. *J Virol Methods*, 2005;126:75–80.

84. Wright R, Stringer J. Rapid testing strategies for HIV-1 serodiagnosis in high-prevalence African settings. *Am J Prev Med*, 2004;27:42–48.

85. Abrao Ferreira P, Gabriel R, Furlan T, et al. Anti-HIV-1/2 antibody detection by Dot-ELISA in oral fluid of HIV positive/AIDS patients and voluntary blood donors. *Braz J Infect Dis*, 1999;3:134–138.

86. Margodo de Moura Machedo J, Kayita J, Bakaki P, et al. IgA antibodies to human immunodeficiency virus in serum, saliva and urine for early diagnosis of immunodeficiency virus infection in Uganda infants. *Pediatr Infect Dis J*, 2003;22:193–195.

87. Tiensiwakul P. Urinary HIV-1 antibody patterns by western blot assay. *Clin Lab Sci*, 1998;11:336–338.

88. Hashida S, Hashinaka K, Ishikawa S, et al. More reliable diagnosis of infection with human immunodeficiency virus type 1 (HIV-1) by detection of antibody IgGs to pol and gag proteins of HIV-1 and p24 antigen of HIV-1 in urine, saliva, and/or serum with highly sensitive and specific enzyme immunoassay (immune complex transfer enzyme immunoassay): a review. *J Clin Lab Anal*, 1997;11: 267–286.

89. Martinez P, Torres A, Ortiz de Lejarazu R, et al. Human immunodeficiency virus antibody testing by enzyme-linked fluorescent and western blot assays using serum, gingival-crevicular transudate, and urine samples. *J Clin Microbiol*, 1999;37:1100–1106.

90. de Freitas Oliveira C, Ueda M, Yamashiro R, et al. Rate and incidence estimates of recent human immunodeficiency virus type 1 infections among pregnant women in Sao Paulo, Brazil, from 1991 to 2002. *J Clin Microbiol*, 2005;43:1439–1442.

91. Gupta P, Kingsley L, Sheppard H, et al. High incidence and prevalence of HIV-1 infection in high risk population in Calcutta, India. *Int J STD AIDS*, 2003;14:463–468.

92. Tu X, Litvak E, Pagano M. Issues in human immunodeficiency virus (HIV) screening programs. *Am J Epidemiol*, 1992;136:244–255.

93. Delaporte E, Dupont A, Merlin M, et al. Seroepidemiology of HIV-1 and HIV-2 antibodies in Gabon. *AIDS*, 1988;2:136-7.

94. Ramirez E, Uribe P, Escanila D, et al. Reactivity patterns and infectious status of serum samples with indeterminate western immunoblot tests for antibody to HIV-1. *J Clin Microbiol*, 1992;30:801–805.

95. Janssens W, Buve A, Nkengasong J. The puzzle of HIV-1 subtypes in Africa. *AIDS*, 1997;11:705–712.

96. Simmond P. Polymerase chain reaction. In: Desselberger U, ed. *Medical Virology: A Practical Approach*. Oxford: Oxford University Press, 1995:107–145.

97. Alter H, Laurian Y, Paul D. Transmission of HTLV-III infection from human plasma to chimpanzee, an animal model for AIDS. *Science*, 1984;226:549–552.

98. Ho D, Rota T, Schooley R. Isolation of HTLV-III from cerebrospinal fluid and neural tissues of patients with neurologic syndromes related to the acquired immunodeficiency syndrome. *New Engl J Med*, 1985;313:1493–1497.

99. Ou C, Kwok S, Mitchell S. DNA amplification for direct detection of HIV-1 in DNA of peripheral blood mononuclear cells. *Science*, 1988;239:295–297.

100. Scarlatti G. Mother-to-child transmission of HIV-1: advances and controversies of the twentieth centuries. *AIDS Rev*, 2004;6:67–78.

101. Zijenah L, Moulton L, Iliff P, et al. Timing of mother-to-child transmission of HIV-1 and infant mortality in the first 6 months of life in Harare, Zimbabwe. *AIDS*, 2004;18:273–280.

102. Campbell T, Schneider K, Wrin T, et al. Relationship between in vitro human immunodeficiency virus type 1 replication rate and virus load in plasma. *J Virol*, 2003;77:12105–12112.

103. Kim A, Lauer G, Ouchi K, et al. The magnitude and breadth of hepatitis C virus-specific CD8+ T cells depend on absolute CD4+ T-cell count in individuals coinfected with HIV-1. *Blood*, 2005;105: 1170–1178.

104. Schupabach J. Measurement of HIV-1 p24 antigen by signal-amplification-boosted ELISA of heat-denatured plasma is a simple and inexpensive alternative to tests for viral RNA. *AIDS Rev*, 2002;4: 83–92.

105. Aquino-De Jesus M, Anders C, Miller G, et al. Genetically and epidemiologically related "non-syncytium-inducing" isolates of HIV-1 display heterogeneous growth patterns in macrophages. *J Med Virol*, 2000;61:171–180.

106. Callaway D, Ribeiro R, Nowak M. Virus phenotype switching and disease progression in HIV-1 infection. *Proc Biol Sci*, 1999;266:2523–2530.

107. Fitzgibbon J, Gaur S, Gavai M, et al. Effect of the HIV-1 syncytium-inducing phenotype on disease stage in vertically-infected children. *J Med Virol*, 1998;55:56–63.

108. Nicastri E, Ercoli L, Sarmati L, et al. Five human immunodeficiency virus type 1 phenotypic variants with different MT-2 cell tropisms correlate with prognostic markers of disease. *J Hum Virol*, 1998;1: 90–95.

109. Anastos K, Barron Y, Cohen M, et al. The prognostic importance of changes in CD4+ cell count and HIV-1 RNA level in women after initiating highly active antiretroviral therapy. *Ann Intern Med*, 2004; 140:256–264.

110. Anastos K, Shi Q, French A, et al. Total lymphocyte count, hemoglobin, and delayed-type hypersensitivity as predictors of death and AIDS illness in HIV-1 infected women receiving highly active antiretroviral therapy. *J Acquir Immune Defic Syndr*, 2004; 35:383–392.

111. Kalish L, McIntosh K, Read J, et al. Evaluation of human immunodeficiency virus (HIV) type 1 load, CD4 T cell level and clinical class as time-fixed and time-varying markers of disease progression in HIV-1-infected children. *J Infect Dis*, 1999;180: 1514–1520.

112. Kozinetz C, Matusa R, Ruta S, et al. Alternatives to HIV-RNA and CD4 count to monitor HIV disease progression: a prospective cohort study in Romania. *J Med Virol*, 2005;77:159–163.

113. Lathey J, Hughes M, Fiscus S, et al. Variability and prognostic values of virologic and CD4 cell measures in human immunodeficiency virus type 1-infected patients with 200-500 CD4 cells/mm³ (ACTG 175). AIDS Clinical Trials Group Protocol 175 Team. *J Infect Dis*, 1998;177:617–624.

114. Zhou J, Kumarasamy N. TREAT Asia HIV Observation Database. Predicting short-term disease progression among HIV-infected patients in Asia and the Pacific Region: preliminary results from the TREAT Asia HIV Observational Database (TAHOD). *HIV Med*, 2005;6:216–223.

115. Kamga I, Kahi S, Develioglu L, et al. Type 1 interferon production is profoundly and transiently impaired in primary HIV-1 infection. *J Infect Dis*, 2005;192:303–310.

116. Mildvan D, Spritzler J, Grossberg SE, et al. Serum neopterin, an immune activation marker, independently predicts disease progression in advanced HIV-1 infection. *Clin Infect Dis*, 2005;40(6): 853–858.

117. Shimizu Y, Miyazaki Y, Ibuki K, et al. Induction of immune response in macaque monkeys infected with simian-human immunodeficiency virus having the TNF-alpha gene at an early stage of infection. *Virology*, 2005;343(2):151–161.

118. Chikwem J, Mohammed I, Oyebode-Ola T. Prevalence of human immunodeficiency virus (HIV) infection in Borno State of Nigeria. *East African Med J*, 1988;65:342–346.

119. Harry T, Ekenna O, Chikwen J, et al. Seroepidemiology of human immunodeficiency virus infection in Borno State of Nigeria by sentinel surveillance. *J Acquir Immune Defic Syndr*, 1993;6:99–103.

120. Harry T, Kyari O, Mohammed I. Prevalence of human immunodeficiency virus-infection among pregnant women attending ante-natal clinic in Maiduguri, north-eastern Nigeria. *Trop Geogr Med*, 1992;44:238–241.

121. Olusanya O, Lawoko A, Blomberg J. Seroepidemiology of human retroviruses in Ogun State of Nigeria. *J Infect Dis*, 1990;22:155–160.

122. Olaleye D, Ekweozor C, Sheng Z, et al. Evidence of serological cross-reactivities with human immunodeficiency virus types 1 and 2 and human T-lymphotropic virus. *Int J Epidemiol*, 1995;24:198–203.

123. Federal Ministry of Health. *Technical Report on 2000 HIV/Syphilis Sero-prevalence and STD Syndromes Sentinel Survey among PTB and STD Patients in Nigeria*. Abuja: Federal Ministry of Health, 2001.

124. Federal Ministry of Health. *The 2001 National HIV/Syphilis Sentinel Survey among Pregnant Women Attending Antenatals Clinic in Nigeria*. Abuja: Federal Ministry of Health, 2001.

125. Federal Ministry of Health. The 2003 National HIV Sero-prevalence Sentinel Survey. Federal Ministry of Health, 2003.

126. UNAIDS. WHO Epidemiological Fact Sheets on HIV/AIDS and Sexually Transmitted Infections. Geneva: UNAIDS, 2004.

THE MOLECULAR EPIDEMIOLOGY OF HIV

Seema Thakore Meloni,* Akinyemi Ojesina,*†
and David O. Olaleye‡

HIV-1 and HIV-2 are members of the lentivirus subfamily. These retroviruses are approximately 50% related at the nucleotide level (1,2). A major difference in their genetic organization is that *vpu*, an accessory gene, is unique to HIV-1 (3), while the *vpx* gene is found only in HIV-2 (4,5). Of the two viruses, HIV-1 is the more widely distributed, accounting for approximately 95% of all HIV infections worldwide. Phylogenetic analyses of sequences from globally circulating strains of HIV reveal a great deal of genetic diversity. Sequence analyses have shown not only that there is genomic heterogeneity between the various strains worldwide, but also that the diversity is unevenly distributed throughout the HIV-1 genome (2). Furthermore, intrapatient isolates have less diversity than interpatient isolates, but even within a single individual replicating viruses can differ as much as 10% at the nucleotide level (1,2,6). Given this extensive variability, the development of a classification scheme for all circulating HIV-1 strains became necessary.

*Department of Immunology and Infectious Diseases, Harvard School of Public Health, Boston, Massachusetts, USA
†AIDS Prevention Initiative in Nigeria, Boston, Massachusetts, USA
‡Department of Virology, College of Medicine, University of Ibadan, University College Hospital, Ibadan, Nigeria

CLASSIFICATION OF HIV STRAINS

Prior to 1992, HIV-1 strains were classified based on their geographic origin, as early phylogenetic analyses indicated that viruses from Europe and North America clustered separately and distinctly from viruses isolated in Africa (7–9). However, as additional sequence data were generated from viruses from around the world, it became obvious that the original classification scheme was insufficient. Further analyses of *env* and *gag* gene sequences indicated the presence of multiple phylogenetic clusters, or clades, that were equidistant from one another (9).

These clades were termed subtypes, which are defined as groups of viruses that closely resemble each other more than they do other subtypes (8,10,11). The viruses originally classified as "European/North American" were re-classified as subtype B, while the African viruses were divided between subtypes A through F, excluding E. Subsequently, subtypes G, H, J, and K were also identified (9). The nine subtypes were organized into one large group of viruses called the group M (major) HIV-1 viruses (9). In 1994, highly divergent HIV-1 viruses that did not cluster with any of the known group M subtypes were identified in Cameroon. These isolates were considered a separate group of viruses, group O (outlier) (12). In 1998, group N (non-M/non-O) viruses were identified in a few individuals from Cameroon (13). Overall, group M viruses account for most HIV infections, while group N and group O viruses are relatively rare. But it must be noted that there is limited detection of group N and O infections because of a lack of specific serological and Western blot profiles available to detect these viruses. This point becomes significant when we consider that because they are not as well detected as group M viruses and may be circulating in larger numbers than we have been able to ascertain, group N and O infections may have a significant impact as antiretroviral regimens become less effective (14).

Group M viruses can be further divided into sub-subtypes (9). Based on full-length sequence data, subtype A has been subdivided into A1, A2 (15), and A3 (16,17), and subtype F into F1 and F2 (18,19). It has also been suggested that subtype K should actually have maintained the name F3; however, for historical reasons, it has been left as a separate subtype (9). Similarly, subtypes B and D should have been reclassified as related sub-subtypes, but have been maintained as separate subtypes (9,20).

Like HIV-1, HIV-2 has been classified into subtypes, designated A–H (21–24). Most HIV-2 infections are from subtypes A and B. At present, the other subtypes are considered rare (24). Each of the HIV-2 subtypes is proposed to represent individual cross-species transmission events (24). In a 2004 paper characterizing HIV-2 subtype H, Damond et al. raised the issue that the HIV-2 nomenclature patterns are inconsistent with those developed for HIV-1 and proposed that the current subtypes of HIV-2 be reclassified as groups (24). Furthermore, the authors suggested that since HIV-2 "groups" C–H had been defined based on single isolates, these groups should be referred to as "putative" (24).

Distinctions Between HIV-1 Groups, Subtypes, and Sub-subtypes

HIV-1 groups, subtypes, and sub-subtypes can be distinguished not only on the basis of phylogenetic analyses, but also by using pairwise genetic distance analyses (2,9–11). The genetic distances between the groups are relatively large, with groups M and O differing by 53% in the envelope gene (2). Within each of the subtypes and sub-subtypes identified, a range of genetic diversity has also been noted (15,25–28). Subtypes are genetically equidistant from one another with the intersubtype nucleotide distances ranging from 15% to 22% in the *gag* gene and from 20% to 30% in the *env* gene (7,9,15,29). Intrasubtype distances range from 3% to 10% in the *gag* gene and 5% to 12% in the *env* gene, while inter-sub-subtype diversity ranges from 7% to 12% in the *gag* gene and 11% to 16% in the *env* gene (9,11,15,29).

HIV Recombinants

With the increasing number of full-length HIV sequences available for analysis, it has become obvious that, in addition to groups, subtypes, and sub-subtypes, a number of intersubtype recombinants also exist (9). These recombinants are either defined as circulating recombinant forms (CRFs) or unique recombinant forms (URFs). CRFs are defined as recombinants that share an identical mosaic structure, indicating that they are descendants of the same recombinant events (9,20). By the end of 2005, 19 CRFs had been formally recognized, with the most recent additions CRF18_cpx and CRF19_cpx from Cuba (30,31). In addition, a large number of URFs, identified in single individuals or a restricted cluster of individuals, also have been characterized. There have also been reports of intergroup recombinants, composed of a mosaic of group M and group O viruses (32–34). Thus far, although dual infection with HIV-1 and HIV-2 has been shown in a number of studies, there has been no in vivo evidence of an HIV-1/HIV-2 recombinant (2,35).

Origin of HIV Viruses

The prevailing hypothesis is that the presence of groups M, N, and O of HIV-1 is the result of three independent introductions of simian immunodeficiency viruses from *Pan troglodytes troglodytes* chimpanzees (SIVcpz) into the human population (2,36–40). Based on inferences from phylogenetic tree analyses, it is believed that group M viruses originated from SIVcpz in west-central Africa (41,42). The earliest recorded isolate of HIV-1 came from a plasma sample from 1959, suggesting that the pandemic likely started in the twentieth century (2,43,44). Through various phylogenetic analyses and evolutionary modeling, it was estimated that the transfer of the group M virus into the human population occurred sometime during the early part of the twentieth century (45–47). Once group M viruses entered the human population, they diversified rapidly. Analyses of subtype C sequences, within the group M radiation, have indicated that these viruses arose in the mid- to late 1960s (48). Similar analyses have also been done for group O sequences and it was estimated that they likely entered the human population around 1920 (49).

Phylogenetic analyses of several group N isolates revealed that they contain a recombinant mosaic structure, where the *gag, pol*, 5'-*vif*, and *nef* genes cluster closely with group M and the 3'-*vif*, *vpr, tat, vpu*, and *env* cluster with Cameroonian SIVcpz and the SIVcpzUS strain of unknown origin (40). It is unclear if the recombination event between the group M and SIVcpz strains occurred before or following zoonotic transmission to humans. However, considering that the group N viruses exhibit less diversity than group M and O viruses, it might be argued that the zoonotic transmission of these virus-es occurred more recently relative to the transfer of the group M viruses. That would suggest that the recombination would have occurred prior to the cross-species transmission event. Yet, without direct evidence it cannot be ruled out that the group N viruses represent a recombination event that occurred in a human that was dually infected with an ancestor of HIV-1 group M and a SIVcpz virus (40). If the in-human recombination scenario was the source of the group N viruses, then the date of origin is esti-mated as pre-1930 (46).

HIV-2 is closely related to the SIVs that have been isolated from *Cercocebus atys* sooty mangabeys (SIVsm) from West Africa as well as from several macaques (three *Macaca* species). As HIV-2 is primari-ly found in West Africa, it has been hypothesized that the cross-species transmission event to humans occurred in that region (37,50). As with HIV-1, it has been estimated that the zoonotic transfer of HIV-2 occurred in the first half of the twentieth century (51).

MECHANISMS OF HIV VARIABILITY

Two major viral mechanisms contribute to the diversity of HIV-1: the error-prone nature of the viral reverse transcriptase and viral recombination. By its nature, reverse transcriptase allows the introduc-tion of mutations into the HIV-1 genome. Combined with the absence of exonuclease proofreading activ-ity and the high replication rate of the virus, it is estimated that there is anywhere from one to ten errors per genome per replication cycle (52,53). It is possible that each new provirus that is generated repre-sents a new mutant strain, distinct at a minimum of one base site (43). Retroviral genomes also undergo insertions, deletions, and frameshifts, and are prone to high rates of G-to-A transitions, or hypermuta-tions (53). In vitro studies have demonstrated that the HIV-1 reverse transcriptase has a higher misin-corporation rate than other retroviral reverse transcriptases, being 10-fold and 18-fold more error prone than avian myeloblastosis and murine leukemia viruses, respectively (54,55). Yet the in vivo mutation rates are much lower than those suggested by the in vitro studies (56).

Recombination has been estimated to occur at a rate of 2.8 crossovers per replication cycle (53,57) and is a fundamental property of viruses because of their diploid RNA genome. For recombination between two subtypes to occur, a cell must be dually infected with two distinct viruses. Then, the resulting progeny virions will contain RNA genomes from each of the viruses. During the next round of reverse transcrip-tion, as the reverse transcriptase switches between strands, the resulting cDNA will contain sequence from the two different viruses. Although we have ample evidence indicating that intersubtype recombi-nation occurs, we still do not have significant data on the rates and limitations (58–60). Intrasubtype recombination also occurs and has been demonstrated. A 2005 study examining in vitro recombination showed that the recombination rate between two subtype C viruses resembles that between two subtype B viruses. The rate of recombination between subtype B and subtype C viruses is much lower, however, than the rates seen in intrasubtype recombination (58). These differences were attributed to a three-nucleotide difference in the dimerization initiation signal region between subtype B and C viruses (58).

As previously mentioned, for recombination to occur, a person must be dually infected with two variants of the virus. Dual infections can occur either simultaneously as coinfections or sequentially as superinfections of a second strain following an infection with a primary strain (59,60). In most cross-sectional studies in which cases of dual infections have been detected, it is difficult to determine whether the infections occurred simultaneously. Diagnoses of superinfection are hard to make as well. In prospective studies in which samples are available over time, however, superinfection can be identified. A few reports have documented cases of superinfection both with the same subtypes and with different subtypes (59,61–67). Superinfection has even been seen with viruses from two different groups, where a person previously infected with an HIV-1 group O virus then became superinfected with a group M CRF02_AG virus (68). Two papers even documented cases of people who were infected with three different of HIV-1 strains (69,70); in these cases, however, the investigators were unable to distinguish between coinfection and superinfection.

To date, while in vivo recombination following superinfection with different subtypes has been postulated, no one has been able to show convincingly recombination between a non-recombinant first and superinfecting second strain within a single individual (71). In a 2004 report, Fang et al. documented the generation of an intersubtype recombinant that took place in a patient originally infected with non-recombinant subtype A who was then suspected to have been superinfected with a subtype C strain (71). While the authors were able to show that the resulting recombinant did contain subtype A sequence from the original infecting strain, they did not show the superinfecting subtype C virus prior to recombination (71).

Finally, selection pressures from the infected host, the environment, or the introduction of therapeutics may also contribute to overall viral diversity (53,72). The mechanisms that generate this diversity result in variants that can evade the host immune system, are resistant to drug therapy, may have an altered cell tropism, or may exhibit a variety of other phenomena that can contribute to disease (2).

GEOGRAPHIC DISTRIBUTION OF HIV-1 GROUP M SUBTYPES

Phylogenetic classification of HIV strains has assisted in tracking the diversity of the globally circulating strains (Figure 4-1). It has been shown that the HIV-1 subtypes exhibit a heterogeneous distribution. Overall, subtypes C and A account for most of the current HIV-1 infections, followed by subtype B and the intersubtype recombinants CRF01_AE and CRF02_AG. While subtype B viruses are primarily found in Europe, the Americas, and Australia, subtype C dominates in sub-Saharan Africa and India (7,8,43,72). It has also been documented that the subtype C viruses are spreading exponentially in Brazil and are slowly outcompeting the predominant subtype B viruses in that country (73). Subtype D viruses are predominantly found in Central and East Africa, with a few cases appearing in southern and West Africa (7,74–77). Although a pure subtype E virus has yet to be found, it is part of the CRF01_AE recombinant form. CRF01_AE has been identified in Thailand, the Philippines, China, and Central Africa. Subtype F has been found in Central Africa, South America, and Eastern Europe. Subtype G has

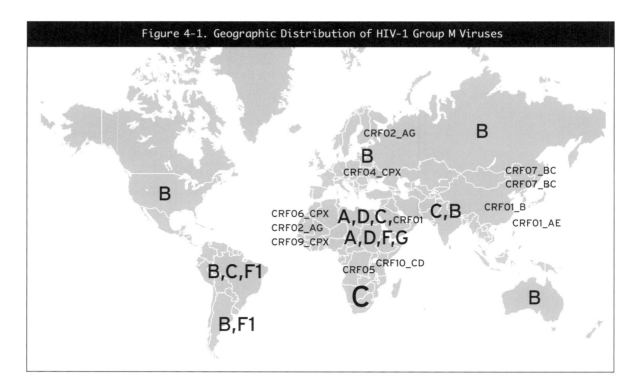

Figure 4-1. Geographic Distribution of HIV-1 Group M Viruses

been reported in West and East Africa as well as Central Europe. Subtype H has only been found in Central Africa. Subtype J was identified in Central America and subtype K was found in the Democratic Republic of Congo and Cameroon. The recombinant virus CRF02_AG is the most prevalent virus in West Africa (8,72,78–82).

Although certain subtypes appear to be restricted geographically, other subtypes are spreading rapidly and co-circulating as the world becomes more of a global community. As immigration and travel increase, there has been a shift in infection patterns; it has been estimated that anywhere from 25% to more than 40% of the new infections in Europe are non-B variants of African and Asian origin (74,83,84). The United States also has an increasing number of non-B infections. For example, in a 2003 report of a well-studied military cohort, 6% of all new infections were because of non-B subtypes (85).

It is difficult to interpret the variations seen in the distribution patterns of the various subtypes. As over two decades have elapsed since the beginning of the HIV epidemic, the global patterns of spread are a result of a long period of evolution, which is nearly impossible to reconstruct. The geographic distribution of the different subtypes has been determined by a number of factors. Primarily, it is believed that founder viruses were introduced into given populations and rapidly diversified. It is interesting to note that, while the rate of HIV spread is not uniform across the globe, there appears to be an inverse correlation between rate of disease spread and the variety of subtypes in a population (7). More specifically, in areas where the rate of spread has been relatively slow and stable, such as Central Africa, there are a number of circulating subtypes in the population, as opposed to southern Africa, which has witnessed an explosive epidemic, but has mainly one predominating subtype. It has been speculated that the large variety of subtypes in Central Africa has been due to the relatively low spread of HIV-1 in the population. Furthermore, it is believed that a number of subtypes can continue to coexist, possibly because of the low crossover between networks of risk groups (7).

IMPLICATIONS OF GENETIC DIVERSITY

The genetic diversity found in HIV is much greater than has been found in any other virus infecting the human population. Whereas with certain viruses a single amino acid change can result in a global pandemic, there can be as much as 10% genetic diversity in the HIV-1 viruses within a single individual (10,86). This diversity has been shown to have an impact on viral phenotype at the level of transmission patterns, pathogenicity, and immunology. In addition, this diversity plays a role in responses to treatment and vaccines.

Studies focusing on the differences between HIV-1 and HIV-2 have shown the clearest evidence of the impact genetic diversity has on the biological phenotype of the virus. While HIV-2 is transmitted through the same modes as HIV-1, the HIV-2 transmission rates are significantly lower, with the most common modes being perinatal and heterosexual (1,87–89). HIV-2 has also been shown to be less pathogenic than HIV-1, with a progression to AIDS significantly longer than that with HIV-1 infection (90,91). In addition, viral load levels are lower with HIV-2 than with HIV-1 (92,93), which likely contributes to the lower pathogenicity of HIV-2. A 2006 in vitro study comparing the viral kinetics of HIV-1 with those of HIV-2 also indicated that, unlike HIV-1, which continuously produces virions at a steady state, HIV-2 had an initial burst of replication and then retired to a latent state with an absence of virion production (94). Interestingly, HIV-2 isolates have also been shown to be more promiscuous in their use of coreceptors; however, the significance of this ability to use additional coreceptors is unclear (95).

Just as with the studies comparing HIV-1 and HIV-2, various reports have shown differences between HIV-1 group M subtypes with regard to important biological characteristics. Evidence has suggested a relationship between subtype and modes of transmission. Studies in South Africa (96), Finland (97), Thailand (98,99), and Australia (100) found that most subtype B strains were associated with homosexual transmission while non-B strains were associated with heterosexual transmission. Similarly, in a study of U.S. military personnel, Brodine et al. found that people infected with non-subtype B HIV were more likely to report heterosexual contact than those with subtype B infection (85). Finally, a study of injection drug users in Thailand found a significantly higher transmission probability associated with subtype E than with subtype B (101), suggesting the certain viruses may be more efficient at certain transmission modes.

It had previously been suggested that certain subtypes were more effectively transmitted through mucosal routes than others and that perhaps certain properties of non-B subtypes facilitate transmission of HIV through the heterosexual route (102), perhaps explaining the exponential spread of disease in parts of Asia and Africa. Furthermore, it has been proposed that since HIV-1 subtype B strains had primarily been transmitted and passaged parenterally and through rectal intercourse, it might have undergone a period of "counterselection," where it lost the genetic sequence material that would have enhanced its capacity to be transmitted through a heterosexual route while other non-B subtypes did not experience this negative selection (102,103). It must be noted, however, that these original findings have subsequently been challenged (104–107), underscoring the difficulty of elucidating the role of subtypes in transmission.

Infection with certain subtypes has also been associated with increased risk of vertical transmission. A study conducted on mother-child pairs in Tanzania revealed that mothers infected with HIV-1 subtype A, subtype C, and intersubtype recombinants were more likely to transmit virus to their infants than mothers infected with subtype D (108). A previous study by the same group found that among perinatally transmitted C/D recombinant viruses, the V3 regions (*env*) were always from subtype C and never from subtype D, suggesting that viruses containing subtype D-V3 may have reduced fitness compared to viruses with subtype C-V3 (109). Conversely, a study conducted in Kenya indicated that women infected with subtype D were more likely to transmit than women who had any other sequence combinations in the *env* and *gag* (110).

Various studies have demonstrated differences among the HIV-1 subtypes with regard to disease progression. Kanki et al. found that women infected with a non-A subtype were eight times more likely to develop AIDS than those infected with subtype A (111). Similarly, Kaleebu et al. reported that subjects with subtype A had a slower progression to disease than those with subtype D (26,112). One study conducted in Brazil even found a difference in disease progression within a subtype (113,114). Specifically, individuals infected with serotype B-Br (Brazilian B) progressed to AIDS more slowly than individuals with non-Brazilian serotype B infections (113). Conversely, a cross-sectional study in London that compared HIV-1–infected African immigrants and non-African Londoners found no difference in progression by subtype (115).

Clinical and immunological differences also have been found between subtypes. In Kenya, where subtypes A, C, and D were all co-circulating within the same population, Neilson et al. found that higher plasma RNA levels and lower CD4+ counts were significantly associated with subtype C infection (116). In a prospective study conducted at a methadone treatment clinic in Thailand, people infected with CRF01_AE were found to have higher viral loads in early infection than those infected with subtype B (117). This difference decreased over time, however, to the point that the viral loads were similar at 12, 18, and 24 months post-seroconversion (117). Similarly, a study in our laboratory indicated that women infected with CRF02_AG had a significantly higher viral load during the early stage of infection than women not infected with CRF02_AG (118). Kaleebu et al. found that subjects infected with subtype D had a lower average CD4+ T cell count over the period of follow-up than those infected with subtype A (112). Conversely, a study in Thailand found no major differences in the degree of immunosuppression or the rates of opportunistic infections between people infected with subtype B' (Thai B) or CRF01_AE (119). Finally, infection with multiple subtypes has also been associated with higher viral load and lower CD4+ T cells counts (120).

A few reports suggest that the different subtypes may vary with regard to chemokine coreceptor usage and tissue tropism. It had been well documented that coreceptor use evolves during subtype B infection from use of CCR5 in the earlier stages of infection to use of CXCR4 during late stages of disease. While in vitro studies have shown that subtype A and CRF01_AE viruses have a similar evolution in coreceptor usage as subtype B viruses, subtype C and D viruses do not (121–124).

Subtype variation has also been associated with different levels of interaction with HIV-2. For instance, Sarr et al. showed that the in vivo interaction between HIV-1 and HIV-2 is influenced by HIV-1 subtype (125). They found that the prevalence of A3 viruses was significantly higher in dually infected individuals than in women who were singly infected with HIV-1 (125). Some cross-sectional studies have failed to demonstrate biological or clinical differences in genetically diverse viral strains. Alaeus et al. found no difference in the rate of CD4+ decline, clinical progression, or plasma HIV-1 RNA levels between individuals infected with subtypes A, B, C, or D (126). Laurent et al. found no difference in survival, clinical disease progression, or CD4+ decline between those infected with CRF02_AG and those infected with other viral strains (127). In addition, in a 2002 study comparing differences between subtypes A and D in mother-to-child transmission, subtype did not appear to influence infant survival (128).

Several in vitro studies have shown that subtypes differ on genetic components that might affect transcriptional efficiency. Subtype C viruses were shown to contain an extra NF-κB site in the long terminal repeat (LTR) region. The presence of the additional binding site is believed to render subtype C more responsive to p65/RelA than subtype B, which has two NF-κB binding sites (129). Subsequently, HIV-1 subtype C isolates were shown to have an elevated responsiveness to TNF-α, which correlated with increased NF-κB copy number (130). In a related study, subtype E LTRs were shown to have only one functional NF-κB site (131). Based on these in vitro results, it was suggested that the presence of an additional NF-κB site might confer an adaptive advantage on subtype C viruses, particularly in regions in which incidence of sexually transmitted infections that stimulate the production of pro-inflammatory cytokines are high (130).

Viral fitness is the relative replicative adaptation of a virus species to its environment, especially in the presence of a competitor (132,133). It depends not only upon the ability of the virus to replicate, but also on its longevity, its potential for transmission, and its ability to cause disease (134). It is not clear whether viruses of different subtypes and sub-subtypes have differing levels of replicative capacity. Several studies have conducted ex vivo assays to determine the relative fitness of two viruses. For example, in dual competition analyses, it was shown that subtype B viruses were capable of outcompeting subtype C viruses in infecting HIV-uninfected cells (135). A similar analysis, comparing CRF02_AG isolates to other subtype A isolates, indicated that CRF02_AG appears to be more fit in an ex vivo setting (136). Similarly, competition assays comparing HIV-2 to HIV-1 group M and group O viruses showed that the group M viruses were most fit, with HIV-2 isolates 100-fold less fit than all the group M viruses and group O viruses 100-fold less fit than HIV-2 (137). Although it is important to take caution in interpreting in vitro data from individual isolates, it is interesting to note that the order in replicative and transmission fitness of the isolates in the Arien et al. study closely mimic the distribution of subtypes in the global epidemic (137).

Finally, another important reason to characterize and understand genetic diversity is that knowledge of the predominant HIV-1 subtypes, sub-subtypes, and CRFs in a given population may be important in designing effective HIV vaccines (138). Although the importance of matching a vaccine candidate to regional circulating strains is yet unclear, incorporation of local strains might maximize the efficacy of a potential vaccine candidate (138).

As mentioned earlier, several studies could not detect differences between subtypes with regard to various disease parameters. The reasons for these discrepancies are still under investigation. It is worth noting that a number of the studies that did not find associations between subtype and correlates of disease and pathogenesis were compromised by a cross-sectional design. Overall, given the complexity of HIV genetic diversity, it is possible that a single characteristic such as subtype will not entirely account for the differences in transmission and pathogenesis. Rather, it might be one of many virologic, immunologic, and host factors that contribute to a particular phenotype or outcome.

Viral Diversity and Antiretrovirals

There is increasing evidence in the literature that subtype diversity might influence susceptibility and resistance to antiretroviral therapy (ART). Although the *pol* gene is the most conserved region of HIV-1, with a variation of approximately 10% (139,140), it possesses sufficient variability to allow for phylogenetic classification of all subtypes and CRFs (141). The *pol* gene encodes three enzymes: protease; reverse transcriptase; and integrase. Antiretrovirals (ARVs) that target reverse transcriptase and protease belong to three classes—nucleoside analogue reverse transcriptase inhibitors (NRTIs); non-NRTIs (NNRTIs); and protease inhibitors (PIs).

Significance of Diversity for Therapy

Widespread use of highly active antiretroviral therapy (HAART) has greatly reduced morbidity and mortality among HIV-infected people in industrialized nations (142). ART is increasingly playing a major role in controlling the pandemic as many developing countries have recently launched treatment programs (143–145), allowing more people access to drugs. A major obstacle to the efficacy of such large-scale treatment programs is the inevitable development of drug-resistance mutations (DRMs). These mutations consist of two varieties: a primary resistance mutation that reduces the susceptibility of the virus to drugs by itself, while a secondary mutation requires the presence of another mutation or mutations to exert its resistant phenotype (146). The development of drug resistance limits treatment options, facilitates viral rebound, and ultimately leads to immunologic decline and the development of opportunistic infections. In addition to the selective pressure from therapy, drug resistance may also be acquired through the transmission of drug-resistant HIV strains. This phenomenon, known as primary drug resistance, has a prevalence of 6% in Switzerland (147), 11% in the United Kingdom (148), 18% in Australia (149), and 6% to 21% in the United States (56).

Genetic variation within the reverse transcriptase and protease may greatly influence viral replication and fitness as well as susceptibility to therapy and the development of drug resistance (146). The evolutionary dynamics within individuals involves the interplay between advantageous natural selective forces and deleterious mutations, resulting in the formation of a heterogeneous ensemble of genetically distinct, yet related variants called quasispecies. Strains with higher replicative advantage in the face of these factors will outcompete the other quasipecies to become the dominant virus in the individual. ART modulates this balance by suppressing the replication of the majority of the quasispecies, including, in most cases, the dominant strain, while sparing some variants that possess mutations that enable them to replicate in the face of drug pressure. These initially "less fit" drug-resistant variants then become the predominant viral strains within the individual's quasispecies population. It is important to note, however, that although many drug-resistant viruses are less fit than wild-type strains, the effect of resistance on fitness depends on the drug used. For example, some NNRTI mutations, such as K103N and Y181C, do not reduce viral fitness significantly, and the variants containing these mutations rapidly become the dominant quasispecies in treated patients (150,151).

Although the relationship between genetic diversity and clinical outcome is complex, various studies have demonstrated that the clinical response of non-subtype B viruses to the available ARVs is similar to that seen in subtype B infection (152–154). Various studies have described genotypic and phenotypic resistance in non-subtype B infections (144,152–158). Most of the studies described the lack of major drug-resistance-conferring mutations, but a high prevalence of secondary mutations; one 2005 study reported considerable overlap between subtype B resistance mutations and mutations associated with at least one non-B subtype (144). The non-subtype B sequences included subtypes A, C, D, F, and G as well as CRF01_AE and CRF02_AG. Each of the 55 known subtype B drug-resistance mutations occurred in at least one non-B isolate, and 44 (80%) of these mutations were significantly associated with ART in at least one non-B subtype. Conversely, 61 of 67 mutations associated with ART in at least one non-B subtype were also associated with ART in subtype B isolates.

Studies examining the relationship between HIV subtype and response to ART have been limited by small samples sizes, leading to general comparisons of subtype B to other subtypes grouped together. It is conceivable that the widespread use of ARVs will exert extra selective pressure on viral reverse transcriptase and protease and that this pressure will result in the development of different mutations by subtype. It is also possible that preexisting polymorphisms may determine the precise mutation pathways used by the viruses to achieve drug resistance; that is, some codons are closer to a resistance phenotype than others even if the amino acid involved is identical.

Impact of Evolutionary Forces on Drug Resistance

Development of drug resistance depends on the extent of viral replication during therapy, the ease of acquiring a particular mutation or set of mutations, recombination, the effect of mutations on drug susceptibility, the presence of viral reservoirs, and viral fitness (159,160). It is unclear whether resistant viruses are pathogenic or would get transmitted at different rates than those with reduced replicative capacity. Following therapy, mutations that confer drug resistance lead to an initial decrease in fitness (124,161). With continued drug pressure, however, secondary or compensatory mutations that partially restore the activity of viral enzymes may result in a rebound in viral fitness.

Drug-resistant viruses are able to persist in CD4+ T lymphocytes, follicular dendritic cells, macrophages, and various other cells and tissues long after initiation of therapy (162). These reservoirs serve as potential sources of viral particles for the circulating viral pool. In addition, even when viruses are at undetectable levels, low-level replication and viral evolution are likely still occurring. Studies have shown that the replication of zidovudine-resistant HIV-1 increases multiplicatively during therapy, and it has been suggested that an intentional increase in mutation rate leading to lethal mutagenesis of the HIV-1 genome may be another viable approach to ART (161).

Subtype-Specific Polymorphisms and the Pathways to Resistance
Subtype-specific polymorphisms, defined as specific mutations occurring in the majority of sequences from a particular subtype, may play functional roles in determining the mutation pathway to drug resistance. The degeneracy of the genetic code may mean that different mutational pathways are possible even when the codon encodes the same amino acid. This relationship between codons that specify the same amino acid but achieve a different pattern of amino acid substitution by a single nucleotide change has been termed quasi-synonymy (163). Quasi-synonymous mutations within the virus may dictate different mutational pathways, which may have bearing on the development of drug resistance and viral escape from the immune response (139,144,163). Figure 4-2 shows an example of subtype-specific codon differences and predictions of how they may influence mutational routes to the development of drug resistance (144). The amino acid valine at position 179 in the reverse transcriptase is encoded by GTT in subtype B and by GTG in CRF02_AG and subtype G. Although these valine codons are synonymous, a single nucleotide change at the first position to adenine results in isoleucine (ATA) and methionine (ATG), respectively. Similarly, a single nucleotide change to adenine at the second codon position results in formation of glutamate for CRF02_AG and subtype G, while subtype B viruses encode aspartate at the same position. Thus, subtype B viruses are more likely to have V179I mutations while CRF02_AG viruses are more predisposed to forming V179M mutations in response to NNRTIs (164).

The Immune Response and Pol Diversity
Recent studies have demonstrated some interplay between the selective pressures exerted by ART on reverse transcriptase and protease and the emergence of viral escape mutants secondary to CD8+ T lymphocyte (CTL)-mediated immune pressure (165–167). Karlsson et al. demonstrated that among individuals who had developed PI mutations, the wild-type epitope was strongly recognized and bound by CTLs, while the mutant epitope (V82A mutation) was poorly recognized by the wild-type–specific CTL (165). V82A is a common PI mutation (146), suggesting that it may act both as a CTL and PI escape mutant. Within reverse transcriptase, the V179I mutation confers intermediate levels of nevirapine resistance (146) and has been reported to reduce HLA-B35 recognition and binding affinity (168). In addition, Mason et al. demonstrated that common drug resistance mutations sustained or even enhanced the antigenicity and immunogenicity of common HIV-1 *pol* CTL epitopes presented by com-

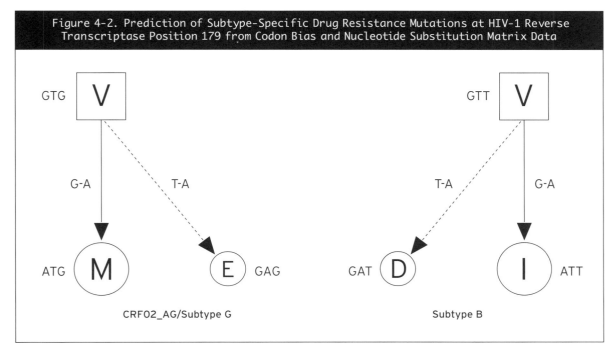

Figure 4-2. Prediction of Subtype-Specific Drug Resistance Mutations at HIV-1 Reverse Transcriptase Position 179 from Codon Bias and Nucleotide Substitution Matrix Data

Resistance mutations may be influenced by quasi-synonymy and genetic cost of mutations. Examples of predicted mutations at position V179 in RT are shown. The wild type amino acids are enclosed within quadrilaterals, while mutant amino acids are enclosed with ovals. The predicted relative abundance of mutants is proportional to the size of the oval. The preferred codon bias is indicated adjacent to each amino acid. Codon usage was determined from consensus sequences from our samples and subtype B consensus. The thickness of the arrows indicates the ease of substitution. G-A substitutions are more likely to occur than T-A substitutions. CRF02_AG and subtype G viruses are predicted to preferentially develop V179M and V179E mutations in RT while subtype B viruses will develop V179I and V179D mutations under drug pressure.

mon HLA molecules (165). These findings suggest that certain viral signatures may be under both drug- and immune-driven selective pressures that could be exploited to combat the HIV-1.

Emerging data support the hypothesis that some subtype-specific polymorphisms in various HIV-1 genes, including *pol*, may be immune escape variants that have persisted in the populations where these epitopes and subtypes predominate (164,169). HIV-1 subtypes are predominant in different regions of the world (74), and many epitopes have ethno-geographic bias (170). It is therefore also possible that differences in HLA frequencies between populations will contribute to this phenomenon.

Subtypes and Vaccines

Whether a candidate vaccine against HIV-1 should be based on the dominant subtypes within a given geographic region has been the subject of much speculation and debate. To address the issue appropriately, one must consider the relationship between the HIV-1 genetic subtypes and immune responses. Since effective neutralizing antibodies appear to function across genetic subtypes (171–173), it has been argued that a vaccine targeting the humoral immune response by focusing on genetic subtypes seems illogical. A vaccine that targets more conserved regions of the genome and that is cross-protective might be more efficacious. As Moore et al. (10) point out, given that subtype designations were not made based on antigenic or immunogenic properties of the virus and do not correspond to neutralization serotypes,

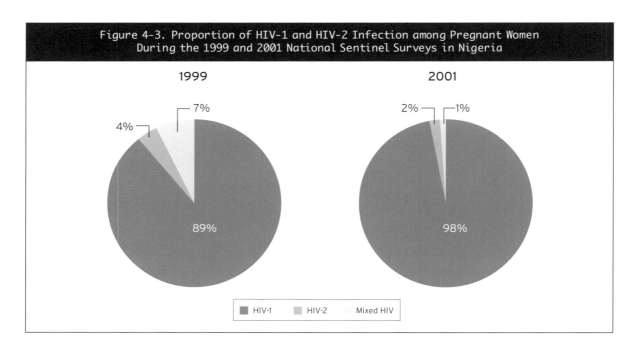

Figure 4-3. Proportion of HIV-1 and HIV-2 Infection among Pregnant Women During the 1999 and 2001 National Sentinel Surveys in Nigeria

it might not be as relevant to generate a subtype-specific vaccine, but it might not be as relevant to generate a subtype-specific vaccine, but rather one that is broadly cross-reactive (71).

Many researchers are still interested in generating subtype-appropriate vaccines for given regions. The belief is that a subtype-specific vaccine candidate might increase the number of potentially cross-reactive epitopes by augmenting the level of similarity between the vaccine and the endemic virus. For those designing subtype-specific vaccines, there are two major approaches: the isolate-based approach and the consensus or ancestral-sequence–based approach (86). The first approach involves selection of an isolate from the geographic region to which the vaccine is directed, while the second approach requires the construction of either a consensus or ancestral sequence using all available sequence data and an evolutionary model (86). When considering the possibility of using an isolate-based vaccine, researchers must decide not only which subtype to use, but also which geographic region from which an isolate should be drawn. Given the great diversity within subtypes and the fact the geographic restrictions of viruses are slowly disappearing, this is a difficult choice. The use of a polyvalent vaccine containing isolates as well as group M consensus sequence is a promising approach (86). A number of multiclade vaccines are now under evaluation.

MOLECULAR EPIDEMIOLOGY OF HIV IN NIGERIA

Both HIV-1 and HIV-2 circulate in Nigeria (174–178). Serologic data from HIV screening centers and published results in the early to mid-1980s showed slightly higher rates of HIV-2 infection than HIV-1 infection (174,175,179–182). The HIV-1 infection rate steadily increased during the late 1980s, however, accounting for approximately 60% of infections during the late 1980s and early 1990s; since then, HIV-1 has accounted for more than 95% of total HIV infections and almost 99% of all AIDS cases (Figure 4-3). While the pattern of the two types of HIV infection in the country can be partly explained by the higher infectivity and transmission efficiency of HIV-1 (183,184), widespread use of rapid testing procedures without follow-up confirmatory Western blotting and inadequately trained personnel for HIV testing may also account for the reportedly low rate of infection of HIV-2 in the country (Kanki P, *personal communication*).

The initial indication that HIV strains circulating in Nigeria may differ from the HIV-1 subtype B viruses that circulate in Western Europe and North America came from the work of Olaleye et al., which showed differential amplification rates of fragments of the HIV genome using primers designed from the HIV-1 subtype B genome (184). Initial sequence analysis of the *env* gene of the isolate designated HIV-1 IbNg (for Ibadan, Nigeria) showed it to be a variant of HIV-1 subtype A (185). Later work indicated that the IbNg isolate was, in fact, a recombinant of HIV-1 subtypes A and G. In addition, another HIV-1 strain from an infected person in Jos, while subtype G based on sequencing of the *env* gene (186), was also found to be a recombinant of subtypes A and G following full-length sequencing. Collectively, these subtype A and G recombinants are classified as CRF02_AG.

The identification of an HIV-1 subtype A variant from the southwest region and a subtype G virus from the north-central region led to the initial speculation of regional differences in the distribution of HIV-1 subtypes in the country (184,185). Subsequently studies found HIV-1 subtype G in most parts of northern Nigeria, but CRF02_AG and subtype A were found in the middle southern parts (82). However, these studies were seriously limited by their small sample size, as well as the relatively low specificity of subtyping due to use of HMA or peptide assays for genotyping.

In recent years, more efforts have been committed to identifying the various HIV-1 subtypes circulating throughout the country. A 1998 study found serologic evidence of HIV-1 group O in the southeastern and northeastern parts of Nigeria (187). Also, using a peptide-based subtyping assay, Odaibo et al. reported circulation of HIV-1 subtypes A, B, and C, and group O in different parts of the country (188,189). Genotypic analyses of samples previously subtyped using the peptide assay have confirmed the circulation of subtypes A, B, and C in Nigeria (190).

Unlike most previous HIV-1 subtyping studies, which were based on samples collected from hospital patients, genotyping of HIV-1 isolates from a community-based HIV project in Oyo State established the HIV subtypes among asymptomatic and symptomatic people at the community level (191). Sequence analyses based on consensus sequences from *env* and *gag* gene fragments of approximately 100 HIV-1 isolates collected from 2001 to 2003 showed the presence of several HIV-1 variants, including multiple CRFs. Approximately 35% of the isolates were CRF02_AG, and another 35% were subtype G. Interestingly, a number of the subtype G samples clustered as a distinct group, previously described as G' (80,82,191,192). Further analysis of several of these samples using full-length sequence data revealed that some people were in fact infected with full-length G' viruses (193).

Other CRFs and subtypes were identified for the first time in Nigeria, including CRF06_cpx, CRF01_AE, CRF11_cpx, and A3. The results of the study also indicated some differences in the distribu-

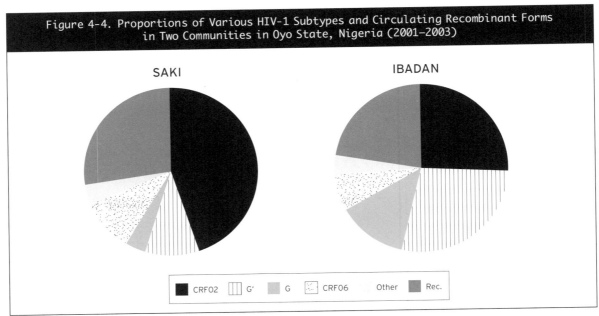

Figure 4-4. Proportions of Various HIV-1 Subtypes and Circulating Recombinant Forms in Two Communities in Oyo State, Nigeria (2001–2003)

SAKI

IBADAN

Legend: CRF02 · G' · G · CRF06 · Other · Rec.

Abbreviations: CRF: circulating recombinant form; Rec.: recombinant

tion of the two major subtypes, G and CRF02_AG, between the two communities. Detection of subtype G in Ibadan was twice that in Saki, a city about 200 kilometers away (Figure 4-4). In similar studies, multiple HIV-1 subtypes and CRFs were found in other parts of the country (194,195).

Although the biological consequences of HIV diversity are not well understood, the implication for diagnosis, ART, and vaccine development are enormous. It is known that the antigens of most of the HIV testing kits are primarily targeted to detect HIV-1 subtype B, the major circulating strain in North America and Western Europe. These test kits may not accurately detect infections due to some non-B subtypes of the virus (196). The problem may even be greater with primer mismatch in the molecular detection or amplification of HIV nucleic acid fragments or genes (184). It is now well established that recombinant forms of HIV are common in Nigeria (191), which may influence the prevalence of drug resistance as data from a study in Ibadan and Saki, in Oyo State, show that the complex CRF06_cpx harbors more DRMs than other subtypes found in antiretroviral-naive individuals (164).

Drug Resistance Mutations in Nigeria

The same study of antiretroviral-therapy–naive HIV-1–infected subjects in Ibadan and Saki found a significant degree of primary and secondary DRMs in the reverse transcriptase and protease, as well as polymorphisms at positions of previously characterized DRMs (164). For instance, 6 of 35 (15%) reverse transcriptase sequences harbored primary NRTI/NNRTI mutations, including M41L, V118I, Y188H, P236L, and Y318F. Notably, three of these individuals were infected with viruses that clustered with CRF06_cpx in the reverse transcriptase. In addition, three of the four CRF06_cpx reverse transcriptase samples harbored primary DRMs, compared with 11% of the other variants combined (p = 0.011). This level of primary drug resistance is high for a drug-naive cohort, but it is noteworthy that half the sequences with drug-naive DRMs are CRF06_cpx, which constitutes only about 10% of viruses in Nigeria (164,191). These findings suggest the possibility that CRF06_cpx sequences harbor natural polymorphisms that are drug resistant rather than acquired after therapy initiation. It is possible, however, that individuals with these DRMs were infected with drug-resistant viruses, possibly from individuals not adherent to therapy, or on suboptimal ARV regimens.

No primary DRMs were observed in protease. Secondary DRMs, however, were observed in all protease sequences. Three secondary PI resistance mutations — L10I/V, M36I, and L63P — were detected. The K20I and M36I secondary PI mutations were found in all subjects, regardless of subtype, while all the subtype G viruses harbored the V82I polymorphism in the protease. Similar patterns have been found in the other parts of the country (197,198). This subtype-specific polymorphism at a DRM site raises concerns about second-line and salvage-therapy regimens, which typically contain PIs.

CONCLUSION

The global HIV epidemic exhibits a great deal of genomic heterogeneity. A number of groups, subtypes, sub-subtypes, and recombinants have been identified and characterized. Interestingly, the distribution of the various strains is also heterogeneous, with the greatest diversity represented in sub-Saharan Africa. The worldwide spread of the various subtypes can primarily be attributed to the increased travel and movement of populations. Various studies indicate that the subtypes differ in biological properties, but many of the findings are still controversial and require further research. It is conceivable that future studies that make more accurate distinctions between subtypes and sub-subtypes may better clarify findings regarding the association between viral genotype and biological phenotype. This diversity has some obvious implications for ART as well as vaccine development. The further characterization of the predominant HIV-1 subtypes, sub-subtypes, and CRFs in a given population will enhance our understanding of viral diversity critical to the informed design of interventions, therapies, and vaccines. Although the importance of matching a vaccine candidate to regional circulating strains is yet unclear, incorporation of local strains might maximize the efficacy of a potential vaccine candidate.

Analyses of the sequence diversity in Nigeria have revealed that the number of variants circulating in the country is increasing. Furthermore, it has become apparent that a growing number of infections are due to recombinant forms of the virus, and one of the recombinants, CRF06_cpx, is associated with primary drug resistance mutations. These factors should be taken into consideration as treatment regimens are designed for a given population. Continued monitoring will enhance our understanding of the scope of diversity in Nigeria as well as the role that diversity plays in the ongoing epidemic.

REFERENCES

1. Kanki PJ, Peeters M, Gueye-Ndiaye A. Virology of HIV-1 and HIV-2: implications for Africa. *AIDS*, 1997;11(Suppl B):S33–S42.

2. McGrath KM, Hoffman NG, Resch W, et al. Using HIV-1 sequence variability to explore virus biology. *Virus Res*, 2001;76:137–160.

3. Cohen EA, Terwilliger EF, Sodroski JG, et al. Identification of a protein encoded by the vpu gene of HIV-1. *Nature*, 1988;334:532–534.

4. Henderson LE, Sowder RC, Copeland TD, et al. Isolation and characterization of a novel protein (X-ORF product) from SIV and HIV-2. *Science*, 1988;241:199–201.

5. Kappes JC, Morrow CD, Lee SW, et al. Identification of a novel retroviral gene unique to human immunodeficiency virus type 2 and simian immunodeficiency virus SIVMAC. *J Virol*, 1988;62:3501–3505.

6. Kuiken CL, Lukashov VV, Baan E, et al. Evidence for limited within-person evolution of the V3 domain of the HIV-1 envelope in the Amsterdam population. *AIDS*, 1996;10:31–37.

7. Janssens W, Buve A, and Nkengasong JN. The puzzle of HIV-1 subtypes in Africa. *AIDS*, 1997;11:705–712.

8. McCutchan FE. Understanding the genetic diversity of HIV-1. *AIDS*, 2000;14:S31–S44.

9. Robertson DL, Anderson JP, Bradac JA, et al. HIV-1 nomenclature proposal: a reference guide to HIV-1 classification. In: Kuiken CL, Foley B, Hahn BH, et al., eds. *Human Retroviruses and AIDS: A Compilation and Analysis of Nucleic and Amino Acid Sequences.* Los Alamos, New Mexico: Los Alamos National Laboratory; 2000:492–505.

10. Moore JP, Parren PW, Burton DR. Genetic subtypes, humoral immunity, and human immunodeficiency virus type 1 vaccine development. *J Virol*, 2001;75:5721–5729.

11. Robertson DL, Anderson JP, Bradac JA, et al. HIV-1 nomenclature proposal. *Science*, 2000;288:55–56.

12. Gurtler LG, Hauser PH, Eberle J, et al. A new subtype of human immunodeficiency virus type 1 (MVP-5180) from Cameroon. *J Virol*, 1994;68:1581–1585.

13. Simon F, Mauclére P, Roques P, et al. Identification of a new human immunodeficiency virus type 1 distinct from group M and group O. *Nat Med*, 1998;4:1032–1037.

14. Quinones-Mateu ME, Ball SC, and Arts EJ. Role of human immunodeficiency viruse type 1 group O in the AIDS pandemic. *AIDS Rev*, 2000;2:190–202.

15. Gao F, Vidal N, Li Y, et al. Evidence of two distinct subsubtypes within the HIV-1 subtype A radiation. *AIDS Res Hum Retroviruses*, 2001;17:675–688.

16. Meloni ST, Kim B, Sankalé JL, et al. Distinct human immunodeficiency virus type 1 subtype A virus circulating in West Africa: sub-subtype A3. *J Virol*, 2004;78:12438–12445.

17. Meloni ST, Sankalé JL, Hamel DJ, et al. Molecular epidemiology of human immunodeficiency virus type 1 sub-subtype A3 in Senegal from 1988 to 2001. *J Virol*, 2004;78:12455–12461.

18. Triques K, Bourgeois A, Saragosti S, et al. High diversity of HIV-1 subtype F strains in Central Africa. *Virology*, 1999;259:99–109.

19. Triques K, Bourgeois A, Vidal N, et al. Near-full-length genome sequencing of divergent African HIV type 1 subtype F viruses leads to the identification of a new HIV type 1 subtype designated K. *AIDS Res Hum Retroviruses*, 2000;16:139–151.

20. Peeters M. Recombinant HIV sequences: their role in the global epidemic. In: Kuiken CL, Foley B, Hahn B, et al., eds. *Human Retroviruses and AIDS 2000: A Compilation and Analysis of Nucleic Acid and Amino Acid Sequences.* Los Alamos, New Mexico: Theoretical Biology and Biophysics Group, Los Alamos National Laboratory, 2000:139–154.

21. Gao F, Yue L, Robertson DL, et al. Genetic diversity of human immunodeficiency virus type 2: evidence for distinct sequence subtypes with differences in virus biology. *J Virol*, 1994;68:7433–7447.

22. Chen Z, Luckay A, Sodora DL, et al. Human immunodeficiency virus type 2 (HIV-2) seroprevalence and characterization of a distinct HIV-2 genetic subtype from the natural range of simian immunodeficiency virus-infected sooty mangabeys. *J Virol*, 1997;71:3953–3960.

23. Yamaguchi J, Devare SG, Brennan CA. Identification of a new HIV-2 subtype based on phylogenetic analysis of full-length genomic sequence. *AIDS Res Hum Retroviruses*, 2000;16:925–930.

24. Damond F, Worobey M, Campa P, et al. Identification of a highly divergent HIV type 2 and proposal for a change in HIV type 2 classification. *AIDS Res Hum Retroviruses*, 2004;20:666–672.

25. Anderson JP, Rodrigo AG, Learn GH, et al. Testing the hypothesis of a recombinant origin of human immunodeficiency virus type 1 subtype E. *J Virol*, 2000;74:10752–10765.

26. Kaleebu P, Ross A, Morgan D, et al. Relationship between HIV-1 env subtypes A and D and disease progression in a rural Ugandan cohort. *AIDS*, 2001; 15:293–299.

27. Mboudjeka I, Bikandou B, Zekeng L, et al. Genetic diversity of HIV-1 group M from Cameroon and Republic of Congo. *Arch Virol*, 1999;144:2291–2311.

28. Sankalé JL, Hamel D, Woolsey A, et al. Molecular evolution of human immunodeficiency virus type 1 subtype A in Senegal: 1988–1997. *J Hum Virol*, 2000; 3:157–164.

29. Dowling WE, Kim B, Mason CJ, et al. Forty-one near full-length HIV-1 sequences from Kenya reveal an epidemic of subtype A and A-containing recombinants. *AIDS*, 2002;16:1809–1820.

30. Casado G, Thomson MM, Sierra M, et al. Identification of a novel HIV-1 circulating ADG intersubtype recombinant form (CRF19_cpx) in Cuba. *J Acquir Immune Defic Syndr*, 2005;40:532–537.

31. Thomson MM, Casado G, Posada D, et al. Identification of a novel HIV-1 complex circulating recombinant form (CRF18_cpx) of Central African origin in Cuba. *AIDS*, 2005;19:1155–1163.

32. Peeters M, Liegeois F, Torimiro N, et al. Characterization of a highly replicative intergroup M/O human immunodeficiency virus type 1 recombinant isolated from a Cameroonian patient. *J Virol*, 1999;73:7368–7375.

33. Takehisa J, Zekeng L, Ido E, et al. Human immunodeficiency virus type 1 intergroup (M/O) recombination in cameroon. *J Virol*, 1999;73:6810–20.

34. Yamaguchi J, Bodelle P, Vallari AS, et al. HIV infections in northwestern Cameroon: identification of HIV type 1 group O and dual HIV type 1 group M and group O infections. *AIDS Res Hum Retroviruses*, 2004;20:944–57.

35. Curlin ME, Gottlieb GS, Hawes SE, et al. No evidence for recombination between HIV type 1 and HIV type 2 within the envelope region in dually seropositive individuals from Senegal. *AIDS Res Hum Retroviruses*, 2004;20:958–963.

36. Vanden Haesevelde MM, Peeters M, Jannes G, et al. Sequence analysis of a highly divergent HIV-1-related lentivirus isolated from a wild captured chimpanzee. *Virology*, 1996;221:346–350.

37. Sharp PM, Bailes E, Chaudhuri RR, et al. The origins of acquired immune deficiency syndrome viruses: where and when? *Philos Trans R Soc Lond B Biol Sci*, 2001;356:867–876.

38. Diop O, Gueye A, Ayouba A, et al. Simian immunodeficiency viruses and the origin of HIVs, In: Essex M, Mboup S, Kanki PJ, Marlink RG, Tlou SD, eds. *AIDS in Africa*. 2nd ed. New York: Kluwer Academic/Plenum Publishers, 2002:104–120.

39. Paraskevis D, Lemey P, Salemi M, et al. Analysis of the evolutionary relationships of HIV-1 and SIVcpz sequences using bayesian inference: implications for the origin of HIV-1. *Mol Biol Evol*, 2003;20: 1986–1996.

40. Roques P, Robertson DL, Souquiere S, et al. Phylogenetic characteristics of three new HIV-1 N strains and implications for the origin of group N. *AIDS*, 2004;18:1371–1381.

41. Gao F, Bailes E, Robertson DL, et al. Origin of HIV-1 in the chimpanzee Pan troglodytes troglodytes. *Nature*, 1999;397:436–441.

42. Peeters M, Toure-Kane C, Nkengasong JN. Genetic diversity of HIV in Africa: impact on diagnosis, treatment, vaccine development and trials. *AIDS*, 2003;17:2547–2560.

43. Burke D, McCutchan F. Global distribution of human immunodeficiency virus-1 clades, In: DeVita VT, Hellman S, Rosenberg SA, eds. *AIDS: Biology, Diagnosis, Treatment and Prevention*. Philadelphia, Pennsylvania: Lippincott-Raven Publishers, 1997: 119–126.

44. Zhu T, Korber BT, Nahmias AJ, et al. An African HIV-1 sequence from 1959 and implications for the origin of the epidemic. *Nature*, 1998;391:594–597.

45. Hillis DM. Origins of HIV. *Science*, 2000;288: 1757–1759.

46. Korber B, Muldoon M, Theiler J, et al. Timing the ancestor of the HIV-1 pandemic strains. *Science*, 2000;288:1789–1796.

47. Yusim K, Peeters M, Pybus OG, et al. Using human immunodeficiency virus type 1 sequences to infer historical features of the acquired immune deficiency syndrome epidemic and human immunodeficiency virus evolution. *Philos Trans R Soc Lond B Biol Sci*, 2001;356:855–866.

48. Travers SA, Clewley JP, Glynn JR, et al. Timing and reconstruction of the most recent common ancestor of the subtype C clade of human immunodeficiency virus type 1. *J Virol*, 2004;78:10501–10506.

49. Lemey P, Pybus OG, Rambaut A, et al. The molecular population genetics of HIV-1 group O. *Genetics*, 2004;167:1059–1068.

50. Chen Z, Telfier P, Gettie A, et al. Genetic characterization of new West African simian immunodeficiency virus SIVsm: geographic clustering of household-derived SIV strains with human immunodeficiency virus type 2 subtypes and genetically diverse viruses from a single feral sooty mangabey troop. *J Virol*, 1996;70:3617–3627.

51. Lemey P, Pybus OG, Wang B, et al. Tracing the origin and history of the HIV-2 epidemic. *Proc Natl Acad Sci USA*, 2003;100:6588–6592.

52. Preston BD, Poiesz BJ, Loeb LA. Fidelity of HIV-1 reverse transcriptase. *Science*, 1988;242:1168–1171.

53. Subbarao S, Schochetman G. Genetic variability of HIV-1. *AIDS*, 1996;10:S13–S23.

54. Roberts JD, Bebenek K, Kunkel TA. The accuracy of reverse transcriptase from HIV-1. *Science*, 1988;242: 1171–1173.

55. Katz RA, Skalka AM. Generation of diversity in retroviruses. *Annu Rev Genet*, 1990;24:409–445.

56. Mansky LM, Temin HM. Lower in vivo mutation rate of human immunodeficiency virus type 1 than that predicted from the fidelity of purified reverse transcriptase. *J Virol*, 1995;69:5087–5094.

57. Zhuang J, Jetzt AE, Sun G, et al. Human immunodeficiency virus type 1 recombination: rate, fidelity, and putative hot spots. *J Virol*, 2002;76:11273–11282.

58. Chin MP, Rhodes TD, Chen J, et al. Identification of a major restriction in HIV-1 intersubtype recombination. *Proc Natl Acad Sci USA*, 2005;102:9002–9007.

59. Hu DJ, Subbarao S, Vanichseni S, et al. Frequency of HIV-1 dual subtype infections, including intersubtype superinfections, among injection drug users in Bangkok, Thailand. *AIDS*, 2005;19:303–308.

60. Smith DM, Richman DD, Little SJ. HIV superinfection. *J Infect Dis*, 2005;192:438–444.

61. Altfeld M, Allen TM, Yu XG, et al. HIV-1 superinfection despite broad CD8+ T-cell responses containing replication of the primary virus. *Nature*, 2002;420:434–439.

62. Blackard JT, Cohen DE, Mayer KH. Human immunodeficiency virus superinfection and recombination: current state of knowledge and potential clinical consequences. *Clin Infect Dis*, 2002;34: 1108–1114.

63. Jost S, Bernard MC, Kaiser L, et al. A patient with HIV-1 superinfection. *N Engl J Med*, 2002;347:731–736.

64. Ramos A, Hu DJ, Nguyen L, et al. Intersubtype human immunodeficiency virus type 1 superinfection following seroconversion to primary infection in two injection drug users. *J Virol*, 2002;76: 7444–7452.

65. Smith DM, Wong JK, Hightower GK, et al. Incidence of HIV superinfection following primary infection. *JAMA*, 2004;292:1177–1178.

66. Smith DM, Wong JK, Hightower GK, et al. HIV drug resistance acquired through superinfection. *AIDS*, 2005;19:1251–1256.

67. Yang OO, Daar ES, Jamieson BD, et al. Human immunodeficiency virus type 1 clade B superinfection: evidence for differential immune containment of distinct clade B strains. *J Virol*, 2005;79:860–868.

68. Plantier JC, Lemee V, Dorval I, et al. HIV-1 group M superinfection in an HIV-1 group O-infected patient. *AIDS*, 2004;18:2444–2446.

69. Gerhardt M, Mloka D, Tovanabutra S, et al. In-depth, longitudinal analysis of viral quasispecies from an individual triply infected with late-stage human immunodeficiency virus type 1, using a multiple PCR primer approach. *J Virol*, 2005;79: 8249–8261.

70. van der Kuyl AC, Kozaczynska K, van den Burg R, et al. Triple HIV-1 infection. *N Engl J Med*, 2005;352: 2557–2559.

71. Fang G, Weiser B, Kuiken C, et al. Recombination following superinfection by HIV-1. *AIDS*, 2004;18: 153–159.

72. Osmanov S, Pattou C, Walker N, et al. Estimated global distribution and regional spread of HIV-1 genetic subtypes in the year 2000. *J Acquir Immune Defic Syndr*, 2002;29:184–190.

73. Salemi M, de Oliveira T, Soares MA, et al. Different epidemic potentials of the HIV-1B and C subtypes. *J Mol Evol*, 2005;60:598–605.

74. Wainberg MA. HIV-1 subtype distribution and the problem of drug resistance. *AIDS*, 2004;18(Suppl 3):S63–S68.

75. Bikandou B, Takehisa J, Mboudjeka I, et al. Genetic subtypes of HIV type 1 in Republic of Congo. *AIDS Res Hum Retroviruses*, 2000;16:613–619.

76. Kandathil AJ, Ramalingam S, Kannangai R, et al. Molecular epidemiology of HIV. *Indian J Med Res*, 2005;121:333–344.

77. Toure-Kane C, Montavon C, Faye MA, et al. Identification of all HIV type 1 group M subtypes in Senegal, a country with low and stable seroprevalence. *AIDS Res Hum Retroviruses*, 2000;16: 603–609.

78. Andersson S, Norrgren H, Dias F, et al. Molecular characterization of human immunodeficiency virus (HIV)-1 and -2 individuals from Guinea-Bissau with single or dual infections: predominance of a distinct HIV-1 subtype A/G recombinant in West Africa. *Virology*, 1999;267:312–330.

79. Carr J, Laukkanen T, Salminen M, et al. Characterization of subtype A HIV-1 from Africa by full genome sequencing. *AIDS*, 1999;13:18189–18126.

80. Cornelissen M, vandenBurg R, Zorgdrager F, et al. Spread of distinct human immunodeficiency virus type 1 AG recombinant lineages in Africa. *J Gen Virol*, 2000;81:515–523.

81. Montavon C, Toure-Kane C, Liegeois F, et al. Most env and gag subtype A HIV-1 viruses circulating in West and West Central Africa are similar to the prototype AG recombinant virus IBNG. *J Acquir Immune Defic Syndr*, 2000;23:363–374.

82. Peeters M, Esu-Williams E, Vergne L, et al. Predominance of subtype A and G HIV type 1 in Nigeria, with geographical differences in their distribution. *AIDS Res Hum Retroviruses*, 2000;16: 315–325.

83. Spira S, Wainberg MA, Loemba H, et al. Impact of clade diversity on HIV-1 virulence, antiretroviral drug sensitivity and drug resistance. *J Antimicrob Chemother*, 2003;51:229–240.

84. Thompson J, Gibson T, Plewniak F, et al. The ClustalX windows interface: flexible strategies for multiple sequence alignment aided by quality analysis tools. *Nuc Acids Res*, 1997;24:4876–4882.

85. Brodine SK, Starkey MJ, Shaffer RA, et al. Diverse HIV-1 subtypes and clinical, laboratory and behavioral factors in a recently infected US military cohort. *AIDS*, 2003;17:2521–2527.

86. Gaschen B, Taylor J, Yusim K, et al. Diversity considerations in HIV-1 vaccine selection. *Science*, 2002; 296:2354–2360.

87. Kanki P. Epidemiology and natural history of human immunodeficiency virus type 2. In: DeVita VT, Hellman S, Rosenberg SA, eds. *AIDS: Biology, Diagnosis, Treatment and Prevention*. Philadelphia, Pennsylvania: Lippincott-Raven Publishers, 1997: 127–135.

88. Kanki P, Sankalé JL, Mboup S. Biology of human immunodeficiency virus type 2 (HIV-2). In: Essex M, Mboup S, Kanki PJ, Marlink RG, Tlou SD, eds. *AIDS in Africa*. 2nd ed. New York: Kluwer Academic/Plenum Publishers, 2002: 73–103.

89. Kanki PJ. Biologic features of HIV-2. An update. *AIDS Clin Rev*, 1991;17–38.

90. Marlink R, Kanki P, Thior I, et al. Reduced rate of disease development after HIV-2 infection as compared to HIV-1. *Science*, 1994;265:1587–1590.

91. Marlink RG, Ricard D, M'Boup S, et al. Clinical, hematologic, and immunologic cross-sectional evaluation of individuals exposed to human immunodeficiency virus type-2 (HIV-2). *AIDS Res Hum Retroviruses*, 1988;4:137–148.

92. Kanki P, M'Boup S, Marlink R, et al. Prevalence and risk determinants of human immunodeficiency virus type 2 (HIV-2) and human immunodeficiency virus type 1 (HIV-1) in West African female prostitutes. *Am J Epidemiol*, 1992;136:895–907.

93. Popper SJ, Sarr AD, Travers KU, et al. Lower human immunodeficiency virus (HIV) type 2 viral load reflects the difference in pathogenicity of HIV-1 and HIV-2. *J Infect Dis*, 1999;180:1116–1121.

94. Marchant D, Neil SJ, McKnight A. Human immunodeficiency virus types 1 and 2 have different replication kinetics in human primary macrophage culture. *J Gen Virol*, 2006;87:411–418.

95. Morner A, Bjorndal A, Albert J, et al. Primary human immunodeficiency virus type 2 (HIV-2) isolates, like HIV-1 isolates, frequently use CCR5 but show promiscuity in coreceptor usage. *J Virol*, 1999;73:2343–2349.

96. van Harmelen J, Wood R, Lambrick M, et al. An association between HIV-1 subtypes and mode of transmission in Cape Town, South Africa. *AIDS*, 1997;11:81–87.

97. Liitsola K, Holmstrom P, Laukkanen T, et al. Analysis of HIV-1 genetic subtypes in Finland reveals good correlation between molecular and epidemiological data. *Scand J Infect Dis*, 2000;32: 475–480.

98. Kalish ML, Korber BT, Pillai S, et al. The sequential introduction of HIV-1 subtype B and CRF01 in Singapore by sexual transmission: accelerated V3 region evolution in a subpopulation of Asian CRF01 viruses. *Virology*, 2002;304:311–329.

99. Ou CY, Takebe Y, Weniger BG, et al. Independent introduction of two major HIV-1 genotypes into distinct high-risk populations in Thailand. *Lancet*, 1993;341:1171–1174.

100. Herring BL, Ge YC, Wang B, et al. Segregation of human immunodeficiency virus type 1 subtypes by risk factor in Australia. *J Clin Microbiol*, 2003;41: 4600–4604.

101. Hudgens MG, Longini IM Jr., Vanichseni S, et al. Subtype-specific transmission probabilities for human immunodeficiency virus type 1 among injecting drug users in Bangkok, Thailand. *Am J Epidemiol*, 2002;155:159–168.

102. Soto-Ramirez LE, Renjifo B, McLane MF, et al. HIV-1 Langerhans' cell tropism associated with heterosexual transmission of HIV. *Science*, 1996;271: 1291–293.

103. Kanki P, Essex M. Virology. In: Mayer K, Pizer H, eds. *The AIDS Pandemic: Impact on Science and Society.* Boston: Elsevier Academic Press, 2005:13–35.

104. Dittmar MT, Simmons G, Hibbitts S, et al. Langerhans cell tropism of human immunodeficiency virus type 1 subtype A through F isolates derived from different transmission groups. *J Virol*, 1997;71:8008–8013.

105. Hu DJ, Buve A, Baggs J, et al. What role does HIV-1 subtype play in transmission and pathogenesis? An epidemiological perspective. *AIDS*, 1999;13:873–881.

106. Pope M, Frankel SS, Mascola JR, et al. Human immunodeficiency virus type 1 strains of subtypes B and E replicate in cutaneous dendritic cell-T-cell mixtures without displaying subtype-specific tropism. *J Virol*, 1997;71:8001–8007.

107. Pope M, Ho DD, Moore JP, et al. Different subtypes of HIV-1 and cutaneous dendritic cells. *Science*, 1997; 278:786–788.

108. Renjifo B, Fawzi W, Mwakagile D, et al. Differences in perinatal transmission among human immunodeficiency virus type 1 genotypes. *J Hum Virol*, 2001;4: 16–25.

109. Renjifo B, Gilbert P, Chaplin B, et al. Emerging recombinant human immunodeficiency viruses: uneven representation of the envelope V3 region. *AIDS*, 1999;13:1613–1621.

110. Yang C, Li M, Newman RD, et al. Genetic diversity of HIV-1 in western Kenya: subtype-specific differences in mother-to-child transmission. *AIDS*, 2003; 17:1667–1674.

111. Kanki PJ, Hamel DJ, Sankale JL, et al. Human immunodeficiency virus type 1 subtypes differ in disease progression. *J Infect Dis*, 1999;179:68–73.

112. Kaleebu P, French N, Mahe C, et al. Effect of human immunodeficiency virus (HIV) type 1 envelope subtypes A and D on disease progression in a large cohort of HIV-1-positive persons in Uganda. *J Infect Dis*, 2002;185:1244–1250.

113. Santoro-Lopes G, Harrison LH, Tavares MD, et al. HIV disease progression and V3 serotypes in Brazil: is B different from B-Br? *AIDS Res Hum Retroviruses*, 2000;16:953–958.

114. Murphy G, Belda FJ, Pau CP, et al. Discrimination of subtype B and non-subtype B strains of human immunodeficiency virus type 1 by serotyping: correlation with genotyping. *J Clin Microbiol*, 1999;37: 1356–1360.

115. Del Amo J, Petruckevitch A, Phillips A, et al. Disease progression and survival in HIV-1-infected Africans in London. *AIDS*, 1998;12:1203–1209.

116. Neilson JR, John GC, Carr JK, et al. Subtypes of human immunodeficiency virus type 1 and disease stage among women in Nairobi, Kenya. *J Virol*, 1999; 73:4393–4403.

117. Hu DJ, Vanichseni S, Mastro TD, et al. Viral load differences in early infection with two HIV-1 subtypes. *AIDS*, 2001;15:683–691.

118. Sarr AD, Eisen G, Gueye-Ndiaye A, et al. Viral dynamics of primary HIV-1 infection in Senegal, West Africa. *J Infect Dis*, 2005;191:1460–1467.

119. Amornkul PN, Tansuphasawadikul S, Limpakarn-janarat K, et al. Clinical disease associated with HIV-1 subtype B' and E infection among 2104 patients in Thailand. *AIDS*, 1999;13:1963–1969.

120. Sagar M, Lavreys L, Baeten JM, et al. Infection with multiple human immunodeficiency virus type 1 variants is associated with faster disease progression. *J Virol*, 2003;77:12921–12926.

121. Tscherning C, Alaeus A, Fredriksson R, et al. Differences in chemokine coreceptor usage between genetic subtypes of HIV-1. *Virology*, 1998;241:181–188.

122. Bjorndal A, Sonnerborg A, Tscherning C, et al. Phenotypic characteristics of human immunodeficiency virus type 1 subtype C isolates of Ethiopian AIDS patients. *AIDS Res Hum Retroviruses*, 1999;15:647–653.

123. Paraskevis D, Hatzakis A. Molecular epidemiology of HIV-1 infection. *AIDS Rev*, 1999;1:238–249.

124. Fenyo EM. The role of virus biological phenotype in human immunodeficiency virus pathogenesis. *AIDS Rev*, 2001;3:157–168.

125. Sarr AD, Sankale JL, Hamel DJ, et al. Interaction with human immunodeficiency virus (HIV) type 2 predicts HIV type 1 genotype. *Virology*, 2000;268:402–410.

126. Alaeus A, Lidman K, Bjorkman A, et al. Similar rate of disease progression among individuals infected with HIV-1 genetic subtypes A–D. *AIDS*, 1999;13:901–907.

127. Laurent C, Bourgeois A, Faye MA, et al. No difference in clinical progression between patients infected with the predominant human immunodeficiency virus type 1 circulating recombinant form (CRF) 02_AG strain and patients not infected with CRF02_AG, in Western and West-Central Africa: a four-year prospective multicenter study. *J Infect Dis*, 2002;186:486–492.

128. Eshleman SH, Guay LA, Fleming T, et al. Survival of Ugandan infants with subtype A and D HIV-1 infection (HIVNET 012). *J Acquir Immune Defic Syndr*, 2002;31:327–330.

129. Montano MA, Novitsky VA, Blackard JT, et al. Divergent transcriptional regulation among expanding human immunodeficiency virus type 1 subtypes. *J Virol*, 1997;71:8657–8665.

130. Montano MA, Nixon CP, Ndung'u T, et al. Elevated tumor necrosis factor-alpha activation of human immunodeficiency virus type 1 subtype C in Southern Africa is associated with an NF-kappaB enhancer gain-of-function. *J Infect Dis*, 2000;181:76–81.

131. Montano MA, Nixon CP, Essex M. Dysregulation through the NF-kappaB enhancer and TATA box of the human immunodeficiency virus type 1 subtype E promoter. *J Virol*, 1998;72:8446–8452.

132. Clavel F, Race E, Mammano F. HIV drug resistance and viral fitness. *Adv Pharmacol*, 2000;49:41–66.

133. Domingo E, Escarmis C, Menedez-Arias L, et al. Viral quasispecies and fitness variation, In: Domingo E, Webster R, and Holland J, eds. *Origin and Evolution of Viruses*. San Diego, California: Academic Press, 1999:141–161.

134. Quinones-Mateu ME. Is HIV-1 evolving to a less virulent (pathogenic) virus? *AIDS*, 2005;19:1689–1690.

135. Ball SC, Abraha A, Collins KR, et al. Comparing the ex vivo fitness of CCR5-tropic human immunodeficiency virus type 1 isolates of subtypes B and C. *J Virol*, 2003;77:1021–1038.

136. Njai H, Arien K, Clybergh C, et al. Higher replicative capacity of HIV-1 circulating recombinant form over its parental subtypes: implications for the predominance of CRF02_AG in west and west central Africa. *12th Conference on Retroviruses and Opportunistic Infections*, Boston, Massachusetts, February 22–25, 2005 (abstract 330).

137. Arien KK, Abraha A, Quinones-Mateu ME, et al. The replicative fitness of primary human immunodeficiency virus type 1 (HIV-1) group M, HIV-1 group O, and HIV-2 isolates. *J Virol*, 2005;79:8979–8990.

138. Ellenberger DL, Li B, Lupo LD, et al. Generation of a consensus sequence from prevalent and incident HIV-1 infections in West Africa to guide AIDS vaccine development. *Virology*, 2002;302:156–163.

139. Kantor R, Katzenstein D. Polymorphism in HIV-1 non-subtype B protease and reverse transcriptase and its potential impact on drug susceptibility and drug resistance evolution. *AIDS Rev*, 2003;5:25–35.

140. McClure MA, Johnson MS, Feng DF, et al. Sequence comparisons of retroviral proteins: relative rates of change and general phylogeny. *Proc Natl Acad Sci USA*, 1988;85:2469–2473.

141. Hue S, Clewley JP, Cane PA, et al. HIV-1 pol gene variation is sufficient for reconstruction of transmissions in the era of antiretroviral therapy. *AIDS*, 2004;18:719–728.

142. Yeni PG, Hammer SM, Hirsch MS, et al. Treatment for adult HIV infection: 2004 recommendations of the International AIDS Society-USA Panel. *JAMA*, 2004;292:251–265.

143. Idigbe EO, Adewole TA, Eisen G, et al. Management of HIV-1 infection with a combination of nevirapine, stavudine, and lamivudine: a preliminary report on the Nigerian antiretroviral program. *J Acquir Immune Defic Syndr*, 2005;40:65–69.

144. Kantor R, Katzenstein DA, Efron B, et al. Impact of HIV-1 subtype and antiretroviral therapy on protease and reverse transcriptase genotype: results of a global collaboration. *PLoS Med*, 2005;2:e112.

145. Laurent C, Diakhate N, Gueye NF, et al. The Senegalese government's highly active antiretroviral therapy initiative: an 18-month follow-up study. *AIDS*, 2002;16:1363–1370.

146. Shafer RW. *Genotypic Testing for HIV-1 Drug Resistance*. 2003. Accessed at http://hivdb.stanford.edu/modules/lookUpFiles/pdf/GenotypicResistance.pdf.

147. Yerly S, Vora S, Rizzardi P, et al. Acute HIV infection: impact on the spread of HIV and transmission of drug resistance. *AIDS*, 2001;15:2287–2292.

148. Analysis of prevalence of HIV-1 drug resistance in primary infections in the United Kingdom. *BMJ*, 2001;322:1087–1088.

149. de Ronde A, van Dooren M, van Der Hoek L, et al. Establishment of new transmissible and drug-sensitive human immunodeficiency virus type 1 wild types due to transmission of nucleoside analogue-resistant virus. *J Virol*, 2001;75:595–602.

150. Bacheler LT, Anton ED, Kudish P, et al. Human immunodeficiency virus type 1 mutations selected in patients failing efavirenz combination therapy. *Antimicrob Agents Chemother*, 2000;44:2475–2484.

151. Richman DD, Havlir D, Corbeil J, et al. Nevirapine resistance mutations of human immunodeficiency virus type 1 selected during therapy. *J Virol*, 1994;68:1660–1666.

152. Bocket L, Cheret A, Deuffic-Burban S, et al. Impact of human immunodeficiency virus type 1 subtype on first-line antiretroviral therapy effectiveness. *Antivir Ther*, 2005;10:247–254.

153. Frater AJ, Beardall A, Ariyoshi K, et al. Impact of baseline polymorphisms in RT and protease on outcome of highly active antiretroviral therapy in HIV-1-infected African patients. *AIDS*, 2001;15:1493–1502.

154. Johnson VA, Brun-Vezinet F, Clotet B, et al. Drug resistance mutations in HIV-1. *Top HIV Med*, 2003;11:215–221.

155. Adje-Toure C, Bile CE, Borget MY, et al. Polymorphism in protease and reverse transcriptase and phenotypic drug resistance of HIV-1 recombinant CRF02_AG isolates from patients with no prior use of antiretroviral drugs in Abidjan, Cote d'Ivoire. *J Acquir Immune Defic Syndr*, 2003;34:111–113.

156. Becker-Pergola G, Kataaha P, Johnston-Dow L, et al. Analysis of HIV type 1 protease and reverse transcriptase in antiretroviral drug-naive Ugandan adults. *AIDS Res Hum Retroviruses*, 2000;16:807–813.

157. Konings FA, Zhong P, Agwara M, et al. Protease mutations in HIV-1 non-B strains infecting drug-naive villagers in Cameroon. *AIDS Res Hum Retroviruses*, 2004;20:105–109.

158. Vicente AC, Agwale SM, Otsuki K, et al. Genetic variability of HIV-1 protease from Nigeria and correlation with protease inhibitors drug resistance. *Virus Genes*, 2001;22:181–186.

159. Rambaut A, Posada D, Crandall KA, et al. The causes and consequences of HIV evolution. *Nat Rev Genet*, 2004;5:52–61.

160. Kellam P, Larder BA. Retroviral recombination can lead to linkage of reverse transcriptase mutations that confer increased zidovudine resistance. *J Virol*, 1995;69:669–674.

161. Chen R, Quinones-Mateu ME, Mansky LM. Drug resistance, virus fitness and HIV-1 mutagenesis. *Curr Pharm Des*, 2004;10:4065–4070.

162. Blankson JN, Persaud D, Siliciano RF. The challenge of viral reservoirs in HIV-1 infection. *Annu Rev Med*, 2002;53:557–593.

163. Kijak GH, Currier JR, Tovanabutra S, et al. Lost in translation: implications of HIV-1 codon usage for immune escape and drug resistance. *AIDS Rev*, 2004;6:54–60.

164. Ojesina A, Sankalé J, Odaibo G, et al. Subtype-specific patterns in HIV-1 reverse transcriptase and protease in Oyo State, Nigeria: implications for drug resistance and host response. *AIDS Res Hum Retroviruses*, 2006;in press.

165. Karlsson AC, Deeks SG, Barbour JD, et al. Dual pressure from antiretroviral therapy and cell-mediated immune response on the human immunodeficiency virus type 1 protease gene. *J Virol*, 2003;77: 6743–6752.

166. Mason RD, Bowmer MI, Howley CM, et al. Antiretroviral drug resistance mutations sustain or enhance CTL recognition of common HIV-1 Pol epitopes. *J Immunol*, 2004;172:7212–219.

167. Yusim K, Kesmir C, Gaschen B, et al. Clustering patterns of cytotoxic T-lymphocyte epitopes in human immunodeficiency virus type 1 (HIV-1) proteins reveal imprints of immune evasion on HIV-1 global variation. *J Virol*, 2002;76:8757–8768.

168. Kawana A, Tomiyama H, Takiguchi M, et al. Accumulation of specific amino acid substitutions in HLA-B35-restricted human immunodeficiency virus type 1 cytotoxic T lymphocyte epitopes. *AIDS Res Hum Retroviruses*, 1999;15:1099–1107.

169. Moore CB, John M, James IR, et al. Evidence of HIV-1 adaptation to HLA-restricted immune responses at a population level. *Science*, 2002;296: 1439–1443.

170. Winkler C, O'Brien S. Effect of genetic variation on HIV transmission and progression to AIDS. In: Essex M, Mboup S, Kanki PJ, Marlink RG, Tlou SD, eds. *AIDS in Africa*. 2nd ed. New York: Kluwer Academic/Plenum Publishers, 2002:52–73.

171. Gorny MK, Williams C, Volsky B, et al. Human monoclonal antibodies specific for conformation-sensitive epitopes of V3 neutralize human immunodeficiency virus type 1 primary isolates from various clades. *J Virol*, 2002;76:9035–9045.

172. Quinnan GV Jr., Zhang PF, Fu DW, et al. Expression and characterization of HIV type 1 envelope protein associated with a broadly reactive neutralizing antibody response. *AIDS Res Hum Retroviruses*, 1999;15:561–570.

173. Pestano GA, Hosford KS, Spira AI, et al. Seroreactivity of analogous antigenic epitopes in glycoprotein 120 expressed in HIV-1 subtypes A, B, C, and D. *AIDS Res Hum Retroviruses*, 1995;11: 589–596.

174. Olaleye D, Bernstein L, Ekwezor C, et al. Prevalence of human immunodeficiency virus type 1 and 2 infections in Nigeria. *J Infect Dis*, 1993;167:710–714.

175. Olaleye D, Ekweozor C, Sheng Z, et al. Evidence of serological cross-reactivities with human immunodeficiency virus types 1 and 2 and human T-lymphotropic virus. *Int J Epidemiol*, 1995;24:198–203.

176. Federal Ministry of Health. *Technical Report on 2000 HIV/Syphilis Sero-prevalence and STD Syndromes Sentinel Survey among PTB and STD Patients in Nigeria*. Abuja: Federal Ministry of Health, 2001.

177. Federal Ministry of Health. *The 2001 National HIV/Syphilis Sentinel Survey among Pregnant Women Attending Ante-natal Clinics in Nigeria*. Abuja: Federal Ministry of Health, 2001.

178. National AIDS/STDs Control Programme. The 2003 National HIV Sero-prevalence Sentinel Survey. Federal Ministry of Health, 2004.

179. Chikwem J, Mohammed I, Oyebode-Ola T. Prevalence of human immunodeficiency virus (HIV) infection in Borno State of Nigeria. *East Afr Med J*, 1988;65:342–346.

180. Harry T, Ekenna O, Chikwen J, et al. Seroepidemiology of human immunodeficiency virus infection in Borno State of Nigeria by sentinel surveillance. *J Acquir Immune Defic Syndr*, 1993;6:99–103.

184. Harry T, Kyari O, Mohammed I. Prevalence of human immunodeficiency virus-infection among pregnant women attending ante-natal clinic in Maiduguri, north-eastern Nigeria. *Trop Geogr Med*, 1992;44:238–241.

182. Olusanya O, Lawoko A, Blomberg J. Seroepidemiology of human retroviruses in Ogun State of Nigeria. *J Infect Dis*, 1990;22:155–160.

183. Abbott R, Ndour-Sarr A, Diouf A, et al. Risk determinants for HIV infection and adverse obstetrical outcomes in pregnant women in Dakar, Senegal. *J Acquir Immune Defic Syndr*, 1994;7.

184. Olaleye D, Sheng Z, Ekweozor C, et al. Genetic screening of HIV-1 strains from seropositive individuals in Nigeria by PCR amplification techniques using different sets of primer pairs and probes. *Biosci Res Comm*, 1995;7:83–87.

185. Howard T, Olaleye D, Rasheed S. Sequence analysis of the glycoprotein 120 coding region of a new HIV type 1 subtype A strain (HIV-1IbNG from Nigeria. *AIDS Res Hum Retroviruses*, 1994;10:1755–1757.

186. Abimiku A, Stern T, Zwandor A. Subtype G HIV type 1 isolates from Nigeria. *AIDS Res Hum Retroviruses*, 1994;10:1581–1583.

187. Kabeya CM, Esu-Williams E, Eni E, et al. Evidence for HIV-1 group O infection in Nigeria. *Lancet*, 1995; 346:308.

188. Odaibo G, Olaleye D, Ruppach H, et al. Multiple presence and heterogeneous distribution of HIV-1 subtypes in Nigeria. *Biosci Res Comm*, 2001;13: 447–458.

189. Odaibo G, Olaleye D, Ruppach H, et al. Epidemiological evidence of recent introduction of HIV-1 subtypes B and O into Nigeria. *Biosci Res Comm*, 2003;15:141–146.

190. Olaleye D, Sankalé J, Odaibo G, et al. Circulating HIV-1 subtypes and recombinants in South Western Nigeria. *XIII International Conference on AIDS and STIs in Africa*, Nairobi, Kenya, 2003 (abstract ThuPs989353).

191. Sankalé J, Odaibo G, Langevin S, et al. Molecular epidemiology of HIV-1 in Oyo State, Nigeria: CRF02_AG does not constitute the majority of circulating strains. *14th International Conference on AIDS and STIs in Africa*, Abuja, Nigeria, December 4–9, 2005 (abstract ThOrD159).

192. McCutchan FE, Carr JK, Bajani M, et al. Subtype G and multiple forms of A/G intersubtype recombinant human immunodeficiency virus type 1 in Nigeria. *Virology*, 1999;254:226–234.

193. Meloni S, Sankalé JL, Odaibo G, et al. A Nigeria-specific cluster of HIV-1 subtype G is sustained in full-length genome sequencing. *14th International Conference on AIDS and STIs in Africa*, Abuja, Nigeria, December 4–9, 2005 (abstract ThOrD157).

194. Agwale S, Zeh C, Robbins K, et al. Molecular surveillance of HIV-1 field strains in Nigeria in preparation for vaccine trials. *Vaccine*, 2002;20:2131–2139.

195. Idoko J, Njoku O. Molecular epidemiology of HIV-1 in north central Nigeria. *13th International Conference on AIDS and STIs in Africa*, Nairobi, Kenya, 2003.

196. Odaibo G, Ibeh M, Olaleye D. Reliability of HIV testing in Africa. *2nd IAS Conference on HIV Pathogenesis and Treatment*, Paris, France, 2003 (abstract 1234).

197. Agwale SM, Tanimoto L, Womack C, et al. Primary antiretroviral resistance and molecular diversity of HIV-1 in antiretroviral therapy patients enrolled into Nigerian national ART programme. *3rd IAS Conference on HIV Pathogenesis and Treatment*, Rio de Janeiro, Brazil, July 24–27, 2005 (abstract WePe4.1C12).

198. Lar P. HIV subtype and drug resistance patterns among drug-naive infected persons in Jos, Nigeria. *2005 International Meeting of the Institute of Human Virology*, Baltimore, Maryland, December 2004 (abstract 69).

5

THE ROLE OF SEXUALLY TRANSMITTED INFECTIONS IN HIV TRANSMISSION

Folasade T. Ogunsola*

Sexually transmitted infections (STIs) are a major cause of acute illness, infertility, long-term disability, and death worldwide. In 1999, the World Health Organization (WHO) estimated that 340 million new cases of four curable STIs — syphilis, gonorrhea, chlamydia, and trichomoniasis — occurred in men and women aged 15 to 49 years (1). Apart from contributing significantly to morbidity and mortality, STIs are often associated with increased sexual transmission of HIV.

STIs traditionally include all contagious infections in which the principal mode of transmission is sexual contact with mucous membranes and/or skin surfaces. Initially, only a few infections — such as syphilis and gonorrhea — were considered to be sexually transmitted (2). The WHO has since broadened this definition, however, to include more than 20 bacteria, viruses, fungi, and protozoa (1,3) (Table 5-1). Bacterial infections that are primarily transmitted sexually include syphilis (*Treponema pallidum*); gonorrhea (*Neisseria gonorrhoeae*); lymphogranuloma venereum (*Chlamydia trachomatis*); chancroid (*Haemophilus ducreyi*); and non-specific urethritis and cervicitis (*Ureaplasma urealyticum* and *Mycoplasma genitalium*). Common sexually transmitted viruses include human immunodeficiency virus, herpes simplex type 2, various strains of human papillomavirus, hepatitis B virus, hepatitis C virus, human herpes virus type 8, and human T-cell lymphotrophic virus.

*Department of Medical Microbiology and Parasitology, College of Medicine, University of Lagos, Lagos, Nigeria

Table 5-1. Causes of Sexually Transmitted Infections Other than HIV

Etiologic Agent/ Syndrome	Clinical Features	Laboratory Diagnosis	Treatment	Epidemiology	Contact Tracing Priority
Bacteria					
Treponema pallidum Syphilis	1° Genital ulcer (chancre) 2° Mucous patches, skin rashes 3° Systemic infection, organ involvement	RPR, TPHA, serology	Penicillin	Sexually transmitted, intrauterine, vertical transmission	High
Neisseria gonorrhoeae Gonorrhea	Asymptomatic in most women, urethral discharge, dysuria	MCS, NAAT	Ciprofloxacin	Mainly sexual	High
Haemophilus ducreyi Chancroid	Genital ulcer	Clinical, culture (difficult)	Erythromycin	Sexual	High
Chlamydia trachomatis serotypes D-K and L1–L3 *Lymphogranuloma venereum* Non-gonococcal urethritis	Urethral and cervical discharge	Clinical, ELISA, DFA,* NAAT*	Doxycycline	Sexual, intrapartum, perinatal	High
Ureaplasma urealyticum/ Mycoplasma genitalium Non-gonococcal urethritis	Urethral and cervical discharge	Clinical, culture difficult. NAAT (not commercially available)	Erythromycin	Sexual	Moderate
Anaerobes, including *Mobiluncus* spp. and *Gardnerella vaginalis* (bacterial vaginosis)	Vaginal discharge with a peculiar odor	Little or no lactobacilli, Clue cells on gram stain or wet mount, ph>4.5, potassium hydroxide	Flagyl	?Sexual	Moderate
Klebsiella granulomatis (Donovanosis)	Beefy, genital ulcers that bleed easily	Clinical, microscopy of scrapings, biopsy	Trimethoprim-sulfamethoxazole, azithromycin	Sexual; no reported cases in Nigeria; common in South Africa	High
Viruses					
Herpes simplex virus type 2	Genital ulcers	Clinical, cell culture, serology, NAAT*	Genital hygiene, Acyclovir	Sexual/ intrapartum	Moderate
Herpes simplex virus type 1	Oral and other non-genital ulcers; implicated more in genital disease	Same as in herpes simplex virus type 2	Same as in herpes simplex virus type 2	Most acquired non-sexually	Moderate
Human papillomavirus	Genital and anal warts, anogenital cancers	Clinical, PAP smear, biopsy	Podophylotoxin, imiquimod; for warts, cryotherapy; for cancer, surgery, chemotherapy, and irradiation	Sexual	Low
Molluscum contagiosum virus type 1 in children and type 2 in adults		Clinical	Curettage, podophyllotoxin, imiquimod	Sexual	Low
Hepatitis B virus Hepatitis	Jaundice, tender hepatomegally	Clinical, serology	Lamivudine, interferon-alpha**	Bloodborne, mainly MSM	
Hepatitis A virus Hepatitis	Jaundice, tender hepatomegally	Clinical, serology		Fecal-oral, mainly MSM	
Human T-cell lymphotrophic virus type I	Lymphoid cancer, tropical spastic paresis	Serology, histology		Sexual	

Etiologic Agent/ Syndrome	Clinical Features	Laboratory Diagnosis	Treatment	Epidemiology	Contact Tracing Priority
Viruses *(continued)*					
Hepatitis C virus	Hepatitis	Serology	Ribivarin, interferon-alpha**	Bloodborne ?sexual	
Human herpes virus 8/ Kaposi's sarcoma	Dark purple lesions on the palate, arms	Clinical, histology	Chemotherapy	> 40% cases in Africa	
Epstein-Barr virus	Mononucleosis, cancer	Serology, histology	Chemotherapy		
Parasites					
Trichomonas vaginalis Trichmoniaisis	Itchy, greenish vaginal discharge	Microscopy, culture	Flagyl	Common	Moderate
Giardia lamblia Giardiasis Gay bowel syndrome	Bulky fatty stool, gastroenteritis	Microscopy	Flagyl	Fecal-oral, sexual especially in MSM	
Other Infections (Less common infections and those for whom sexual transmission is not well defined)					
Shigella spp.	Diarrhea	MCS	Quinolones	Fecal-oral, sexual especially in MSM	
Campylobacter spp.	Diarrhea	MCS	Quinolones	Fecal-oral, sexual especially in MSM	
Entamoeba histolytica	Diarrhea	Microscopy	Flagyl	Fecal-oral, sexual especially in MSM	
Phthirus pubis	Pubic lice	Clinical	1% permethrin cream, malathion	Close contact	
Sarcoptes scabei	Scabies	Clinical	5% permethrin cream, lindane cream, or ivermectin orally	Close contact	
Candida albicans	Vaginal thrush	Clinical, microscopy, culture	Miconazole, nystatin	Mainly non-sexual, ?sexual	

*not usually done or not available
**Tenofovir with HIV coinfection
Abbreviations: DFA: direct fluorescent assay; **ELISA:** enzyme-linked immunosorbent assay; **MCS:** microscopy, culture, and sensitivity; **MSM:** men who have sex with men; **NAAT:** nucleic acid amplification test; **RPR:** Rapid Plasma Reagin screening test; **TPHA:** Treponema pallidum hemagglutination assay

Parasitic STIs include *Trichomonas vaginalis*, *Giardia lamblia*, and ectoparasites such as *Phthirius pubis* (body lice) and *Sarcoptes scabei*.

The concurrent high prevalence and rapid increase of HIV and other STIs among sex workers in Africa and in Asia suggest an epidemiologic association between STIs and HIV transmission (4–6). Studies have shown that STI rates tend to rise before HIV rates climb (7). STIs such as gonorrhea and chlamydia increase HIV shedding from the genital tract (6,8,9), which suggests that STIs may enhance the infectivity of HIV-infected people. Some data also suggest that STIs increase susceptibility to HIV (10,11), although that causal relationship is more tenuous (12). Moreover, by suppressing normal host immune responses, HIV infection both increases susceptibility to and lengthens the clinical course of STIs (13). This relationship between STIs and HIV appears stronger with genital ulcer diseases than with non-genital ulcer diseases such as gonorrhea. Nonetheless, the presence of an untreated STI—ulcerative or non-ulcerative—can increase the risk of both acquisition and transmission of HIV tenfold. Improvement in the management of STIs can reduce the incidence of HIV infection in the general population by about 40% (14). Prevention and treatment of STIs are therefore critical components of HIV prevention and treatment strategies.

The interrelationship between HIV and STIs has been well recognized in Nigeria. A survey among STI patients in 2000 showed that sexual activities and STI prevalence are particularly common in the 20-to-29 age group, and that sexual exposure to STIs and HIV typically begins between the ages of 10 and 19 (15). Similarly, the national median HIV prevalence among STI patients rose steadily from 4.6% in 1991 to 15.0% in 1995, with a slight decline to 11.5% in 2000. This chapter, therefore, will examine selected STIs and their possible roles in HIV transmission, the epidemiology and relative importance of these STIs to HIV transmission in Nigeria, and current preventive strategies.

EPIDEMIOLOGY AND PUBLIC HEALTH BURDEN OF STIS

Public Health Concerns

For many years experts have recognized the public health effects of STIs, which include severe medical, psychological, economic, and social consequences for millions of infected individuals. Left untreated, STIs can lead to a range of pathologies, including pelvic inflammatory disease, infertility, wastage, ectopic pregnancies, urethral stricture, congenital infections, anogenital cancers, and premature death. This public health burden varies significantly between developed and developing countries and is borne most heavily by such vulnerable groups as women, children, and the urban poor. In developing countries, STIs rank fifth among the most common diseases for which adults seek health care (3). STIs tend to be underreported in developing countries, including Nigeria, however, so the full extent of disease burden is not known (3).

The most significant consequence of STIs is pelvic inflammatory disease (PID) in young women. In this population, PID is particularly catastrophic both medically and socially, as it can cause chronic pelvic pain and infertility. The World Bank estimates that PID and salpingitis account for 94% of all STI-related morbidity. The social impact of PID is likely felt most strongly in African countries where female infertility is stigmatized and infertile women risk divorce and ill treatment from in-laws (16).

The interdependence of the STI and HIV epidemics has underscored the public health importance of STIs. Unfortunately, HIV shares similar risk profiles with other STIs and, like other STIs, HIV is common in developing countries. UNAIDS estimates that at least 95% of the 40 million people infected with HIV live in developing countries, with as many as 6 million in Nigeria alone (17,18).

The Magnitude of the Problem

The epidemiology of STIs is a function of the interplay of several factors, including sexual practices, health-care–seeking behavior, transmissibility of individual pathogens, duration of infectiousness, antimicrobial resistance, and the presence of other coinfections. Demographics and social conditions—which affect the availability of sexual health education, diagnostic facilities, and effective treatments—also play important roles (16,19). STIs tend to be more prevalent in developing countries and among urban residents, unmarried individuals, and young adults. Females tend to be infected at younger ages than males, most likely reflecting differences in the age at which they become sexually active, as well as the relative rates of transmission from one gender to the other.

The WHO estimates that in 1999 there were 12 million syphilis cases, of which more than two-thirds were in sub-Saharan Africa, South Asia, and Southeast Asia. Gonorrhea accounted for 62.4 million cases, while *C. trachomatis* accounted for 92 million cases. The incidence of *T. vaginalis*, which is endemic globally, was more common in lower socioeconomic classes and accounted for 172 million cases (1,20). The global incidence of other STIs, especially viral STIs, has not been well documented, however. Nevertheless, it is generally believed that human papillomavirus and herpes simplex virus infections are widespread. Furthermore, hepatitis B virus is considered an STI in the industrialized world but not in Africa and Asia, where it is endemic (21–23).

TYPES OF SEXUALLY TRANSMITTED INFECTIONS

Bacterial STIs

Treponema Pallidum

Syphilis is a highly infectious systemic disease caused by the microaerophilic spirochete *Treponema pallidum*. The reported incidence of syphilis in the developed world declined substantially after the introduction of penicillin in the 1940s. In Western Europe, syphilis rates peaked just after World War II and fell to below 5 per 100,000 in most countries (24,25). Rates remained stable until the mid-1980s when they once again began to climb with the onset of the HIV epidemic (1,26). This resurgence was seen mainly among men who have sex with men (MSM).

In Nigeria, antibodies against yaws—an endemic, non-venereal treponemal infection—made serologic diagnosis of syphilis unreliable before the 1950s. Yaws may also protect against syphilis infection, as syphilis prevalence rates tended to be low in areas of yaws endemicity (2,27). Thus, the WHO mass treatment campaigns to eradicate yaws in the 1950s (27) may have actually increased susceptibility to syphilis in many developing countries, although this supposition has never been confirmed (2,28).

In sub-Saharan Africa, approximately 10% of pregnant women harbor syphilis, with prevalence rates ranging from 2.5% in Burkina Faso to 17.4% in Cameroon (29,30). In Nigeria, national prevalence data on pregnant women in 2003 suggested that syphilis is uncommon, with a national prevalence of 0.3% (17). The prevalence was lowest in the southwest (0.1%) and highest in the northeast (0.6%). In contrast, a study targeting sexually active females aged 12 to 49 years in a rural community in southern Nigeria recorded a prevalence rate of 3.0% (31)—about 10 times the national average.

Several factors may account for the low syphilis rates in Nigeria:

- the national figures are obtained from women attending antenatal care programs in public health care institutions and there may be a selection bias for those with relatively good health-care–seeking behavior;
- there is considerable antibiotic use and abuse in Nigeria, as antibiotics are easily purchased (32); and
- it is possible that there are still endemic non-venereal treponemes that afford some cross-protection to venereal treponeme infection. Expanded community-based studies are needed to understand better the varied aspects of syphilis epidemiology in Nigeria.

Transmission of *T. pallidum* is mainly sexual, although transmission may also occur transplacentally from mother to child (congenital syphilis), during moist kissing, or during inoculation injuries. The risk of acquiring syphilis from an infected partner ranges from 10% to 60% during primary infection (33). The disease is most contagious in the first two years after initial infection when large quantities of the spirochete can be found in lesions. Most patients are rarely infectious after four years of infection (33).

Syphilis occurs in three stages. The incubation period typically lasts two to four weeks but may range from 3 to 90 days (34). The primary stage of infection is characterized by a painless indurated ulcer/chancre that develops at the site of inoculation in the genital, mouth, or other areas. The chancre may go unnoticed; in some cases, no chancre develops (33). Chancres usually heal within two to eight weeks but may persist in HIV-infected individuals and other immunocompromised individuals.

If left untreated, this stage is followed by a more generalized infection typically characterized by disseminated mucocutaneous lesions on the palms of the hands and the soles of the feet. Other common lesions associated with this secondary stage include condylomata, muqueuses (mucous patches), and a patchy alopecia described as "moth-eaten alopecia." There may be fever and general malaise, as well as mild hepatitis. The secondary stage becomes clinically obvious about six weeks after infection when large numbers of treponemes are present in the tissue, bloodstream, and lymph nodes. Treponemes can also be found in the central nervous system in 35% of cases. An immune complex glomerulonephritis may occur at this stage because of the high antigen-antibody load (33).

A latent period often occurs between the secondary and tertiary stages, during which the infection has no clinical symptoms, although serologic reactions are positive. During latency, the patient remains infectious; the immune response remains brisk, however, suggesting that the infection is not quiescent. In the late latency stage, the patient is relatively resistant to re-infection, although *T. pallidum* may still be transmitted transplacentally.

The tertiary stage of syphilis occurs years later in approximately one-third of untreated individuals. This stage is characterized by granulomas and vasculitis in several organs. Most commonly affected are the central nervous system (neurosyphilis); the heart and arteries (cardiovascular syphilis); and the skin, muscle, and bones (gummatous syphilis) (33,34).

Presumptive diagnosis of syphilis is by serologic detection of antibodies against non-treponemal antigens. In Nigeria, both the rapid plasma reagin (RPR) and the Venereal Disease Research Laboratory (VDRL) tests are regularly used. These tests have a high level of false positive results because they do not differentiate between previous and current infections; therefore, specific confirmatory tests should be performed before patients are diagnosed as positive (35). The most common confirmatory test, the *Treponema pallidum* hemagglutination test (TPHA), detects antibodies to treponemal antigens in patient plasma or sera. This test is not widely available in many laboratories in developing countries, however, including Nigeria (35).

Under ideal circumstances, a positive RPR is accurate in 80% to 86% of primary infections, 100% of secondary infections, 80% of latent infections, and 71% to 73% of late-stage syphilis (35). As a result, the WHO has determined that in resource-poor countries where no TPHA is available, the benefits of treating all RPR-positive people far outweigh the risks of treating those for whom the RPR was a false positive (35). Treatment for syphilis is benzathine penicillin, although doxycycline and tetracycline are appropriate alternatives for individuals who cannot take penicillin (35,36).

In HIV-infected people, diagnosis of syphilis requires a high index of suspicion. The clinical course is often more protracted and aggressive with atypical florid lesions, more systemic involvement, and a higher probability of neurosyphilis with uveitis (33,37,38). This unusual clinical presentation is often compounded by confounding serologic responses to syphilis and other antigens, which are more common in early HIV disease, when polyclonal B cell stimulation more typically occurs (39–41). In HIV-associated syphilis, penicillin is still the drug of choice, and HIV-infected people generally have good responses. Bacteriostatic drugs such as doxycycline and erythromycin are best avoided because of their high relapse rate in some HIV-infected people (42). It is recommended that therapy should be prolonged to increase the possibility of cure, especially in patients with neurosyphilis (33). Prevention of syphilis can be achieved through condom use or abstinence; there is currently no vaccine.

Neisseria Gonorrhoeae

Neisseria gonorrhoeae, a gram-negative intracellular diplococcus bacterium, is transmitted mainly through vaginal, oral, or anal contact. Intrapartum infection may also occur and results in gonococcal ophthalmia neonatorum. In women, the bacterium usually causes asymptomatic cervicitis, urethritis, and proctitis, although a small number may experience a thick vaginal discharge or dysuria. Women constitute the main reservoir of infection, although some community surveys have found a large pool of asymptomatic men (43). Because women are largely asymptomatic, most prevalence figures derive from men.

In men, infection is usually symptomatic, with an anterior urethritis that results in a painful, burning sensation in the urethra during micturation associated with a purulent urethral discharge. *N. gonorrhoeae* can also cause a symptomatic rectal infection in MSM (44).

Urethral discharge is the most common symptom among men in sub-Saharan Africa, and *N. gonorrhoeae* accounts for 53% to 80% of all cases (45–47). In a recent polymerase-chain-reaction–based study in 659 men from seven West African countries, *N. gonorrhoeae* was the most common STI, accounting for

61.9% of cases. In addition, men with *N. gonorrhoeae* were more likely to have multiple infections, especially with *T. vaginalis* and *C. trachomatis*. Although no similar study has been conducted in Nigeria, there is no reason to believe the picture would differ significantly from those in other West African countries.

Serious sequelae follow ascending gonococcal infection of the genitals in both men and women. In women, salpingitis and PID are complications that may lead to infertility and ectopic pregnancies. Posterior urethritis, if untreated, may result in urethral stricture and chronic prostatitis. This usually presents with chronic lower back pain and occasional discharge. Gonorrhea has also been associated with male infertility and azospermia (49–51). There are no national data on the prevalence of gonorrhea in Nigeria, however, because of the difficulty in isolating the organism in laboratories. Several issues further complicate a true estimation of the prevalence of gonorrhea in Nigeria: many people do not go to the hospital for diagnosis and treatment (32); the high expense prohibits many laboratories from preparing selective media for the isolation of the gonococcus; and clinicians rarely request culture for *N. gonorrhoeae* because they manage most cases syndromically.

Diagnosis of gonorrhea is by culture on selective media. Culture has been shown to be more sensitive for urethral cultures than with endocervical cultures; however, the sensitivity of culture is affected by prior antibiotic use, the condition under which the samples are transported, and duration of transport. In Nigeria, widespread antibiotic use affects the sensitivity of culture, and figures obtained in many studies are likely gross underestimations (52). More recently, nucleic acid amplification tests have been developed for diagnosis. Although polymerase chain reaction (PCR) is more sensitive than culturing (53), it is at present too expensive to be used for routine purposes. Other amplification methods include the ligase chain and the Amplicor PCR assay, which can detect gonorrhea from swabs, as well as urine with a sensitivity of 90% to 97% and a specificity of 100% (53,54). Strand displacement amplification, which can also detect gonorrhea from self-administered vaginal swabs, has a low sensitivity (77%) when used on female urine (55).

Penicillin has been the traditional treatment of choice for gonorrhea, but because of its widespread resistance, the recommended treatment now includes ciprofloxacin, ceftriaxone, and spectinomycin (1). Treatment of gonorrhea is the same in HIV-positive and HIV-negative patients. In Nigeria, penicillin has long ceased to be used because of the high prevalence of penicillinase-producing *N. gonorrhoeae* (46,56). the first-line drug for treating gonorrhea is ciprofloxacin (57).

Haemophilus Ducreyi

An estimated 7 million people worldwide have chancroid, with most cases occurring in developing countries. Chancroid's true prevalence in developing countries is not known, however, because of the absence of simple, affordable diagnostic methods (58). Diagnosis can be made by culture of exudates from the base of the ulcer or from bubo aspirates. Non-cultural methods include enzyme immunoassays and PCR, both of which have higher sensitivities than culture. Although no studies specifically address the prevalence of *H. ducreyi* in the general population of Nigeria, existing studies suggest that the infection may be common (59), with an 86% seroprevalence among sex workers (60). Culture methods are insensitive and lead to unrealistically low rates. The advent of PCR, however, has revolutionized the diagnosis of chancroid worldwide, even though it is neither available nor affordable in most African countries. Elsewhere in Africa, prevalence rates of 11% and 56% have been recorded (61,62).

A small gram-negative bacillus, *H. ducreyi*, is the etiologic cause of chancroid. The infection is found worldwide and is typically associated with low socioeconomic status (62). The incubation period is from one day to several weeks. It is a common cause of genital ulcer disease in Africa and tropical countries. Extragenital lesions on the breasts and fingers are uncommon except in immunocompromised individuals. These ulcers tend to be single in men, while women often have multiple lesions. In the developed world, *H. ducreyi* usually occurs in small, localized outbreaks (63,64). Diagnosis is usually clinical because culturing is difficult, although gram-stained smears from the base of the ulcer or from an aspirate of the inguinal bubo may show the characteristic "school of fish" appearance that is suggestive of chancroid (65). A single oral dose of azithromycin or ceftriaxone is an effective therapy, as is a seven-day course of erythromycin, although reduced susceptibility to antibiotics has been reported in some strains (66). There is no vaccine to prevent chancroid infection.

Chlamydia Trachomatis

Chlamydia trachomatis, an obligate intracellular parasite with a unique reproductive mechanism, is the causative organism of a range of STIs. It is also responsible for non-sexually transmitted infections such as trachoma, a leading cause of blindness in the developing world. On the basis of its surface antigens, it can be divided into multiple serovars, or serologic variants. Genital infections are primarily caused by serovars D–K, with D–F being the most prevalent. Serovars F and G appear to be responsible for many asymptomatic infections and serovar F is most often associated with upper genital infection (5).

Chlamydia trachomatis is the most prevalent STI in both developed and developing countries, with 92 million cases worldwide (1). Its true incidence is unknown, however, as more than 70% of women and approximately 50% of men also have asymptomatic infection (1,15).

In women, chlamydia causes a cervicitis that is asymptomatic in 60% to 80% of the cases (1,16). This lack of symptoms means women frequently remain untreated, develop ascending infections, and consequently PID. Chlamydia, the leading cause of PID, is associated with increased risk for infertility (67). Unfortunately, chlamydia infection is common among female adolescents (68–70), the group most vulnerable to the consequences of PID. In men, chlamydia can cause non-gonococcal urethritis and an acute proctitis (71).

Serovars L1–L3 are responsible for lymphogranuloma venereum, which is common in developing countries. This infection presents initially as a papule or herpes-like ulcer that is usually asymptomatic or resolves before recognition (25). It then spreads to the inguinal lymph nodes, which become tender and swollen and later break down to form large ulcers (72).

Diagnosis of *C. trachomatis* infection involves detection of the organism itself, its antigen, or its genetic material from the endocervix, vagina, urethra, or urine. It cannot be cultured on cell-free media and requires expertise and equipment for tissue culture that are not commonly available in laboratories in

Nigeria and other resource-poor countries. Moreover, the sensitivity of tissue culture is low, ranging from 65% to 80% (73), and there is high variability in the sensitivities of systems in use. Tests that detect chlamydial antigens — such as direct fluorescence antibody test and enzyme immunoassay — have specificities between 96% and 99%. They are expensive, however, and therefore not generally available except in research laboratories. There is also a high level of false positive results, especially in areas of low prevalence. These assays cannot be used to detect rectal infection with chlamydia (74). As with other STIs, the introduction of nucleic acid amplification tests has revolutionized the diagnosis of chlamydia. These include ligase chain reaction, Roche Amplicor PCR, and strand displacement amplification. These assays have the advantages of high sensitivity and specificity, as well as the ability to detect chlamydia from a variety of clinical infections in both symptomatic and asymptomatic people (75–78). Treatment requires doxycycline for seven days; however, this approach leaves a large reservoir of asymptomatic individuals and their partners untreated.

Given the number of chlamydia infections globally and the dire clinical consequences of infection, a preventive vaccine for adolescent women is urgently needed to significantly reduce the incidence of *C. trachomatis* infection. Currently, no such vaccine exists; however, the U.S. Preventive Services Task Force recommends that clinicians routinely screen all sexually active women younger than 25 for chlamydial infection because of their increased risk (79). This strategy presents resource-poor countries with a significant problem because of the cost of widespread screening.

Mycoplasma and Ureaplasma
Mycoplasmas and ureaplasmas belong to an unusual class of self-replicating bacteria that lack cell walls and require cholesterol for membrane function and growth. *Ureaplasma urealyticum*, *Mycoplasma hominis*, and *Mycoplasma genitalis* are agents of non-gonoccocal urethritis and cervicitis. There is considerable evidence to suggest that mycoplasmas activate the immune system, stimulate cytokine production, and induce oxidative stress, resulting in increased HIV replication and accelerated progression to AIDS (80,81).

The contribution of genital mycoplasma to non-gonococcal urethritis has been the subject of debate, as several mycoplasmas — such as *M. hominis* and *M. fermentans* — are commensals of the male lower genital tract. *M. genitalium*, which appears to be a major pathogen in the genital tract, is a common cause of non-gonococcal urethritis in men and has been isolated more frequently from the sexual partners of infected women (82). *M. genitalium* also has consistently been found more often in people with non-gonococcal urethritis than in asymptomatic controls (83,84). In West Africa, it is responsible for approximately 10% of non-gonococcal urethritis, with symptoms that are indistinguishable from those of *C. trachomatis* and *T. vaginalis*. There is also increasing evidence that *M. genitalium* causes mucopurulent cervicitis in women (85) and that it may cause endometritis (67,86), tubal infection, ectopic pregnancy, and tubal infertility (87). Nonetheless, routine diagnosis remains difficult, as no commercial diagnostic tests are available (16). Treatment consists of either doxycycline for seven days (83) or azithromycin (88).

In some studies, *M. genitalium* has been implicated as a cause of urethritis in men, and it accounted for 14% of all cases of non-gonococcal urethritis seen in men attending an STI clinic in Ibadan. (16,89,90). A well-designed case-controlled study in West Africa could not prove a pathogenic role for *U. urealyticum* (41). *U. urealyticum* can be differentiated from *M. genitalium* by its very small size and strong urease positivity. Clinical infections cannot be distinguished from those caused by *C. trachomatis*, such that diagnosis is usually by exclusion in developing countries. *U. urealyticum* is typically treated with macrolides or tetracycline (16,90).

Klebsiella Granulomatis

A gram-negative bacterium, *Klebsiella granulomatis* (formally *Calymmatobacterium granulomatis*) is responsible for a chronic genital ulcer characterized by beefy ulcers that bleed easily when touched. Although it is common in South Africa, India, Jamaica, and Brazil, its prevalence in most countries is low—between 0% and 4.1% (91,92,93).

Clinically, *K. granulomatis* causes four types of lesions: ulcerogranulomatous, hypertrophic, necrotic, and sclerotic. Ninety percent of lesions are in the genital area, with 10% in the inguinal area. The exact incubation period is unknown but is most likely around 50 days (94). Diagnosis often depends on a high level of suspicion and is by identification of the typical Donovan's bodies within large mononucleocytes in giemsa or silver-stained smears obtained from tissue or biopsy samples (95). This infection is common neither in Nigeria nor the rest of West Africa, and no report appears in the Nigerian literature. Recommended treatments include trimethoprim-sulfamethoxazole and azithromycin (35,96).

Bacterial Vaginosis

Bacterial vaginosis is a common and recurrent disorder of the lower genital tract in women of childbearing age, especially those who are sexually active. The infection is characterized by the replacement of normal lactobacilli-predominant vaginal flora with *Gardnerella vaginalis*, anaerobic bacteria, and genital mycoplasma and may be accompanied by increased vaginal pH (97,98). It can be diagnosed easily using a combination of clinical and simple laboratory criteria (97,98). The prevalence ranges from 17.7% in pregnant women to 40% in sex workers (99–101). Studies have shown that 20% to 51% of women in sub-Saharan Africa are affected (102). In a recent study in Ibadan, it was found to be the third most common genital tract infection among sex workers after candidiasis and HIV (103).

Although not normally considered an STI, bacterial vaginosis is common in populations with a high prevalence of STIs and is associated with an increased risk of acquiring HIV (104). Some evidence for sexual transmission has been obtained from studies involving women who have sex with women, in whom there is usually a concordance in vaginal flora (whether normal or abnormal). Though bacterial vaginosis was previously considered to be non-inflammatory in nature, more recent data suggest that it stimulates the production of pro-inflammatory cytokines, thus providing a plausible mechanism by which disruption of the vaginal flora may increase HIV acquisition (106). The first-line regimen for the treatment of bacterial vaginosis is metronidazole for seven days; a single dose can also be used but is less effective (107).

Viral STIs

Viral STIs are common but not typically included in national surveillance figures. Those recognized as sexually transmitted include herpes simplex type 2 (HSV-2); human papillomavirus; and hepatitis B virus (HBV). Sexual transmission of hepatitis A virus (HAV); hepatitis C virus (HCV); hepatitis D virus (HDV); human herpes virus-8 (HHV-8); and human T-cell lymphotrophic virus type I (HTLV-I) has also been described (1,3).

Herpes Simplex Viruses

Ten to thirty percent of adults worldwide are infected with HSV-2; 25% to 90% are infected with HSV-1 (108). Most HSV-1 cases are acquired non-sexually as children, although the prevalence of HSV-1 genital infection is increasing in Europe and in the United States as a result of orogenital sex (109). HSV-2 is acquired predominantly through sexual transmission, with a higher prevalence in high-risk populations and women, although most cases go undiagnosed (109,110). HSV-2 is the most common cause of genital ulcer disease in the developed world, with an estimated incidence of 500,000 annually in the United States (111).

HSV-2 appears to be more prevalent in Africa than previously believed, though few data are available, as many people do not present in the hospital. In a study of the effects of STIs on HIV incidence in Kenya, a baseline seroprevalence rate of 72.7% was detected among HIV-negative women (4). A 43.5% incidence rate was also reported in Uganda (56).

HSV-1 and HSV-2 infections are characterized by vesicles that later evolve into pustules and shallow ulcers of different sizes and shapes. They vary in severity from mild and unrecognized, to widespread and painful herpetic lesions, especially in the immunocompromised (112,113). Primary lesions typically resolve in approximately three weeks without therapy, while recurrences may occur every 5 to 12 days. Lesions may be extensive across the perineum, causing so much debilitating pain that the person requires hospitalization (112,114).

HSV-2–infected genital lesions can be identified by light microscopy using the Tzanck smear (scrapings from the base of the ulcer can be stained with Wright–Giemsa stain), but the test has poor sensitivity and specificity (115,116). Serologic tests can distinguish between HSV-1 and HSV-2 by identifying type-specific viral glycoproteins (117).

As there is currently no cure for HSV, the goal of therapy is to hasten resolution of the lesions and to reduce infectivity. Oral acyclovir, an inhibitor of viral DNA polymerase, is the most commonly used chemotherapeutic agent; however, newer agents, such as valacyclovir and famciclovir, have longer half-lives and are more bioavailable when given orally (118). Drug-resistant strains may also occur (119,120). In patients with HIV infection, treatment time may be increased and prolonged (109,118,120). There is no vaccine for HSV.

Importantly, HSV infection is a significant risk factor for the transmission of HIV (108). HSV-2 may increase local HIV replication in the vagina, thereby enhancing HIV transmission (121). In addition, HSV-2, like other genital ulcer diseases, results in infiltration of activated CD4+ cells, thereby increasing a person's susceptibility to infection (122). Moreover, the ulcerative nature of HSV infection itself may provide an important site of entry for HIV, thus facilitating transmission.

Human Papillomaviruses

Human papillomaviruses (HPV) include more than 80 DNA viruses that are the common causes of warts. HPV can cause cancer of the cervix, vulva, vagina, penis, and anus (123). The prevalence of HPV is difficult to evaluate because of the asymptomatic nature of infection in most people and the absence of serologic tests (123). Not all HPVs are sexually transmitted. HPV types 6 and 11 cause genital warts but are not often associated with cervical cancers, while HPV types 16 and 18, though frequently asymptomatic, are oncogenic (124). Furthermore, types 16, 18, 31, and 33 are often associated with dysplastic changes of the cervical mucosa. High-risk types of HPV are virtually a prerequisite for all cervical cancers and dysplasias, as well as more than 90% of anogenital malignancies (125).

Lesions vary in size and shape from flat and inconspicuous to verrucous, pedunculated, or large cauliflower-like lesions called condyloma accuminata. Diagnosis is usually clinical through cytological studies (the Pap smear); biopsy may be used to assess mucosal lesions. HPV cannot yet be grown in culture, and type-specific serologic tests are still under development (123).

The true incidence of HPV infection is unknown; nonetheless, most adults are likely infected, although only a small proportion of infected individuals develop warts or cancer. Seroprevalence studies have shown much higher HPV infection rates in women than in men even when men were at greater behavioral risk, suggesting gender-based difference in susceptibility to HPV infection (126).

Hepatitis Viruses

The sexual transmission of hepatitis A, B, and C viruses has been described (1,22). HBV is endemic in Africa and is largely acquired in childhood (22,23). Although sexual transmission of HBV has been described, especially in MSM, it is not believed to contribute significantly to the epidemiology of HIV in Nigeria and the rest of sub-Saharan Africa. The epidemiologic trends of HAV and HCV also suggest that sexual transmission may occur; more important is the negative impact of coinfection with HCV on HIV disease progression (22).

Hepatitis B is a non-enveloped DNA virus belonging to the Hepadnaviridae family. It causes an inflammation of the liver, and its incubation period usually ranges from 45 to 180 days. The infectious period begins before symptoms develop and continues until the infected person has eliminated the virus from his or her body (22). An acute phase follows the incubation period; patients in this phase generally feel unwell and may experience jaundice, aches and pains, nausea and vomiting, and abdominal pain. After the acute phase, those who are unable to eliminate the virus from their body enter into the chronic phase. Chronically infected people are often asymptomatic but remain infectious for life, although the risk of transmitting HBV to others varies considerably from person to person. These carriers are also at increased risk of developing cirrhosis and hepatocellular carcinoma (22).

It is estimated that HBV infects 2 billion people worldwide, of which 350 million are chronic carriers (127). HBV is endemic in sub-Saharan Africa, Southeast Asia, and South America, where it is a major problem because of its role in the development of hepatocellular carcinoma and liver cirrhosis. More than 50 million chronic carriers of HBV are found in Africa, with a 25% mortality risk. In sub-Saharan Africa, carrier rates range from 9% to 20% (127).

HBV is spread through infectious body fluids such as blood, saliva, semen, and vaginal fluids. Sexual transmission of HBV occurs through unprotected sex, though HBV may be more likely to be transmitted during anal intercourse, which occurs in both heterosexual and homosexual relationships with all the inherent risks of HIV, HBV, and other STIs (128). Unfortunately, because both anal intercourse and MSM are highly stigmatized—and therefore not acknowledged—in many countries, including Nigeria, it is difficult to quantify the contribution of anal intercourse to the incidence of HBV infection.

In Nigeria, most studies to detect HBV surface antigen (HBsAg) were carried out in the 1980s and early 1990s. Prevalence rates among blood donors ranged from 5.1% in Ibadan to 26% in Benin (129,130). Community-based studies among adults in Enugu and Zaria showed similar prevalence rates: 9.1% and 10%, respectively (21,131). Other studies throughout Africa have shown that horizontal transmission in childhood is likely the most important means of spread of HBV (132,133), while vertical transmission is low. The importance of horizontal transmission was further confirmed by the Zaria study, in which 59% of healthy children under the age of five showed evidence of exposure to HBV, with the presence of either HBsAg or anti-HBV surface antibodies (21). Another study found that 87% of Nigerians had been exposed to HBV by the age of 40, and that the risk of exposure was higher in rural settings than in urban settings. An interesting observation of the study was that there was no significant correlation between HBV infection and blood transfusion in rural settings (131).

In addition, prisoners—apart from having the highest HBsAg prevalence rates—were also more likely to carry antibodies to the HBV core antigen (anti-HBc). It is likely that these high rates can be attributed in part to sexual transmission, because same-sex relationships have been documented among prisoners worldwide (131), and anecdotal reports suggest that same-sex relationships are also common in Nigerian prisons. Studies are urgently required to determine the risk factors for acquisition of HBV—and other STIs—in prisons to enable better intervention strategies to be designed.

Diagnosis of both acute and chronic HBV infection is by serology, although a liver biopsy may also be useful in determining disease stage. Vaccines to prevent HBV are highly effective and have now been incorporated into Nigeria's national immunization program. A yeast-derived recombinant HBV vaccine is given at birth, one month, and six months. Interferon-alpha can also be used to treat chronic HBV. A meta-analysis has suggested that interferon-treated patients were more likely to achieve hepatitis B core antigen (HBcAg) seroconversion (loss of HBcAg and acquisition of antibody to the HBVe antigen, or anti-Hbe) and clear hepatitis B DNA (HBVDNA) (133). Furthermore, relapse rates are few, and post-treatment seroconversions continue to occur for up to 10 years post-therapy in Western patients (133,134). Lamivudine, a nucleoside analogue, has been introduced for the treatment of HBV (135), but resistance to this drug has been reported (136). In hepatitis–HIV coinfection, tenofovir-containing antiretroviral regimens are recommended.

HCV, an RNA virus belonging to the Flaviviridae family, is primarily bloodborne, although sexual transmission is also strongly suspected. An estimated 170 million people are infected worldwide (137). In Nigeria, no population-based study of HCV has been carried out. In a seroprevalence study of 150 patients, however, 14% tested positive for HCV antibodies, while 29.3% were positive for HBV. Anti-HCV was positively associated with a history of blood transfusion and heterosexual exposure to partners at risk. HCV is clinically indistinguishable from other viral hepatitis infections, but there is a high rate of subclinical infections, with only 15% to 25% of cases being icteric (138). The incubation period ranges from 14 days to 120 days (139). Following acute hepatitis infection, 85% of people go on to develop chronic HCV infection (140). Approximately one-third of HIV-infected people are coinfected with HCV because of the common bloodborne route of infection (140). Among coinfected patients, the level of viremia is elevated and the rate of disease progression is accelerated (141). Treatment of HCV is combination therapy with interferon-alpha and ribavirin, regardless of the person's HIV status; however, HCV treatment success rates are approximately 50% during HCV mono-infection and only 25% during HCV/HIV coinfection (142). No vaccine has been developed for HCV infection (143).

Human Herpes Virus Type 8

HHV-8 is significantly associated with Kaposi's sarcoma (KS), as it is found in a latent form in endothelial spindle cells in all types of KS: classic, endemic, and AIDS-related or epidemic KS (144). The classic and endemic types tend to run an indolent course, involving primarily the skin of the lower extremities and feet. AIDS-related KS is more aggressive, however, with a high rate of systemic involvement (145). KS lesions, even in HIV-infected patients, are usually asymptomatic and tend to appear over a range of CD4+ cell counts, though they become more common as immune function is lost. Although lesions usually appear as slightly raised or nodular dark-colored tumors, they may vary from barely visible to large, disfiguring tumors (144). In AIDS-related KS, lesions are commonly located in the oral cavity and on the face, lower extremities, and feet. Gastrointestinal involvement is also common.

The transmission routes of HHV-8 are unclear, although homosexual transmission has been suggested and seems plausible for several reasons. First, clustering of KS was observed in young, sexually active MSM during the early AIDS epidemic (144). Second, high seroprevalence rates appear in MSM with HIV or other STIs (146). Third, KS has been isolated from semen and prostate tissue (147). The evidence for heterosexual transmission of HHV-8 is less convincing (146,148,149). Non-sexual transmission of HHV-8 is also likely, as HHV-8 has been recovered from saliva (150), and high seroprevalence rates have been reported in children (151,152).

In Lagos, a seroprevalence study found HHV-8 antibodies in 26.5% of study subjects (153), a figure much lower than those found in East and Central Africa (154–156). HHV-8 was more common in sex workers and in people with an STI than in the general population (19%). There was a significant association between HHV-8 seropositivity and having multiple sexual partners or at least one STI, providing additional evidence of sexual transmission of HHV-8 (153).

Despite its systemic presentation, KS does not usually lead to death in people with HIV unless there is pulmonary involvement. Highly active antiretroviral therapy (HAART) is usually accompanied by regression of KS tumors in HIV-infected people, but specific antiviral chemotherapy may be used alone or in addition to HAART. Traditionally, combination therapy with adriamycin, bleomycin, and vinblastine has achieved response rates of 24% to 60% in patients with pulmonary disease (157). More recently, single-agent chemotherapeutic drugs—such as doxorubicin, paclitaxel, and vinorelbine—have been introduced with better response rates and a lower incidence of toxicity (144).

Parasitic STIs

Trichomonas Vaginalis

Trichomonas vaginalis is caused by a pear-shaped flagellate motile protozoan with an undulating membrane. A few days after exposure, symptoms of vulval irritation, dysuria, and dyspareunia with a purulent vaginal discharge develop. On examination, there is often erythema of the vulva and vaginal mucosa (123). In many cases, there is an elevated pH and a positive whiff test, which may represent an associated bacterial vaginosis. Generally, there are no sequelae, although *T. vaginalis* infection has been associated with premature rupture of the membranes and preterm delivery (158,159).

Recent evidence suggests that trichomoniasis may be an important cause of non-gonococcal urethritis. When PCR was used to evaluate the prevalence of trichomoniasis among men with non-gonococcal urethritis, *T. vaginalis* was found in 19.9% (160). Approximately 8% to 50% of patients with *T. vaginalis* had concomitant infections; coinfection with gonorrhea and trichomoniasis was almost as common as coinfection with gonorrhea and chlamydia. Several risk factors for acquisition of *T. vaginalis* were identified, including multiple sexual partners, a history of a previous STI, and coinfection with *N. gonorrhoeae* (160).

Similarly, in a study of West African men with urethral discharge, *T. vaginalis* was found to be the cause of non-gonococcal, non-chlamydial urethritis in 15% of cases (47). Among a subset of people with gonorrhea, *T. vaginalis* was a more frequent coinfection than chlamydia, further confirming its role as a significant pathogen. This study, however, did not include Nigerian men, although previous studies have shown that *T. vaginalis* was the cause of urethritis in 5% to 11% of Zimbabwean and Nigerian men with non-gonococcal urethritis (161–163). More recently, *T. vaginalis* was diagnosed in 45% of male partners of infected women in Ibadan (164).

Diagnosis of *T. vaginalis* is by microscopy of a wet mount in which motile flagellated trichomonads can be seen. Wet mounts have a sensitivity of 70% to 80% in experienced hands (166), but are adversely affected by duration of time between sample collection and examination. Treatment of *T. vaginalis* is with metronidazole (57).

Table 5-2. Determinants of Risk for Sexually Transmitted Infections

Individual Determinants

1. Knowledge and Awareness
- Knowledge of STIs, risks, and sequelae
- Condom effectiveness
- Condom availability
- Location and types of available services
- STI test availability

2. Attitudes, Motivations, and Intentions
- Attitudes toward condom use and safer sex
- Motivations to use condoms or to abstain from sex
- Intentions to use condoms or to abstain from sex

3. Beliefs and Perceptions
- Perceived vulnerability to STIs
- Perceived social norms regarding safer sex (also peer norms)
- Beliefs in one's ability to change
- Cultural and religious beliefs about sexual practices

4. Skills
- Communication skills
- Ability to negotiate safer sex and condom use
- Sexual assertiveness skills

Environmental Determinants

1. Economic
- Funding for services, education, and awareness raising
- Socioeconomic status—income, education, and employment

2. Organizational
- Availability of condoms
- Availability of health care services
- Availability of well-organized STI services for prevention and treatment

3. Societal
- Community attitudes about safer sex (abstinence, condom use, religious and cultural beliefs)
- Stigmatization of marginalized communities, such as migrants, refugees, sex workers, and men who have sex with men
- Accessibility of services

4. Policy
- Laws and regulations to protect against discriminization, human rights for women, and policies encouraging education of such groups as adolescents and men who have sex with men
- Age of consent
- Age of legal access to condoms

SOCIAL AND ECONOMIC DETERMINANTS OF STI EPIDEMIOLOGY

Sexual behavior is linked to the social conditions under which people live and work. These conditions have a bearing on people's thinking and attitudes, and they represent the "causes behind the causes" of poor health (167). Such social conditions influence the many risk determinants for STI infection, including age, gender, partner preference and number, and health-care–seeking and protective behavior.

The environmental determinants of behavior include cultural norms and practices, demographics, socioeconomic status, availability and quality of health care services, peer opinions, social pressures, societal attitudes and prejudices, and access to services (Table 5-2). STI prevalence tends to be higher among urban residents, unmarried individuals, and young adults. STIs tend to occur at a younger age in females than in males, which may be explained by differences in patterns of sexual activity and the relative rates of transmission from one gender to the other (1). Other high-risk groups include sex workers, refugees, and highly mobile people such as long-distance truck drivers and migrants.

Individual determinants are influenced by factors such as low self-esteem, lack of information, lack of skill in condom use, the inability to negotiate safer sex, and lack of knowledge about the risks of different sexual behaviors (109). These factors are most obvious among youth, whose STI prevalence rates are among the highest. Adolescence is a period of dynamic change, representing the transition from childhood to adulthood and marked by emotional, physical, and sexual maturation. Age is therefore an important risk determinant in terms of both risky behavior and increased biologic susceptibility to infection, especially among adolescent females (169).

Habits formed during adolescence have major repercussions in adulthood, and it is easier to prevent the acquisition of bad habits than to break them once they are formed. Globally, puberty is occurring earlier for both boys and girls, and the age at which people marry is rising. This leaves a widening gap of time during which young adults may be engaging in premarital sex (168). Most young people throughout the world will engage in sexual intercourse by age 20. A survey of STI clinics in 2000 showed that sexual debut occurs in Nigeria between the ages of 10 and 19 years, with the average age of 17 years (15). This is not limited to urban communities; even in rural Nigerian communities, girls as young as 12 are sexually active (50,60). These disturbing trends are further compounded by the fact that many developing countries place a premium on fertility, encouraging women to bear children at a young age.

The young are more likely to have multiple partners either sequentially or concurrently. They are also less likely to buy or to use condoms, and they tend to have a low awareness of the risks of STIs (170). These tendencies are often because of either a lack of money or a feeling of modesty, as most African communities equate sexual activity in the young with promiscuity (171). In developing countries an estimated one-third of all STIs occur in people aged 13 to 20 years (50). Furthermore, youth often fail to seek medical care for STIs, as STI clinics are frequently geared toward older patients and adolescents feel uncomfortable accessing their services (172). This failure to seek treatment is worse in Africa, where adolescents visiting clinics may risk being reported to their parents by concerned community members. This lack of confidentiality also limits uptake of care and may lead to further transmission of STI and HIV, as well as to the development of long-term sequelae.

Many sexually active young people do not use contraception, and among those who do, many experience higher contraceptive failure and are more likely to discontinue use than older people (168). While condoms are a key contraceptive method for youth, many young people view condoms unfavorably, as they are often seen as a symbol of distrust between partners and are thought to reduce intimacy and sexual pleasure (168,173,174).

Women are biologically more vulnerable to STIs than men (56,175). This vulnerability is compounded by women's unequal social status, which in many communities makes them economically dependent on men. Such dependence often leads to feelings of powerlessness and low self-esteem. As a result, women tend to become sexually active at younger ages than men and are less likely to negotiate safer sexual practices (1,170). Indeed, many women do not have a say in sexual relations, although absolute fidelity is expected from them. This societal demand holds true for both married and unmarried women. Moreover, women may be less likely to seek medical care not only because their infections are often asymptomatic, but also because of poor economic resources and a sense of modesty (176–178). Polygamy and the early marriage of girls also contribute to the vulnerability of women. Rape of young girls is not uncommon, as frequently reported in the newspapers. Little formal documentation of this trend appears in the Nigerian scientific literature, however, because of the extreme taboos surrounding the issue.

The role of men as transmitters of STIs is not well documented in the Nigerian scientific literature, as most studies have generally focused on commercial sex workers or women attending antenatal or family planning clinics. In many African countries, polygamy is accepted and men frequently have extramarital affairs. Some occupations further expose men to increased risk of acquiring and transmitting STIs. These include occupations that separate men from their families, such as out-of-state transfers in the military or police, or jobs that require frequent travel, which increases the likelihood that the men will engage in sexual relations with sex workers or "girlfriends" at each stop. Those exposed to STIs by long-distance truck drivers and migrant males include sex workers, restaurant owners who provide girls for the truck drivers, food vendors, hawkers, traders, and brothel owners (179). In some settings, food vendors and hawkers may carry out clandestine sex work to augment their meager incomes. Migrant workers also constitute a high-risk group because of their sporadic condom use. Moreover, frequent travelers may avoid the health services of the regions in which they travel because they are unfamiliar with those services (179). These kinds of social dynamics are major factors in the spread of STIs, including HIV, in many developing countries.

One's choice of sexual partner also determines the level of risk for acquiring an infection. STIs have traditionally been attributed to heterosexual contact in Africa (180). Interventions have focused on sex workers and women, with few or no programs targeting men specifically. This is unfortunate, as male partners of women tend to have the final say on whether the woman may attend a health clinic.

The topic of MSM has met with resounding silence in Africa. In many Western countries, this group is at high risk of acquiring and transmitting STIs, including HIV (181,182). While the number of MSM is not known in Nigeria, the concept of same-sex relationships is not new to the country. Among the Hausa in northern Nigeria, for example, such men are called *dan daudu*, or "men who are wives of men"; many also marry and have children. Men in these bisexual relationships may be important bridges for the transmission of HIV and other STIs. In addition, there are largely unrecognized communities of MSM in Nigeria that have only recently begun to organize themselves into such advocacy groups as Alliance Rights Nigeria, whose membership numbers more than 10,000. Unless these groups are also targeted for intervention, a large community of men at high risk — heterosexual, bisexual, and homosexual alike — will be left out of the STI prevention equation.

Socioeconomic determinants are intrinsically linked to inequities in health. They help to explain why poor and marginalized people become sick and die sooner than people in better social positions. Poverty, limited educational opportunities, and a lack of access to medical care and appropriate therapies often lead to migration out of rural communities and into large cities. Many of these transplanted individuals ultimately end up in urban slums that are all too often characterized by a lack of critical amenities such as water, electricity, housing, schools, and health care services. The poor in such settings — particularly women, who have limited opportunities in the job market — must often exchange sex for money, security, food, and shelter. At the same time they may have regular male partners who provide some security, they may also have clients to whom they sell sex. These clients include married men, students, expatriates, long-distance truck drivers, and migrants who can then transmit STIs to people who would not otherwise have been at high risk for STIs. Further compounding the issue, most slums have no or severely limited health centers, and the communities tend to use traditional medicine healers who do not understand the dynamics of STIs and HIV.

RELATIONSHIP BETWEEN HIV AND OTHER STIS

The STI and HIV epidemics are interdependent. As noted earlier, several studies have demonstrated a strong association between both ulcerative and non-ulcerative STIs and HIV infection (10,18). There is also biologic evidence that the presence of an STI increases shedding of HIV, and that STI treatment reduces HIV shedding (6,183). Therefore, STI control may contribute substantially to HIV prevention.

The Role of Genital Ulcer Disease
Genital ulcer disease has been identified as a major risk factor associated with heterosexual transmission of HIV in Africa. Genital ulcer disease increases the transmission of and susceptibility to HIV by breaching the protective barrier of the genital mucosa, modulating the mucosal immune response, recruiting activated HIV target cells to the mucosa, and increasing viral shedding from infected cells (6,8,111). In the countries most affected by HIV, the prevalence of genital ulcer disease among men and women with STIs was 45% to 68% and 13% to 68%, respectively (184). In contrast, the prevalence of genital ulcer disease was much lower in West Africa, where HIV prevalence rates are also relatively low (183), further suggesting that the presence of genital ulcer disease may be associated with increased transmission of HIV. Moreover, a model simulation of the transmission dynamics in Uganda has suggested that genital ulcer disease was responsible for 80% to 97% of HIV infections in that country (183).

Epidemiologic data also shows a strong association between syphilis and HIV. Syphilis appears to increase the efficiency of HIV transmission three- to fivefold by inducing HIV expression in infected monocytes and by promoting the expression of CCR5, a co-receptor for HIV (185,186). Syphilis, because it causes a genital ulcer, also disrupts the dermal and mucosal protective barriers, thereby increasing susceptibility to HIV. Syphilis coinfection promotes HIV shedding as well, thereby increasing infectivity of the virus (185).

In Nigeria, the true impact of genital ulcer disease on the HIV transmission rate is unknown, as the prevalence and causes of genital ulcer disease are not known. Recent national figures suggest that syphilis is uncommon, though independent studies in the community hint at higher figures (17,31). Furthermore, chancroid appears to be common (59,60), and genital herpes has been found to be especially significant in some African countries (56).

The Role of Non-Genital Ulcer Disease
Prevalence figures of non-ulcerative STIs, such as gonorrhea and chlamydia, are limited or absent for much of Nigeria. Evidence to support the role of non-ulcerative STIs in HIV transmission is less convincing than those for non-genital ulcer disease. Nonetheless, gonorrhea and chlamydia have been

shown to promote the recruitment of HIV-infected T-lymphocytes and macrophages, resulting in increased vaginal shedding of HIV RNA in semen (187). This recruitment of inflammatory cells is a normal immune response to infection and is considerably reduced with treatment of the gonococcal infection (187). *T. vaginalis* infection also increases the transmission of HIV by increasing the vaginal shedding of virus (160), although HIV has no effect on the incidence, prevalence, duration, or recurrence of *T. vaginalis* infection (165). Furthermore, coinfection of a genital tract infection with trichomoniasis was independently associated with HIV seroconversion (18).

HIV CONTROL THROUGH STI PREVENTION AND MANAGEMENT

The strong association between both ulcerative and non-ulcerative STIs and HIV infection suggests that STI management may contribute substantially to HIV prevention and control. Aside from the obvious ethical reasons for averting infections, the economic arguments for prevention are substantial. The actual cost of treating STIs extends far beyond the finite cost of diagnosing and treating the infections themselves, as it includes avoidance of the long-term sequelae of untreated STIs. While certain fundamental prevention strategies must be applied universally in the prevention of STIs, it is also important to note that some STIs, such as HSV-2 and HPV, can be transmitted even during condom-protected intercourse from the skin around the genitalia, while others, such as syphilis and gonorrhea, can also be transmitted during oral sex.

Effective interventions can be delivered at different levels — whether individual, group, or community — and they can address the full range of risk determinants simultaneously. It is also important to identify successful strategies that can achieve a national approach and to determine ways of replicating success stories from the developed world and other African countries. For interventions to succeed, the interdependence of health and other social conditions must be considered, and social barriers such as poverty and stigma must be overcome.

Ghana, for example, launched a program promoting public dialogue on HIV and other STIs in 2000. Mass media campaigns were integrated with local interventions to promote abstinence, faithfulness, and condom use. Public figures such as politicians and religious leaders were actively involved. Two years later, condom sales had risen from 18.8 million to 34.8 million, reports of fidelity had grown, and the number of men reporting condom use had increased considerably. These changes occurred significantly more often among those who had been exposed to the messages than those who had not (188). Peer educator programs, youth centers, safe houses for vulnerable women and children, community outreach efforts, and mass media campaigns also have been used successfully in several African countries (189–192).

STI control programs have been targeted at three levels: individuals (partner notification and risk counseling); groups (group counseling and health education, youth awareness programs, and sex education in schools); and communities (through community development, formation of local organizations, legislation to criminalize discrimination, allocation of community resources to educational programs, and stabilization of the infrastructure and environment for professional development).

Among all these intervention strategies, the common aims are to increase condom use, to reduce the number of sexual partners, to encourage abstinence, to increase awareness of STIs, and to provide adequate and effective diagnosis and treatment. STI and HIV management can be further divided into primary (pre-exposure) and secondary (post-exposure) interventions. In most instances, the main focus is on primary prevention interventions that will ultimately influence sexual behavior and will thus reduce the incidence of STIs. Peer opinions, economic pressures, societal attitudes and prejudices, and the availability of such resources as condoms also affect access to services (189) and subsequently influence STIs.

Strategies to Modify Sexual Behavior

Behavioral skills training is important because of its effect on self-efficacy—a person's beliefs about his or her ability to carry out a chosen health behavior and the effort he or she must invest in the face of difficulties and resistance (190). The first stage in modifying sexual behavior is therefore to increase awareness and to impart knowledge about safer sexual practices. Awareness counseling must then be followed by development of the necessary skills to put into effect this newly acquired information. Such a strategy relies on the premise that when people fully understand the implications of their actions, they will modify their behavior in appropriate and sustainable manners. Modifying sexual behavior is thus the key factor in reducing the incidence of STIs, and behavior-change strategies must address multiple determinants of risk (Table 5-2).

All members of the population should be targeted, whether they are considered to be at low or high risk, because knowledge across the population reduces stigma. Special attention should be given to youth, sex workers, migrants, military and police force, refugees, and long-distance truck drivers. The information imparted to these groups must be basic and accurate. Messages must use clear, unambiguous language and be tailored to the specific needs of the target population. Such information should take into account the epidemiology of the STIs prevalent in the community, sexual preferences, types of risk behavior practiced, and cultural and social practices that may put people at risk or prevent them from using educational and medical services.

The importance of STI screening must be emphasized because of the asymptomatic nature of many infections. The fear of infertility has been found to be a more powerful incentive for practicing safer sex than the fear of acquiring STIs, particularly among youth (189). Therefore, it is critical to reiterate that STIs are a major cause of infertility. Target populations should also be informed of the protective value of barrier methods, such as condoms. The locations of available STI clinics and related medical services should be provided. Individuals must also be reassured that their privacy and confidentiality will be maintained at the clinics. These messages may be individualized or disseminated during group sessions. A review of various intervention strategies showed that targeting groups appeared to result in more people adopting risk-averse behavior than targeting individuals (189). In Nigeria, this may be a useful strategy at outreach meetings, because it creates a condition of anonymity, thus removing the risk of being seen attending an STI clinic. Individual interventions may occur later, as trust develops between the health provider and the patient.

As sexual activity, or at least sexual awareness, occurs very young in children, sex education should begin in primary school. For this age group, sex education can take the form of short messages or short stories that carry a moral message (191). In adolescents, it has been shown that messages promoting risk reduction work better than those promoting abstinence (189). The issue of sex education is a controversial one in Nigeria, because it is felt that discussing sexual behavior in the classroom encourages sexual activity. Nonetheless, a review of 35 studies worldwide showed conclusively that sex education programs did not increase sexual activity (192). It is important to carry out well-designed studies to determine if this also holds true in Nigeria, however.

Today's youth are visually oriented, having come of age in an era of television and computers. Thus, videos showing the effects of HIV and other STIs on individuals and populations send powerful messages and complement more traditional styles of education. Programs that address both sexual and nonsexual determinants of risk tend to be more effective than programs that address only one group of determinants. It is therefore important to determine the reasons for sexual risk-taking and to then select the best programs (193). The choice of the person to deliver prevention messages is critical. Research has shown that people tend to listen better to peers and to community leaders (194,195) because these are the people they trust and consider to be like themselves (168,196). Successful educators build the individual's sense of competency and teach the necessary skills to practice safer sex. To achieve their full effectiveness, however, these messages must be augmented regularly (190).

Condom Promotion

Abstinence and condom use are the two most common approaches to STI prevention. Other proposed methods have thus far not proved to be better than condoms.

Although condom use is effective in preventing transmission of HIV and other STIs (194), several studies have shown that youth do not often use condoms (168). Two case-controlled interventions that promoted safer sex among youths aged 14 to 19 years are highlighted. In one study, peer educators distributed condoms; in the second study, vocational skills were taught and small loans distributed to enable them start their own businesses as a means of building self-esteem. Both methods led to safer sexual practices among the adolescents. Participants in both programs reported an increase in abstinence and monogamy and a decrease in STIs. In addition, youths in the intervention areas were better informed about ways to prevent HIV transmission than those in the control group. The interventions did not lead to greater use of contraception or condoms for dual protection, however, showing that the poor uptake of contraception or condoms among youths is not due to ignorance (197).

Access to Health Care

Ideally, access to health care should take place in a culturally acceptable setting and should be as close as possible to target communities. It is also important to integrate STI clinics into the community's regular medical facilities, rather than separating them, to avoid the unnecessary stigma. In Nigeria, primary health centers are the obvious choices to provide STI-related services. They are situated in all local government areas and are accessible to a large number of people. They also offer other services besides STI care, which helps to obscure the reason someone is attending the clinic. Unfortunately, however, there are not enough primary health centers to cover all the people needing services. For example, to serve the needs of 15 million people, Lagos has one primary health center in each of its 20 local government areas—approximately one center for every 750,000 people. Thus, providing adequate medical access and care is impossible, and many clinics are often not accessible to high-risk populations, many of whom live in urban slums and are forced to self-medicate or use alternative healers.

This inadequacy has led to a proliferation of small private clinics aimed at serving as many people as possible. Many people also receive treatment directly from pharmacies, traditional medicine healers, traditional birth attendants, and other non-medical personnel who are not licensed to diagnose and treat patients (198). To reverse this trend and to increase the number of people using government medical facilities will be difficult. A more practical approach might be to train and empower those who already provide these services, such as pharmacists and doctors in private clinics, and, in settings without doctors, traditional birth attendants. Local pharmacists as well as nongovernmental organizations interested in preventing the transmission of HIV and other STIs could also be encouraged to offer STI education, counseling services, and syndromic management. The benefits of this approach are that the health care of more people will be better managed and both HIV incidence and the complications of related STIs will be reduced. The challenge is how to balance the risk-benefit ratio of proper training against the harm that untrained medical providers may inadvertently cause.

At a first glance, these alternatives may not seem acceptable. They must be weighed, however, against the need to reach the millions of Nigerians who do not visit a health center, or who cannot be reached by the formal health sector. Many already use alternative sources for their health care and have identified the settings they find culturally and socially acceptable. To solve this problem will require well-organized investigations and planning to identify all viable options and to establish the framework that will enhance a good referral system for complicated cases. Thus, the task now before the medical community will be how to ensure that these alternative sources provide quality health care.

In addition to the current limitations already mentioned, young people avoid many of the formal health care settings because of their social connotations. Various strategies to provide non-threatening, conducive environments where young people can learn about reproductive health, get counseling, and have access to recreational facilities have been proposed. These include provision of youth-friendly services, youth centers, and school-linked health care facilities (192). In Nigeria, youth-friendly services offered within existing health care facilities seek to improve the access to, and quality of, existing reproductive health services, by making them more welcoming and acceptable to adolescents. They tend to have friendly young health personnel and offer literature designed for the adolescent reader (189,190,192). These services have generally failed, however, as they were not able to attract enough youth away from local pharmacies (189,190). Youth centers, on the other hand, are centers in which youth congregate. They are usually set up by nongovernmental organizations to offer a variety of recreational and vocational services, with or without health care services, and provide non-threatening and non-judgmental environments in which young people can learn about HIV and other STIs and discuss other social problems. Integrating health care services that incorporate STI counseling and treatment into such centers may be another option. To optimize their appeal, such centers should be run by young adults whom adolescents consider trendy or "cool." They should be people that adolescents would like to emulate as role models and who are unlikely to be moralistic and judgmental toward their young clients. The impact of these non-clinical services on accessing health care, safer sexual practices, and STI and HIV incidences in youth will need further evaluation.

Traditionally, female sex workers have been the focus of various interventions in Nigeria, and many nongovernmental organizations work with them. A few others work with other high-risk groups, such as youth, long-distance truck drivers, the military, and the police. Other high-risk groups — such as unmarried men, MSM, migrant workers, refugees, and seafarers — have been largely ignored thus far, although their role in the transmission of HIV and other STIs is well recognized (179,180).

Strengthening Syndromic Management

Syndromic diagnosis and treatment are now standard care for STIs at the primary health care level, largely because of the inadequacy of current diagnostic facilities and the need to better reach people in their communities. Effective management of STIs prevents the development of complications and sequelae, decreases the spread of infection in the community, and provides opportunities for HIV prevention (199,200). While syndromic management is generally cost-effective, it also has limitations. For example, cervicitis, caused mainly by gonorrhea and chlamydia, cannot easily be predicted (201). To solve this, scoring mechanisms have been devised (202), although they were found to be complicated and were not recommended for routine use in developing countries. In addition, there is a high chance of over-treatment, and many asymptomatic cases of gonorrhea and chlamydia may be missed (201). Most importantly, it does not allow for continuous evaluation of antibiotic sensitivity patterns to detect resistant strains. There is thus a need for continuing validation of diagnostic and treatment algorithms and etiologic management.

Etiologic Management

Etiologic management of STIs should remain the gold standard of care, as it is better than syndromic management for estimating disease burden, detecting resistant strains as they arise, and ruling out the issue of treating uninfected people. It is also more objective. In many developing countries, however, poor laboratory facilities make etiologic management of STIs nearly impossible because of inadequate resources and the limited access many people have to these centers. Despite these limitations, it is crucial that etiologic management or at least periodic microbiologic assessment of prevalent STIs be established. Secondary institutions, such as general and district hospitals, and tertiary institutions, such as university teaching hospitals, federal medical centers, and research institutions, may be designated to carry out these functions and serve as referral centers for recurrent cases, validation of treatment algorithms, and periodic confirmation of STI etiologies.

For secondary and tertiary institutions to fulfill their roles as etiologic management sites, more attention must be paid to laboratories in terms of ensuring adequate funding, updated equipment, proper organizational structure, and highly skilled staff. Staff should be trained continually in the newest diagnostic methodologies and equipment. In recent times, the federal government of Nigeria has been working on strengthening laboratories and designating some as centers of excellence. In addition, the AIDS Prevention Initiative of Nigeria has established STI/HIV reference laboratories at Lagos University Teaching Hospital, the Nigerian Institute of Medical Research, University College Hospital in Ibadan, Jos University Teaching Hospital, and the University of Maiduguri Teaching Hospital. These research laboratories, together with designated federal and state government laboratories, can form the focal point for referral STI centers. Governments and corporate organizations should be further encouraged to sponsor the refurbishment and maintenance of existing laboratories as well as to help invest in new ones.

Screening Services, Including Partner Notification

Many people infected with STIs are asymptomatic and may not seek help from the formal health sector. It is important, therefore, that they be sought out. Screening programs can be integrated into health care centers. Decisions about which infections to screen for and which diagnostic tests to use will depend on the regional epidemiology of the STIs in question, as well as the cost, availability, sensitivity, and specificity of the diagnostic assays. In locations without access to laboratory tests, screeners may consider syndromic algorithms as well as the person's history of risk behavior and past exposure to STIs. Screening is routinely carried out on some categories of people, such as pregnant women and potential blood donors, who are screened for syphilis as well as for HIV. Screening can also be conducted as part of mass campaigns to high-risk groups; however, it is important to counsel people, ensure they understand fully what they are consenting to, and maintain their confidentiality.

An integral part of STI management and prevention is partner notification (189). There are three types of partner notification: patient referral, in which the patient sends in his or her partner without the provider requesting names or addresses; provider referral, in which the provider contacts the partners directly; and patient and provider referrals. Provider referrals have been shown to be more effective than the other two approaches, although they are more expensive. This approach may not be culturally sensitive, however, and patients should be encouraged rather than pressured into bringing in their partners.

Targeted interventions have better success the more aware a population is of the risks of transmission of HIV and other STIs; therefore, population-based interventions should run concurrently through mass awareness programs such as rallies, mass media outlets, and posters.

Periodic Mass Treatment

Improved STI treatment services targeted at an entire population have been shown to significantly reduce HIV incidence (203–205). Such programs may be most effective in communities with a low but rising prevalence of HIV. There is limited evidence from randomized controlled trials to suggest STI treatment as an effective HIV prevention strategy. The three community-based trials conducted in Africa—one in Tanzania and two in Uganda—to determine the value of various STI intervention strategies on HIV incidence yielded conflicting results. The Mwanza, Tanzania, trial set out to improve diagnosis and treatment of STIs in the general population and to determine their impact on the incidence of HIV. A 38% reduction in HIV incidence was observed after two years of community-wide STI treatment (205). In contrast, the Rakai, Uganda, study employed intermittent home-based treatment of STIs but showed no impact on HIV incidence (56). The differences in study results may be attributable in part to the fact that the Rakai HIV epidemic was already mature, thereby leaving little room for improvement based on an STI intervention. The Kamali study, based on syndromic treatment and behavior change interventions in 18 rural communities in Uganda, supported the findings of the Rakai trial (206). Further research into community-based STI interventions for the prevention of incident HIV infections is clearly needed.

Proponents of mass control strategies suggest that mass interventions, such as that used in the Mwanza study, help to destigmatize HIV and other STIs. Such a broad approach, however, may limit the resources available to curb STIs in high-risk groups as resources are stretched over large populations of low-risk groups with little measurable impact on the incidence rate (207). Effective resource management in such initiatives becomes even more critical in resource-limited communities, which also tend to be those with the highest STI prevalence rates.

Those in favor of targeting high-risk groups point out that significant resources are used to target low-risk groups in population-based strategies that could better be used in high-risk groups. They also argue for evidence-based targeted interventions that are tailored to the needs of individual communities and that are based on the epidemiology of the prevalent STIs, as well as the recognized risk groups. For example, the Rakai study showed that genital herpes was the most prevalent genital ulcer disease and was an important risk factor for HIV transmission. The interventions adopted in the trial did not specifically treat HSV infection, however, and were therefore unlikely to have any significant effect on its incidence. This may ultimately explain the poor correlation between STI control and HIV transmission (56,208). Unfortunately, interventions that target a specific STI tend to stigmatize the targeted group. In Nigeria, as well as in other African countries, most interventions to date have targeted sex workers and their clients, giving the impression that those are the only populations at risk.

There are, however, other compelling reasons why STI treatment services should be strengthened and extended to larger populations. The available evidence suggests that when an intervention is accepted it can substantially improve the quality of other STI-related services. In all three STI intervention studies, there was a substantial reduction in the incidence of STIs. Furthermore, the Kamali study showed an increase in condom use, a marker of improved health protective behavior, while periodic mass treatments were also found to be effective in limiting STI transmission to partners of infected people (206).

Vaccines

With the exception of viral STIs, most STIs can be treated with antibiotics. Drug resistance is a major problem in treating *N. gonorrhoeae* (52,207), however, and it is increasingly seen with other organisms, such as *H. ducreyi* (66). Preventive strategies, especially vaccines, are therefore becoming more attractive. Thus far, only vaccines against the viral STIs are available or in the pipeline. An HBV vaccine has been available for more than 20 years, and HBV is the only STI for which there is a vaccine. Yet despite the endemicity of HBV in Nigeria, an HBV vaccine has only just been introduced into its national immunization program (209). A prophylactic HPV vaccine against the serogroups most likely to cause cancer is not yet commercially available, though initial reports suggest it is highly effective (210). An HIV vaccine would be extremely desirable, because the virus easily develops resistance to antiretrovirals, full compliance to dosage regimens is difficult to achieve, antiretrovirals are expensive, and antiretrovirals cause unpleasant side effects (211). Considerable research has gone into the area of vaccine development, but an HIV vaccine may still be decades away.

The possibility that vaccines will be developed against other STIs is limited, as vaccine production is so expensive only a small number of companies undertake it. Moreover, these companies have little profit incentive to design and develop STI vaccines, as they are usually needed in developing countries that cannot afford to pay premium prices (212). In addition, most STIs are not life-threatening and can be prevented by behavior modification, providing little additional incentive to commit large amounts of resources to developing STI vaccines.

Microbicides

Microbicides are substances that can significantly reduce the transmission of HIV and other STIs when applied topically to genital and/or anal surfaces. Importantly, microbicides can complement existing prevention methods and future vaccines. Although current microbicides may not be as effective as condoms, they are more likely to be used, because acceptability studies have shown that they are well accepted as lubricants and appear to heighten sexual pleasure (213). Furthermore, women can use microbicides without having to seek the permission of their partners (214). It has been estimated by modeling studies that a partially effective microbicide used in half of coital acts by 20% of women at risk would prevent 2.5 million transmissions of HIV or other STIs in three years, while a microbicide with a 40% efficacy against both HIV and other STIs that is used 50% of the time (without condom use) would prevent an additional 40% of infections (215).

More than 500 candidate microbicides are now in various stages of development. Most are designed to block HIV infection by directly inactivating the virus or by interrupting its attachment, entry, or replication (216). Microbicides have several advantages over condoms. They allow women to make choices regarding safer sex without having to negotiate with their partners. Moreover, because microbicides provide a chemical rather than a physical barrier, they do not interfere with sexual pleasure and so should be more acceptable (217). Additionally, microbicides are likely to be relatively inexpensive over-the-counter products with a broad spectrum of action against HIV and other STIs. Some may also have contraceptive properties. Furthermore, microbicides may have an indirect impact on perinatal transmission of HIV by decreasing the prevalence of STIs and HIV RNA levels in sexually active women (218). Microbicides may also prove to be more acceptable to youth and augment safer sex practices, although this has yet to be formally studied. Two microbicides—6% Cellulose Sulphate gel (a sulphated polymer) and SAAVY (C-31G)—are currently undergoing randomized, placebo-controlled phase III clinical trials in Lagos, Ibadan, and Port Harcourt. These trials are expected to end by early 2007.

CONCLUSION

Much more research needs to be done to elucidate the epidemiology of the various STIs in Nigeria. Few data exist on the etiology of genital ulcer diseases, for example, and the increased use of syndromic management will make it more difficult to determine individual prevalence rates. As most people do not access formal health care sectors for STI treatment, it is crucial to adopt more community-based strategies that use non-conventional care providers to ensure effective coverage. The potential for abuse exists when non-medical personnel are empowered to conduct minimal treatment procedures. Yet this disadvantage must be balanced against the benefits of diagnosing and treating more people with STIs with the subsequent benefits in controlling the spread of HIV. The promise of new technologies and the strengthening of research, diagnostic, and treatment capabilities through collaboration with international donors have increased the potential for more sophisticated research and an increased understanding of the interplay between STIs and HIV transmission in Nigeria.

REFERENCES

1. World Health Organization. *Global Prevalence and Incidence of Selected Curable Sexually Transmitted Infections: Overview and Estimates.* Geneva: World Health Organization, 2001.

2. Arya OP, Osoba AO, Bennett FJ. *Tropical Venereology.* 2nd ed. Edinburgh: Churchill Livingstone, 1988.

3. McGee ZA, Pavia AT. Is the concept "agents of sexually transmitted disease" still valid? *Sex Transm Infect,* 1991;18:69–71.

4. Kaul R, Kimani J, Nagelkerke NJ, et al. Monthly antibiotic chemoprophylaxis and incidence of sexually transmitted infections and HIV-1 infection in Kenyan sex workers. A randomized controlled trial. *JAMA,* 2004;291:2555–2562.

5. Flemming D Wasserheit J. From epidemiological synergy to public health policy and practice: the contribution of other sexually transmitted diseases to sexual transmission of HIV infection. *Sex Transm Infect,* 1999;75:3–17.

6. Cohen MS, Hoffman IF, Royce RA, et al. AIDSCAP Malawi Research Group. Reduction of concentration of HIV-1 in semen after treatment of urethritis: implications for prevention of sexual transmission of HIV-1. *Lancet,* 1997;349:1868–1873.

7. Osman GI Smolkowski E, Noell J. Mathematical modeling of epidemic transmission. Implications for syphilis control programmes. *Sex Trans Dis,* 1996; 23:30–39.

8. Ghys PD, Fransen K, Diallo MO, et al. The associations between cervicovaginal HIV shedding, sexually transmitted diseases and immunosuppression in female sex workers in Abidjan, Cote d'Ivoire. *AIDS,* 1997;11:F85–F93.

9. Corbett EL, Steketee RW, Kuile FO, et al. HIV-1/ AIDS and the control of other infectious diseases in Africa. *Lancet,* 2002;359:2177–2187.

10. Cameron DW, Simonsen JN, D'Costa LJ, et al. Female to male transmission of human immunodeficiency virus type 1: risk factors for seroconversion in men. *Lancet*, 1989;2:403–407.

11. Plummer FA, Simonsen JN, Cameron DW, et al. Cofactors in male-female sexual transmission of human immunodeficiency virus type 1. *J Infect Dis*, 1991;163:233–239.

12. Cohen MS, Miller WC. Sexually transmitted diseases and human immunodeficiency virus infection: cause, effect, or both? *Int J Infect Dis*, 1998;3:1–4.

13. Kaul R, Kimani J, Nagelkerke NJ, et al. Risk factors for genital ulcerations in Kenyan sex workers: the role of human immunodeficiency virus type 1 infection. *Sex Transm Dis*, 1997;24:387–392

14. Bunnell RE, Dahlberg L, Rolfs R, et al. High prevalence and incidence of sexually transmitted diseases in urban adolescent females despite moderate risk behaviour. *J Infect Dis*, 1999;180:1624–1631.

15. United Nations Population Division, 2000.

16. Donovan B. Sexually transmissible infections other than HIV. *Lancet*, 2004;363:545–556.

17. Federal Ministry of Health. Technical Report. *2003 National HIV Seroprevalence Sentinel Survey*. Abuja: Federal Ministry of Health, 2004.

18. Laga M, Manoka A, Kivuvu M, et al. Non-ulcerative sexually transmitted disease as a risk factors of HIV-1 transmission in women: results from a cohort study. *AIDS*, 1993;7:95–102.

19. Aral SO. Determinants of STD epidemics: implications for phase appropriate intervention strategies. *Sex Transm Infect*, 2002;78(Suppl 1):S3–S13.

20. Bowden FJ, Garnett GP. *Trichomonas vaginalis* epidemiology: parameterising and analysing a model of treatment interventions. *Sex Transm Infect*, 2000; 76:248–256.

21. Fakunle YM, Abdurrhaman MB, Whittle HC. Hepatitis B virus infection in children and adults in northern Nigeria: a preliminary survey. *Trans R Soc Trop Med Hyg*, 1981;75:626–629.

22. World Health Organization. Hepatitis WHU/CDS/CSR/LYO/2002. Hepatitis Department of Communicable Disease Survey and Response. Geneva: World Health Organization, 2002.

23. Doganci T, Uysal G, Kir T, et al. Horizontal transmission of hepatitis B in children with chronic hepatitis B. *World J Gastroenterol*, 2005;11:418–420.

24. Costello DC, Wangel AM, et al. Validation of the WHO diagnostic algorithm and development of an alternative scoring system for the management of women presenting with vaginal discharge in Malawi. *Sex Transm Infect*, 1998;74(Suppl 1):S50–S58.

25. Garcia-Lechuz JM, Rivera M, Catalan P, Sanchez Carillo C, Rodriguez-Creixems M, Bouza E. Differences in curable STDs between HIV and non-HIV population in Spain. *AIDS Patient Care STDs*, 1999;13:175–177.

26. Doherty L, Fenton KA, Jones J, et al. Syphilis: old problem, new strategy. *BMJ*, 2002;325:153–156.

27. World Health Organization. World Health Organization Treponematosis Research. Report of a WHO Scientific Group. Technical Report Series, 455. Geneva: World Health Organization, 1970.

28. Wilcox RR. Changing patterns of treponemal disease. *Br J Vener Dis*, 1974;50:169–171.

29. Meda N, Sangare L, Lankoande S, et al. The HIV epidemic in Burkina Faso: current status and the knowledge level of the population about AIDS, 1994–95. *Rev Epidemiol Sante Publique*, 1998;6:14–23.

30. Mbopi Keou FX, Mbu R, Mauclere P, et al. Antenatal HIV prevalence in Yaounde, Cameroon. *Int J STD AIDS*, 1998;9:400–402.

31. Brabin L, Kemp J, Obunge OK, et al. Reproductive tract infections and abortions among adolescent girls in rural Nigeria. *Lancet*, 1995;345:300–304.

32. Agbaje EO, Uwakwe LO. Irrational use of antimicrobial agents in Surulere local government area of Lagos state, Nigeria. *Nigeria Q J Med*, 2003;13:1–2.

33. Tramont EC. Syphilis in AIDS era. *N Engl J Med*, 1987;316:1600–1601.

34. Chapel TA. The variability of syphilitic chancres. *Sex Transm Dis*, 1978;5:68.

35. World Health Organization. *WHO Guidelines for the Management of Sexually Transmitted Infections*. Geneva: World Health Organization, 2001.

36. Olumide YM, Mohammed T. Early diagnosis and management of sexually transmitted infections in the prevention and control of HIV/AIDS. *Arch Ibadan Med*, 2004;5:14–26.

37. Zaidman GW. Neurosyphilis and retrobulbar neuritis in patients with AIDS. *Ann Opthamol*, 1986;18:200–237.

38. Kamling RT, Villalobos R, Lalina M. Recurrent syphilitic uveitis. *N Engl J Med*, 1989;320:62.

39. Hicks CB, Benson PM, LuptonGP, et al. Seronegative secondary syphilis in a patient infected with the human immunodeficiency virus (HIV) with Kaposi sarcoma. *Ann Intern Med,* 1987;107: 492–495.

40. Radolf JD, Kaplan RP. Unusual manifestation of secondary syphilis and abnormal hormonal response to *T. Pallidum* antigen in a homosexual man with asymptomatic HIV. *Infect J Am Acad Dermatol Dis,* 1988;18:423–427.

41. Mandutto KS, Knot TJ, Norgard MV. Monoclonal antibodies directed against major histocompatibility complex antigens bind to the surface of *T. Pallidum* isolated from infected rabbits and humans. *Cell Immunol,* 1986;101:633–642.

42. Duncan WC. Failure of erythromycin to cure secondary syphilis in a patient infected with the HIV virus. *Arch Dermatol,* 1989;125:82.

43. Grosskurth H, Mayaud P, Mosha F, et al. Asymptomatic gonorrhoea and chlamydia infection in rural Tanzania. *BMJ,* 1996;312:277–280.

44. Donovan B, Bodsworth NJ, Rohrschelm R, et al. Characteristics of homosexually active men with gonorrhoea during an epidemic. *Int J STD AIDS,* 2001;12:437–443.

45. Goeman J, Meheus A, Piot P. L'épidémiologie des maladies sexuellement transmissibles dans les pays en développement a l'ere du SIDA. *Ann Soc Belg Med Trop,* 1991;71:81–113.

46. Mabey D. The diagnosis and treatment of urethritis in developing countries. *Genitourin Med,* 1994;70: 1–2.

47. Pepin J, Sobe F, Deslandes S, et al. Etiology of urethral discharge in West Africa: the role of *Mycoplasma genitalium* and *Trichomonas vaginalis.* *Bull World Health Organ,* 2001;79:118–126.

48. Muir DG, Belsely MA. Pelvic inflammatory disease and its consequences in developing countries in the developing world. *Am J Obstet Gynecol,* 1980;138: 913–928.

49. Osoba AO. Sexually transmitted diseases in tropical Africa: a review of present situation. *Brit J Ven Dis,* 1981;57:89–94.

50. Alausa O, Osoba AO. The role of sexually transmitted disease in male infertility in tropical Africa. *Niger Med J,* 1978;8:225–229.

51. Ojengbede OA, Omonria WE, Ladipo OA. Screening for obstruction of the vas deferens in Nigerian men with azoospermia using the alpha-glucosidase reaction in semen. *Afr J Med Med Sci,* 1992;21:79–81.

52. Bakare RA, Oni AA, Arowojolu AO, et al. Efficacy of pefloxacin in acute gonococcal urethritis. *Afr J Med Med Sci,* 1997;26:185–186.

53. Crotchfelt KA, Welsh LE, DeBonville D, Rosenstraus M, Quinn TC. Detection of *Neisseria gonorrhoeae* and *Chlamydia trachomatis* in genitourinary specimens from men and women by a coamplification PCR assay. *J Clin Microbiol,* 1997;35: 1536–1540.

54. Turner CF, Rogers SM, Miller JM, et al. Untreated gonococcal and chlamydial infection in probability sample of adults. *JAMA,* 2002;287:726–733.

55. van Der Pol B, Ferrero DV, Buck-Barrington L, et al. Multicenter evaluation of the BDProbeTec ET system for detection of *Chlamydia trachomatis* and *Neisseria gonorrhoeae* in urine specimens, female endocervical swabs, and male urethral swabs. *J Clin Microbiol,* 2001;39:1008–1016.

56. Wawwer MJ, Sewakambo NK, Serwadda D, et al. Control of sexually transmitted diseases for AIDS prevention in Uganda: a randomised community trial. *Lancet,* 1999;353:525–535.

57. Federal Ministry of Health. *Nigeria Syndromic Management of Sexually Transmitted Diseases: A Manual for Health Workers.* 2nd ed. Abuja: Federal Ministry of Health, 2001;57.

58. World Health Organization. *An Overview of Selected Curable Sexually Transmitted Diseases.* Geneva: World Health Organization, 1995.

59. Fawole OJ, Okesola AO, Fawole AO, Genital ulcer diseases among sexually transmitted diseases clinic attendees in Ibadan in Nigeria, *Afr J Med Sci,* 2000; 29:17–22.

60. Dada AJ, Ajayi AO, Diamondstone L, et al. A serosurvey of *Haemophillus ducreyi,* syphilis and herpes simplex virus type 2 and their association with HIV among female sex workers in Lagos, Nigeria. *Sex Transm Dis,* 1998;25:237–242.

61. Totten PA, Kuypers JM, Chen CY, et al. Etiology of genital ulcer disease in Dakar, Senegal, and comparison of PCR and serologic assays for detection of *Haemophilus ducreyi. J Clin Microbiol,* 2000;38: 268–273.

62. Gaisin A, Heaton CL. Chancroid: alias the soft chancre. *Int J Dermatol*, 1975;14:188–197.

63. Hammond GW, Schutch M, Scatliff J, et al. Epidemiologic, clinical, laboratory and therapeutic features of an urban outbreak of chancroid in North America. *Rev Infect Dis*, 1980;251:867–679.

64. Blackmore CA, Limpakarnjanarat K, Rigao-Perez JG, et al. An outbreak of chancroid in orange County, California: descriptive epidemiology and disease-control measures. *J Infect Dis*, 1985;151: 840–844.

65. Hannah P, Greenwood JR, Isolation and rapid identification of *Haemophilus ducreyi*. *J Clin Microbiol*, 1982; 16:861–864.

66. Ison CA, Dillon JA, Tapsall JW. The epidemiology of global antibiotic resistance among *Neisseria gonorrhoeae* and *Haemophilus ducreyi*. *Lancet*, 1998; 351(Suppl III):S8–S11.

67. Simms I, Stephenson JM. Pelvic inflammatory disease epidemiology: what do we know and what we need to know? *Sex Transm Infect*, 2000;76:80–87.

68. Bunnell RE, Dahlberg L, Rolfs R, et al. High prevalence and incidence of sexually transmitted diseases in urban adolescent females despite moderate risk behavior. *J Infect Dis*, 1999;180:1624–1631.

69. Burstein GR, Gaydos CA, Diner-West M, et al. Incident *Chlamydia trachomatis* infections among inner-city adolescent females. *JAMA*, 1998;280: 521–526.

70. Cook RL. St. George K, Lassak M, et al. Screening for *Chlamydia trachomatis* infection in college women with a polymerase chain reaction assay. *Clin Infect Dis*, 1999;28:1002–1007.

71. Stamm WE. *Chlamydia trachomatis* infections of the adult. In: Holmes KK, Sparling PF, Mardh PA, et al, eds. *Sexually Transmitted Diseases*. New York: McGraw-Hill, 1999;407–422.

72. Bauwens JE, Orlander H, Gomez MP, et al. Epidemic *Lymphogranuloma venereum* during epidemics of crack cocaine use and HIV infection in the Bahamas. *Sex Transm Dis*, 2002;29:253–259.

73. Marrazzo JM, Celum CL, Hillis SD, et al. Performance and cost effectiveness of selective screening criteria for *Chlamydia trachomatis* infection in women: implications for a national chlamydia control strategy. *Sex Transm Dis*, 1997;24:131–141.

74. Sales V, Miller MA, Libman M. False positive enzyme immunoassay test results for *Chlamydia trachomatis* because of contact of the collection swab with agar. *Sex Transm Dis*, 1998;25:418–420.

75. Lee HH, Chernesky MA, Schachter J, et al. Diagnosis of *Chlamydia trachomatis* genitourinary infection in women by ligase chain reaction assay of urine. *Lancet*, 1995;345:213–216.

76. Watson EJ, Templeton A, Russel I, et al. The accuracy of screening tests for *Chlamydia trachomatis*: a systematic review. *J Med Microbiol*, 2002;51: 1021–1031.

77. Chernesky MA. Nucleic acid tests for the diagnosis of sexually transmitted diseases. *FEMS Immunol Med Microbiol*, 1999;24:437–446.

78. Cheng H, Macaluso M, Vermund SH, et al. Relative accuracy of nucleic acid amplification tests and culture in detecting chlamydia in asymptomatic men. *J Clin Microbiol*, 2001;39:3927–3937.

79. U.S. Preventive Services Task Force. Screening for chlamydial infection: recommendations and rationale. *Am J Prev Med*, 2001;20(Suppl):S90–S94.

80. Blanchard A, Montagnier L. AIDS-associated mycoplasmas. *Annu Rev Microbiol*, 1994;48:687–712.

81. Wang RY, Shih JW, Weiss SH, et al. *Mycoplasma penetrans* infection in male homosexuals with AIDS: high seroprevalence and association with Kaposi's sarcoma. *Clin Infect Dis*, 1993;17:724–729.

82. Simms I, Eastick K, Mallinson H, et al. Associations between *Mycoplasma genitalium*, *Chlamydia trachomatis*, and pelvic inflammatory disease. *Sex Transm Infect*, 2003;79:154–156.

83. Taylor-Robinson D, Furr PM. Update on sexually transmitted mycoplasmas. *Lancet*, 1998;351(Suppl III):S12–S15.

84. Horner PJ, et al. Association of *Mycoplasma genitalium* with acute non-gonococcal urethritis. *Lancet*, 1993;342:582–585.

85. Manhart LE, Critchlow CW, Holmes KK, et al. Mucopurulent cervicitis and *Mycoplasma genitalium*. *J Infect Dis*, 2003;187:650–657.

86. Cohen CR, Manhart LE, Bukusi EA, et al. Association between *Mycoplasma genitalium* and acute endometritis. *Lancet*, 2002;359:765–766.

87. Clausen HF, Fedder J, Drasbek M, et al. Serological investigation of *Mycoplasma genitalium* in infertile women. *Hum Reprod*, 2001;16:1866–1874.

88. Taylor-Robinson D. *Mycoplasma genitalium*: an update. *Int J STD AIDS*, 2002;145–151.

89. Bakare RA, Oni AA, Umar US, Kehinde AO, Fayemiwo SA, Fasina NA. Ureaplasma urealyticum as a cause of non-gonococcal urethritis: the Ibadan experience. *Niger Postgrad Med J*, 2002;9:140–145.

90. Braithwaite AR, Figueroa JP, Ward E. A comparison of prevalence rates of genital ulcers among patients attending a sexually transmitted disease clinic in Jamaica. *West Indian Med J*, 1997;46:67–71.

91. Morrone A, Toma L, Franco G, Latini O. Donovanosis in developed countries: neglected or misdiagnosed disease? *Int J STD AIDS*, 2003;14: 288–289.

92. O'Farrell N, Hoosen AA, Coetzee K, et al. Genital ulcer disease in women in Durban, South Africa. *Genitourin Med*, 1991;322–326.

93. Greenblatt RB, Diernst RB, Pund ER, et al. Experimental and clinical *Granuloma inguinale*. *JAMA*, 1939; 113:1109–1116.

94. O'Farrell N. Donovanosis. *Sex Transm Inf*, 2002;78: 452–457.

95. U.S. Centers for Disease Control and Prevention. Sexually transmitted diseases treatment guidelines. *MMWR*, 2002;51:RR6.

96. Amsel R, Totten PA, Spiegel CA, et al. Nonspecific vaginitis: diagnostic criteria and microbial and epidemiologic associations. *Am J Med*, 1983;74:14–22.

97. Hillier SL. Diagnostic microbiology of bacterial vaginosis. *Am J Obstet Gynecol*, 1993;169:455–459.

98. Tosun I, Aydin F, Kaklikkaya N, Yazici Y. Frequency of bacterial vaginosis among women attending for intrauterine device insertion at an inner-city family planning clinic. *Eur J Contracept Reprod Health Care*, 2003;8:135–138.

99. Dan M, Kaneh N, Levin D, *et al.* Vaginitis in a gynaecologic practice in Israel: causes and risk factors. *Isr Med Assoc J*, 2003;5:629–632.

100. Riedner G, Rusizoka M, Hoffmann O, et al. Baseline survey of STDS in a cohort of female bar workers in Mbeya Region, Tanzania. *Sex Transm Infect*, 2003;79:382–387.

101. Begum A, Nihifar S, Akther K, et al. Prevalence of selected reproductive tract infections among pregnant women attending an urban maternal and childcare unit in Dhaka, Bangladesh. *J Health Popul Nutr*, 2003;21:112–116.

102. Laurent C, Seck K, Coumba N, et al. Prevalence of HIV and other STDs and risk behaviors of unregistered sex workers in Dakar, Senegal. *AIDS*, 2003;17: 1811–1816.

103. Bakare, et al. Pattern of STDs among commercial sex workers in Ibadan, Nigeria. *Afr J Med Sci*, 2002; 31:243–247.

104. Taha TE, Hoover DR, Dallabetta GA, et al. Bacterial vaginosis and disturbances of vaginal flora: association with increased acquisition of HIV. *AIDS*, 1998; 12:1699–1706.

105. Martin HLJ, Richardson BA, Nyange PM, et al. Vaginal lactobacilli, microbial flora, and risk of human immunodeficiency virus type 1 and sexually transmitted disease acquisition. *J Infect Dis*, 1999; 180:1863–1868.

106. Sturm-Ramirez K, Gaye-Diallo A, Eisen G, Mboup S, Kanki PJ. High levels of tumor necrosis factor-alpha and interleukin-1beta in bacterial vaginosis may increase susceptibility to human immunodeficiency virus. *J Infect Dis*, 2000;182:467–473.

107. Swedberg J, Steiner JF, Deiss F, et al. Comparison of single-dose versus one-week course of metronidazole for symptomatic bacterial vaginosis. *JAMA*, 1985;254:1046–1049.

108. Lafferty WE, Downy L, Celum C, et al. Herpes virus type 1 as a cause of genital herpes: impact on surveillance and prevention. *J Infect Dis*, 2000;181: 1454–1457.

109. Brugha R, Keersmaekers K, Renton A. Genital herpes infection: a review. *J Epidemiol*, 1997;26:698–709.

110. Siegal FP, Lopez C, Hammer GS, et al. Severe acquired immunodeficiency in male homosexuals manifested by chronic perianal ulcerative herpes simplex lesions. *N Engl J Med*, 1981;305:1439–1444.

111. Stamm WE, Handsfield HH, Rompalo AM, et al. The association between genital ulcer disease and acquisition of HIV in homosexual men. *JAMA*, 1998; 260:1409–1433.

112. Whitely R, Barton N, Collins E, et al. Mucocutaneous herpes simplex virus infection in immunocompromised patient: a model for evaluation of topical antiviral agent. *Am J Med*, 1982;73:236–240.

113. Maier JA, Bergman A, Rose MG. Acquired immunodeficiency syndrome manifested by chronic primary genital herpes. *Am J Obstet Gynecol*, 1986;155: 756–758.

114. Englund JA, Zimmerman ME, Swierkosz EM, et al. Herpes simplex virus resistant to acyclovir: a study in a tertiary care center. *Ann Intern Med*, 1990;112: 416–422.

115. Nahass GT, Goldstein BA, Zhu WY, Serfling U, Penneys NS, Leonardi CL. Comparison of Tzanck smear, viral culture and DNA diagnostic methods in detection of herpes simplex and varicella-zoster infection. *JAMA*, 1992;268:2541–2544.

116. Spruance SL, Overall JC Jr, Kern ER, et al. The natural history of recurrent herpes simplex labialis: implications of antiviral therapy. *N Engl J Med*, 1977; 29:69.

117. Hulto C, Arvin A, Jacobs R, et al. Intrauterine herpes simplex virus infections. *J Paediatr*, 1987;110:97.

118. Augenbraun MH. Genital skin and mucous membrane lesions. In: Mandell GL, Bennett JE, Dolin R, eds. *Mandell, Douglas, and Bennett's Principles and Practice of Infectious Diseases.* 6th ed. Philadelphia: Elsevier Churchill Livingstone, 2005:1339–1346.

119. Erlich KS, Jacobson MA, Koehla JE, et al. Foscarnet therapy for severe acyclovir-resistant herpes simplex virus type-2 infections in patients with the acquired immunodeficiency syndrome (AIDS): an uncontrolled trial. *Ann Intern Med*, 1989; 110:710–713.

120. Schacker T, Ryncarz AJ, Goddard J, et al. Frequent recovery of HIV-1 from genital herpes simplex virus lesions in HIV-1 Infected men. *JAMA*, 1998; 280:61–66.

121. Solomon AR, Rasmussen SE, Varami J, et al. The Tzanck smear in the diagnosis of cutaneous herpes simplex. *JAMA*, 1984;251:633–635.

122. Hook EW III, Cannon RO, Nahmias AJ, et al. Herpes simplex virus infection as a risk factor for human immunodeficiency virus infection in heterosexuals. *J Infect Dis*, 1992;165:251–255.

123. McCormack WM. Vulvovaginitis and cervicitis. In: Mandell GL, Bennett JE, Dolin R, eds. *Mandell, Douglas, and Bennett's Principles and Practice of Infectious Diseases.* 6th ed. Philadelphia: Elsevier Churchill Livingstone, 2005:1357–1372.

124. Stone KM, Karem KL, Sternberg MR, et al. Seroprevalence of human papillomavirus type 16 in the United States. *J Infect Dis*, 2002;186:1369–1402.

125. Guillano AR, Harris R, Sedjo R, et al Incidence prevalence and clearance of type specific human papillomavirus infections: the young women's health study. *Lancet*, 2001;357:1831–1836.

126. Walboomers JMM, Jacobs MV, Manos MM, et al. Human papillomavirus is a necessary cause of invasive cervical disease. *J Pathol*, 1999;189:12–19.

127. Kiire CF. The epidemiology and prophylaxis of hepatitis B in sub-Saharan Africa: a view from tropical and subtropical Africa. *Gut*, 1996;38(Suppl 2): S5–S12.

128. Halperin DT. Heterosexual anal intercourse: prevalence, cultural factors, and HIV infection and other health risks, Part I. *AIDS Patient Care STDS*, 1999;13: 717–730.

129. Smith JA, Francis TI, Uriri R. HbsAg in blood donors in Ibadan, Nigeria: prevalence and genetic studies. *Ghana Med J*, 1972;11:43–49.

130. Halim NKD, Offor E, Ajayi OI. Epidemiologic study of the seroprevalence of hepatitis B surface antigen (HBsAg) and HIV-1 in blood donors. *Niger J Clin Pract*, 1999;2:42–45.

131. Amazigo UO, Chime AB. Hepatitis B virus infection in rural and urban populations of eastern Nigeria: prevalence of serologic markers. *East Afr Med J*, 1990;67:539–544.

132. Mutimer DJ, Olomu A, Skidmore S, et al. Viral hepatitis in Nigeria-sickle cell disease and commercial blood donors. *Q J Med*, 1994;87:407–411.

133. Craxi A, Di Bona D, Camma C. Interferon-alpha for HBcAg-positive chronic hepatitis B. *J Hepatol*, 2003; 39(Suppl 1):S99–S105.

134. Lok AS, Chung HT, Liu VW, Ma OC. Long-term follow-up of chronic hepatitis B patients treated with interferon alfa. *Gastroenterol*, 1993;105:1833–1838.

135. Martinson FEA, Kristen AW, Royce RA, et al. Risk factors for horizontal transmission of hepatitis B virus in a rural district in Ghana. *Am J of Epid*, 1998; 147:478–487.

136. Galan MV, Boyce D, Gordon SC. Current pharmacotherapy for hepatitis B infection. *Expert Opin Pharmacother*, 2001;2:1289–1298.

137. Andreone P, Caraceri P, Grazi GL, et al. Lamivudine treatment for acute hepatitis B after liver transplantation. *J Hepatol*, 1998;29:985–989.

138. Lauer GM, Walker BD. Hepatitis C virus infection. *N Engl J Med*, 2001;345:41–52.

139. Farci P, Alter HJ, Wong D, et al. A long term study of hepatitis C virus replication in non-A, non-B hepatitis. *N Engl J Med*, 1991:325:98–104.

140. Graham CS, Baden LR, Yu E, et al. Influence of human immunodeficiency virus on the course of hepatitis C virus infection: a meta-analysis. *Clin Infect Dis*, 2001;33:562–569.

141. Bica J, McGovern B, Dhar R, et al. Increasing mortality due to end stage liver disease in patients with human immunodeficiency virus. *Clin Infect Dis*, 2001;32:492–497.

142. Chung RT, Evans SR, Yang Y, et al. Immune recovery is associated with persistent rise in HCV RNA, infrequent test flares and is not impaired by HCV in co-infected subjects. *AIDS*, 2002;16:1915–1923.

143. Dienstag JL. Chronic viral hepatitis. In: Mandell GL, Bennett JE, Dolin R, eds. *Mandell, Douglas, and Bennett's Principles and Practice of Infectious Diseases*. 6th ed. Philadelphia: Elsevier Churchill Livingstone, 2005:1441–1464.

144. Gates A, Trubowitz PR, Volberding PA. Malignancies in human immunodeficiency virus infection. In: Mandell GL, Bennett JE, Dolin R, eds. *Mandell, Douglas, and Bennett's Principles and Practice of Infectious Diseases*. 6th ed. Philadelphia: Elsevier Churchill Livingstone, 2005:1601–1618.

145. Zeigler J, Templeton AC, Vogel CL. Kaposi's sarcoma: a comparison of classical, endemic and epidemic forms. *Semin Oncol*, 1984;11:47–52.

146. Martin JN, Ganem DE, Osmond DH, Page-Shafer KA, Macrae D, Kedes DH. Sexual transmission and the natural history of human herpesvirus 8 infection. *N Engl J Med*, 1998;338:948–954.

147. Monini P, de Lellis L, Fabris M, et al. Kaposi's sarcoma-associated herpesvirus DNA sequences in prostate tissue and human semen. *N Engl J Med*, 1996;334:1168–1172.

148. Cannon MJ, Dollard SC, Smith DK, et al. Blood-borne and sexual transmission of human herpesvirus 8 in women with or at risk for human immunodeficiency virus infection. *N Engl J Med*, 2001;344:637–643.

149. Whitby D, Smith NA, Matthews S, et al. Human herpesvirus 8: seroepidemiology among women and detection in the genital tract of seropositive women. *J Infect Dis*, 1999;179:234–236.

150. Pauk J, Huang ML, Brodie SJ, et al. Mucosal shedding of human herpesvirus 8 in men. *New Engl J Med*, 2000;343:1369–1377.

151. Gessain A, Mauclere P, van Beveren M, et al. Human herpesvirus 8 primary infection occurs during childhood in Cameroon, Central Africa. *Int J Cancer*, 1999;81:189–192.

152. Biggar RJ, Whitby D, Marshall V. Human herpesvirus 8 in Brazilian Amerindians: a hyperendemic population with a new subtype. *J Infect Dis*, 2000;181:1562–1568.

153. Eltom MA, Mbulaye SM, Dada AJ, et al. Transmission of human herpesvirus 8 by sexual activity among adults in Lagos, Nigeria. *AIDS*, 2002;16:2473–2478.

154. Engels EA, Sinclair MD, Biggar RJ, et al. Latent class analysis of human herpesvirus 8 assay performance and infection prevalence in sub-Saharan Africa and Malta. *Int J Cancer*, 2000;88:1003–1008.

155. Dada AJ, Ajayi AO, Diamondstone L, et al. A serosurvey of *Haemophilus ducreyi*, syphilis, and herpes simplex virus type 2 and their association with human immunodeficiency virus among female sex workers in Lagos, Nigeria. *Sex Transm Dis*, 1998;25:237–242.

156. Plancoulaine S, Abel L, van Beveren M, et al. Human herpesvirus 8 transmission from mother to child and between siblings in an endemic population. *Lancet*, 2000;356:1062–1065.

157. Ireland-Gill A, Espina B, Akil B, et al. Treatment of acquired immunodeficiency syndrome-related Kaposi's sarcoma using bleomycin containing combination chemotherapy regimes. *Semin Oncol*, 1992;2(Suppl 5):32–36.

158. Minkoff H, Grunebaum AN, Schwarz RH, et al. Risk factors for prematurity and premature rupture of the membranes: a prospective study of the vaginal flora in pregnancy. *Am J Obstet Gynecol*, 1984;150:965–972.

159. Klebanoff MA, Carey JC, Hauth JC, et al. Failure of metronidazole to prevent preterm delivery among pregnant women with asymptomatic *Trichomonas vaginalis* infection. *New Engl J Med*, 2001;345:467–493.

160. Schwebke JR. Update of trichomoniasis. *Sex Transm Infect*, 2002;78:378–379.

161. Latif AS, Mason PR, Marowa E. Urethral trichomoniasis in men. *Sex Transm Dis*, 1987;14:9–11.

162. Sogbetun AO, Osoba AO. Trichomonal urethritis in Nigerian males. *Trop Geogr Med*, 1974;26:319–324.

163. Pillay DG, Hoosen AA, Vezi B, Moodley C. Diagnosis of *Trichomonas vaginalis* in male urethritis. *Trop Geogr Med*, 1994;46:44–45.

164. Bakare RA. Prevalence of *Trichomonas vaginalis* among the sexual partners of women with Trichomoniasis in Ibadan. *Afr J Clin Exp Microbiol*, 2003;4:107–113.

165. Cu-Uvin S, Ko H, Jamieson DJ, et al. Prevalence, incidence and persistence or recurrence of Trichomoniasis among human immunodeficiency virus (HIV) positive women and HIV negative women at high risk of HIV infection. *Clin Infect Dis*, 2002;34:1406–1411.

166. DeMeo LR, Draper DL, McGregor JA, et al. Evaluation of a deoxyribonucleic acid probe for the detection of *Trichomonas vaginalis* in vaginal secretions. *Am J Obstet Gynecol*, 1996;174:1339–1342.

167. The president of Chile and the WHO director-general launch global commission to tackle the "causes behind the causes of ill-health." News release by the World Health Organization, March 18, 2005. Accessed at www.who.int/mediacentre/news/releases/2005/pr13/en.

168. James-Traore T, Magnami N, Murray N, et al. In: Finger B, Lapetina M, Pribila M, eds. *Intervention Strategies that Work for Youths: Summary of the FOCUS on Young Adults*. Arlington, Virginia: Family Health International YouthNet Program, 2002.

169. Brabin L. Clinical management and prevention of sexually transmitted diseases: a review focusing on women. *Acta Trop*, 2000;75:53–70.

170. Olayinka BA, Osho AA. Changes in attitude, sexual behavior and the risk of HIV/AIDS in southwest Nigeria. *East Afr Med J*, 1997;74:554–560.

171. Ojwang SBO, Maggwa ABN. Adolescent sexuality in Kenya. *East Afr Med J*, 1991;58:74–81.

172. Brabin L. Providing accessible health care for adolescents with sexually transmitted diseases. *Acta Tropica*, 1996;62:209–216.

173. Fetters T, Munkonze F, Solo J. *Investing in Youth: Testing Community Based Approaches for Improving Adolescent Sexual and Reproductive Health*. Lusaka: CARE Zambia and Population Council, 1999.

174. Adeokun LA, Ladipo OA, Odutolu O, et al. Bridging the knowledge gap through HIV surveillance in four markets in Ogbomoso and Ibadan, Nigeria. *Archives of Ibadan Medicine*, 2005;5:59–65.

175. Emonyi IW, Gray RH, Zenilman J, et al. Seroprevalence of herpes simplex virus type 2 (HSV-2) in Rakai district, Uganda. *E Afr Med J*, 2000;77:428–430.

176. U.S. Centers for Disease Control and Prevention. HIV transmission among black women — North Carolina, 2004. *MMWR*, 2005;54:89–94.

177. Zabin LS, Clark SD Jr. Why they delay: a study of teenage family planning clinics. *Fam Plann Perspect*, 1981;13:205–217.

178. McNamara R. Female genital health and the risk of HIV transmission. New York: HIV and Development Programme, United Nations Development Programme, 2005;3.

179. UNAIDS. *Report on the Global HIV/AIDS Epidemic*. Geneva: UNAIDS, 2002.

180. UNAIDS. *Report on the Global AIDS Epidemic*. Geneva: UNAIDS, 2004.

181. U.S. Centers for Disease Control and Prevention. Unrecognized HIV infections, risk behaviors and perceptions among young black men who have sex with men in 6 US cities, 1994–1998. *MMWR*, 2002;51:733–736.

182. U.S. Centers for Disease Control and Prevention. HIV/STD risks in young men who have sex with men who do not disclose their sexual orientation — 6 U.S. cities, 1994–2000. *MMWR*, 2003;52:81–85.

183. Robinson NJ, Mulder DW, Auvert B, Hayes RJ. Proportion of HIV infections attributable to other sexually transmitted diseases in a rural Ugandan population: simulation model estimates. *Int J Epidemiol*, 1997;26:180–189.

184. Hayes RJ, Schulz KF, Plummer FA. The co-factor effect of genital ulcers on the per-exposure risk of HIV transmission. *J Trop Med Hyg*, 1995;98:1–8.

185. Theus SA, Harrich DA, Gaynor R, et al. *Treponema pallidum*, lipoproteins, and synthetic lipoprotein analogues induce human immunodeficiency virus type 1 gene expression in monocytes via NF-kappa B activation. *J Infect Dis*, 1999;177:941–950.

186. Sellati TJ, Wilkinson DA, Sheffield JS, et al. Virulent *Treponema pallidum*, lipoprotein, and synthetic lipopeptides induce CCR5 on human monocytes and enhance their susceptibility to infection by human immunodeficiency virus type 1. *J Infect Dis*, 2000;181:283–293.

187. Moss GB, Overbaugh J, Welch M, et al. Human immunodeficiency virus DNA in urethral secretions in men: association with gonococcal urethritis and CD4 cell depletion. *J Infect Dis*, 1995;172:1469–1474.

188. John Hopkins Bloomberg School of Public Health Center for Communication Programs. *Stop AIDS Love Life* in Ghana "Shatters the Silence." *Impact*, February 2003;1–2.

189. Ellis S, Grey A. Prevention of sexually transmitted infections (STIs): a review of reviews into the effectiveness of non-clinical interventions. *Evidence Briefing*, 1st edition, January 2004.

190. Wong ML. Behavioral interventions in the control of human immunodeficiency virus and other sexually transmitted diseases—a review. *Ann Acad Med Singapore*, 1995;24:602–607.

191. Marinho AO. Getting the AIDS message to the youth. *Arch Ibadan Med*, 2005;5:65–67.

192. Kirby D, Coyle K. School-based programs to reduce sexual risk-taking behavior. *Child Youth Serv Rev*, 1997;19:415–436.

193. Kirby D. Effective approaches to reducing adolescent unprotected sex, pregnancy, and childbearing. *J Sex Res*, 2002;39:51–57.

194. Speizer I, Heller G, Brieger W. *Survey Findings from the West African Youth Initiative Project: Final Evaluation of Peer Educator Intervention.* New York: Rockefeller Foundation, 2000.

195. Speizer IS, Tambashe BO, Tegang SP. An evaluation of the "Entre Nous Jeunes" peer educator program for adolescents in Cameroon. *Stud Fam Plann*, 2001;32:339–351.

196. Brieger WR, Delano GE, Lane CG, et al. West African Youth Initiative: outcome of a reproductive health program. *J Adolesc Health*, 2001;294:36–46.

197. U.S. Centers for Disease Control and Prevention. Update: barrier protection against HIV infection and other sexually transmitted diseases. *MMWR*, 1993;42:589–597.

198. Okonofua FE, Ogonor JI, Omorodion FI, et al. Assessment of health services for treatment of sexually transmitted infections among Nigerian adolescents. *Sex Transm Dis*, 1999;26:184–190.

199. World Health Organization. Simplified approaches for sexually transmitted disease (STD) control at the primary health care (PHC) level. *Report of a Working WHO Group.* Geneva: World Health Organization, 1984;24–28.

200. World Health Organization. *Guidelines for the Management of Sexually Transmitted Infections.* Geneva: World Health Organization, 2001.

201. Thomas T, Choudri S, Kariuki C, et al. Identifying cervical infection among pregnant women in Nairobi, Kenya: limitations of risk assessment and symptom based approaches. *Genitourin Med*, 1996;72:334–338.

202. Obunge OK, Brabin L, Dollimore N, et al. A flow-chart for managing sexually transmitted infections among Nigerian adolescent females. *Bull World Health Organ*, 2001;79:301–305.

203. Sangani P, Rutherford G, Wilkinson D. Population-based interventions for reducing sexually transmitted infections, including HIV infection. *The Cochrane Database of Systematic Review*, 2004;3.

204. O'Farrell N. Targeted interventions required against genital ulcers in African countries worst affected by HIV infection. *Bull World Health Organ*, 2001;79:569–577.

205. Mayaud P, Mosha F, Todd J, et al. Improved treatment services significantly reduce the prevalence of sexually transmitted diseases in rural Tanzania: results of a randomized controlled trial. *AIDS*, 1997;11:1873–1880.

206. Kamali A, Quigley M, Nakinyingi J, et al. Syndromic management of sexually transmitted infections and behaviour interventions on transmission of HIV-1 in rural Uganda: a community randomised trial. *Lancet*, 2003;361:645–652.

207. Osoba AO. Overview of penicillinase producing *Neisseria gonorrhoeae* in Africa. *Afr J Ven Dis*, 1986;2:51–55.

208. O'Farrell N. Increasing prevalence of genital herpes in developing countries: implications for heterosexual HIV transmission and STI control programmes. *Sex Transm Infect*, 1999;75:377–384.

209. Nasidi A, Harry TO, Vyazov SO, et al. Prevalence of hepatitis B virus markers in representative areas of Nigeria. *Int J Epidemiol*, 1986;15:274–276.

210. Koutsky LA, Ault KA, Wheeler CM, et al. A controlled trial of a human papillomavirus type 16 vaccine. *N Engl J Med*, 2002;347:1645–1651.

211. Schambelan M, Benson CA, Carr A, et al. Management of metabolic complications associated with antiretroviral therapy for HIV-1 infection: recommendations of an International AIDS Society–USA Panel. *J Acquir Immune Defic Syndr*, 2002; 31:257–275.

212. Batson A. Win-win interactions between the public and private sectors. *Nat Med*, 1998;4(Suppl 5): S487–S491.

213. Bentley ME, Fullem AM, Tolley EE, et al. Acceptability of a microbicide among women and their partners in a 4-country phase I trial. *Am J Public Health*, 2004;94:1159–1164.

214. Woodsong C. Covert use of topical microbicides: Implications for acceptability and use. *Int Fam Plan Perspect*, 2004;30:94–98.

215. Coplan PM, Mitchnick M, Rosenberg ZF. Regulatory challenges in microbicide development. *Science*, 2004;304:1911–1912.

216. Stone A. Microbicides: a new approach to preventing HIV and other sexually transmitted infections. *Nat Rev Drug Discov*, 2002;1:977–985.

217. Pool R, Whitworth J, Green G, et al. Ambivalence, sexual pleasure and the acceptability of microbicidal products in southwest Uganda. *AIDS*, 2000;14: 2058–2059.

218. *Strengthening Collaboration in Microbicide Development.* Report of a meeting sponsored by the International Working Group on Microbicides, November 2000.

6

THE PATHOPHYSIOLOGY AND CLINICAL MANIFESTATIONS OF HIV/AIDS

Idris Mohammed* and
Abdulsalami Nasidi†

AIDS was first clinically identified and described in 1981 in patients presenting with symptoms of severe immunosuppression in the United States (1–3). While the clinical presentations varied among these initial cases, they shared enough features to justify their being treated as part of a syndromic disease caused by a single pathogen. This syndrome was characterized by immune abnormalities resulting from infection and destruction of CD4+ T-lymphocytes, which immunologically compromised the infected person. The term "acquired immune deficiency syndrome" (AIDS) was coined to describe the disease, since the causative agent was not yet known. Prolonged infection resulted in disease with protean clinical manifestations that differed to some degree from country to country and from region to region. Clinicians and scientists realized this new disease had a wide spectrum of signs and symptoms. This variable disease presentation resulted from the capacity of the virus to infect nearly every organ or system, particularly during the more advanced stages of disease.

The emergence of HIV/AIDS was mired in pervasive ignorance, mystery, fear, and stigma, frequently out of proportion to the reality of the situation. As a result, most African countries resisted advocacy and research, making it difficult to engage in informed discussions that would have otherwise promoted awareness of the disease. This was particularly true for Nigeria, where nei-

---

*Department of Medicine, Federal Medical Centre, Gombe, Gombe State, Nigeria
†Federal Ministry of Health, Abuja, Nigeria

ther the transmission modes nor the possible prevention measures could be openly discussed (4). It was against such a background that Nigerians failed to appreciate the need for the education, research, social reorientation, and behavioral change necessary for understanding the disease and planning actions to curtail the epidemic. This explains in part why Nigerians were slow to appreciate the reality of HIV/AIDS, delaying studies even on knowledge, attitudes, and practices until many years later (5–7).

DEFINITION OF AIDS

When first identified, the new syndrome lacked an agreed-upon, accurate definition, and its causative agent was unknown. Therefore, the U.S. Centers for Disease Control and Prevention (CDC) suggested that a combination of opportunistic infections and immunosuppression were indicative of AIDS. Once the causative agent, HIV, was identified, the definition was revised appropriately. The CDC and the World Health Organization (WHO) developed simplified diagnostic criteria that considerably eased the difficulties African physicians encountered in diagnosing HIV-related disease from a clinical standpoint. This definition was based on the presence of certain "indicator" diseases, backed by laboratory evidence of HIV infection (8) (Table 6-1).

At a WHO-sponsored meeting in Bangui in 1985, African scientists agreed upon another definition of AIDS, largely to enable surveillance and to promote a better understanding and diagnosis of the disease. Like the earlier definition, this clinical case definition, known as "The Bangui Definition," promoted more reliable diagnosis of AIDS by identifying certain major and minor clinical features of HIV disease with or without laboratory evidence of HIV infection (Table 6-2).

Although the Bangui Definition was eventually found to be insensitive, at the time it enhanced the diagnostic ability of health workers in developing countries. Many resource-poor sub-Saharan African countries could not even afford the equipment and reagents needed for accurate HIV diagnosis. Yet these were the very countries where such diagnosis was — and still is — needed most because of the enormous burden of HIV/AIDS. Initially, many health care providers were uncomfortable with the imprecise definition of disease; fortunately, significant clinical research during the early HIV epidemic made it possible to revise the definition by introducing more accurate laboratory diagnostic tests. The CDC developed new criteria, which led to an improved clinical classification system (Table 6-3).

Simplification of methods to identify HIV/AIDS provides easily comprehensible data to clinicians with little training in understanding and interpreting the complicated CDC disease staging algorithm.

Table 6-1. CDC Classification System of HIV Disease

Group		Clinical Stage
I.		Acute HIV infection
III.		Asymptomatic HIV infection
IV.		Persistent generalized lymphadenopathy
IV.		Other diseases
	Subgroup A	Constitutional symptoms
	Subgroup B	Neurologic disease
	Subgroup C	Secondary infectious diseases
	Subgroup D	Secondary neoplasms
	Subgroup E	Other conditions

Modified from the original U.S. Centers for Disease Control and Prevention classification for HIV disease.

and little time to devote to complicated diagnoses, as they are usually treating hundreds of patients. Several "simple" laboratory tests were recommended to help African health workers make a reasonably accurate diagnosis of HIV infection in the absence of high-technology facilities; to some extent,

Table 6-2. World Health Organization/Bangui AIDS Case Definition

Major Signs	Minor Signs
• Weight loss > 10% body weight	• Persistent cough > 1 month • Pruritic rash
• Chronic diarrhea > 1 month duration	• Recurrent herpes zoster • Oropharyngeal candidiaisis
• Prolonged fever > 1 month duration infection	• Chronic progressive herpes simplex
	• Generalized lymphadenopathy

Any two major signs, or one major plus two minor signs, constitute an AIDS diagnosis.

these simple tests and modified screening algorithms helped achieve the intended objective. An accurate characterization of the disease manifestations and a positive HIV antibody test result enabled reliable AIDS diagnoses. In some settings, though, several of the recommended laboratory tests fell short of the expected accuracy; instead of confirming the diagnosis of HIV and/or AIDS, they gave inconsistent and irreproducible results.

As a result of the limited diagnostic capacity in Africa, it was agreed that two positive enzyme-linked immunosorbent assay (ELISA) results using different assay methods were acceptable as confirmatory evidence of HIV infection. In Nigeria, the Federal Ministry of Health decided to establish regional laboratories with equipment and training to confirm ELISA-positive results using the Western blot technique.

Table 6-3. The Modified U.S. Centers for Disease Control and Prevention (CDC) Classification of HIV Infection and Disease

Clinical Stage I	**Asymptomatic disease** Asymptomatic/acute HIV infection, persistent generalized lymphadenopathy
Clinical Stage II	**Early (mild) disease** Weight loss ≥ 10% of body weight; minor mucocutaneous manifestations (seborrheic dermatitis, prurigo, fungal nail infection, recurrent oral ulceration, and angular cheilitis); recurrent respiratory tract infections, such as bacterial sinusitis
Clinical Stage III	**Intermediate (moderate) disease** Weight loss ≥ 10% of body weight; chronic unexplained diarrhea ≥ one month; oral candidiasis (thrush); oral hairy leukoplakia; pulmonary tuberculosis within the past year; severe bacterial infection, such as pneumonia and pyomyositis
Clinical Stage IV	**Late (severe) disease AIDS** HIV-wasting syndrome as defined by the CDC; *Pneumocystis carinii* pneumonia; toxoplasmosis of the brain; cryptosporidiosis with diarrhea ≥ one month; extrapulmonary cryptosporidiosis; cytomegalovirus disease other than in liver, spleen, or lymph nodes; herpes simplex virus infection; mucocutaneous ≥ one month or visdermal of any duration; progressive multifocal leukoencephalopathy; disseminated endemic mycosis, such as histoplasmosis and coccidioidomycosis; candidiasis of the esophagus, trachea, bronchi, or lungs; atypical mycobacteriosis; disseminated, nontyphoidal salmonella septicemia; extrapulmonary tuberculosis; lymphoma, Kaposi's sarcoma; HIV encephalopathy as defined by the CDC.

In 1986, federal health authorities established four centers, only one of which attained acceptable diagnostic competence. This limitation made it impossible to verify the prevalence of HIV infection in Nigeria at that time, and progress in this area was made only years later, after more centers with adequate diagnostic competence were established.

THE HIV LIFECYCLE

In 1983, and 1984, respectively, U.S. and French researchers isolated and described the causative agent of AIDS, with each group calling the virus a different name: human T-cell lymphotropic virus type III (HTLV-III) or lymphadenopathy-associated virus (LAV) (9,10). Ultimately, the International Taxonomic Association resolved this issue by naming the causative agent human immunodeficiency virus (HIV). The identification and characterization of HIV, apart from enhancing our understanding of the pathophysiology of AIDS, also allowed the development of appropriate diagnostic tests to measure HIV-induced antibodies in the serum, a critical step in diagnosing AIDS. Later virologic studies identified antiretroviral (ARV) therapies to treat this unique and chronic viral infection.

HIV is an enveloped RNA virus whose basic structure consists of an outer bilayer of lipid and glycoprotein and an inner core containing two single RNA strands bound together by a *gag*-derived protein, p24. The outer membrane of HIV contains specific structural elements that play important roles in infectivity and disease progression. The most important of these is the viral envelope glycoprotein 120 (gp120), which is necessary for HIV's interaction with host cell receptors on cells, including CD4+ lymphocytes, macrophages, and monocytes. For this reason, early attempts to develop an HIV vaccine were based on trying to induce production of antibodies directed against gp120. Gp120 is closely associated with the envelope transmembrane viral protein, gp41, which is involved in viral–cell membrane fusion. Both gp41 and gp120 are essential for infectivity.

Gp120 interacts with the CD4+ receptor on the surface of susceptible cells. However, gp120 attachment also requires the presence of chemokine co-receptors, such as CXCR4 or CCR5, which facilitate the process of cell binding and entry. Typically, T-cell-tropic (T-tropic) HIV viruses use the CXCR4 receptor and are syncytium-inducing (SI) viruses, whereas macrophage-tropic (M-tropic) viruses use the CCR5 receptor and are non-syncytium–inducing (NSI) viruses. Other minor chemokine co-receptors—such as CCR1, CCR2, CCR3, and CCR4—may also facilitate the entry of HIV into CD4+ bearing cells (11–16).

To understand how HIV infection progresses from asymptomatic to clinical disease, it is necessary to consider possible modes of virus infection and the mechanisms of progression that result in damage to the immune system. The diversity of HIV-related illnesses requires consideration of these factors to understand the clinical presentation of HIV/AIDS. Thus, it is important to understand the complex mechanism of HIV replication at the cellular level, from the initial stage of attachment of a viral particle to a cell of the immune system—such as lymphocytes and monocytes—to the replication and budding of new viruses from that cell (Figure 6-1). These cellular events lead to the production of massive numbers of new viral particles, death of the infected cells, and ultimately the destruction of the immune system, which leads to the development of AIDS.

The HIV lifecycle can be divided into eight stages: binding or attachment; entry into the susceptible cell and subsequent uncoating of the virion; reverse transcription, in which the viral genetic material (RNA) is reverse transcribed into a DNA, or proviral form; integration, in which the viral DNA is inserted into the host cell DNA; synthesis of viral RNA, in which the proviral DNA is transcribed to make multiple viral RNA copies; translation, which involves the synthesis of viral proteins; assembly and budding, in which the new virions complete forma-

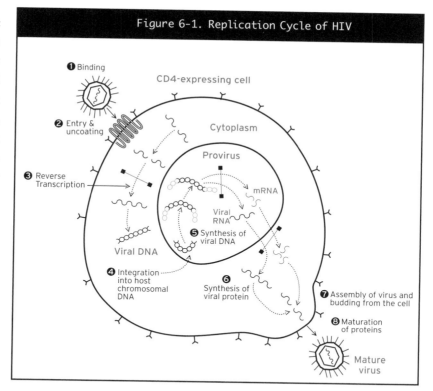

Figure 6-1. Replication Cycle of HIV

tion and exit the host cell; and maturation, which involves the processing of viral proteins and is required for the virus to become infectious. This cascade of events has been studied and described in detail (17,18).

Stage 1: Viral Binding

On the surface membrane of all living cells are complex protein structures that may serve as "receptors." A receptor is often compared to a lock into which a specific key or "ligand" will fit. HIV binds to at least two specific receptors on the host cell: the primary receptor, called the CD4+, and a secondary receptor, a chemokine co-receptor, such as CXCR4 or CCR5, as described earlier.

HIV infection of a lymphocyte begins with attachment of the virus, via its gp120, to the cell membrane through both of these "ligand-receptor" interactions. Tight attachment of the viral particle to receptors on the cell's membrane activates other proteins that enable viral fusion with the cell membrane.

Stage 2: Entry and Uncoating

Once the virus has fused with the host cell, the viral core and its associated RNA enter the cell. In order for the genetic material of the virus to reproduce, the coating that surrounds the RNA, or nucleocapsid, must be dissolved. A partial uncoating of the nucleocapsid occurs, resulting in the release of viral RNA into the cytoplasm of the host cell.

Table 6-4. The WHO System for Clinical Staging of HIV Infection and Disease

1. Candidiasis of the esophagus, trachea, bronchi, or lungs
2. Cryptococcosis (extrapulmonary)
3. Cryptosporidiosis (with diarrhea)
4. Cytomegalovirus infection (other than liver, spleen, or lymph nodes)
5. Herpes simplex virus infection
6. Kaposi's sarcoma in people younger than 60 years
7. Brain lymphoma (primary)
8. Lymphoid interstitial pneumonitis/pulmonary lymphoid hyperplasia (LIP/PLH) in a child
9. *Mycobacterium-avium* complex infection
10. *Pneumocystis carinii* pneumonia
11. Progressive multifocal leukoencephalopathy
12. Toxoplasmosis (of the brain)

Stage 3: Reverse Transcription

Conversion of the viral genetic material (RNA) to DNA occurs through the action of an enzyme—reverse transcriptase—that HIV produces. Reverse transcriptase reads the sequence of viral RNA that enters the host cell and transcribes the sequence into a complementary DNA sequence, which can then use the cellular machinery to make viral proteins and additional copies of viral RNA. Without this process, the virus cannot replicate.

The process of reverse transcription is unique to retroviruses as a result of their reverse transcriptase; thus, multiple nucleoside reverse transcriptase inhibitors (NRTIs) and non-nucleoside reverse transcriptase inhibitors (NNRTIs) have been developed for use as ARVs to treat HIV infection. These ARVs are not as effective in treating HIV-2 infection and disease, however, because of differences in the HIV-2 reverse transcriptase (19–24). Current ARVs also suffer from the drawback that a single nucleotide mutation within the *pol* gene can yield a virus resistant to the ARV.

In the case of HIV, the process of reverse transcription is error-prone; thus, a small number of mutations are introduced in the HIV genome each time it replicates. This error-prone process results in the extreme heterogeneity of HIV (25). At the cellular level, the viruses produced after each round of replication are not identical to the original infecting virions. This variation of HIV within an individual and between HIV isolates from distinct geographic regions has a profound impact on the diagnosis and treatment of HIV, as well as the design and development of potential HIV vaccines.

Stage 4: Integration into Host Chromosomal DNA

During this stage, viral DNA is randomly inserted into the host cell DNA by the viral enzyme integrase. This stage of the HIV lifecycle has enabled the design and development of a new class of ARVs known as integrase inhibitors (26–29); several are still in the testing phase and none is in clinical use currently. Once the viral DNA is integrated into the host genetic material, it can remain there in a latent state for many years. The ability of HIV to persist in this latent state poses a major barrier to eradicating or curing HIV.

Stage 5: Synthesis of Viral DNA

Upon activation of infected cells, viral DNA is transcribed along with the host DNA into messenger RNA (mRNA). The mRNA codes for the production of viral proteins and enzymes. The new viral RNA also serves as the genetic material for the next generation of viruses. Once produced, the viral mRNA is transported out of the nucleus and into the cytoplasm of the host cell.

Stage 6: Translation and Production of Viral Proteins

Translation of viral mRNA results in the production of polypeptide sequences. Each section of the mRNA corresponds to a protein or enzyme that serves as a building block used to construct new HIV particles.

Stage 7: Assembly of Virus and Budding from the Host Cell

This stage of the viral infection is the formation of a new virus particle, or virion, which is preceded by the assembly of functional viral proteins such as the envelope and core proteins (gp120, gp41, and Gag) and necessary viral enzymes (reverse transcriptase, protease, and integrase). Viral polypeptides must be cleaved into smaller parts by the viral protease enzyme. Inhibitors of this viral protease, termed protease inhibitors, block the ability of the protease to cleave the viral polypeptide into functional enzymes or proteins; thus, protease inhibitors interfere with the production of new HIV particles, although they do not prevent infection of the cell in the first place.

When viral RNA and associated proteins are packaged and released from the cell surface as viral particles, they take with them a small portion of the cellular membrane that also contains viral surface proteins. These viral proteins then become the "envelope" of the new viral particles. As described earlier, these envelope proteins then bind to the receptors on other immune cells, thereby facilitating continued infection. If this process of viral replication occurs in CD4+ lymphocytes in a progressive and uncontrolled manner, HIV will eventually destroy them and progressively deplete their numbers. These infected CD4+ cells may also become functionally defective and inefficient in executing their central immunoregulatory functions. An additional consequence of CD4+ cell depletion is the development of opportunistic infections or malignancies that would otherwise not occur in immunocompetent individuals, as the CD4+ cell count is depleted to less than 200 cells/mm^3.

It is well documented that HIV can be cytotoxic to infected CD4+ lymphocytes (30–32). This immune-mediated cytotoxic effect probably involves inhibition of T-cell regeneration in the thymus. For example, T-cell proliferative responses to HIV are quickly lost and the repertoire of antigen recognition diminishes with time. The use of ARVs has provided evidence, however, that some of these immune cells, particularly CD4+ T-lymphocytes, can be reconstituted and become functionally effective once more (33–35). It has been suggested that Africans may have an activated immune system because of chronic exposure or infection with other pathogens, resulting in an unusual susceptibility to HIV infection, which may play a significant role in a more rapid progression of AIDS (7,36,37).

Stage 8: Maturation

The final step in the viral lifecycle, maturation, is required in order for the virus to become infectious. Shortly after budding from the host cell, the protease enzymes in the new viral particle become active and cleave the polypeptides into their appropriate functional subunits, or proteins and enzymes. This processing step results in the generation of a mature and infectious virion.

CLINICAL COURSE OF HIV DISEASE

The pathophysiologic features described in this section refer mostly to ARV-naive individuals, which is what is usually seen in most African settings. While most people are considered typical progressors, with a median incubation period of eight to ten years, a small portion of HIV-infected people are rapid progressors, while still others are long-term non-progressors (29,38).

Primary HIV infection

Primary infection with HIV occurs two to six weeks after infection, a period in which it is extremely difficult to make a specific diagnosis by standard laboratory assays. During this period, viral antigen or RNA detection is required since antibody responses to viral proteins are slower to develop post-infection. Various clinical studies show that many infected people experience flu-like symptoms during primary infection, which they may ignore partly because of the self-limiting and mild nature of those symptoms. Clinical symptoms of primary infection, when recognized, may include mild fever, muscle aches and pains, fatigue, headaches, enlargement of the lymph nodes, rashes, a sore throat, and mild diarrhea. A minority of infected subjects may present with other symptoms suggestive of meningeal, pulmonary, or gastrointestinal involvement (38).

In Nigeria, most of the laboratory and clinical findings associated with primary infection are nonspecific and may mimic other clinical conditions caused by various pathogens. Measurement of levels of HIV-infected peripheral blood lymphocytes, plasma HIV RNA, and HIV p24 antigens—made possible by advances in such sensitive applications as the polymerase chain reaction (PCR)—have greatly facilitated the diagnosis of primary HIV infection (29,38). The fact that early ARVs may delay progression from asymptomatic to symptomatic HIV disease makes early diagnosis of the infection highly desirable.

Asymptomatic Infection

Many HIV-infected persons are asymptomatic for a long time. This stage has a number of important implications for the epidemiology of HIV infection. A lack of awareness and a poor laboratory investigative infrastructure are major impediments to the characterization of the entire disease process, from primary exposure and infection through development of pathophysiologic and clinical features, to relevant diagnostic investigations. Thus, effective control and therapeutic measures (including ARV treatment) that may delay disease progression were slow to be introduced in Nigeria. Fortunately, studies on the course of HIV disease progression have been performed in other African countries.

Symptomatic Infection

Advanced HIV infection predisposes people to many opportunistic infections seen commonly in African patients. The most common of these infections are caused by *Mycobacteria*, exemplified best by *M. tuberculosis*. Tuberculosis develops either by reactivation of latent infection, or primary infection that progresses rapidly in HIV-infected people (39–41). The incidence of tuberculosis in Africa had been declining before the emergence of HIV/AIDS, when the incidence of tuberculosis infection began to increase dramatically. The association between HIV disease and tuberculosis is significant, and some clinicians screen all patients with a diagnosis of tuberculosis for HIV co-infection.

Other opportunistic infections associated with advanced HIV disease include candidiasis caused by *Candida albicans* and other *Candida sp*, *Cryptococcal* infections, *Pneumocystis carinii* pneumonia (PCP), cytomegalovirus infections, cryptosporidiosis, and herpes virus infections (42–47). Not surprisingly, patients tend to have multiple opportunistic infections. HIV infection may also occur in association with hepatitis B or C virus infection (48–50). A number of malignancies—including Kaposi's sarcoma, cervical cancer, brain lymphomas, and non-Hodgkin's lymphoma—are also associated with advanced HIV disease (51–54). HIV-infected people with low CD4+ lymphocytes also have an increased incidence of other microbial infections.

Clinical Presentation of HIV Disease

Progression from HIV infection to disease is often insidious, but once sufficient immunologic damage and immunosuppression have occurred, a variety of signs and symptoms appear, depending on the clinical severity and immunopathology of the disease. Nonetheless, the disease course is variable, and patients may present with mild, moderate, or severe manifestations. Diarrhea is a common clinical sign, resulting in rapid wasting, particularly in Central Africa, East Africa, and southern Africa, where this symptomatic complex was initially referred to as "slim disease." In Africa, emaciation or body wasting is often associated with HIV disease, even without formal documentation of HIV infection. AIDS is a clinical syndrome of diseases that results from the profound immunosuppression that permits opportunistic infections to replicate in an uncontrolled manner. This syndromic nature of HIV disease complicates the clinical diagnosis of AIDS, as similar signs and symptoms may be found in a number of other infectious diseases.

Symptomatic HIV disease results from prolonged untreated infection. ARVs and other therapies to prevent and treat the opportunistic infections associated with symptomatic disease have been developed, but their cost renders them beyond the reach of most HIV-infected Africans. Clinical awareness and appropriate diagnostic support are also required in dealing effectively with the disease. Despite the potential of the infection to cause multisystem disease, the manifestations are described according to organ or system, for easier understanding and better appreciation of HIV-associated illnesses.

Skin Manifestations

Dermatologic disease or pathology is almost invariably observed during HIV symptomatic disease. These vary from mild pruritus with or without rashes, to severe coalescent mucocutaneous rashes, such as the kind seen in patients with Stevens-Johnson syndrome. Among people whose behavior places them at high risk, the persistence of skin lesions should lead to a suspicion of HIV infection (55). Similarly, the appearance of herpes simplex or herpes zoster infections in the skin should always prompt testing for HIV infection. These infections may be associated with oral ulcers, sometimes severe enough to cause large and deep mucocutaneous lesions. Orolabial lesions may also occur. Some patients develop Kaposi's sarcoma (56), a disease caused by human herpesvirus 8. HIV-associated Kaposi's sarcoma is more severe than the endemic African form, which is usually a mild, slow-growing, and fungating tumor. The histological features of the two are broadly similar, however, as both are multicentric tumors with fibroblastic elements (57).

Candidiasis is another significant cause of oral and skin manifestations in many people with HIV (58). Apart from oral lesions, there may be hyperkeratosis of the skin in patients co-infected with *Candida albicans*. Anal warts may be due to human papilloma virus (HPV) or candida infection, while some patients develop generalized mycoses and dermatitis. Another significant oral manifestation of HIV infection is hairy leukoplakia, a persistent white lesion around tongue margins, caused by co-infection with Epstein-Barr virus (59,60). Other skin manifestations of HIV disease include peripheral small arterial lesions, such as angiomatosis, seborrheic dermatitis, and folliculitis (55).

Gastrointestinal Disease

Chronic diarrhea lasting many months is one of the earliest HIV-associated symptoms described in Africa. It can result in progressive weight loss and related metabolic (electrolyte) disturbances. Diarrhea in people with AIDS may be caused by several pathogens, including *Giardia lamblia*, *Salmonella* sp., *Campylobacter* sp., and *Shigella* sp. (61,62). As the patient's clinical condition worsens, other pathogens may be isolated, including cytomegalovirus, *Cryptosporidium*, *Toxoplasma gondii*, *Mycobacteria*, *Cyclosporidia* sp., *Isosporidia* sp., and *Candida* sp. (61–68). Diarrhea may also occur as a result of gastrointestinal cyclosporidiosis, isosporidiosis, and infection by other *Coccidia* sp. (66). The prevalence of these pathogens in Africans with HIV-related diarrhea is difficult to determine, because their isolation requires expensive laboratory equipment not readily available on most of the African continent.

Toxoplasmosis is a protozoan infection that primarily infects the gastrointestinal tract, the central nervous system, and the respiratory tract. Other organs or systems, however, may be involved, although to a lesser extent and with milder clinical manifestations. HIV-associated *Toxoplasma gondii* is isolated in 34% to 80% of asymptomatic individuals, including children and pregnant women in some parts of Africa (69,70).

Hepatic Disease

Clinically relevant involvement of the liver is not common during the early stages of HIV infection, even though mild "hepatitis-like" self-limiting symptoms may occur in some people with acute or primary infection with HIV. Chronic active hepatitis in people with HIV is a progressive illness that is often difficult to treat. Although the transmission modes of HIV and hepatitis viruses are similar, co-infection with hepatitis C virus is both more common and serious in terms of morbidity than co-infection with hepatitis B virus (48–50,71,72). There is no evidence that HIV infection per se is directly oncogenic to primary liver cells; thus, any increase in the number of people with primary liver cancer in Nigeria and other African countries may be due to increased incidence of infection by hepatitis B and C viruses and/or improved diagnostic capabilities. Certain ARV therapies may also act on hepatitis viruses and therefore slow the progression of HIV co-infection with hepatitis B or C viruses (48–50). ARVs may also exacerbate liver disease in people co-infected with HIV and hepatitis C virus, however, through increased hepatotoxicity (48,49).

Respiratory Disease

The respiratory tract may be involved in various ways during symptomatic HIV disease. Upper respiratory infections may occur early in some patients, caused by common respiratory pathogens, such as *Haemophilus influenzae, Staphylococcus aureus,* and *Klebsiella pneumoniae.* Respiratory disease may also be caused by opportunistic infections as a result of prolonged HIV infection. Patients with HIV-related pneumonia or pneumonitis often present with cough, fever, and shortness of breath, which may become severe as the disease progresses.

Limited facilities and poor manpower capacity make diagnosis of *Pneumocystis carinii* pneumonia (PCP) difficult in most resource-poor African nations (42,73–75). Although sputum tests are easy to perform and are routinely done, they do not yield the necessary accuracy for diagnosis. Moreover, the more reliable and sensitive investigative techniques used for diagnosing PCP—such as PCR—are not generally available in sub-Saharan countries because of their high costs and the lack of adequate laboratory expertise. Therefore, they are neither in routine use nor satisfactorily standardized. Additionally, the signs and symptoms of PCP may closely mimic those of pneumonia from causes other than HIV infection. This may partly explain why PCP has not been reported commonly in Nigerians or other Africans with HIV disease.

In terms of numbers, complications, and severity, co-infection with *Mycobacterium tuberculosis* is one of the most common and serious respiratory diseases in people with symptomatic HIV disease (76–78). Pulmonary tuberculosis is the most common form. The diagnosis of tuberculosis is simple, as sputum examination may be all that is required in most patients when a positive smear stained with Ziel-Nielsen shows acid-alcohol-fast bacilli. Other diagnostic methods can increase the sensitivity to nearly 100% (79). In some cases, HIV-infected people suspected of having tuberculosis on clinical or radiological grounds may be sputum negative, in which case it may be necessary to employ other rigorous diagnostic procedures, such as sputum culture or PCR. Patients with suspected HIV-associated tuberculosis and possible brain lesions of other etiologies should undergo computerized tomographic (CT) scanning and magnetic resonance imaging (MRI) to rule out brain tumors.

The incidence of tuberculosis is significantly higher in HIV-infected people than in those without infection (39–41,80). The clinical presentation of tuberculosis is the same regardless of association with HIV infection; however, the disease severity may be higher in people with immunodeficiency. For instance, those with tuberculosis may present with bilateral hilar adenopathy, interstitial fibrosis, collapse/consolidation, pleural effusions, and cavitating disease. Tuberculosis associated with HIV infection may also affect the cardiovascular system and present as pericarditis with or without effusions. Central nervous system infection by *Mycobacteria* may cause meningitis, while ascites may occur in gastrointestinal involvement. Disseminated tuberculosis is a serious condition predisposing to miliary presentation, polyarthritis, osteolytic lesions, and paravertebral abscess.

Hematologic Disease

The cardiovascular system may be directly affected in a number of ways during symptomatic disease, with manifestations ranging from minor peripheral immune-complex–mediated vascular lesions to septicemia. Common hematologic disturbances in HIV-infected people include anemia, thrombocytopenia, lymphopenia, lymphocytosis, and mild lymphadenopathy. Lymphopenia results from persistent HIV infection, concomitant with progressive destruction of CD4+ lymphocytes. As depletion of CD4+ cells continues, the imbalance between CD4+ and CD8+ lymphocytes progresses, often reversing the CD4+/CD8+ cell ratio. The reversed ratio is attributable largely to severe depletion of CD4+ cells, rather than an absolute rise in CD8+ lymphocyte numbers.

Persistent generalized lymphadenopathy (PGL) is one of the earliest clinically recognized features of symptomatic HIV disease. For this reason, it was one of the first illnesses used to diagnose AIDS before definitive laboratory indices were developed. PGL is thought to result from progressive and rapid turnover of infected lymphocytes in the lymph nodes (81). The lymph nodes are clinically indistinguishable from other causes of lymph node enlargement, underscoring the need to exclude other causes, such as tuberculosis and lymphomas.

Lymphomas and Kaposi's sarcoma are among the opportunistic tumors that occur in HIV-associated disease. Both Hodgkin's and non-Hodgkin's lymphoma may occur in patients with HIV disease, the most common forms being diffuse large-cell lymphomas with widespread extranodal involvement (54). Moreover, an association exists between HIV-related lymphomas and Epstein-Barr virus, as well as human herpesvirus type 8 (52,54,82). HIV-related Hodgkin's lymphoma occurs late during HIV disease and is more advanced than autonomous Hodgkin's disease.

Central Nervous System Disease

Numerous central nervous system (CNS) manifestations of HIV disease occur, as well as peripheral neuropathies, neuronitis, and mononeuritis. Neuropsychiatric manifestations also arise in people with HIV-related CNS disease (83,84). Dementia is common in patients with advanced HIV disease and is often known as AIDS dementia complex (83,84). While the exact mechanisms by which HIV causes CNS manifestations remain unclear, the virus infects and is cytopathic to neuronal cells (85–89). In addition, some patients present with features of meningeal irritation or meningitis because of opportunistic infections by *Mycobacterium tuberculosis*, *Cryptococcus* sp., *Streptococcus pneumoniae*, *Meningococcus* sp., or *Toxoplasma gondii*. Primary brain lymphoma, characterized by focal or multifocal neurologic deficits, is another clinical CNS manifestation of HIV disease, the diagnosis of which is facilitated by CT and MRI scans (54). Progressive multifocal leukoencephalopathy occurs in association with human polyoma JC virus (90). Other CNS pathologies include astrocytomas and ependymomas, although these are rare. Bacteremia due to co-infection with *Streptococcus pneumonia* or *Escherichia coli* may cause meningitis, thereby increasing mortality among HIV-infected people with severe immune dysfunction (91).

HIV INFECTION IN NIGERIA

The minister of health announced Nigeria's first confirmed case of HIV infection in 1986, followed by a formal report from the National Institute of Medical Research, the one institution with the appropriate facilities to confirm HIV infection at the time. Studies that began soon afterward demonstrated that the HIV seroprevalence rate in the general population ranged between 0.15% and 1.3% (92–95). The authors of these initial publications concluded that the incidence of HIV infection in Nigeria was low, and that Nigeria was the African country least affected by HIV at the time. The same researchers also reported that the highest incidence of infection was among female sex workers and their patrons, commercial blood donors, long-distance truck drivers, and those with sexually transmitted infections. A one-year follow-up study by one group showed a 9.81% rise in seroprevalence among sex workers and concluded that the rate of HIV infection would increase sharply within a few years unless appropriate preventive measures were taken (96). Unfortunately, the lower rates of infection found among "low-risk" groups is these early studies contributed to the country's denial about its growing epidemic.

Since these early studies, the estimated seroprevalence of HIV infection in Nigeria has risen to 5.0% overall (97). Considering the size of Nigeria's population, this means that as many as six million Nigerians may be infected with HIV. Thus, although no longitudinal investigations of rising HIV prevalence were carried out at the time, by the late 1990s it had become clear that Nigeria's epidemic had changed from one concentrated in high-risk populations to a more generalized epidemic, resulting in an epidemic that resembled those in Central Africa and southern Africa (98).

One of the problems that delayed early action on the HIV epidemic in Nigeria was the lack of political and financial commitment at the highest level. The National Expert Advisory Committee on AIDS, which the minister of health instituted in 1986, was full of ivory-tower clinicians and scientists and short on social workers, counselors, health education specialists, media and communications experts, and people living with HIV/AIDS. No community, religious, or traditional leaders were involved—a serious omission in Nigeria. Real progress began only in 2000, when a new political leadership placed HIV/AIDS at the top of the national agenda, with President Olusegun Obasanjo himself chairing a new National Action Committee on AIDS (NACA). The president also personally led advocacy campaigns, a significant undertaking in Nigeria, making citizens appreciate the serious nature of the epidemic and the need to take preventive measures. For the first time, the government provided substantial funding for multimedia communication and research. The levels of denial, shame, stigma, discrimination, and similar negative perceptions of HIV/AIDS decreased, making way for more honest and open discussions of the epidemic. In 2001, the government also committed to providing a heavily subsidized ARV program.

With published data on HIV in Africa relatively sparse, the paucity of scientific information, particularly on the pathophysiology and clinical manifestations of infection, has continued. In Nigeria, such data are especially limited, as research has generally been a low priority, leading to a lack of funding for scientific investigations (99). Most of the early seroprevalence studies on HIV/AIDS in Africa were carried out in East Africa, Central Africa, and southern Africa. Nigeria's need for additional research to characterize the pathophysiology HIV infection and disease progression has grown critical.

Initially, sentinel surveillance was conducted with considerable difficulty in Nigeria, leading to insufficient data on which to plan or base intervention strategies. For many years seroepidemiology remained the only method for ascertaining HIV prevalence in Africa, though a few sophisticated investigations were also carried out (100); at same time, many African clinicians questioned whether seroepidemiology or clinical epidemiology should be used to estimate prevalence. Despite being asymptomatic, HIV-infected people have laboratory abnormalities, many of which may be nonspecific in nature. For instance, some may have moderately low hemoglobin levels, neutropenia, lymphopenia, and other hematologic abnormalities, such as low platelet counts (101). In much of Africa, including Nigeria, the inability to run confirmatory tests for HIV infection has contributed to the rapid spread of HIV infection. Inexpensive, simple assays, such as ELISA, are now available in Africa, but monitoring the progress of HIV disease, with or without ARV treatment, requires more complex and expensive assays that tend not to be generally available, such as quantitating the amount of virus in the blood, or viral load. Thus, many people perceived the overall threat of HIV/AIDS to be low until a critical threshold of "visible" HIV infections or AIDS cases became evident in society.

The response to HIV/AIDS in Africa is accentuated by large-scale poverty, limited access to education, inadequate health care, and poor health care systems. As resources become available for ARVs, the requisite needs for adequate infrastructure and human capacity will slow the scale-up efforts. Furthermore, the migration of many highly qualified professionals from poor developing countries ravaged by the HIV pandemic to countries in North America and Europe compounds the problem (102,103).

The early studies in Nigeria showed that the HIV seroprevalence rate was highest among the 16-to-30-year age group (94). One epidemiologic study revealed that within one year (1987 to 1988), the seroprevalence rose from 0.2% to 1% (96). It was widely believed that HIV first arrived in Nigeria several years after high rates of HIV infection were reported from Central Africa, then regarded as the focus of the infection (104,105). The clinical manifestations and disease progression of HIV/AIDS in Nigeria resemble those found in other African countries.

MANAGEMENT AND CONTROL

Early in the HIV epidemic, no drugs were capable of reducing HIV replication, slowing disease progression, or prolonging the life of people with HIV. Consequently, the management of HIV/AIDS was extremely difficult and frustrating. Effective ARVs became available only much later. Yet unlike developed countries, the resource-poor countries of Africa could not—and most still cannot—afford to procure or regularly supply the drugs to people with HIV/AIDS to prolong their lives. In addition, facilities for clinical and laboratory diagnosis were—and in many countries remain—poor or nonexistent, so even when ARVs were affordable and available, treatment safety and efficacy could not be properly monitored. Ignorance, discrimination, stigmatization, denial, and poverty remain major factors driving the HIV/AIDS epidemic and hindering effective control measures.

ARV therapy has, no doubt, provided greater hope for longer lasting survival and improved quality of life (106,107). Apart from their high cost, however, the need for combination therapy—a minimum of three drugs—may be problematic. In addition, the treatment is not always tailored toward individual patient responses to the particular drugs being used. For many years, effective ARVs were unavailable, and when they became available, it was difficult to make decisions about their use in Nigeria, as was the case in much of sub-Saharan Africa. These drugs have progressively become more available largely on account of reduced costs brought about by allowing developing countries to manufacture generic formulations. Intervention by international agencies and donor countries has contributed significantly to the campaign to make ARVs more affordable to the people in poor developing countries who are the most in need of these drugs. On a number of occasions, ARVs have not reached the individuals for whom they were intended. Instead, officials responsible for distributing or administering them have diverted them inappropriately, charging patients more for the drugs.

Logistical problems, political considerations, and the weakness and incapacity of the health systems have further compromised the fair and equitable distribution of ARVs in many African countries. In some developing countries, ARV access has been subject to political considerations; rather than allowing clinical or professional criteria to determine which people received ARVs, governments have withheld drugs from people perceived as their political opponents. Education of clinicians on the multiple combinations of the drugs most appropriate for individual patients or access to these combinations continues to be problematic, impeding rapid progress in treatment and control of the infection. The infrastructure is still poor and the capacity to monitor ARV therapy inadequate. Moreover, patient education, acceptance, and adherence continue to hinder treatment efforts. Many infected people are reluctant to be tested for HIV, even after they develop signs of HIV disease. When they agree to be tested, they are often reluctant to reveal their HIV status because of the stigma. In Nigeria, all these constraints are gradually giving way to more openness and a better understanding of HIV/AIDS. At the same time, caregivers and physicians are becoming more familiar with combination ARV therapy, and facilities for diagnosis and monitoring treatment continue to improve.

Management and control of the HIV pandemic and disease progression depend heavily on international assistance to poor developing countries. Rich developed countries were slow to come to the rescue of sub-Saharan Africa. Even after realizing the gravity of the socioeconomic damage and the sharp rise in disease burden from HIV/AIDS, these countries offered assistance that has not been able to make a significant difference to the affected countries. The more recent establishment of large-scale intervention initiatives — such as the Global Fund for HIV/AIDS, Tuberculosis and Malaria; the Millennium Development Goals; and the Global Alliance for Vaccines and Initiatives — are laudable (108–110). Logistical problems and incapacity in poor countries are hampering progress, however, making timely attainment of the intended goals unlikely (111–114). Some countries, including the United States, have already served notice that the Millennium Development Goals must be re-focused or even abandoned.

CONCLUSION

The general clinical and pathogenesis features of HIV infection and disease are no different in Nigeria than in other African countries. Although the early epidemic was thought to be less pronounced in Nigeria than elsewhere in Africa, the country's estimated 5% prevalence rate is equivalent to the current estimates for the rest of the continent. This underscores the need for increased prevention efforts and support services, including access to ARV treatment and care.

The clinical and diagnostic limitations that have hindered progress in understanding the pathophysiologic basis and clinical manifestations of HIV infection are diminishing. Improved infrastructures and capacity are infusing the health care system, and increased access to HIV/AIDS education, prevention, and treatment is reducing stigmatization and encouraging a more open approach to the crisis. This new positive approach to HIV/AIDS in Nigeria provides hope for efforts to curb the epidemic and control the disease.

REFERENCES

1. Gottlieb MS, Schroff R, Schanker HM, et al. *Pneumocystis carinii* pneumonia and mucosal candidiasis in previously healthy homosexual men: evidence of a new acquired cellular immunodeficiency. *N Engl J Med,* 1981;305:1425–1431.

2. Siegal FP, Lopez C, Hammer GS, et al. Severe acquired immunodeficiency in male homosexuals, manifested by chronic perianal ulcerative herpes simplex lesions. *N Engl J Med,* 1981;305:1439–1444.

3. Masur H, Michelis MA, Green JB, et al. An outbreak of community-acquired *Pneumocystis carinii* pneumonia: initial manifestation of a cellular immune dysfunction. *N Engl J Med,* 1981;305:1431–1438.

4. Chikwem JO, Chikwem SD, Ola TO. Evaluation of public awareness and attitudes to acquired immune deficiency syndrome. *Niger Med Pract,* 1988;16(5/6):159–162.

5. Adebamowo CA, Ezeome ER, Ajuwon JA, et al. Survey of knowledge, attitude and practice of Nigerian surgery trainees to HIV-infected persons and AIDS patients. *BMC Surgery,* 2002;2: 23–41.

6. Salihu N, Olaseha I, Adeniyi JD, et al. Knowledge and attitude of physicians and nurses about AIDS in Sokoto, Nigeria. *Int J Health,* 1998;36:26–28.

7. Clerici M, Declich S, Rizzardini G. African enigma: key player in human immunodeficiency virus pathogenesis? *Clin Diagn Lab Immunol,* 2001;8(5):864–866.

8. Ezedinachi EN, Ross NW, Meremike M, et al. The impact of an intervention to change health workers' HIV/AIDS attitudes and knowledge in Nigeria: a controlled trial. *Public Health,* 2002:116:106–112.

9. World Health Organization. Acquired immunodeficiency syndrome (AIDS). 1987 revision of CDC/WHO case definition of AIDS. *Wkly Epidemiol Rec,* 1988;63:1–7.

10. Barre-Sinoussi F, Chermann JC, Rey F, et al. Isolation of a T-Lymphotropic retrovirus from a patient at risk for acquired immune deficiency syndrome (AIDS), 1983. *Rev Invest Clin,* 2004;56(2):126.

11. Gallo RC, Montagnier L. The discovery of HIV as the cause of AIDS. *New Engl J Med,* 2003;349(24):514–515.

12. Montano M, Williamson C. Molecular biology of HIV-1. In: Essex M, Mboup S, Kanki PJ, Marlink RG, Tlou SD, eds. *AIDS in Africa.* 2nd ed. New York: Kluwer Academic/Plenum Publishers, 2002:11–33.

13. He J, Chen Y, Farzan M, et al. CCR3 and CCR5 are coreceptors for HIV-1 infection of microglia. *Nature,* 1997;385:645–649.

14. Tien PC, Chiu T, Latif A, et al. Primary subtype C HIV-1 infection in Harare, Zimbabwe. *J Acquir Immune Defic Syndr Hum Retrovirol,* 1999;20:147–153.

15. Lee B, Doranz BJ, Rana S, et al. Influence of the CCR2-V64I polymorphism in human immunodeficiency virus type 1 coreceptor activity and on chemokine receptor function of CCR2b, CCR3, CCR5, and CXCR4. *J Virol,* 1998;72:7450–7458.

16. van Rij RP, de Roda Husman AM, Brouwer M. Role of CCR2 genotype in the clinical course of syncytium-inducing (SI) or non-SI human immunodeficiency virus type 1 infection and in the time to conversion to SI virus variants. *J Infect Dis,* 1998;178:1806–1811.

17. Michael NL, Louise LG, Rohrbauch AL, et al. The role of CCR5 and CCR2 polymorphism in HIV-1 transmission and disease progression. *Nat Med,* 1997;3:1160–1162.

18. Gomez C, Hope TJ. The ins and outs of HIV replication. *Cell Microbiol,* 2005;7(5):621–626.

19. Cann AJ, Karn J. Molecular biology of HIV: new insights into the virus lifecycle. *AIDS*, 1989;3 (Suppl 1):S19–S34.

20. Shih CK, Rose JM, Hansen GL, et al. Chimeric human immunodeficiency virus type 1/type 2 reverse transcriptases display reversed sensitivity to nonnucleoside analog inhibitors. *Proc Natl Acad Sci USA*, 1991;88(21): 9878–9882.

21. Rodes B, Holguin A, Soriano V, et al. Emergence of drug resistance mutations in human immuno-deficiency virus type 2-infected subjects under-going antiretroviral therapy. *J Clin Microbiol*, 2000; 38(4):1370–1374.

22. Auwerx J, Stevens M, Van Rompay AR, et al. The phenylmethylthiazolylthiourea nonnucleoside reverse transcriptase (RT) inhibitor MSK-076 selects for a resistance mutation in the active site of human immunodeficiency virus type 2 RT. *J Virol*, 2004; 78(14):7427–7437.

23. Perach M, Rubinek T, Hizi A. Resistance to nucleo-side analogs of selective mutants of human immun-odeficiency virus type 2 reverse transcriptase. *J Virol*, 1995;69(1):509–512.

24. Buckheit RW Jr, Watson K, Fliakas-Boltz V, et al. SJ-3366, a unique and highly potent nonnucleoside reverse transcriptase inhibitor of human immunod-eficiency virus type 1 (HIV-1) that also inhibits HIV-2. *Antimicrob Agents Chemother*, 2001;45(2): 393–400.

25. Hizi A, Tal R, Shaharabany M, et al. Specific inhibi-tion of the reverse transcriptase of human immun-odeficiency type 1 and type 2 by nonnucleoside inhibitors. *Antimicrob Agents Chemother*, 1993;37(5): 1037–1042.

26. Buckheit RW Jr, White EL, Fliakas-Boltz V, et al. Unique anti-human immunodeficiency virus activ-ities of the nonnucleoside reverse transcriptase inhibitors calanolide A, costatolide, and dihydro-costatolide. *Antimicrob Agents Chemother*, 1999;43(8): 1827–1834.

27. Corbett JW, Ko SS, Rodgers JD, et al. Expanded-spectrum nonnucleoside reverse transcriptase inhibitors inhibit clinically relevant mutant vari-ants of human immunodeficieny virus type 1. *Antimicrob Agents Chemother*, 1999;43(12):2893–2897.

28. Lamarre D, Croteau G, Wardrop E, et al. Antiviral properties of palinavir, a potent inhibitor of the human immunodeficiency virus type 1 protease. *Antimicrob Agents Chemother*, 1997;41(5):965–971.

29. Pilcher CD, Eron JJ, Galvin S, et al. Acute HIV revisited: new opportunities for treatment and pre-vention. *Clin Invest*, 2004;113(7):937–945.

30. Dyer JR, Eron JJ, Hoffman IF, et al. Association of CD4 T cell depletion and elevated blood and semi-nal plasma human immunodeficiency virus type 1 (HIV-1) RNA concentrations with genital ulcer disease in HIV-1-infected men in Malawi. *J Infect Dis*, 1998;177:224–227.

31. McCune JM, Hanley MB, Cesar D, et al. Factors influencing T-cell turnover in HIV-1 seropositive patients. *J Clin Invest*, 1999;105:R1–R8.

32. Sibanda EN, Stanczuk G, Kasolo F. HIV/AIDS in Central Africa: pathogenesis, immunological and medical issues. *Int Arch Allergy Immunol*, 2003;132.

33. Autran B, Carcelian G, Li TS, et al. Positive effects of combined antiretroviral therapy on CD4+ T-cell homostasis and function in advanced HIV disease. *Lancet*, 1997;227:112–116.

34. Lederman MM, Connick E, Landay A, et al. Immunologic responses associated with 12 weeks of combination antiretroviral therapy consisting of zidovudine, lamivudine and ritonavir. *J Infect Dis*, 1998;178:70–79.

35. Plana M, Garcia F, Gallart T, et al. Immunological benefits of antiretroviral therapy in the very early stages of asymptomatic chronic HIV-1 infection. *AIDS*, 2000;14:1921–1933.

36. Lawn SD, Butera ST, Folks TM. Contribution of immune activation to the pathogenesis and trans-mission of human immunodeficiency virus type 1 infection. *Clin Microbiol Rev*, 2001;14:753–777.

37. Mohammed I, Williams EE. Acquired immune deficiency syndrome. *Nig Med Pract*, 1987;14:41–55.

38. Fauci AS. Host factors and pathogenesis of HIV 1 induced disease. *Nature*, 1996;384:529–534.

39. U.S. Centers for Disease Control and Prevention. Nosocomial transmission of multi-drug-resistant tuberculosis among HIV-infected persons. Florida and New York, 1988–1991. *MMWR*, 1991;40:595–591.

40. Edlin BR, Tokars JL, Grieco MH, et al. An outbreak of multidrug-resistant tuberculosis among hospi-talized patients with the acquired immunodefi-ciency syndrome. *N Engl J Med*, 1992;326:1514–1521.

41. Daley CL, Small PM, Schecter GF, et al. An outbreak of tuberculosis with accelerated progression among persons infected with the human immunodeficiency virus. An analysis using restriction-fragment-length polymorphisms. *N Engl J Med*, 1992;326:231–235.

42. Thomas CF, Limper AH. *Pneumocystis* pneumonia. *N Eng J Med*, 2004;350:2487–2498.

43. Deayton JR, Sabin CA, Johnson MA, et al. Importance of cytomegaloviraemia in risk of disease progression and death in HIV-infected patients receiving highly active antiretroviral therapy. *Lancet*, 2004;363:2116–2121.

44. Fisk DT, Meshnick S, Kazanjian PH. *Pneumocystis carinii* pneumonia in patients in the developing world who have acquired immunodeficiency syndrome. *Clin Infect Dis*, 2003;36:70–78.

45. Specter SA, Hsia K, Crager M, et al. Cytomegalovirus (CMV) DNA load is an independent predictor of CMV disease and survival in advanced AIDS. *J Virol*, 1999;73(8):7027–7030.

46. Allen AI, Martin-Mazuelos E, Lozano F, et al. Correlation of fluconazole MICs with clinical outcome in cryptococcal infection. *Antimicrob Agents Chemother*, 2000;44(6):1544–1548.

47. Denkers EY, Gazzinelli RT. Regulation and function of T-cell-mediated immunity during *Toxoplasma gondii* infection. *Clin Microbiol Rev*, 1998;11(4):569–588.

48. Chung R, Kinm A. HIV/hepatitis B and coinfection: pathogenic interactions, natural history and therapy. *Antivir Chem Cheomother*, 2001;12:73–91.

49. Konopnicki D, Mocroft A, de Bit S, et al. Hepatitis B and HIV: prevalence, AIDS progression, response to highly active antiretroviral therapy and increased mortality in the EuroSIDA cohort. *AIDS*, 2005;19(6):593–601.

50. Sherman KE, O'Brien J, Gutierrez AG, et al. Quantitative evaluation of hepatitis C virus RNA in patients with concurrent human immunodeficiency virus infections. *J Clin Microbiol*, 1993;31:2679–2682.

51. Gatphoh ED, Zamzachin G, Devi SB, et al. AIDS related malignant disease at regional institute of medical sciences. *Indian J Pathol Microbiol*, 2001;44:1–4.

52. Ablashi DV, Chatlynne LG, Whitman JE Jr, Cesarman E. Spectrum of Kaposi's sarcoma-associated herpesvirus, or human herpesvirus 8, diseases. *Clin Microbiol Rev*, 2002;15(3):439–464.

53. Weissenborn SJ, Funke AM, Hettmich M, et al. Oncogenic human papillomavirus DNA loads in human immunodeficiency virus-positive women with high-grade cervical lesions are strongly elevated. *J Clin Microbiol*, 2003;41(6):2763–2767.

54. Ng VL, McGrath MS. HIV-associated lymphomas. In: Cohen PT, Sande MA, Volbering PA, eds. *The AIDS Knowledge Base*. 3rd ed. Philadelphia: Lippincott Williams & Wilkins, 1999:381–385.

55. Valle S-L. Dermatologic findings related to human immunodeficiency virus infection in high risk individuals. *J Amer Acad Dermatol*, 1987;17:951

56. Safar B, Johnson KG, Myskowski PL, et al. The natural history of Kaposi's sarcoma in the acquired immune deficiency syndrome. *Ann Intern Med*, 1985;103(5):744–750.

57. Tappero JW, Conant MA, Wolfe SF, et al. Kaposi's sarcoma. Epidemiology, pathogenesis, histology, clinical spectrum, staging criteria and therapy. *J Am Acad Dermatol*, 1993;28(3):371–395.

58. Feigal DW, Katz MH, Greenspan D, et al. The prevalence of oral lesions in HIV-infected homosexual and bisexual men: three San Francisco epidemiology cohorts. *AIDS*, 1991;5:519.

59. Mabruk MJ, Antonio M, Flint SR, et al. A simple and rapid technique for the detection of Epstein-Barr virus DNA in HIV-associated hairy leukoplakia biopsies. *J Oral Pathol Med*, 2000;29:118–122.

60. Triantos D, Leao JC, Porter SR, et al. Tissue distribution of Epstein-Barr virus genotypes in hosts coinfected by HIV. *AIDS*, 1998;12:2141–2146.

61. Sharma SK, Kadhiravan T, Banga A, et al. Spectrum of disease in a series of 135 hospitalised HIV-infected patients from north India. *BMC Infect Dis*, 2004;4:52.

62. Johnson JF, Sonnenberg A. Efficient management of diarrhea in the acquired immunodeficiency syndrome (AIDS): a medical decision analysis. *Ann Intern Med*, 1990;112:942–948.

63. Conlon CP, Pinching AJ, Perera CU, et al. HIV-related enteropathy in Zambia: a clinical, microbiological, and histological study. *Am J Trop Med Hyg*, 1990;42:83–88.

64. Sewankambo N, Mugerwa RD, Goodgame R, et al. Enteropathic AIDS in Uganda. An endoscopic, histological and microbiological study. *AIDS*, 1987;1: 9–13.

65. Henry MC, De Clercq D, Lokombe B, et al. Paracytological observations of chronic diarrhea in suspected AIDS adult patients in Kinshasa (Zaire). *Trans R Soc Trop Med Hyg*, 1986;80:309–310.

66. Goodgame RW. Understanding intestinal spore-forming protozoa: Cryptosporidia, Microsporidia, Isospora and Cyclosporia. *Ann Intern Med*, 1996;124: 429–141.

67. Colebunders R, Lusakumuni K, Nelson AM, et al. Persistent diarrhea in Zambian AIDS patients: an endoscopic and histological study. *Gut*, 1988;29: 1687–1691.

68. Drobniewski F, Kelly P, Carew A, et al. Human microsporidiosis in African AIDS patients with chronic diarrhea. *J Infect Dis*, 1995;171:515–516.

69. Doehring E, Reiter-Owona I, Baur O, et al. *Toxoplasma gondii* antibodies in pregnant women and their newborns in Dar es Salaam, Tanzania. *Am J Trop Med Hyg*, 1995;52:546–548.

70. Guebre-Xabia M, Nurulign A, Gebre-Hiwot A, et al. Sero-epidemiological survey of *Toxoplasma gondii* infection in Ethiopia. *Ethiop Med J*, 1993;31:201–208.

71. Nelson KE, Thomas DL. Reciprocal interaction of human immunodeficiency virus and hepatitis C virus infections. *Clin Diag Lab Immunol*, 2001;8(5): 867–870.

72. Matthews-Greer JM, Caldito GC, Adley SD, et al. Comparison of hepatitis C viral loads in patients with or without human immunodeficiency virus. *Clin Diagn Lab Immunol*, 2001;8(4):690–694.

73. Hopewell PC. *Pneumocystis carinii* pneumonia: diagnosis. *J Infect Dis*, 1988;157(6):1

74. Davey RT, Jr, Masur H. Recent advances in the diagnosis, treatment and prevention of *Pneumocystis carinii* pneumonia. *Antimicrob Agents Chemother*, 1990; 34(4):499–504.

75. Rous P, Lavrard I, Poirot JI, et al. Usefulness of PCR for detection of *Pneumocystis carinii* DNA. *J Clin Microbiol*, 1994;32:2324–2326.

76. Sepkowitz KA, Raffalli J, Riley L, et al. Tuberculosis in the AIDS era. *Clin Microbiol Rev*, 1995;8: 180–199.

77. Smole SC, McAleese F, Ngampasutola J, et al. Clinical and epidemiological correlates of genotypes within the *Mycobacterium avium* complex defined by restriction and sequence analysis of hsp65. *J Clin Microbiol*, 2002;4(9):3374–3380.

78. Thomson VO, Dragsted UB, Baur J, et al. Disseminated infection with *Mycobacterium genavense*: a challenge to physicians and microbiologists. *J Clin Microbiol*, 1999; 37(2):3901–3905.

79. Walker D, McNerney R, Mwembo MK, et al. An incremental cost-effectiveness analysis of the first, second and third sputum examination in the diagnosis of pulmonary tuberculosis. *Int J Tuberc Lung Dis*, 2000;4:246–251.

80. Bandera A, Gori A, Catozzi L, et al. Molecular epidemiology study of exogenous re-infection in an area with a low incidence of tuberculosis. *J Clin Microbiol*, 2001;39(6):2213–2218.

81. Schnittman AM, Fauci AS. Human immunodeficiency virus and acquired immune deficiency syndrome: an update. *Adv Intern Med*, 1994;39:305–354.

82. Foreman KE, Bacon PE, His ED, Nickoloff BJ. In situ polymerase chain reaction-based localization studies support role of human herpesvirus-8 as the cause of two AIDS-related neoplasms: Kaposi's sarcoma and body cavity lymphoma. *J Clin Invest*, 1997; 99(12):2971–2978.

83. Atkinson JH, Grant I. Natural history of neuropsychiatric manifestations of HIV disease. *Psychiatr Clin North Am*, 1994;17:17–33.

84. Atwood WJ, Berger JR, Kaderman R, et al. Human immunodeficiency virus type 1 infection of the brain. *Clin Microbiol Rev*, 1993;6(4):7211–7220.

85. Power C, McArthur JC, Nath A, et al. Neuronal death induced by brain-derived human immunodeficiency virus type 1 envelope genes differs between demented and nondemented AIDS patients. *J Virol*, 1998;72(11):9045–9053.

86. Zheng J, Ghorpade A, Niemann D, et al. Lymphotropic virions affect chemokine receptor-mediated neural signalling and apoptosis: implications for human immunodeficiency virus type 1-associated dementia. *J Virol*, 1999;73(10):8256–8267.

87. Brooke S, Chan R, Howard S, Sapolsky R. Endocrine modulation of the neurotoxicity of gp120: implications for AIDS-related dementia complex. *Proc Natl Acad Sci USA*, 1997;94(17):9457–9462.

88. Conant K, Garzino-Demo A, Nath A, et al. Induction of monocytes chemoattractant protein-1 in HIV-1 Tat-stimulated astrocytes and elevation in AIDS dementia. *Proc Natl Acad Sci USA*, 1998;95(6): 3117–3121.

89. Iskander S, Walsh KA, Hammond RR. Human CNS cultures exposed to HIV-1 gp120 reproduce dendritic injuries of HIV-1-associated dementia. *J Neuroinflammation*, 2004;10:7.

90. Shwartz SA, Nair PN. Current concepts in human immunodeficiency virus infection and AIDS. *Clin Diagn Lab Immunol*, 1999;6(3):295–385

91. Afessa B, Morales I, Weaver B. Bacteremia in hospitalised patients with human immunodeficiency virus: a prospective cohort study. *BMC Infect Dis*, 2001;1:3.

92. Chikwem JO, Mohammed I, Oyebode T, et al. Prevalence of human immunodeficiency virus (HIV) infection in Borno State of Nigeria. *E Afr Med J*, 1988;65(5):342–346.

93. Williams EE, Mohammed I, Chikwem JO, et al. HIV-1 and HIV-2 antibodies in Nigerian populations with high- and low-risk behavior patterns. *AIDS*, 1990;4(10):1041–1042.

94. Harry TO, Kyari O, Mohammed I. Prevalence of human immunodeficiency virus infection among pregnant women attending antenatal clinic in Maiduguri, north-eastern Nigeria. *Trop Geogr Med*, 1992;44:238–241.

95. Harry TO, Ekenna O, Chikwem JO, et al. Seroepidemiology of human immunodeficiency virus infection in Borno State of Nigeria by sentinel surveillance. *J Acquir Immun Deficiency Syndr*, 1993;6: 99–103.

96. Chikwem JO, Mohammed I, Ola T. Human immunodeficiency virus type 1 (HIV-1) infection among female prostitutes in Borno State of Nigeria: one year follow-up. *East Afr Med J*, 1989;66(11):752–756.

97. Federal Ministry of Health. *HIV/Syphilis Sero-Prevalence and STD Syndromes Sentinel Survey among PTB and STD Patients in Nigeria*. Abuja: Federal Ministry of Health, 2003.

98. Mann J. Worldwide epidemiology of AIDS. In: Fleming AF, Carbello M, eds. *The Global Impact of AIDS*. New York: Alan R. Liss Inc., 1988:3–7.

99. Kanki P. Viral determinants of the HIV/AIDS epidemic in West Africa. *BMJ, West Africa Edition*, 2004: 7(2):69–71.

100. Piot P, Bartos M. The epidemiology of HIV and AIDS. In: Essex M, Mboup S, Kanki PJ, Marlink RG, Tlou SD, eds. *AIDS in Africa*. 2nd ed. New York: Kluwer Academic/Plenum Publishers, 2002:72–101.

101. Dominquez A, Gamallo G, Garcia R, et al. Pathophysiology of HIV related thrombocytopenia: an analysis of 41 patients. *J Clin Pathol*, 1994;47:999.

102. Hagopian A, Thompson MJ, Fordyce M, et al. The migration of physicians from sub-Saharan Africa to the United States of America: measures of the African brain drain. *Hum Resour Health*, 2004;2:17.

103. Coombes R. Developed world is robbing African countries of health staff. *BMJ*, 2005;330:923.

104. Vandpitte J, Verwilghen R, Zachee P. AIDS and cryptococcosis (Zaire 1977). *Lancet*, 1983;1:925–26.

105. Bygbjerg IC. AIDS in a Danish surgeon (Zaire 1976). *Lancet*, 1983;1:925

106. Weidle PJ, Timothy DM, Alison DG, et al. HIV/AIDS treatment and HIV vaccines for Africa. *Lancet*, 2002;359:2261–2267.

107. Jordan R, Gold L, Cummins C, et al. Systematic review and meta-analysis of evidence for increasing numbers of drugs in antiretroviral combination therapy. *BMJ*, 2002;324(7340):757.

108. United Nations. *United Nations Millennium Development Goals (MDG)*. Geneva: United Nations, 2000.

109. More funds for health: the challenge facing recipient countries. *Bull World Health Organ*, 2002;80:164–165.

110. Mozyuski P. Global Fund calls for increased HIV funding. *BMJ*, 2005;331:533.

111. Dyer O. UN predicts that millennium development goals will be missed by a wide margin in Africa. *BMJ*, 2005;330:1350.

112. Mayor S. Poorer countries will not meet health targets, warns WHO. *BMJ*, 2005;331:7.

113. Wyss K. An approach to classifying human resources constraints to attaining health-related Millennium Development Goals. *Hum Resour Health*, 2004;2:11.

114. Figures J. The road to reform: look to the neighbours. *BMJ*, 2005;331:170–171.

7 SOCIAL AND CULTURAL FACTORS AFFECTING THE HIV EPIDEMIC

Lawrence Adeokun*

The complexity of the HIV/AIDS epidemic stems from its links with all aspects of society and culture. Social and cultural factors affect not only viral transmission, but also the success of prevention strategies and the compassion with which people living with the virus are treated. A clear understanding of those factors therefore becomes a point of departure for planning the control of the epidemic.

KEY ASPECTS OF THE EPIDEMIC

Three aspects of the HIV epidemic shape the role of social and cultural factors in its propagation and, in turn, modify the culture of the people as they respond to the epidemic: the known modes of transmission; the ways in which the biomedical imperatives of AIDS shape the popular imagery of the epidemic; and the immediate social and cultural responses to the epidemic.

Known Modes of Transmission

Heterosexual transmission accounts for as many as 95% of HIV infections in Nigeria, where having multiple sexual partners has been a major behavioral factor fueling the epidemic. Consequently,

*Association for Reproductive and Family Health, Ibadan, Nigeria

customs and social practices that produce sexual networks have been the major focus of behavioral surveillance. Details of sexual practices such as dry sex also have received attention, with the assumption that men prefer dry sex (1), leading to trauma that can facilitate HIV transmission (2–4).

Other transmission modes are nonetheless intimately linked to culture as well. High fertility preferences, elevated female infection rates, and low levels of voluntary counseling and testing (VCT) make mother-to-child transmission of HIV an inevitable element of the unfolding epidemic. Inadequate levels of prenatal care and poor delivery services render blood transfusions to pregnant women common. The patchy distribution of HIV screening services expose significant segments of the urban poor and rural populations to unscreened blood. Homosexual transmission may also play a role, as there are anecdotal reports of men having sex with men within traditional and religious frameworks or in response to demands created by sex tourism in the metropolitan centers. Homosexual practices have also been reported for incarcerated populations (5). Finally, nonsexual traditional practices—particularly male and female circumcision and the custom of creating facial and body markings with shared, non-sterile skin-piercing implements—expose significant numbers of people to infection as well.

Imagery of the Epidemic Based on Biomedical Features

The initial characterization of HIV infection as fatal helped both to define the epidemic and to shape people's responses to those infected and affected by it. This characterization aided the scare tactics employed for creating mass awareness of the epidemic. Although it is now known that antiretrovirals can help people with HIV achieve long-term survival, the subtle distinction between managing and curing a condition eludes the understanding of most people, including policy makers.

The dominance of sexual transmission of HIV and the corollary that frequent episodes of sexually transmitted infections (STIs) facilitate HIV transmission are largely responsible for the stigma of promiscuity attached to HIV infection even when people are not sexually infected. The continent as a whole faced the stigmatization of AIDS, increasing the reluctance of many African governments to acknowledge the severity of the epidemic openly (6,7) and, until recently, to make HIV prevention and management major priorities (8).

In addition, the long latency between HIV infection and the development of AIDS-related conditions reduces the likelihood that people will associate a particular sexual contact with the time of transmission (9). It also compromises the role of VCT in helping to prevent transmission.

Social and Cultural Responses to the Epidemic

People's beliefs about disease causation ultimately influence their health-care–seeking behavior and efforts to protect themselves from infection. Many Nigerians believe that the origins of ailments are not as simple as modern medicine posits. According to Caldwell, Orubuloye, and Caldwell, the syncretic nature of African religion—the beliefs that events are multicausal and that the timing of death is predestined—resulted in an initial underreaction to AIDS (6). A fatalistic attitude allowed some people to remain in denial about the epidemic. Orubuloye and Oguntimehin demonstrated that this indifference to the prospect of death produces a high risk-taking sexual culture among men and little behavior change in response to HIV prevention interventions (10).

The reluctance to talk about sex within marriages and between generations also has delayed the public health response to a sexually transmitted epidemic. Many Nigerians believe that fertility-associated diseases are in a special category, treatable by indigenous practitioners. Wasting, a dominant feature of AIDS, also is perceived as linked to witchcraft. The alien image of AIDS adds to its stigma and encourages the perception of AIDS as retribution for those who engage in immoral activities.

In addition, the country's high levels of infant and childhood mortality draw attention away from complications arising from the secondary epidemic of pediatric AIDS and the need to make prevention of mother-to-child transmission (PMTCT) a robust element of HIV/AIDS control programs.

FEATURES OF THE NIGERIAN EPIDEMIC

Sentinel Data Quality and the Role of Migration

Information about the patterns of the Nigerian epidemic comes from sentinel surveys conducted between 1991 and 2001 (11,12). The difficulty of applying the sentinel data to the general population arises from the nature of the sentinel groups and the large size and population of Nigeria. Nevertheless, the broad pattern of HIV infection that emerges in these surveys gives a clear idea of the similarities between the Nigerian epidemic and those of more mature epidemics in eastern and southern Africa (13). Apart from the usual sentinel groups—women receiving antenatal care, sex workers, people with tuberculosis, and STI patients—voluntary and involuntary migration connected with local and international travel, refugee movements, and army movements have emerged as major factors in the spread of the virus across countries, borders, and regions. The culture of mobility is basic to human existence and development.

It took a decade after that first reported case in 1986 for Nigeria's HIV prevalence rate to reach 4.5%. The relative delay of the emergence of a Nigerian epidemic—compared to the eastern and southern African regions (14)—has been attributed to a number of reasons, including differences in levels of male circumcision and in the practice of polygamy.

It is tempting to speculate that sexual networks differ significantly from region to region. But according to Orubuloye et al., people in Yorubaland are thought to have as many sex partners as those in eastern and southern African countries with severe HIV epidemics (15). According to Caldwell et al., a declining degree of polygamy in southern and eastern Africa allows males to marry earlier, and the length of postpartum sexual abstinence is notably shorter in those regions than in Nigeria (16). These changes, however, have not produced the postulated declines in male non-marital sex and sexual networking.

In 1992 the researchers speculated that Nigeria's lower HIV prevalence might be due to its near-universal practice of male circumcision at infancy. The rareness of male circumcision in other parts of Africa also has been suggested as a reason for the spread of HIV in those areas (17). Whatever the validity of the circumcision hypothesis, it has since become clear that the pace of the epidemic is now no less relentless in Nigeria than in other regions of sub-Saharan Africa.

Variations in Nigeria's HIV/AIDS Prevalence Rates

The geographic variations in Nigeria's HIV prevalence rates suggest two likely explanations (11,12). First, previous hubs of STIs—such as in the tin-mining area of Plateau and in the petroleum industry of the Delta region—are primed for the rapid spread of HIV. According to Carael and Makinwa, the large-scale presence of other STIs may account for the rapid spread of HIV in some regions (16). Second, urban areas and the network of roads that link them throughout the country have produced arteries of infection that stand out from the more remote rural areas of the country. Both explanations are firmly rooted in the phenomenon of migratory movements between areas with depressed economies and areas of economic prosperity. It is related to the preponderance of male migration, which produces a low sex ratio in places of origin and a high sex ratio at the destinations.

Immediate Research and Programmatic Responses

Social Surveillance

Against the background of the stigma attached to AIDS, the limitations of sentinel survey data, and the overall pessimism about the quick development of a cure, the initial research response focused on the social surveillance of the epidemic. In this context, the role of social and cultural factors was viewed as largely negative. Investigators assumed that an understanding of the negative cultural factors would help correct or eradicate those factors. While this approach has helped raise AIDS awareness, based largely on scare tactics, it has not contributed significantly to the attitude and behavior changes needed to halt the spread of infection or to help individuals and communities cope with the consequences of the epidemic.

It is becoming clear that the culture has positive factors that can be harnessed to make behavior change communication (BCC) interventions plausible and effective. The exploitation of these factors in a number of ongoing projects has formed the basis of a tentative, yet evidence-based conclusion that the positive aspects of culture will increasingly become better researched as people move away from the image of HIV as incurable to a more balanced view—that with a combined strategy of well-considered BCC, VCT, and antiretroviral programs, HIV can be survived for long periods and the epidemic can be brought under control.

Condom Use

Advocating condom use appears logical, but prejudices relating to the role of the condom in family planning appear to be plaguing its promotion as a tool for HIV prevention. Integrating dual protection into family planning services and involving men in dual protection appear to address some of the concerns about condom use (18). The next logical step has been to combine information, education, and communication (IEC) interventions with carefully planned BCC programs targeted at specific groups that offer the right social, economic, and cultural setting for such interventions. The groups that have been most responsive—and that have the greatest potential impact on the epidemic—are market populations, students, out-of-school youths, and health providers in the private sector. These may not be the conventional "risk groups" of the early stages of the epidemic, but they do provide access to significant proportions of the general population who are at risk and urgently in need of behavior change at the disseminated phase of the epidemic.

In short, all biosocial and biomedical aspects of the epidemic are linked to the culture within which people live and die. While social research has thus far focused on negative factors, only a balanced view of the role of social and cultural factors can form the basis of an evenhanded strategy for HIV prevention and management. The next section briefly sketches out a framework for integrating both the positive and the negative social and cultural features.

THE SOCIOCULTURAL FRAMEWORK

Features of the Culture

The features of a culture derive from the components of the demographic and socioeconomic composition of the population. The most important demographic and socioeconomic features are age, sex, residence, education, marital status, and religion, family/social units, and ethnic identity. These features influence the spatial and sexual mobility of people, their exposure to infection, and their health-care–seeking and managing responses.

Age is a changing characteristic with direct impact on sexuality through biological processes as well as social devices. The onset of sexual feelings, the timing of marriage, the sexual debut, and the ability to cope with the demands of sexuality all relate to the age of the individual. Equally powerful is the effect of the link between age and cultural patterns on the level of culture change and cultural shifts (19). The young are, in the right atmosphere, receptive to new lifestyles and ideas.

Sex forms the basis of allocating roles, privileges, and positions open to members of a community. This typecasting of individuals by gender starts from birth. Most societies share these roles and rights in such a way as to subjugate females to males. The sexual domain is marked by some of the most adverse inequities between the sexes, including unequal sexual negotiating powers. The different timing of marriage by sex, the practice of polygamy, and the age gap between spouses within polygamous unions all sustain these inequities (20). So total is the dominance of men that women may be considered to have only duties and responsibilities and no rights (21). Yet the roles of women in the domestic domain make them major assets for caregiving in times of health emergencies (22,23).

In the context of both the age and sex of individuals, Carael and Makinwa have suggested that the tendency for females' first intercourse to occur at a relatively young age in part explains the spread of HIV among female youths (16).

Residence in urban or rural areas helps determine people's economic and social options, opportunities, and limitations. It also creates the context for developing the coping mechanisms for sexual needs, satisfaction, and consequences. Expansion in the entertainment industry resulted in the creation of the drinking bars, brothels, and rooming houses in large towns where rural-urban migrants, single men, and married men all have access to sex for cash. In effect, both urban and rural areas offer challenges and opportunities for HIV prevention and management.

Education, one of the most potent acquired socioeconomic characteristics, is by itself not always the predictor of risk exposure (24). In combination with other lifestyle issues—such as opportunity for travel, type of employment, and access to cash income—though, it is closely related to the dynamics of HIV infection, prevention, and management in a population. In effect, both a negative and a positive feedback loop operate between education and the epidemic.

The type of marriage may influence the sexual practices within each type and thus affect the potential exposure to the risk of HIV infection within marriage. The link operates through differential age at marriage between monogamous and polygamous women, the length of postpartum sexual abstinence, and lactational amenorrhea. Although a strong negative relationship exists between polygamy and community fertility (25), it has been difficult to establish any significant differences in HIV prevalence with the type of marriage. This is hardly surprising since serial monogamy is an alternative to having multiple sexual partners (26).

According to Caldwell, Orubuloye, and Caldwell, polygamy for the Ekiti Yoruba means a reduction of the access of some males to mates and an occasion for engaging in premarital and extramarital sexual activities (27). Those male sexual needs are met by sex workers in urban areas and by a significant number of divorced, separated, or widowed women. In addition, certain living and cultural arrangements facilitate the sexual access of young family members to the wives of older relatives (15) or the access of visitors to wives of hosts (28). All these devices are likely predictors of exposure to sexual networks and to HIV infection.

Within polygamy or outside of marriage, young girls are often the preferred and possibly the easier targets of older men. The public health implication shows up in the differential levels of infection between young males and young females in some populations (29).

Religion plays a major role in both social behavior and health belief systems. Religion and modernization are modifying some of the sexual excesses of males within traditional sexual codes, yet this modification may be contributing to an increase in the use of sex workers.

Other features of family formation have a potential impact on the epidemic. In the past, the universality of marriage and the early timing of marriage served as safety nets for reducing the incidence of premarital sex and promiscuity (30). Mate selection processes are now less autocratic and allow greater sexual experimentation between consenting adults than in the past. Even religious dogma and values have failed to reverse the trend (6,24). The ease with which children born out of wedlock can receive legal status is a major factor driving this liberal mate selection process. In effect, having multiple sexual partners may not be seen in terms of loose morals but as an integral part of mate selection. Adapting the process to HIV prevention may be more feasible than its drastic modification or condemnation.

The formation of social units — such as the family, trade groups, and ad hoc self-help groups — is based on combinations and permutations of these demographic and social parameters. Some units, such as the family, are formed after elaborate rituals and processes, while others are temporal and easy to form and dissolve as occasion demands. These social units provide the setting within which the interaction of culture, sexuality, and risk of HIV infection takes place. So complex are these interactions that an assumption of a static and predictable role of social and cultural factors in the epidemic is likely to be invalid. As with other social and demographic variables, the epidemic can alter the structure and functionality of a family, yet the family is also the frontline unit for caring for people infected with or affected by HIV.

Ethnic identity is the medium through which all the social and economic variables are filtered, and individuals make decisions that they believe confirm that identity. In Nigeria, with a population of more than 130 million and 247 ethnic groups (31), it is unhelpful to assume that cultural practices affecting sexual and reproductive health are monolithic and universal to all ethnic groups. Such practices as bride wealth (32) and postpartum abstinence can vary significantly between, and in some cases, within the major Nigerian ethnic groups (33). What is needed therefore is a brief exploration of the ways in which cultural changes from within and without can be used to design constructive roles in HIV prevention.

Changing Culture from Without and from Within

In the course of modifying culture and the relationship between the sexes, the actors often justify the new norms in terms of the benefits they confer on society in general. That way, the new patterns of behavior associated with the new norms are not classified as deviant (34). Moderating influences can have a range of sources; in general, influences from without are more potent than those from within the society.

The Place of Global Acculturation

Ramel has suggested that the spectacular human development over the past 10,000 years can be ascribed entirely to a cultural rather than genetic evolution (35). Apart from the localized changes in culture, the post–World War II period has witnessed dramatic changes in the economy, civil rights, women's rights, and the associated sexual freedom. These changes include new emerging norms about the desirability of marriage, the optimal timing of children, and the involvement of fathers in child-bearing and of mothers in breadwinning (36). The sexual freedom came with new codes and mores regarding sexual negotiation between the sexes, with the most remarkable being the visibility of commercial sex work in different cultures and at different strata of society. The oldest profession became an open profession. The role of education has been pivotal to these changes, and the horizontal spread of information through mass media may be accelerating the cultural evolution and a concomitant loss of cultural diversity.

Cultural Classification, Hybridization, and Parental Control

Some degree of cultural change and hybridization is taking place in Nigeria, especially in the sexual behavior of youths as they attempt to combine elements of Western sexual norms with traditional sexual norms. This development can produce significant variation in sexual identities different from those that are based on traditional values or easily explained in terms of modernization and religious values (37).

The hybridization of sexual culture can be traced to the loss of parental control as society has moved from a subsistence economy to a patchy market economy. To explain the causes of adolescent pregnancy in Cameroon, Ilinigumugabo et al. have postulated that the social pressures once placed on adolescents to control their sexual behavior have been greatly reduced due to youth attending schools far from home and to new behavior modes promoted by school peers and the mass media (38). Under the new autonomy of the young, poverty has led some girls to exchange sexual relations for gifts.

Globalization and Poverty

Not all culture changes and influences are beneficial. Globalization can be cited as the primary cause of disease distribution and incidence of modern epidemics (39). An associated phenomenon is that the drugs needed to treat emerging and re-emerging diseases are priced beyond the reach of people in poor countries, often the most in need of affordable treatments. Globalization presents both challenges and opportunities, however, that can be harnessed to balance some of the inequities in periods of health emergencies such as the HIV epidemic (40).

Family Planning, Economic Downturns, and the Collapse of Health Systems

The decline in fertility in sub-Saharan Africa is a product of significant changes in cultural values relating to family formation and aspirations. A rising age at marriage, an increase in contraceptive use, improved school attendance among girls, and changes in cultural norms and family relationships have contributed greatly to the fertility decline (41). Some of these reproductive behavior gains have produced a side effect: the delay in marriage has created a period of heightened risk of premarital sexuality. The line of protection that family planning and dual protection can offer in an epidemic is compromised by the decay of health systems in response to the global economic downturn of the past decades and the persistent effect in the rising level of poverty in sub-Saharan Africa.

Family planning services have been targeted mainly at married women who have had their husband's consent. The needs of youth, men, and women not in a union have been neglected. Consequently the institutional and resource framework with which to respond to the HIV/AIDS emergency has been lacking. This vacuum has aggravated the negative links between culture and the epidemic.

The Idealized View of Sex Culture

Some contradictions arise in the conceptualization of sexual culture in societies experiencing rapid modernization. On the one hand, traditional sexual codes are supposed to be strong and strict for the young female. Orubuloye et al. argue, however, that extensive premarital and extramarital sexual activity is deeply rooted in traditional culture, and is supported largely by women's long period of postpartum abstinence, which men use as an occasion to engage in extramarital sexual affairs (42). Traditional society allows young, unmarried men to enjoy premarital sex, and about three-quarters of postpubertal males, married or unmarried, can be without current access to a wife or sexual activity because of prolonged postpartum female sexual abstinence (27). The fact that males are not correspondingly more affected by the HIV epidemic makes an examination of the basis of male sexual codes necessary.

Male Sexual Codes

The differential male sexual code is premised on the prevailing notion that male sexuality cannot be contained or confined to a single woman. In a 1994–95 survey, Orubuloye et al. found that 41% of urban men, 59% of rural men, 27% of urban women, and 36% of rural women hold this view of male sexual needs (20). Half of the urban wives and three-quarters of the rural wives surveyed believed that greater love within marriage could curb the extramarital escapes of men. One-third believed that the fear of AIDS could effect behavioral changes in the men. This male sexual code is consistent with the earlier view of Yoruba marriage by Caldwell and Caldwell as deemphasizing husband-wife emotional relationships and marital female sexuality (43). Modern education and Christian values may play a part in the development of emotional ties within marriage and the reduction in promiscuity. Promoting such emotional content within marriage is certainly consistent with HIV prevention. It is also a potential behavior change outcome that IEC/BCC interventions should take into account.

Clarification of Sexual Networks

Another strand of the social surveillance of HIV/AIDS has been the clarification of the sexual networks of high-risk groups. The initial assumption was that the impact of sexual networking on the epidemic would significantly differ between those that involved sex workers and those that involved other members of the general population (44). It was conceded, however, that the economic returns to young women from commercial sex were so high and the social sanctions so weak that it was unlikely that the tide of inflow into commercial sex work could be stemmed, AIDS or no AIDS. In effect, the lucrative nature of commercial sex work broke down some of the gender codes of sexual behavior by granting young women the option of exploiting their bodies to greater economic effect and survival.

MIGRATION AND HIV/AIDS IN NIGERIA

The mobility of people is an integral part of human development, transforming the demographic, social, and economic circumstances of populations. This same mobility, however, becomes an agent for the spread of epidemics. Given that the etiology of HIV/AIDS is well known and that the disease is associated with particular, known transmission sites and routes, the study of the mobility of the populations that come into contact with such sites can help determine the actual patterns of transmission and can contribute to the formation of HIV prevention and control strategies (45). This principle informed the study of the transfer of first outbreak of malaria in the 1960s and 1970s and later HIV from high-incidence areas to low-incidence areas via the human vector (46–48). This principle has also affected the attention focused on the links between migration and the spread of HIV from the early hot spots of infection to other areas.

In a review of scientific and other literature during the 1990s that links migration and mobility with the spread of STIs, including HIV, in West and Central Africa, Lydie and Robinson (49) came to several conclusions that have relevance for the Nigerian epidemic:

- With the exception of Senegal, countries with high emigration and immigration rates tend to have high levels of HIV infection;
- The main destinations of West African immigrants are Senegal, Nigeria, and Côte d'Ivoire;
- Both the risk of infection and the rate of HIV transmission vary among migrants; and
- Little exists in the literature that substantiates hypotheses about a strong association between migration and HIV-positive status.

These conclusions can enhance our understanding of the dynamics of the Nigerian epidemic and the development of appropriate prevention strategies. First, before the emergence of the HIV epidemic, parts of Nigeria—especially in the southwest (now northern Oyo State)—had more than half a century of migrant labor (50), trading, and commercial sex contacts with Ghana and Côte d'Ivoire, two West African countries that turned out to be the region's earliest hot spots for HIV.

Second, these migratory contacts persist to the extent that major northern Yoruba towns such as Ejigbo, Ogbomoso, and Iwo have transport depots where "commuting migrants" can take international road transport at affordable prices whenever they want. These transport nodes in southwest Nigeria certainly provide points of potential contact for the type of research that Lydie and Robinson suggest (49).

Third, migrants tend to be in their most economically productive years and in the most sexually active and mobile age groups.

And fourth, it can be deduced from the patchy literature on these migratory waves that, with the exception of refugees, most of the classic risk groups linked with HIV spread are represented in the migrant population—migrant laborers, long-distant truck drivers, itinerant traders, and sex workers.

The West African HIV/AIDS Corridor

Decosas suggests that international migration has shaped the profile of the HIV epidemic in West Africa (14). Côte d'Ivoire, the main country of immigration, has by far the highest HIV prevalence along the West Coast. That country has distinct foci of infection in Abidjan and in the agro-industrial centers of Daloa and Bouaké. According to Kouamé, migrants made up 40% of the population of Abidjan (51). More than half of the sex workers in Abidjan are from Ghana. This dominance of commercial sex activities by Ghanaians may in part explain why Ghana became a focus of HIV-2 in the early stages of the

West African epidemic. By 1993, HIV seroprevalence in the Abidjan region was estimated at more than 10% for the general population and at least 80% for sex workers.

Decosas and others observed that 25% of Côte d'Ivoire's total population comprised migrants from other countries (52). Sex workers were brought in to meet the sexual needs of plantation workers, with each woman serving about 25 men. This pattern of sexual networking must have contributed to that country's elevated HIV prevalence rates, which are higher than estimated for sex workers in less adverse situations (53).

Another potentially significant channel of transmission is through migrants returning to Nigeria after long periods of residence on cocoa farms in both Ghana and Côte d'Ivoire and gold-mining activities in Ghana. The economic and political crises in these countries in the past two decades probably aided the transfer of large number of returnees and an appreciable number of HIV-infected people from those countries. Nigeria has other cross-border contacts with Cameroon and Niger, but none carries the same potential epidemiologic significance as those along the West Coast.

In-Country Population Movement and HIV/AIDS in Nigeria

Nigeria's significant in-country flows between regions and between rural and urban areas have implications for the spread of HIV. Such movements can be effective in reducing urban-rural differentials in HIV prevalence. In connection with the geographic spread of Guinea worm, Watts observed that Yoruba women are highly mobile and travel widely (45). Travel during festivals and celebrations and the seasonal circulation of migrant farm laborers and their families may result in the long-distance transmission of Guinea worm infection. In the same way, the movement of traders and workers within Nigeria—between cities and the rural areas and between poor regions and areas of commercial activities, such as in the petroleum mining sector—contribute to the significance of the link between migration and HIV transmission and its prevention and management.

Ososanya and Brieger's study of migratory movements between Igbo-Ora and Lagos among 377 residents aged 15 to 49 years found that 62.3 percent were female and 81.7% had traveled an average of 3.6 times to Lagos in the preceding six months (54). One in fifty traveled with their spouses. Almost half of the respondents had sexual partners in Lagos, and just over one-third of those had more than one. One in twelve respondents reported a history of STIs. Of these, nearly three-quarters attributed the infections to non-spouses. Just over one-quarter of the respondents or their partners used condoms. Condom use increased with education, and single migrants were more likely than married ones to use condoms. In focus groups, greed for economic gain, the existence of sexual networks, peer approval, and crowded housing conditions in Lagos were suggested as factors encouraging risky sexual behavior. Women traders were described as being especially able to conduct numerous clandestine affairs. The same surely can be true of men, except they may be more blatant as they are away from home and are subject to less rigorous sanction if their behavior is discovered

In a study of another Yoruba village, Ago Are, Ajuwon and others were able to show that even small villages along main trade routes have female sex workers in residence (55). Most of their clients are commercial drivers and migrant farm laborers. The authors observed that both premarital and extramarital sex, although against local custom, were common in their study site. Like Orubuloye et al. (15) they attributed the practice of extramarital sex to other customs such as postpartum abstinence, wife inheritance, frequent informal divorces, and polygamy. In effect, the breach of one set of cultural values is made possible by another set that facilitates the breach. Holidays, festivals, and the presence of return migrants from the city also encourage casual sexual encounters that can be critical in the introduction of HIV into rural areas.

Much larger settlements along Nigerian transport arteries such as Ilorin (56) have elaborate infrastructures that sustain the sex trade (15). The low education and high mobility of most of the drivers and transport workers who patronize the sex workers place these men at a disadvantage for accessing information. In addition, many long-haul drivers have unprotected casual and commercial sex. These men include both homosexuals and heterosexuals, and they often take drugs and suffer high STI rates (57).

Peacekeeping and HIV Infection
Peacekeeping operations by Nigerian soldiers in Liberia, Sierra Leone, Côte d'Ivoire, the former Yugoslavia, and Somalia at various times have produced other distinct strands of net transfer of infection from these countries to Nigeria. The lifestyle of peacekeeping officers is characterized by high levels of multiple sexual partners, low condom use, and exposure to blood transfusions in the line of duty. After an initial period of secrecy surrounding the extent of the HIV/AIDS problem in the military and among returning peacekeeping forces, the Nigerian military is addressing the spread of HIV among soldiers (58). The coming out of soldiers living with HIV/AIDS has raised awareness of the impact of peacekeeping expeditions on the spread of HIV. It has also helped shape the public policy on HIV in Nigeria. The privileged position of the military means that policies made for it set standards to which the public HIV/AIDS policy can aspire, such as the introduction of a free antiretroviral program for infected soldiers (59).

Nigerian police officers also have been involved in peacekeeping operations, mostly within Nigeria but occasionally abroad. Their sexual lifestyles are no less risky than those of soldiers (60). They maintain modest levels of condom use and high rates of STIs, take advantage of modern medical treatment, and report good rates of partner notification when infected but low rates of notifying their spouses about infection episodes.

Sex Tourism by Nigerian Females Traveling To Europe
A combination of the popularity of air travel and the downturn of the Nigerian economy has produced an increase in sex tourism to some European countries by young Nigerian females, including well-educated yet unemployed females easily drawn into foreign sex work. Oladepo and Brieger found that 29.2% of university students in their study had sexual relations during travel outside of Nigeria (61). Sex tourism has potential implications for the spread of HIV, the development of coinfections with HIV-1 and HIV-2, and an increase in the range of HIV subtypes found in Nigeria. Given the better education of those involved, however, they may be able to monitor their health, maintain a higher level of

condom use, and experience less frequent episodes of STIs. These circumstances will likely limit the public health significance of sex tourism for the Nigerian epidemic. Yet a large cluster of HIV-infected returning female sex tourists into an area of origin could have a devastating effect on the course of the epidemic in the area.

International Travel and Tuberculosis

HIV-positive people coinfected with tuberculosis are more likely to die from tuberculosis than from any other condition. The popularity of air travel and exposure to tuberculosis on long international flights is also a potential link between migration and HIV infection, morbidity, and mortality from AIDS (62).

Male Migration and Sexuality

The impact of male labor migration affects both the sexuality of mobile males and the females with whom they have sex. While conditions in Nigeria are not as dramatic as in parts of eastern and southern Africa (63), the relatively high incidence of female-headed households and low sex ratios create similar conditions in the fishing and mining communities of the country's Delta and Middle Belt regions. The migrant men include fishermen, traders, farmers, and refugees. Decosas estimates that 3% of West African men live in camps and temporary accommodations while away from their families and communities (14). These migrants have sex with sex workers while traveling and living in temporary places of residence. Those who contract HIV then transmit the virus to other short- and long-term sex partners at their temporary places of residence and in their places of origin.

Forced Migration and Refugees

The timing of the forced migration of Ghanaians from Nigeria because of the shrinking oil economy and growing political pressure (64,65) was such that it had little impact on the HIV epidemic. Today such a massive transfer of population from one of the foci of HIV infection to another country could precipitate an increase in rates of transmission. This is precisely why the refugee movements from war-affected areas of Liberia and Sierra Leone in the late 1980s and mid-1990s may have introduced new infections as well as new subtypes into the Nigerian population.

Research Implications

For some of the puzzles surrounding the migration-and-HIV-infection hypothesis to be solved Lydie and Robinson have called for research on the migrants' duration of trips, frequency of return visits, living conditions, sexual activities, and behavior before their departure, along the routes, at their final destination, and at the time of their return (49). Behavioral surveillance that could link biomedical HIV surveillance with individual-level data on the migration and medical history would be the best source for this type of information. At the conceptual level, though, the gatekeepers on the migratory routes should receive as much attention as the migrants themselves. The police, military personnel, and custom officers—most of whom are male—are co-actors with women eager to maximize their profit and avoid payment of high official and unofficial tariffs along the borders. These are the sex-for-cash transactions frequently mentioned in anecdotes of traders along the West Africa corridor.

Ironically, the women involved in these transactions may not view themselves as sex workers and may not attach the same significance to their behavior that epidemiologists do. But they are more likely to become involved with multiple sexual partners and less likely either to be in a superior negotiating position with their "mentors" or to be able to negotiate condom use. In effect, the absence of strong evidence-based association between migration and HIV status is no reason to ignore the potential role of cross-border movement and the dynamics of the Nigerian epidemic, especially in the southwest, where the West Coast trade corridor connects with Nigeria.

DISTINGUISHING BETWEEN POSITIVE AND NEGATIVE FACTORS

In making the distinction between positive and negative cultural influences, it is worth re-emphasizing that heterosexual transmission of HIV predominates in Nigeria. The bases of prejudicial sexual customs include liberal sexual codes for males, subordination of females in sexual relations, early marriages, and the reluctance to discuss sex. This reluctance further reinforces the norms and their persistence.

Two points about the exploitation of culture for HIV prevention should be made, however. The first is that there are non-prejudicial customs that can facilitate HIV/AIDS prevention and management. The challenge is to find ways of maximizing their contribution to programs. The second observation is that some cultural factors are often the wrong target of HIV prevention programs because they may be compatible with safer sex behavior (28). Attacks on culture are also not the best entry points into HIV prevention.

Positive Cultural Choices

There are five related requirements for successfully exploring positive cultural values in HIV prevention through effective BCC programs:

- Choosing the most culturally relevant mode of communication;
- Identifying the most suitable platforms for interacting with the target population;
- Diagnosing the hierarchical structure within social groups;
- Using the appropriate protocol that will facilitate but not unduly force cooperation with HIV prevention programs; and
- Devising and testing the health belief model that most closely approximates those of the local population.

Relevant Modes of Communication

With the exception of the Yoruba, who have experience with large pre-industrial agglomerations (66), most traditional communities in Nigeria are small. Political and social organizations in such communities tend to value face-to-face communication, and interactions are highly verbal. In the context of culture and AIDS, community dialogue is one of those non-prejudicial customs that can be employed in

HIV prevention initiatives. Talking in formal groups is a common feature of community decision-making processes that has been moved into the political, religious, and social realms.

Evaluation studies of IEC/BCC programs often identify the utility of health talks to audiences. This principle suggests that verbal interactions in focus groups discussions are particularly useful in consensus building and in generating inter-community dialogue about new ideas, controversies, or innovations. Plays and skits—live or on radio or television—extend the role of verbal communication further. Implicit in the choice of verbal communication is the preference for particular platforms for interacting with target populations.

Suitable Platforms for Interacting with Target Populations

The basis of ethnic and cultural identity in most Nigerian ethnic groups relates to the place of birth. In effect, the settlement is the first platform for interacting with a target population. Lower levels are the compounds into which agnates—or relatives on the father's side—aggregate, and within them are the families and finally the individuals who can exercise varying degrees of autonomy in their dealings, depending on their demographic and socioeconomic characteristics.

The social platforms form a second layer to the settlement platform. The major avenues of interaction are linked to traditional rituals that take place in connection with births, deaths, marriages, and social mobility. Others are linked to commerce, largely conducted in traditional markets.

Different occupations have formal and informal avenues for bringing people into groups, so the traditional role of group identity can be further reinforced by the common aims of the trade group. In this connection, modern health facilities become new platforms for health behavior modifications and the care-seeking needs of the population.

Religious bodies and associations are also gaining in relevance as platforms for molding moral values and character. Religious leaders have regular and intense contacts with millions of Nigerians on a weekly and even daily basis. In some sense, the teachings of these leaders have irrevocably changed the culture of the people. Are these leaders suitable candidates for catalyzing behavior change? Do they have any influence on the sexual life of their followers and are they willing to take on the responsibility?

Early in the epidemic, the prevailing view among religious leaders was that God had sent AIDS as a punishment for sexual sins and other moral failings. One in three religious leaders condemned premarital and extramarital sex and suggested that a reduction in postpartum abstinence and the promotion of monogamy were the answers to stemming the spread of HIV. The different positions religious groups hold about polygamy and contraceptive use show up in their attitudes toward the management of the epidemic. In a 1993 study by Orubuloye et al., about three-quarters of the members of the Protestant Communion reported that the HIV epidemic had prompted them to address sexual behavior more often and with greater intensity in their religious discourse than in the past (67). They were also more predisposed to promote family planning and contraceptive use. In contrast, 80% of Muslim leaders objected to contraceptive use. Others, though, could understand that barrier contraceptives had a place within the HIV prevention strategy if AIDS became a problem. More than a decade later, with AIDS emerging as a major health problem, the position of some religious leaders has changed significantly. Some elements persist, however. The Catholic Church maintains a strong opposition to condom promotion, preferring instead to promote abstinence and fidelity.

That same 1993 study revealed an overall reluctance on the part of religious leaders to take responsibility for conducting a campaign against immoral sexual behavior. Their view was that the government was better equipped to handle that task (67).

The educational institution is a major platform for modernization and, by its demographic composition, a crucial platform for HIV prevention efforts. The variety of institutions also reflects the age-sex compositional differences, which must inform how IEC/BCC programs can be tailored to meet the sexual and reproductive health needs of the cohort represented in each type of institution.

Hierarchical Structure within Social Groups

Traditional societies have a love of ritual in the conduct of business. Project staff members should be aware of the hierarchical structure within different social groups to help them gain entry. The acknowledgment of this hierarchy may be merely symbolic, as in most Yoruba towns where the right of informed consent lies with individual households and families. Or it may be more substantive and a precondition for entry into the population in the more feudal societies in northern Nigeria. When there is an overlay of religious leadership on the traditional hierarchy, getting protocols right is helpful to project implementation.

The framework put in place for social control within the markets remains traditional even though the trade articles have extended beyond the sale of agricultural produce. The king holds the land in trust for the community. The market leaders get elected in an open and transparent way. Subgroups based on age, sex, and articles of trade also form with their own leadership structures. Although interactions appear informal, all members know well the rights and obligations of the leaders.

Other domains—such as the family, the neighborhood, and the village—have similar hierarchical structures. Just as religious leaders set the tone for behavior and give guidance to the formation of attitudes to innovation, these other secular leaders play a vital role in the adoption of change. Fundamental changes involving sexual behavior, alteration of disease beliefs, and the adoption of new health-care–seeking behavior are likely to be effective if they are aligned with—but not necessarily dominated or hijacked by—the leadership for their own ends.

Family Structure and Resilience as Factors in HIV/AIDS Management

The family is probably the most remarkable of the social platforms. Its structure is a product of the sexual and reproductive health outcomes of the people. It is also a product of the impact of migration, type of marriage, and demographic composition of its members. The idealized extended family reported in anthropological and ethnographic studies relied on a variety of sources of resources with which to cope with emergencies. In the view of Caldwell et al., the family typically absorbs the burden of an AIDS-affected member (9). But with the erosion of the cohesion of that extended family structure and the costly nature of caring for a person living with HIV/AIDS (PLWHA); it is doubtful whether this cultural feature of Nigerian life can play a major role in caring for PLWHAs.

Ironically, the age selectivity of HIV/AIDS morbidity and mortality creates gaps in family structures and in the quality of life and coping capacity of surviving members, especially AIDS orphans. An understanding of the strength and weaknesses of the family structure can help program designers shape care support programs to the strengths of that structure.

Trans-Theoretical Health Belief Models as the Bases of BCC Strategies

The quality of an HIV prevention intervention ultimately depends on its compatibility with the target population's health belief systems. Negative links exist between beliefs and the HIV epidemic, such as fatalism about death. Planning for survival, however, is equally culturally acceptable. To work, a health belief model must be built on the attitudes and practices of the target population. One such trans-theoretical health belief model in Oyo State successfully moved participants through four stages, from awareness of the danger posed by HIV/AIDS to actual changes in risky behavior.

The Resources Needed for Exploiting Positive Cultural Values

The obstacles to the full exploitation of positive cultural values can be classified as follows: those relating to the familiarity of project staff to the negative cultural links, those relating to the stigma created in the minds of the target population that make them resist program objectives and require a reorientation and exposure to new information with which to fight stigma, and those relating to the cost-benefit analysis of using the positive approach to linking culture and HIV prevention and management.

Staff Training for Change

Project staff members are often selected because of their familiarity with the culture in which the implementation is taking place. That familiarity often forms the basis of their ready acceptance of the negative connotation given to cultural practices linked to HIV infection. Retraining such staff, however, can make them aware of the potential contributions of a positive approach to cultural practices that can assist in HIV prevention.

Removing Stigma and Resistance to Change

Fear, ignorance, and confusion about the finer details of HIV/AIDS are the major causes of the stigma surrounding HIV infection. Awareness creation is often not enough to erase those emotions. At times the eagerness to create awareness can result in a message distortion, as is the case when the image most people associate with AIDS is death (68). In this atmosphere, the efficacy of the proposed behavior change, the motivation of project staff, and the futility of behavior change in the light of the absence of a cure for AIDS make people resist the superficial prescriptions for behavior change, such as "ABC," which promotes *Abstinence, Being* faithful, and *Condom* use. What is becoming clear is that the objectives and methods of intervention must be credible for people to ascribe to them. To achieve that level of communication calls for a sustained period of training of the target population to allow them to understand the logic and feasibility of the modified practices being suggested to them.

HIV surveillance provides a good example of an intervention in which this approach works. If the limited purpose is to obtain epidemiologic or scientific parameters, then a rapid approach that meets the minimum ethical standards can be used to obtain participation. The person is bled, the laboratory tests are undertaken, and the necessary information is obtained. But if the ultimate aim of such surveillance is to prolong the period of non-infection and survival of infection for participants, then the rapid approach must give way to a period of training, followed by adequate monitoring of behavior over the life of the project so the target population can understand the link between the non-infected status or infection survival and adherence to behavior change guidelines. This approach generates frequent contacts between project staff and the target population and provides occasions for clarification of issues linked to science, policy, and personal problems relating to the project.

The body of knowledge needed, even by a layperson, to cope with the prevention or management of HIV infection is substantial. When project staff members have frequent contacts with the target population, they can present information in a gradual and persuasive manner, helping to lessen the perceived barriers to change and to build the self-efficacy that forms the basis of behavior change. Similarly, with more education, people are less likely to endorse stigmatizing beliefs toward HIV/AIDS (68).

Target populations often construe attempts at promoting changes in sex-related social norms and normative beliefs as subversive. This response is prompted by a shift from idealizing culture to the promotion of change based on the adoption of new cultural values, beliefs, and norms (69). But traditional practices—both sexual and nonsexual—often have their origins in a combination of myths and norms. The disease theory underlying such practices may be nil. Consequently, when beliefs or norms have to be reformulated through the logic of modern science, developing an appropriate trans-theoretical model to guide IEC/BCC interventions is an important first step.

The Concept of "Ewu" in Yoruba Health Belief Modeling

As mentioned earlier, a four-phase trans-theoretical model of behavior change based on the Yoruba concept of "*ewu*" (loosely translated as "hazard" or "danger") developed for HIV prevention projects in Oyo State has been shown to be effective in moving participants from the initial stage of awareness of the danger posed by HIV/AIDS to the expected outcome of changing risky behavior. The second stage of self-risk assessment has been crucial to the transition from that awareness to the third stage of being receptive to information and ideas relating to the prevention and management of HIV infection. People may fear AIDS in much the same way they fear electrocution, but it is only when they are helped to make a competent assessment of their chances of being affected that they take intervention seriously. The expected outcome of effecting behavior change largely depends, however, on the fourth stage, during which participants are trained to attain behavioral self-control (70).

It is worth emphasizing that this trans-theoretical model takes advantage of the gregarious attitude of the Yoruba, their preference for joint action to tackle what might be viewed as personal problems, and their use of the open forum as a way of crossing the conventional protocol that culture sets up to separate the generations and the sexes in other domains of existence.

The marketplace provides a wonderful setting for further subversion of the divisive protocol that stands in the way of learning and of acceptance of innovation relating to safer sexual practices. The monthly meetings of various market groups and trade associations are used precisely for the adoption of innovation and new ideas in their profession. The ten two-hour contacts needed to implement the four-stage trans-theoretical model program have been virtually grafted onto these monthly gatherings. Similarly, the methods of communication have been varied to suit the needs of the stages of the model. As a result of the combined IEC/BCC strategies, an initial cynicism or resentment of plans seen as subversive can give way to recognition of the logic between the prejudicial and non-prejudicial customs upon which the behavior change strategies are based.

Other Options for Culture Change

Prospects for Improved Gender Relations

In attempting to make culture a vehicle of HIV prevention, other profound options have been suggested: The emancipation of women can be a powerful means for promoting and sustaining healthy families and societies. A quantum change in the position of women actively advocated in various global initiatives requires a longer timeframe, however, than is appropriate to tackling an emergency on the scale of the HIV epidemic (71). The positive cultural approach to HIV prevention may also help improve relations between the sexes.

Carael and Makinwa suggest that a reduction in the rate of infection among young females can be attained through "demand reduction," which includes major alterations of norms such as making sex with teenage girls socially unacceptable and providing girls with skills and opportunities that reduce their economic and emotional dependence on men (17). This component of gender relations largely depends on the absorptive capacity of economies. There is little basis for optimism that rapid economic growth in Africa will provide the driving force for gender equity. Yet the participation of women in the market economy, particularly in southwest Nigeria, has produced generations of self-employed and assertive women. Their economic autonomy is a major factor in the design of effective BCC programs among market populations (50,72).

Demographic Transition and Culture Change

The transitions producing the decline in population growth as well as the improvement in health—demographic and health transitions—clearly indicate that cultural shifts can take place with dramatic implications for sexual behavior. Fertility decline depends on changes in sexual and reproductive behavior that are also relevant to the links between culture and HIV infection. As in other parts of Africa (73), delayed marriage, changes in the role of women, and contraceptive use for birth spacing have produced a fertility decline in Nigeria (74).

The Place of Dual Protection in Family Planning

Although it is estimated that AIDS mortality will increase over the next five years to afflict 15.5 million people in the 45 worst-hit countries, only in exceptional cases such as in South Africa will the population decline until 2025 before experiencing population increases. The continued population growth will, according to the most recent UN population projections for 2050, be fueled by estimated higher fertility rates for 16 developing countries, which will alone add 374 million people. The higher estimates are particularly important in the cases of Bangladesh and Nigeria (34). This situation raises a vital question as to the role of family planning not just in the management of population growth but also in HIV prevention in Nigeria.

Thirty years after the introduction of family planning services in Nigeria, the impact on fertility reduction has been limited. About one in eight married women uses a modern method. Half of these women rely on hormonal contraceptives, which are highly effective but offer no protection against STIs, including HIV (74). Consequently, the promotion of barrier methods becomes both an issue of increasing method mix within family planning services and a crucial element in HIV prevention. Unlike the exclusive focus on married women, however, dual protection must be made to reach out to the wider constituency of men and women, single or married, who are not the usual clients of the traditional family planning services. A series of studies in Nigeria demonstrated the feasibility of promoting dual protection in and out of family planning clinics and with the involvement of male partners (18).

CONCLUSION

Sentinel survey data reveal that Nigeria's HIV epidemic is moving from the high-risk-group stage to a disseminated phase in the general population. At the same time, knowledge about the virus has moved out of the AIDS-is-a-killer phase to a recognition that infection can be managed to maintain quality of life and survival of infection. In effect, the literature lags behind by being preoccupied with the formation of exclusive networks of so-called high-risk groups. Other networks in the general population can be as prolific as any, especially in the context of a permissive male sexual culture. In addition, the public health focus has shifted from avoiding transmission to making VCT the basis of access to antiretroviral programs.

Given these changes, a continued focus on the negative features of culture and exposure to risk can become counterproductive if it gives a false sense of safety to those who perceive themselves as being free of negative cultural events. On the other hand, attempts at propagating HIV surveillance and advocating VCT are in their relative infancies. For these efforts to be effective and for VCT to become normative, emphasis must shift from the negative features to the positive features of the culture. The fuller range of social and cultural factors should be exploited in a new phase of aggressive HIV prevention efforts and of coping with the secondary epidemic of pediatric AIDS.

REFERENCES

1. Smith J, McFadyen L, Zuma K, Preston-Whyte E. Vaginal wetness: an underestimated problem experienced by progestogen injectable contraceptive. *Soc Sci Med*, 2002;55(9):1511–1522.

2. Baleta A. Concern voiced over "dry sex" practices in South Africa. *Lancet*, 1998;352(9136):1292.

3. Civic D, Wilson D. Dry sex in Zimbabwe and implications for condom use. *Soc Sci Med*, 1996;42(1):91–98.

4. Brown JE, Ayowa OB, Brown RC. Dry and tight: sexual practices and potential AIDS risk in Zaire. *Soc Sci Med*, 1993;37(8):989–994.

5. Okochi CA, Oladepo O, Ajuwon AJ. Knowledge about AIDS and sexual behaviors of inmates of Agodi prison in Ibadan, Nigeria. *Int Q Community Health Educ*, 2000;19(4):353–362.

6. Caldwell JC, Orubuloye IO, Caldwell P. Under-reaction to AIDS in sub-Saharan Africa. *Soc Sci Med*, 1992;34(11):1169–1182.

7. Nigerians divided on AIDS prevalence. International/case rates. *AIDS Wkly*, Oct 10, 1994;12–13.

8. National Action Committee on AIDS. *National HIV/AIDS Behavior Change Communication Strategy (2004–2008)*. Abuja: National Action Committee on AIDS, 2004.

9. Caldwell J, Caldwell P, Ankrah EM, et al. African families and AIDS: context, reactions and potential interventions. *Health Transit Rev*, 1993;(Suppl 3):S1–S16.

10. Orubuloye IO, Oguntimehin F. Death is pre-ordained, it will come when it is due: attitudes of men to death in the presence of AIDS in Nigeria. In: Caldwell JC, Caldwell P, Anarfi J, et al., eds. *Resistances to Behavioural Change to Reduce HIV/AIDS Infection in Predominantly Heterosexual Epidemics in Third World Countries*. Australia: Australian National University, National Centre for Epidemiology and Population Health, Health Transition Centre, 1999;101–111.

11. Federal Ministry of Health. *Sentinel Surveillance Report*. Abuja: Federal Ministry of Health, 1999.

12. Federal Ministry of Health. *HIV/AIDS Sentinel Sero-Prevalence Survey*. Abuja: Federal Ministry of Health, 2001.

13. Adeokun LA, Twa-Twa J, Ssekiboobo A, Nalwadda R. Social context of HIV infection in Uganda. *Health Transit Rev*, 1995;(Suppl 5):S1–S26.

14. Decosas J. Special report: West Africa. Migration factor makes regional approach essential. *AIDS Anal Afr*, 1995;5(3):8–9.

15. Orubuloye IO, Caldwell JC, Caldwell P. Sexual networking and the risk of AIDS in southwest Nigeria. In: Dyson T, ed. *Sexual Behaviour and Networking: Anthropological and Socio-cultural Studies on the Transmission of HIV*. Liege, Belgium: Editions Derouaux-Ordina, 1992:283–301.

16. Caldwell JC, Caldwell P, Orubuloye IO. The family and sexual networking in sub-Saharan Africa: historic regional differences and present day implications. Health Transition Working Paper No. 5. Canberra, Australia: Australian National University, National Centre for Epidemiology and Population Health, Health Transition Centre, 1990;35.

17. Carael M, Makinwa B. AIDS underlines need for action in sub-Saharan Africa. *Glob Health Environ Monit*, Winter 2000;8(1):3.

18. Adeokun L, Mantell JE, Weiss E, Delano GE, Jagha T. Promoting dual protection in family planning clinics in Ibadan, Nigeria. *Int Fam Plan Perspect*, 2002;28(2):87–95.

19. Lieberson S. A brief introduction to the demographic analysis of culture. *Soc Cult Sect Newsl*, 1992;6(4):21–23.

20. Orubuloye IO, Caldwell JC, Caldwell P. Perceived male sexual needs and male sexual behaviour in southwest Nigeria. *Soc Sci Med*, 1997;44(8):1195–1207.

21. Khan SA. Following in my sister's footsteps. Pakistan. *Real Lives*, Feb 2001;6:17.

22. Oppong, C. Occupational and conjugal inequalities and insecurity: effects on family organization and size. In: Federici N, Mason KO, Sogner S, eds. *Women's Position and Demographic Change*. Oxford, England: Clarendon Press, 1993;339–359.

23. Oppong C. The seven roles and the status of women: outline of a conceptual and methodological approach. (Les sept roles et le status des femmes: l'ébauche d'une approache conceptuelle et methodologique.) In: *Guides anthropologiques et questionnaires pour l'etude des changements demographiques et des roles des femmes.* Geneva: Bureau International du Travail, 1986;93–129.

24. Chang JS. What do education and work mean? Education, nonfamilial work/living experiences and premarital sex for women in Taiwan. *J Comp Fam Stud,* 1996;27(1):13–40.

25. Hern WM. Polygyny and fertility among the Shipibo of the Peruvian Amazon. *Pop Stud,* 1992; 46(1):53–64.

26. Adeokun LA, Nalwadda RM. Serial marriages and AIDS in Masaka district. *Health Transit Rev,* 1997: (Suppl 7):S49–S66.

27. Caldwell JC, Orubuloye IO, Caldwell P. The destabilization of the traditional Yoruba sexual system. *Popul Dev Rev,* 1991;17(2):229–262, 373–375.

28. Gausset Q. AIDS and cultural practices in Africa: the case of the Tonga (Zambia). *Soc Sci Med,* 2001;52(4):509–518.

29. Abdool Karim Q, Abdool Karim SS, Singh B, Short R. Seroprevalence of HIV infection in rural South Africa. *AIDS,* 1992;6(12):1535–1559.

30. Farooq GM, Adeokun LA. Impact of a rural family planning program in Ishan, Nigeria, 1969–1972. *Stud Fam Plann,* 1976;7(6):158–169.

31. Talbot PA. Birth: prenatal and birth ceremonies, etc. In: Talbot PA. *The Peoples of Southern Nigeria: A Sketch of Their History, Ethnology and Languages, with an Abstract of the 1921 Census.* Vol. 2. Ethnology. London: Oxford University Press, 1926:352–423.

32. Isiugo-Abanihe UC. Bridewealth, marriage and fertility in the east-central states of Nigeria *Genus,* 1995;51(3–4):151–178.

33. Adeokun LA. Marital sexual relationships and birth spacing among two Yoruba sub-groups. *Africa,* 1982;52(4):1–14.

34. The United Nations revises its world population predictions upward. (L'ONU revoit à la hausse ses prévisions sur la population mondiale.) *Equilibres et Populations,* 2001;(66):5.

35. Ramel C. Man as a biological species. *Ambio,* 1992;21(1):75–78.

36. Bianchi SM, Casper LM. American families. *Popul Bull,* 2000;55(4):1–44.

37. Carrillo H. Cultural change, hybridity and male homosexuality in Mexico. *Cult Health Sex,* 1999;1(3): 223–238.

38. Ilinigumugabo A, Walla G, Azombo M. *Causes and Consequences of Adolescent Pregnancy in Cameroon.* (Causes et conséquences des grossesses chez les adolescentes au Cameroun.) Research Report Series No. 3. Yaounde, Cameroon: Centre d'Etudes de la Famille Africaine, 1996;4(viii):98.

39. Henry C, Farmer P. Risk analysis: infections and inequalities in a globalizing era. *Development,* 1999;42(4):31–34.

40. Yach D, Bettcher D. The globalization of public health I: threats and opportunities. *Am J Public Health,* 1998;88(5):735–738.

41. Locoh T, Makdessi Y. The decline of fertility: the end of the African exception. (Baisse de la fécondité: la fin de l'exception africaine.) *Chronique du Ceped,* 1995;18:1–4.

42. Orubuloye IO, Caldwell JC, Caldwell P. *Experimental Research on Sexual Networking in the Ekiti District of Nigeria.* Health Transition Working Paper No. 3. Canberra, Australia: Australian National University, National Centre for Epidemiology and Population Health, Health Transition Centre, 1990;19.

43. Caldwell JC, Caldwell P. The function of child-spacing in traditional societies and the direction of change. In: Page HJ, Lesthaeghe R, eds. *Child Spacing in Tropical Africa: Traditions and Change.* Studies in Population. New York: Academic Press, 1981;73–92.

44. Orubuloye IO, Caldwell JC, Caldwell P. The cultural, social and attitudinal context of male sexual behaviour in urban south-west Nigeria. *Health Transit Rev,* 1995;5(2):207–222.

45. Watts SJ. Population mobility and disease transmission: the example of Guinea worm. *Soc Sci Med,* 1987; 25(10):1073–1081.

46. Prothero RM. Migration and AIDS in West Africa. *Geography,* 1996;81(353):374–377.

47. Prothero RM. Malaria and the importance of people. *Dev Pract,* 2001;11(1):86–90.

48. Prothero RM. Population movements and tropical health. *Glob Change Hum Health,* 2002;3(1):20–32.

49. Lydie N, Robinson NJ. West and Central Africa. *Int Mig,* 1998;36(4):469–511.

50. Sudarkasa N. The role of Yoruba commercial migration in West African development. In: Lindsay B, ed. *African Migration and National Development*. University Park, Pennsylvania: Pennsylvania State University Press, 1985;40–63.

51. Kouamé K. Migration and prostitution in the Abidjan region. (Migrations et prostitution dans la région d'Abidjan.) In: Actes du Symposium "SIDA et Migrations," under the direction of Kane F and Trudelle M in collaboration with France Galarneau, in the book of the VIII International Conference on AIDS in Africa, Marrakech, Morocco, December 1993. Quebec: Centre de Coopération Internationale en Santé et Développement, Université Laval, 1994;32–42.

52. Decosas J, Kane F, Anarfi JK, Sodji KD, Wagner HU. Migration and AIDS. *Lancet*, 1995;346(8978): 826–828.

53. Chikwem JO, Ola TO, Gashau W, Chikwem SD, Bajami M, Mambula S. Impact of health education on prostitutes' awareness and attitudes to acquired immune deficiency syndrome (AIDS). *Public Health*, 1988;102(5):439–445.

54. Ososanya OO, Brieger WR. Rural-urban mobility in southwestern Nigeria: implications for HIV/AIDS transmission from urban to rural communities. *Health Educ Res*, 1994;9(4):507–518.

55. Ajuwon AJ, Oladepo O, Adeniyi JD, Brieger WR. Sexual practices that may favor the transmission of HIV in a rural community in Nigeria. *Int Q Community Health Educ*, 1994;14(4):403–416.

56. Araoye MO, Onile BA, Jolayemi ET. Sexual behaviour and condom acceptance among Nigerian drivers. *West Afr J Med*, 1996;15(1):6–10.

57. Nnoli C. Motor-park people shift gear. *WorldAIDS*, 1992;19:10.

58. Raufu A. AIDS scare hits Nigerian military. *AIDS Anal Afr*, 2001;11(5):14.

59. Raufu A. Nigeria promises free antiretroviral drugs to HIV positive soldiers. *Br Med J*, 2002;13;324(7342):870.

60. Akinnawo EO. Sexual networking, STDs, and HIV/AIDS transmission among Nigerian police officers. *Health Transit Rev*, 1995;(Suppl 5):S113–S121.

61. Oladepo O, Brieger WR. AIDS knowledge, attitude and behaviour patterns among university students in Ibadan, Nigeria. *Afr J Med Med Sci*, 1994;23(2): 119–125.

62. TB deaths reach historic levels. *AIDS Wkly*, April 8, 1996;15:14–16.

63. Population Reference Bureau. Male responsibility in today's Africa. Radio script. Washington, DC: Population Reference Bureau, January 1996;32.

64. Cowell A. At a homecoming in Ghana: few amenities, much worry. *New York Times*, February 4, 1983;A1,A4.

65. Adepoju A. Expulsion of illegals from Nigeria: round two. *Migr World Mag*, 1986;14(5):21–24.

66. Mabogunje AL. Migration and urbanization. In: Caldwell JC, ed. *Population Growth and Socioeconomic Change in West Africa*. New York: Published for the Population Council by Columbia University Press, 1975;153–168.

67. Orubuloye IO, Caldwell JC, Caldwell P. The role of religious leaders in changing sexual behaviour in southwest Nigeria in an era of AIDS. *Health Transit Rev*, 1993;(Suppl):S93–S104.

68. Volk JE, Koopman C. Factors associated with condom use in Kenya: a test of the Health Belief Model. *AIDS Educ Prev*, 2001;13(6):495–508.

69. Ortiz-Torres B, Serrano-Garcia I, Torres-Burgos N. Subverting culture: promoting HIV/AIDS prevention among Puerto Rican and Dominican women. *Am J Community Psychol*, 2000;28(6):859–881.

70. de Assis MA, Nahas MV. Motivational aspects of nutritional behavior change programs. (Aspectos motivacionais em programas de mudanca de comportamento alimentar.) *Revista de Nutricao*, 1999;12(1):33–41.

71. International Conference on Population and Development. *Programme of Action Adopted at the International Conference on Population and Development, Cairo, 5–13 September 1994*. New York: United Nations Population Fund, 1996;viii:166.

72. Paiva V. Plenary Lecture II: Issues in Reproductive Health Education. In: Tan ML, Barrios, RT, eds. *Proceedings of the 2nd Regional Consultation on Reproductive Tract Infections in Asia and the Pacific*. Quezon City, Philippines: Health Action Information Network, 1998;46–62.

73. Ouadah-Bedidi Z; Vallin J. The Maghreb: the irresistible fall of fertility. (Maghreb: la chute irrésistible de la fécondité.) *Population et Société*, 2000;359:1–4.

74. National Population Commission and ORC Macro. *Nigeria Demographic and Health Survey 2003*. Calverton, Maryland: National Population Commission and ORC Macro, 2004.

THE IMPACT OF HIV/AIDS ON THE PRIVATE SECTOR

David Canning,* Ajay Mahal,* Olakunle Odumosu,†
and Prosper Okonkwo‡

The economic and social impacts of the HIV/AIDS epidemic have attracted much attention in recent years. The reasons for this attention are not surprising. The scale of the epidemic presents a unique health policy challenge. Already 25 million people worldwide have died, and the number of deaths is certain to rise from its existing rate of 3 million per year. AIDS is now the fourth largest cause of mortality worldwide, ranking just below cardiovascular disease and acute lower respiratory tract infections. In Africa, where more than 70% of all HIV-infected people live, AIDS now accounts for an estimated one-fifth of all deaths, making it the leading cause of mortality on the continent by a wide margin.

The HIV/AIDS epidemic is also characterized by several elements that strongly point to its influence on households, the private sector, and national economies. In particular, HIV causes premature morbidity and mortality among people in their most productive ages, and some researchers suggest that economically better off adults—who are likely to be the most productive—may be at greater risk than those less economically well off (1,2). Increased ill health and mortality among productive

*Department of Population and International Health, Harvard School of Public Health, Boston, Massachusetts
†Nigerian Institute of Social and Economic Research, Ibadan, Nigeria
‡AIDS Prevention Initiative in Nigeria, Ibadan, Nigeria

adults, when combined with the large size of the epidemic, suggest a large negative effect on national economic performance in the context of standard models of economic growth (3).

Bell et al. highlight the fact that high rates of AIDS-related deaths among more educated age groups not only reduce the stock of human capital directly, but do so indirectly as well, because people will have less of an incentive to acquire costly educational capital if they do not expect to live long enough to enjoy substantial gains from acquiring it, and firms will have less of an incentive to train their at-risk workers (4). Future stock of educational capital could also be affected if children whose parents die prematurely due to AIDS face economic bottlenecks in efforts to continue their education. Other researchers have highlighted additional channels—such as a decline in savings of households, firms, and the government that result from increased medical treatment costs associated with HIV/AIDS—that could lead to adverse implications for economic growth (1,5). Savings rates could also decline if people expect to live for fewer years owing to HIV/AIDS and so feel less need for savings to meet their old age consumption needs. Others have contested these findings on the impact of HIV on national economic performance on both theoretical and empirical grounds (6,7).

Notwithstanding the different viewpoints with regard to the adverse *macroeconomic* impacts of AIDS, experts agree on the general direction of the *microeconomic* effects in developing countries, if not the specific circumstances of individual countries. That is, the average household with HIV-positive members, or the individual firm with large numbers of HIV-positive employees, is unlikely to escape the adverse economic impacts of the epidemic in the absence of policy interventions.

With 5% of Nigeria's adult population infected with HIV and prevalence expected to grow further among adults, the potential impact of HIV/AIDS on Nigerian firms is of obvious policy relevance. At this point, we know relatively little about the impact of AIDS on Nigerian firms, or about the strategies they have adopted to ameliorate its impact. The only previous study of Nigerian firms focusing on AIDS that we are aware of is Rosen et al., which examined correlates of firms' behavioral responses in a sample of 232 firms surveyed in 2001 (8). This study highlighted the low level of HIV prevalence among employees, with only 13.6% reporting an AIDS-related death or retirement in the two years preceding the survey, and an even smaller proportion reporting an employee who was HIV positive. Only about a third of the sample companies reported any sort of HIV-prevention activities for their employees, and less than a quarter considered AIDS a threat to their business. Most of the HIV-prevention activities involved educational materials. In general, larger firms, firms that had previously encountered an HIV-positive employee, and firms that had received informational materials from external sources were more likely to have taken even a limited set of actions. In a separate study, Rosen and Simon found evidence of other mechanisms that Nigerian firms adopted to reduce the impacts of HIV: surreptitiously testing employees for HIV and dismissing them if found to be infected, and excluding AIDS-related health conditions from their medical benefits package (9).

While these studies offer valuable contributions, considerable work remains to be done in assessing the impacts of AIDS on Nigeria's private sector, including more detailed analyses of the way firms respond to HIV/AIDS in the workplace and the medical benefits they offer to employees. Moreover, given the fast-growing nature of the epidemic, up-to-date information on available firm responses is important for devising appropriate policy responses. To this end, this chapter seeks to add to the literature on the impacts of HIV/AIDS on the labor and non-labor costs of Nigerian firms by focusing on two Nigerian states—Oyo and Plateau—both target states of the AIDS Prevention Initiative in Nigeria.

Oyo and Plateau states account for only about 6.3% of the total land area of Nigeria, and a roughly similar share of its estimated total population of 135 million in 2003.[1] The two states have geographic variation—with one located in southwestern Nigeria and the other in central Nigeria—and ethnic variation. The adult HIV prevalence rates in the two states are close to the 5.0% national average: 3.9% for Oyo State and 6.3% for Plateau State—or roughly 82,000 HIV-infected adults in Oyo State and 81,000 in Plateau State.[2] Thus our analysis can potentially offer insights for Nigeria as a whole as well.

In this chapter we pose three specific questions important for the development of policy. First, what strategies are Nigerian firms adopting to ameliorate the impacts of HIV/AIDS? Second, given these strategies, how large will the impacts of HIV/AIDS on firms be? And finally, what do existing strategies suggest about the likelihood of Nigerian firms participating in long-term efforts to address HIV/AIDS in Nigeria?

CONCEPTUAL FRAMEWORK AND LITERATURE REVIEW

The direct impacts of HIV on firms can take several different forms. Given that a typical firm's focus is the economic bottom line, in theory at least, it may experience the impacts of AIDS in one, or more, of several ways that affect costs and revenues. Consider labor costs first. There may be increases in per-unit costs of production, owing to reduced per-worker productivity among workers who are unable to work either because they are sick, or because they are caring for friends and family members who have HIV/AIDS (10). Production costs may also increase on account of greater workforce turnover as some of the workers die, and obtaining replacements entails the costs of hiring and training new workers.

In a 1997 study of nearly 1,000 firms in sub-Saharan Africa, Biggs and Shah concluded that the impact of HIV on staff turnover was minimal, although this situation would obviously have changed since the time as the epidemic has grown (11). Biggs and Shah found replacing professional staff to be challenging, with firms taking 24 weeks to replace a deceased professional, compared to two to three weeks for less skilled staff. Other, smaller studies in Benin, Kenya, Rwanda, and Zaire have shown how, at certain stages of the epidemic, HIV infections can be disproportionately concentrated among exactly these skilled workers (10). Other sources of potential cost increases include rising payouts by firms for funeral expenses of employees and their family members, expenses incurred in order to provide health care

---

[1] The 1991 census data on population and geographic area for each state were obtained from the Nigerian Population Commission website at www.nigeriabusinessinfo.com/nigeria-population.htm. The projected population for 2003, owing to the lack of a census since 1991, was obtained from the United Nations website at http://esa.un.org/unpp/p2k0data.asp.

[2] HIV prevalence data was obtained from the National Action Committee on AIDS (NACA) website at www.naca.gov.ng. Estimates of adults with HIV in the two states were based on HIV prevalence rates reported by NACA, combined with age-distribution data from the National Population Commission and projected populations in the two states from the United Nations.

for sick employees and their families, and any termination benefit payouts, several instances of which are available in Africa (10,12–15).

In addition, there may be intangible effects on labor costs of production, if HIV/AIDS affects workers' morale adversely. No study has been completed detailing the impact on morale and productivity in a country with a serious and sustained epidemic. One study of entrepreneurs, however, found that HIV/AIDS led to a loss of focus on the business, while the Thai Business Coalition on AIDS highlighted poor morale as one factor facing businesses who fail to deal with AIDS in the workplace (10).

Then, there are non-labor expenses. For instance, costs of borrowing may increase if credit ratings of firms in a country decline owing either to projected adverse impacts of AIDS, or if individual firms that rely heavily on labor are deemed to be at financial risk. HIV/AIDS has been known to enter the calculus of determining a country's sovereign risk rating, and there is no reason why the same should not be true for individual firms (16). We are unaware of any firm-level studies on this subject. Firms that sell insurance, particularly health and life insurance, may incur increased claims payments as well.

On the demand side, firms may face reduced profits owing to declines in demand and prices. For instance, tourist demand for high HIV prevalence countries may decline if the risk of HIV infection figures into tourists' calculations while planning their visits. More generally, some have posited that, because HIV/AIDS affects mostly young adults who are also the major consumers of goods and services, a rising number of deaths and declining incomes owing to AIDS in this group will reduce demand for firms' products. Others have argued that demand may also decline because of deterioration in the *overall macroeconomic environment* due to AIDS (17).

For individual firms, however, these theoretical effects are likely to be small. For one, domestic demand is likely to be dissipated throughout the economy and on importers of products. If the demand is from foreign markets, especially outside of Africa, where HIV prevalence is much smaller, the impacts will be even less marked. Impacts on customer demand are likely to be more transparent if there are dominant firms, or if AIDS channels demands into specific sectors, such as health. In 1998, the JD Group, South Africa's leading furniture retailer, forecast that changes in demography, presumably due to AIDS, would reduce its customer base by 18% by 2015 (10). And AIDS has certainly led to a rising need for firms supplying health care services and drugs, although its translation into effective demand has typically required the mediation of government subsidies, as in Botswana, Nigeria, South Africa, and elsewhere. Consumer demand may also be influenced if HIV/AIDS affects a firm's brand—a term that encapsulates the value, image, and character of a company—although no direct evidence is available on the subject thus far.

Whether these effects turn out to be substantial depends on the magnitude of the HIV epidemic. For an individual firm, moreover, the impacts also depend on whether it can devise effective strategies to avoid the adverse implications of HIV/AIDS on its profits. Individual firms may be able to further reduce these impacts by HIV screening that enables them to reduce the hiring of workers with HIV, or dismissing them, or prematurely retiring workers who turn out to have AIDS, with limited compensation. Alternatively, firms may cap or otherwise eliminate worker benefits, especially relating to medical care. Existing literature does offer some evidence of strategies along these lines being adopted by firms in

Botswana, Nigeria, South Africa, and Zimbabwe (9). In so doing, these firms impose a negative externality on other firms that are looking to employ from the labor force by increasing the pool of HIV-infected people in it. Yet if screening costs are low enough, firms that are reasonably knowledgeable would act in a similar manner. In the short run, the real economic impact would then be distributional, being borne mainly by HIV-affected households or entities that support people with HIV, whether the government, nongovernmental organizations, or the communities in which people with HIV live.

Practices such as screening for HIV before hiring or dismissal on account of HIV status may be ruled out by cultural norms, business practices, and laws that prevent firms from discriminating against workers—or clients, in the case of insurance companies—by HIV status. These prohibitions may also cause firms to make financial contributions to the health care and funeral expenses of workers or their family members. These limits to actions by firms may be more common among firms that belong to the organized—or the formal—sector as well as among public sector firms (10). Although workers may still feel the burden of increased expenses under these circumstances in the form of lowered salaries, the firms will likely share at least part of this burden (18). Screening and subsequent dismissal, even if feasible, may not be cost-beneficial if the epidemic is concentrated among individuals with scarce skill sets who are hard to replace, such as individuals with managerial and high-end technical skills. Under these circumstances, firms may not be able to escape the impacts of AIDS.

Even if some short-term impacts are unavoidable, firms may adopt longer-term strategies to reduce the impacts of HIV/AIDS. These include shifting to production technologies that are capital intensive, or moving production itself to countries or regions with lower levels of HIV prevalence, although there is little evidence available on this score. Alternatively, firms may sponsor HIV prevention programs for their workers or lobby the government for prevention programs aimed at the general population. Such actions do, to an extent, confer external benefits on competing firms that plan to employ additional workers in future years, and this may result in underinvestment in prevention efforts (18). Thus while prevention programs directed toward the population might be larger-scale if undertaken in coordination with other firms to reduce the disincentives arising from the externalities involved, individual firms would probably prefer to undertake these programs toward their own employees. There is some previous evidence of prevention programs in workplaces in Africa, and Nigeria in particular (8,10). If workers have a high average length of tenure, the HIV-reduction gains resulting from prevention strategies toward its employees can be internal to the firm. The latter is particularly likely when the firms in questions are large and therefore have longer decision-making horizons.

None of these methods of coping suffices to address certain long-run consequences of AIDS. If the population-wide HIV/AIDS epidemic continues to progress, there may come a point where *all* firms face a domestic employee population with a high risk of HIV infection, low skills, and generally poor employability. One could argue whether such a point is ever reached; if it is, firms' shorter-run strategies may not help avoid the longer-run consequences of the epidemic. Whether this really matters depends first on the time horizons of the firms themselves; and second on whether other parties—governments, nongovernmental organizations, and the households themselves—take up measures to reduce HIV infection. The appropriate role of firms in such circumstances becomes thus an issue of policy interest. This discussion is also relevant to the question about how firms can be enrolled in strategies to address the epidemic more generally (10). A number of experts and leaders in the fight against AIDS have argued that firms have a crucial role to play because of the financial resources they command, their attention to efficiency, and their strong record of being able to reach households that are the focus of worldwide efforts against the spread of HIV.

DATA SOURCES

We carried out a survey of enterprises in Oyo and Plateau states. To highlight two different ways in which the epidemic could affect firms, we sampled insurance companies where the impact of HIV/AIDS was most likely to be felt in the form of higher claims payouts. We also sampled a collection of firms not operating in the insurance sector, and here we focused on the potential impacts of HIV/AIDS on costs related to labor inputs.

The sampling of firms outside of the insurance sector was undertaken as follows. Within each state, a sampling frame was constructed and firms were stratified by the number of employees: firms with employee sizes of 10 to 50 people, 51 to 300 people, and more than 300 people were defined as small, medium and large scale, respectively. It was expected that 40 firms would be covered from each state making for a total of 80 firms overall. The share of large, medium, and small firms in the sample was 20%, 40%, and 40%, respectively. All insurance companies in the capital city of each state were surveyed. This ought not to be particularly problematic from the standpoint of the sample being representative, because one ought to expect the regional headquarters to be located in the capital. Information was obtained with the help of a structured questionnaire that was completed with the assistance of trained field workers.

Overall we were able to access 102 enterprises in the organized sector, of which 29 were insurance companies and 73 were involved in activities outside the insurance sector. Of the firms outside the insurance sector, only 70 specified ownership structure, and these were the ones we included in our analysis. Nearly 80% of the reporting firms in the sample belonged to the private sector, as noted in Table 8-1. Our sample of private firms also included a few multinationals—about 5% of the total number of firms in the survey. Not surprisingly, given the potential sensitivity of financial data, not every sampled firm was willing to part with such information, and some refused outright to participate in the

Table 8-1. Sample of Firms by Type of Business, Ownership, and State, 2004				
	Oyo State		Plateau State	
Type of Business	Public	Private	Public	Private
Insurance • General/Life • Health	2 0	17 0	1 0	7 2
Other	8	38	5	19
Total	10	55	6	28

Source: Survey undertaken by the Nigerian Institute of Social and Economic Research. In our analysis we considered the 70 non-insurance firms for which information on public and private ownership was available, as well as 29 insurance companies, for a total of 99 firms.

Table 8-2. Enterprises (Excluding Insurance Companies) by Number of Employees, Wage Bill, and Years of Operation

Characteristic	Oyo State		Plateau State	
	Public	Private	Public	Private
Number	8	38	5	19
Employment	1808 (8)	3,377 (38)	2,093 (5)	1,865 (19)
Average annual wage bill (naira millions)	45.6 (4)	10.9 (27)	17.9 (5)	9.7 (11)
Employment	859 (4)	2,446 (27)	2,093 (5)	818 (11)
Mean years of operation	35.14 (7)	20.14 (37)	20.50 (2)	21.69 (16)

Source: Authors' estimates based on survey data provided by the Nigerian Institute of Social and Economic Research
Note: Numbers in parentheses indicate the number of enterprises that provided the relevant information.

study, as reflected in the sample size, which was 10% lower than what we had originally planned. Thus some of the questions in our survey of firms in Oyo and Plateau states are plagued by non-response. In the following discussion, and where necessary, we take note of problems raised by non-response and the potential biases involved.

Table 8-2 provides additional information about the employee base of our sample of non-insurance firms. The data show that an average firm in the sample had operated for at least 20 years, with the average public firm noticeably larger in terms of employees — 300 versus 92 — and annual wage bill — 30.2 million naira versus 10.6 million naira — than the average private firm.

FINDINGS AND DISCUSSION

Impacts on Costs on Labor in Firms outside the Insurance Sector

Health and related benefits offered by firms to their employees can play a critical role in determining the cost of labor inputs due to HIV/AIDS. Thus, we first inquired of our sample of firms about the health-related benefits that they currently offer their employees. The list of benefits included premium contributions by employers toward insurance, free (or subsidized) provision of health services in firm-owned health facilities or facilities contracted by firms, reimbursements for health expenditures incurred by the employees themselves at outside facilities, and any medical allowances that were paid as part of the salary. We also examined whether employees contributed to insurance premiums, and inquired about the proportion of the total number of employees covered by the insurance schemes referred to previously.

Table 8-3 summarizes the results of our analysis. Most of the organized sector firms in our sample provide some form of financial support to the health needs of their employees. All firms in the public sector reported providing some form of support, at least as medical allowance in salary. However 10% of private sector firms (6 of 57) reported carrying *no responsibility* for health care expenditures of their employees.

A second key finding is that the bulk of the health care support provided by firms is channeled through mechanisms other than formal health insurance; that is, through firm-owned or contracted off-site

Characteristic	Oyo State		Plateau State	
	Public	Private	Public	Private
Number of Firms	8	38	5	19
Health Benefits				
Treatment at on-site clinic (Yes)	6	9	2	4
Pay for treatment at off-site facility (Yes)	1	18	2	7
Pay for health insurance (Yes)	0	2	0	1
Reimburse health expenses (Yes)	3	7	0	7
Medical allowance in salary (Yes)	3	11	4	10
No responsibility for health care (Yes)	0	6	0	0
Other Benefits				
Pay for funeral expenses (Yes)	4	12	5	10
Pay for family support (Yes)	1	2	0	0
One-time death benefits (Yes)	4	11	2	4
Disability payments (Yes)	1	6	1	5
Benefits offered if HIV positive (Yes)	*6 (7)*	*21 (30)*	*4 (5)*	*12 (16)*

Source: Authors' estimates, based on survey data provided by the Nigerian Institute of Social and Economic Research
Note: Numbers in parentheses indicate the numbers of firms offering one or more of the listed health (or non-health) benefits in the corresponding ownership category.

facilities, reimbursements for health expenditures and medical allowances included as part of salary. Less than 5% of all firms (or 3 of 70) firms in the sample reported contributing toward health insurance premiums for their employees, none in the public sector. The available data indicate that private sector firms offer a somewhat wider variety of benefit categories compared to public sector firms, especially health insurance and reimbursements for expenditures incurred by employees at health care facilities.

Table 8-4 presents additional information on expenditures incurred per worker by firms, under the different heads described earlier. Unfortunately, the data are characterized by a high level of non-response. One striking finding is that only 18% of the firms that offered medical benefits reported requiring their employees to make a contribution as well. Where such contributions are made, as indicated in the last row of Table 8-4, they occur primarily in the form of "partial reimbursements" for expenditures incurred by employees on their health care, or in the form of partial coverage for care received at offsite facilities.

Apart from benefits in the form of health expenditures, HIV/AIDS can also impose costs on firms if they end up paying benefits to employees who then die prematurely, disability benefits, funeral expenses, and support to surviving family members. The second panel of Table 8-3 describes benefits offered by firms in this category. Note that public firms are more likely to support funeral expenses—roughly 70%

Characteristic	Oyo State		Plateau State	
	Public	Private	Public	Private
Number	8	38	5	19
Insurance Premiums Paid by Employers *(naira per worker)*	0	1,425 (2)	0	n/a
Total Employees	0	540	0	265
Expenditures on Own Facility *(naira per worker)*	755 (1)	1,577 (2)	n/a	571 (1)
Total Employees	1260 (6)	1727 (9)	619(2)	1,025 (3)
Retainers/Other Private *(naira per worker)*	3,300 (1)	1,200 (1)	n/a	1,500 (1)
Total Employees	202 (1)	2,306 (17)	662 (2)	1,585 (8)
Reimbursement *(naira per worker)*	260 (2)	1,180 (1)	n/a	n/a
Total Employees	1,109 (3)	1,579 (5)	0(0)	1,533 (5)
Medical Allowance *(naira per worker)*	n/a	3,664 (4)	n/a	3,095 (1)
Total Employees	396 (2)	1,039 (10)	1,117 (2)	674 (8)
Employee (% share) • Onsite facility • Offsite facility • Insurance premiums • Reimbursements	n/a n/a n/a 50-70 (2)	0-90 (3) 0-90 (4) 0 (2) 0-60 (5)	0 (1) 0 (1) 0 (1) 100 (1)	0 (2) 10-60 (2) 0 (2) 0 (2)

Table 8-4. Health Expenditures Incurred by Firms

Source: Authors' calculations based on survey data
Note: Numbers in parentheses indicate the number of firms reporting the necessary information.

of public firms, or 9 of 13, reported doing so, compared to about 40% (22 of 57) of private firms. About 46% of the public firms reported offering lump-sum death benefits, compared to 26% of private firms. A roughly similar — though small — proportion of public and private firms provide disability payments.

The previous discussion highlights the following: while not universal, the practice of paying for a substantial variety of health- and non-health benefits for employees of Nigerian firms means that in the absence of mechanisms that exclude HIV-positive personnel from receiving such benefits, the HIV/AIDS epidemic could impose a substantial addition to the labor costs on firms.

Strategies to Avoid the Impact of HIV Through Labor Costs
We inquired first whether the firms in our sample excluded HIV-positive individuals from receiving health benefits. We found that this was generally *not* the case, at least not overtly — more than 70% (43

Table 8-5. Number of Companies Offering Health Insurance to Employees				
Characteristic	Oyo State		Plateau State	
	Public	Private	Public	Private
Number of firms	8	38	5	19
Companies offering health insurance to employees	0	2	0	1
Number of employees covered, 2002	0	540	0	265
Companies covering antiretroviral therapy	0	1	0	1

Source: Authors' calculations, based on survey data

of 58) of all firms currently offering some health (or non-health) benefits described in Table 8-3 would not deny their HIV-positive employees access to benefits available to their HIV-negative employees. The proportion of public sector firms that would continue to offer benefits to their HIV-positive employees was close to 80%, whereas the corresponding proportion for private enterprises was about 70%.

In the absence of risk or experience rating—or if risk rating occurs with some lag—employers may hope to temporarily pass on some of the health care costs associated with AIDS to insurance companies, especially if health insurance covers ARV therapy, as was the case with our sample of firms. Unfortunately, few companies offer formal health insurance to their employees. Only 3 of 70 firms did so, together employing about 9% of the total workforce in the sample of firms considered (Table 8-5). More crucially, it appears reasonable to presume that on the supply side, insurance companies will make up for any extra health care expenditures incurred by employees by charging higher premiums rather than just passively incurring higher claim payments.

Second, firms could avoid these costs by discriminating against individuals with HIV/AIDS—whether in hiring decisions or in termination decisions as suggested by Rosen and Simon (9). Table 8-6 describes firms' responses in Oyo and Plateau States to different questions about the role of health and HIV/AIDS in influencing firms' decisions to hire individuals. Our survey data suggest that about 35 firms (50% of the full sample) have some health-related criterion for hiring individuals, with a greater percentage of public sector firms requiring the meeting of some health standards. Roughly 13% (9 of 70) firms report having separate policies for hiring people with HIV. This number may be biased downward if firms that use a health criterion for hiring also require a medical examination with an HIV test, even when the HIV exam is ostensibly irrelevant to the hiring decision. In our sample, at least two such firms existed, and the actual number may be greater. If there are a significant number of such firms, the proportion of firms for whom HIV status influences hiring will obviously be much greater than revealed by our survey responses.

Firms can also try to avoid the economic burden of HIV/AIDS by prematurely terminating employees with HIV/AIDS. In our sample, 42 firms (or about 60% of the total) reported having policies addressing situations when an employee is unable to work on grounds of poor health; and some 29 firms specifically reported having termination policies linked to health. Termination on grounds solely of HIV status (a discriminatory policy) appears to be quite limited: only 6 (or about 10%) of private sector firms reported having

Table 8-6. Employee Hiring and Termination Practices by Ownership, Health Status, and State, 2004				
Characteristic	Oyo State		Plateau State	
	Public	Private	Public	Private
Number of firms	8	38	5	19
Health-related criteria for hiring (if yes)	5	19	3	8
Hiring affected by HIV status (if yes)	1	4	1	3
Policy if employee cannot work due to ill health (if yes)	4	27	3	8
Any health-related criteria for termination (if yes)	4	16	1	8
Termination affected by HIV status (if yes)	0	5	0	1
Laid-off if someone unable to work (if yes)	1	12	0	5

Source: Authors' calculations, based on survey data
Note: Data refer to the number of firms responding in the affirmative to the question.

termination policies associated with HIV status. Nevertheless, if inability to work is grounds for termination firms may still be able to shed medical and other costs arising from employees with full-blown AIDS. Our survey data reveal that this practice is likely to be more common among private firms, some 17 of whom (or 30% of the total in our sample) reported having a policy of termination if a person were permanently unable to work, in contrast to only one public sector firm that reported having such a policy.

Third, Nigerian firms can potentially avoid adverse economic implications due to AIDS through the adoption of HIV prevention strategies that, by their nature, yield longer-term rewards. Table 8-7 summarizes these findings. Our data reveal that 50% (35 of 70) of the firms in our sample had at least one program with a strong prevention focus—condom distribution, testing and treatment for sexually transmitted infections, voluntary testing, counseling, or information, education and communication initiatives—in place, and several had more than one. It is worth noting that this is a higher proportion of firms than Rosen et al. reported in their study of Nigerian firms in 2003 (8). With the caveat that the samples of the studies may not be directly comparable (one was a national sample, whereas ours focuses on two states), we believe this to be evidence that Nigerian firms may be increasingly waking up to the epidemic and taking steps to address it, at least within their workforce. As in the Rosen et al. study, educational programs were the most common mode of intervention funded by firms in our sample (8). However, nearly 20% (14 of 70) of our sample of firms was involved in more substantive strategies such as condom distribution programs, which is double the proportion reported by Rosen et al. (Table 8-3) (8). Condom distribution programs appeared to be more popular in public sector companies, which is in line with our argument in the introduction, suggesting that larger firms are more likely than smaller ones to find prevention programs beneficial.

Implications for Nigerian Firms outside the Insurance Sector

What does the above discussion imply in terms of the financial impacts of HIV/AIDS on Nigerian firms? In principle, we should expect these costs to be small thus far, both because the Nigerian AIDS epidemic is not as far advanced, say, as the epidemic in Botswana and South Africa, and also because of the ways in which at least some of the firms could potentially avoid the epidemic's impacts.

Only 10 of 70 Nigerian firms in our sample reported an AIDS death among employees in the five years preceding the survey, or about 14%, a proportion that is similar to that reported in Rosen et al. (8). Thus, it is not surprising to find from Table 8-8 that only about 11% of the firms in our sample, or 8 of 70 that responded (all but one in Oyo State), reported that their profits or operations had been affected by HIV/AIDS. Among the five firms whose representatives provided a guess as to the number of HIV-positive employees, the estimated HIV prevalence rate was 1.3%, with AIDS prevalence possibly much lower. Firms reporting the death of an employee because of AIDS also reported being able to replace that employee, and data the firms provided to us reveal that the proportion of employees showing up for work appears to be high, ranging from 90 to 100%.

These findings suggest that it is still early in the AIDS epidemic for any negative financial effects to show up among Nigerian firms. Moreover, strategies adopted by some of these firms to lower their financial liability from workers with HIV/AIDS are likely to have further reduced these already small impacts. For some other firms, if they continue to support employee benefits at their current levels, a significant HIV epidemic among employees could severely affect their economic viability, especially if they are committed to these benefits for legal and/or cultural reasons. Public sector firms may be especially vulnerable on this account.

This does not mean, however, that longer-term effects can be wished away if the epidemic were to greatly expand in magnitude, even with the strategies described earlier. The survey data (not reported in Table 8-8) also reveal that employee departures linked to AIDS have the potential of increasing attrition rates in a non-trivial way: In firms reporting an AIDS case, attrition rates were 50% to 100% higher than other firms. Some 10 firms (14% of the total) also reported an increase in the proportion of workers reporting sick and the number of deaths among employees in the five years preceding the survey. Whether HIV caused these higher attrition and worker absenteeism rates can only be settled by obtain-

Characteristic	Oyo State		Plateau State	
	Public	Private	Public	Private
Number of firms	8	38	5	19
Condom distribution	3	9	1	1
STI diagnosis and treatment	2	6	0	2
Voluntary testing	1	9	0	2
Counseling	1	11	1	3
IEC programs	4	10	2	7
At least one of the above programs	5	19	3	8

Table 8-7. HIV/AIDS Related Services and Prevention Programs at the Workplace, by Ownership, Program, and State, 2004

Source: Authors' calculations based on survey data.
Abbreviations: STI: sexually transmitted infection; **IEC:** information, education, and communication

Characteristic	Oyo State		Plateau State	
	Public	Private	Public	Private
Number of firms	8	38	5	19
HIV affected profits?	1	6	0	1
Estimated HIV positive as percentage of employees	3.0 (1)	1.3 (3)	0	0.5 (1)
Employees with HIV/AIDS during past five years	1	4	1	4
Able to replace employees who have died from AIDS?	1	4	1	4
Percentage of workers showing up for work on average	90% (8)	95% (25)	98.5% (2)	100% (13)
Increasing share of employees leaving for sickness/death?	2	0	0	2
Increasing share reporting sick or funerals during the past five years?	0	4	2	4
Average number of weeks for training new employees	5.5 (4)	10.0 (26)	3.0 (4)	5.3 (10)
HIV as future problem for profits?	1	21	0	2

Table 8-8. Assessing the Impact of HIV/AIDS on Nigerian Firms

Source: Authors' calculations using survey data
Note: Numbers in parentheses indicate firms that reported the information.

ing more information about the HIV status of workers and longitudinal data, which we do not have at present. But if these reported trends are, in fact, attributable to HIV, then higher rates of HIV prevalence in Nigeria in the future — by fueling similar increases in attrition rates and absenteeism across all firms — could mean serious delays in filling vacant positions.

The firms we surveyed are clearly worried about the future impact of HIV/AIDS on their economic bottom line. As the last row in Table 8-8 suggests, three times as many firms report being concerned about the impacts on future profits as the number of firms reporting a current impact of HIV/AIDS on profits (24 versus 8). Keeping in mind the differences in the samples between our sample and that used by Rosen et al., it would appear that a slightly greater proportion of Nigerian firms (24 of 70, or 34%) are worried about the economic impacts of HIV than was the case only a few years ago (24%) (8).

Impacts on Non-Labor Costs: The Insurance Sector

Apart from impacts on the costs of labor, HIV/AIDS could also influence non-labor costs of firms. In the introduction we discussed the potential impacts on credit rating and consequently the borrowing costs of firms. There is little evidence of such impacts in Nigeria thus far, and one might imagine that poor infrastructure, political instability, and the generally weak rule of law to be a much greater influence on risk rating of firms in Nigeria than HIV/AIDS. Instead, we focused on a category of non-labor costs that more directly reflect HIV/AIDS — claim payouts by health and life insurance companies. These are like-

Table 8-9. Insurance Companies Offerings of Health Insurance Policies, 2004		
Business	Oyo State	Plateau State
Individual health policies	19	9
Private employer group policies	19	7
Public employer group policies	13	6
Other	3	1

ly to be important for firms that offer health and life insurance since an advanced HIV/AIDS epidemic could increase claims payments significantly.

To assess the current and potential future impact of HIV/AIDS on Nigerian insurance companies, we carried out a survey of 29 Nigerian insurance companies, only 3 of which were in the public sector. Most of these companies offer health insurance products: 28 had individual health insurance clients, 26 had group policies with private employers, and 19 had group policies with public sector employers.

The primary mechanism used by Nigerian insurance companies to avoid the adverse impacts of HIV/AIDS is the practice of excluding individuals who are HIV positive from obtaining a policy. Twenty of the 29 companies in our sample practiced exclusion restrictions of this type. Most of the companies test individuals for HIV before selling them insurance policies. However, these companies do not exclude HIV-positive individuals who are already policyholders from obtaining benefits. This could leave them potentially financially vulnerable in the short-run to group insurance policyholders who turn out to be HIV positive. On the other hand, if group policyholders are also tested for HIV prior to their being accepted for insurance, or if insurance premiums are risk- and experience-rated, insurance companies can address their financial risk by simply raising premiums for companies with a high number of HIV-positive personnel. Unfortunately, we know too little about the principles underlying the sale of group-insurance policies in Nigeria to say more on the subject.

One way to assess the impact of HIV/AIDS on Nigerian insurance companies is to estimate its impact on insurance company claim payments directly. This is easier said than done; only five companies agreed to share their financial data with us. With these limitations in mind, the data reveal quite substantial surpluses of premiums over claims—about 50%. This finding supports on the surface, at least, the contention that AIDS has not imposed losses on insurance companies. This is not to say that AIDS expenditures are negligible. One of the few insurance companies that supplied us with estimates of claims data associated with AIDS determined that nearly 20% of the overall claims it paid were HIV/AIDS related. The company was also concerned about the future implications of AIDS: it projected that if the share of policyholders with AIDS exceeds a mere one-quarter of a percent among all policyholders, it will not be able to break even.

That said, it is difficult to imagine a situation in which insurance companies bear the brunt of a future HIV/AIDS epidemic on a sustained basis, given the arsenal of strategies at their disposal, such as risk/experience rating in premium setting and exclusion restrictions. More than likely firms outside the insurance sector will feel the impacts, as will households affected by AIDS.

CONCLUSION

Our findings suggest that the AIDS epidemic in Nigeria is not yet advanced enough to have adversely affected the financial state of Nigerian firms, whether in the insurance sector or outside it. With the scale of the epidemic still relatively small, even firms that are pre-committed to providing medical and other employee benefits to their workers regardless of their HIV status may not yet be adversely affected.

Our findings also suggest that strategies adopted by some Nigerian firms to avoid the burden of HIV/AIDS include the testing of applicants and the termination of employees found to be HIV positive. This is unsurprising if somewhat unpalatable behavior, and one that would be expected of optimizing firms (18). However, it does have a distributional impact, shifting the financial burden of HIV/AIDS to households, the government, and nongovernmental entities that support people living with HIV/AIDS; this trend has been experienced in some other African countries as well (9).

If the scale of the AIDS epidemic were to increase dramatically, the distributional impact will be increasingly felt in rising poverty rates among households and fiscal burdens. Moreover, there may be issues about the long-run well-being of firms, especially if the epidemic were to greatly enlarge in Nigeria, so that the pool of workers the firms can draw on may lack adequate levels of education and health. Indeed, this last concern is reflected in the firms' own assessments and their increasing role in HIV-prevention activities directed to their workers.

These issues raise an obvious question: What is the optimal strategy toward involving firms to act in ways that are socially desirable? As noted in the introduction, relying upon individual firms to behave in a socially desirable manner appears difficult, given the external benefits such action confers on other firms. At best the firms are likely to undertake HIV prevention activities among their employees, and this emerges from the Nigerian data as well.

Three types of policy steps have been suggested in the economic literature as a means of encouraging firms to undertake greater HIV prevention activities (10,18). First, there are government subsidies that could be provided to private firms to promote prevention activities and reduce discriminatory behavior. Firms could be offered tax deductions for expenditures incurred on HIV-prevention programs, or for instituting workplace programs that enhance the rights of people with HIV. A more sophisticated strategy could take the form of subsidizing insurance premiums, contingent on the introduction of prevention programs by firms. Because only a small percentage of firms in Nigeria purchase private insurance, the focus would have to be on contributions to social insurance programs. Another possibility would be to offer prioritized access to government ARV programs for firms that follow best practices with regard to prevention and anti-discrimination programs in the workplace. Insurance premiums contingent on prevention programs or better access to ARV programs financed by the government would reduce firms' financial risk exposure from engaging employees with HIV and reduce the incentives for

HIV-related discrimination by employers. Penalties and taxes on firms that neither impose anti-discriminatory norms in the workplace nor promote preventive interventions are another possibility, but we believe that their implementation might be more difficult because of heavier informational requirements on the government, which presumably would have to furnish proof of non-compliance.

Second, the government could itself finance *and* provide prevention services, the typical manner in which HIV prevention programs directed at the general population are currently undertaken. But because employees are concentrated in one place and serve as a captive audience, preventive interventions undertaken at the workplace are particularly cost-effective in reaching an important segment of the adult population. In the Nigerian context, one possibility is for the government, funding agencies, and civil society organizations involved in HIV/AIDS work to supply free condoms and to produce and conduct information, education, and communication campaigns in Nigerian workplaces. Some of this is already occurring, although its scale could be expanded. Such a strategy may be invaluable for firms outside the corporate sector that are unlikely to gain much from increased tax deductions, if they do not pay taxes or already have a low tax burden. In this manner, at least part of the cost of these programs — but not production losses due to employee attendance at education programs — could be borne by groups other than firms. These measures may still require considerable buy-in from firms, especially those that intend to discriminate against employees and potential hires with HIV, and thereby shift the cost to another firm or the individuals themselves.

A third possibility, suggested by Bloom and Sevilla in line with the famous "Coase solution" in economics, is that private entities be assigned *property rights* to HIV prevalence and discrimination, in that they somehow become responsible for its reduction (18). They do not suggest a practical mechanism by which this "internalization" of the externality can be done. However, we can imagine settings whereby policy interventions and programs are promoted not by individual firms but by a collectivity of firms such as Nigerian business associations, both in the corporate sector and in the informal sector, perhaps with some nudging by the government. The obvious advantage of business association involvement is that individual firm interests' would be expressed in the context of the collective interests of associations that may otherwise impose external costs on each other, thereby addressing at least part of the externality.

These possibilities still do not address costs imposed on households by collections of firms, which may choose to collectively discriminate against people with HIV and share related information about current and past employees. This possibility suggests a need for a broader and more active dialogue between business leaders, civil society organizations, and the Nigerian government whereby prevention, care, and elimination of discrimination become part of the national and corporate ethic. Firms do care about brand names and goodwill, and explicit support from civil society (including religious organizations) for firms and business associations undertaking HIV-intervention work could be an important way to enhance their goals in this respect. HIV-related activities of members of the Global Business Council on HIV/AIDS, which includes some of the largest firms in the world, offer a useful model in this regard (10).

ACKNOWLEDGMENTS

We are grateful to a number of individuals and institutions for their encouragement, comments, and material help in undertaking this work. We are especially thankful to Professors Phyllis Kanki and Michael Reich, Dr. Soji Adeyi, and Dr. Wole Odutolu at the AIDS Prevention Initiative in Nigeria. At the Nigerian Institute of Social and Economic Research (NISER) we greatly benefited from the guidance and advice of Dr. D. O. Ajakaiye, Dr. A. Sunmola, Ms. Nancy Nelson-Twakor, Mr. L. N. Chete, and Mr. A. O. Ajala. Dr. A. O. Okesola (Oyo State AIDS Control Programme) and Mr. Bala Mitok Rumtong (Plateau State AIDS Control Programme) provided us with access to data on expenditures on HIV/AIDS. Seminar participants at Harvard and NISER provided several useful comments that benefited this study.

REFERENCES

1. Over M. *The Macroeconomic Impact of AIDS in Sub-Saharan Africa.* Technical Working Paper No. 3. Washington, DC: World Bank, Africa Technical Department, 1992.

2. Yamano T, Jayne TS. Measuring the impacts of working-age adult mortality on small-scale farm households in Kenya. *World Dev,* 2004;32:91–119.

3. Bloom D, Canning D, Sevilla J. The effect of health on growth: a production function approach. *World Dev,* 2004;32:1–13.

4. Bell C, Devarajan S, Gersbach H. *The Long Run Economic Costs of AIDS: Theory and an Application to South Africa.* Washington, DC: World Bank, 2003.

5. Cuddington J. Modeling the macroeconomic effects of AIDS, with an application to Tanzania. *World Bank Econ Rev,* 1993;7:403–417.

6. Bloom D, Mahal A. Does the AIDS epidemic threaten economic growth? *J Econom,* 1997;77:105–124.

7. Young A. The gift of the dying: the tragedy of AIDS and the welfare of future African generations. *Q J Econ,* 2005;120:423–466.

8. Rosen S, Macleod W, Vincent J, Thea D, Simon J. *Why Do Nigerian Manufacturing Firms Take Action on AIDS?* Discussion Paper No. 3. Boston: Center for International Health and Development, Boston University School of Public Health, 2003.

9. Rosen S, Simon J. Shifting the burden: the private sector's response to the AIDS epidemic in Africa. *Bull World Health Organ,* 2003;81:131–137.

10. Bloom D, Mahal A, River Path Associates. HIV/AIDS and the private sector: a literature review. Draft paper. Boston, Massachusetts: Harvard School of Public Health, 2002.

11. Biggs T, Shah M. *The Impact of the AIDS Epidemic on African Firms.* RPED Discussion Paper No. 72. Washington, DC: World Bank, Africa Region, 1997.

12. Bollinger L, Stover J. *The Economic Impact of AIDS in Zambia.* Washington, DC: Futures Group International, 1999.

13. Bollinger L, Stover J, Nalo D. *The Economic Impact of AIDS in Kenya.* Washington, DC: Futures Group International, 1999.

14. Bollinger L, Stover J, Riwa P. *The Economic Impact of AIDS in Tanzania.* Washington, DC: Futures Group International, 1999.

15. Whiteside A, Sunter C. *AIDS: The Challenge for South Africa.* Cape Town, South Africa: Human & Rousseau Tafelberg, 2000.

16. Moody's Investors Service. *South Africa.* New York: Moody's Investors Service, Global Credit Research, 2000.

17. McPherson M, Hoover D, Snodgrass D. The impact on economic growth of Africa of rising costs and labor productivity losses associated with HIV/AIDS. Discussion Paper No. 79. Cambridge, Massachusetts: Harvard Institute for International Development, 2000.

18. Bloom D, Sevilla J. People and profits: on the incentives of business to get involved in the fight against AIDS. Draft paper. Boston, Massachusetts: Harvard School of Public Health, 2003.

THE IMPACT OF HIV/AIDS ON NIGERIAN HOUSEHOLDS

David Canning,* Ajay Mahal,* Olakunle Odumosu,[†]
and Prosper Okonkwo[‡]

The HIV/AIDS epidemic has devastated families in Nigeria emotionally, socially, and financially. In addition to the expenses that infected individuals accrue, each affected family must bear the psychic costs associated with the death and illness of a family member, the breakdown in family structure, and the stigma associated with HIV (1,2). The HIV/AIDS epidemic and its associated morbidity and mortality rates carry a number of implications, such as reduced non-health consumption expenditures among household members (3–5). Another implication may be reduced levels of consumption for children in affected households when they grow up to be adults, if HIV/AIDS leads to lower levels of health and education achievements among them (4,6–9). These effects arise because of the costs of caring for family members with HIV, funeral expenses, and the premature mortality among younger adult members, which potentially constitutes the loss of an earning member of a household, coupled with a lack of adequate mechanisms to cope with these financial shocks (3,4,10–13).

The precise extent of these impacts depends on the nature of coping mechanisms available to households. If financial transfers from other households and the government are accessible, for

Department of Population and International Health, Harvard School of Public Health, Boston, Massachusetts
Nigerian Institute of Social and Economic Research, Ibadan, Nigeria
AIDS Prevention Initiative in Nigeria, Ibadan, Nigeria

Table 9-1. Economic Impact of HIV/AIDS on Households

The most direct impact of HIV/AIDS on households take the form of:
- Consumption (other than health) expenditures;
- Expenditures for medical treatment;
- Income losses to households due to morbidity and premature death of adult members; and
- Psychic costs.

These impacts are exacerbated by:
- Stigmatization and discrimination associated with HIV/AIDS that leads to economic loss, inadequate community and extended family support, and inadequate access to care;
- Regulations that make access to essential drugs more expensive; and
- Loss of assets (such as through property grabbing by others).

Seriously affected households cope with these impacts by:
- Drawing down on savings, selling assets, or borrowing;
- Withdrawing children from schools;
- Reducing consumption of other essential health care;
- Adding to households or dissolving households; and
- Increasing the number of members joining the labor force to supplement declining incomes, while some members devote more time to caregiving for sick members.

These coping mechanisms have a long-run impact on the economic well-being of households, by affecting both human capital accumulation and asset positions.

Civil society and enhanced government support in the form of free (or subsidized) antiretroviral treatment act to ameliorate these impacts. Access to health and life insurance, private transfers from other members of the community, and publicly financed health facilities also help.

example, or if subsidized public health care is available, some of the adverse financial effects may be ameliorated without major adverse consequences for consumption. More often, households must sell productive assets, borrow at high interest rates, or withdraw their children from school to meet their immediate health and non-health expenditure requirements (4,6,14). Thus households may well end up mortgaging future consumption, for themselves and/or their heirs, although wealthier households tend to cope better than poorer ones (6,10,15). Under these circumstances, reduced food consumption as a response to increased health spending (or lowered incomes) may adversely affect nutrition levels with obvious implications for future earning potential (7). Again, if social mechanisms are in place to care for orphans and meet their health and educational needs, whether by the state or other households, the impact on members of HIV-affected households will be that much less severe. Without such mechanisms, households may have to rely on increased savings (and reduced current consumption); and sick parents will incur increased psychic costs relating to the future survival of their children and other dependents. When households weakened by HIV lose their land and have their assets grabbed by others, these adverse effects will obviously be exacerbated (6,16).

Note that the changing composition of the household itself can be thought of as another coping mechanism. If in response to difficulties faced by a given household, young adults previously outside the household join in caregiving or income-generation activities, some of the negative effects may be ameliorated (10). On the other hand, if these responsibilities fall upon elderly individuals, or if the household dissolves, the adverse impacts of HIV may not be so readily escaped (17). Much depends on the nature of the dissolution and social support mechanisms available for orphans and the elderly (10).

These negative economic effects on the households—whether expressed in terms of consumption outcomes or in terms of coping strategies—are likely to be worse the greater the stigmatization of HIV/AIDS. Although this formula was implicit in our earlier discussion, additional losses of incomes and earn-ngs can occur, for instance, because of the loss of a job from the stigma associated with HIV infection, even if the HIV-positive individual is not sick with opportunistic infections associated with HIV/AIDS. Moreover, if drugs for treatment of HIV/AIDS become more expensive, if public subsidies for care provision remain limited, or if health insurance is unavailable, out-of-pocket health care spending can be expected to increase with obvious negative implications for non-health spending and for the coping options available to households (18–20). Clearly, the adverse policy implications of HIV/AIDS for households call for priority policy attention, independent of whether AIDS visibly affects the growth of gross domestic product (GDP), GDP per capita, or some other macroeconomic indicator. Table 9-1 provides lists of the household impacts and the different factors that influence their magnitude.

With 5% of Nigeria's adult population infected with HIV, and in light of the previous discussion, the subject of the impact of HIV/AIDS on Nigerian households carries obvious policy relevance. Unfortunately, we know little about the economic and social challenges that Nigerian households affected by HIV are currently facing. This chapter seeks to address this gap in research by focusing primarily, although not exclusively, on the economic impact of HIV/AIDS on households in Oyo and Plateau, two target states of the AIDS Prevention Initiative in Nigeria.

Although Oyo and Plateau states account for only about 6.3% of the total land area of Nigeria, and a roughly similar share of its projected total population of more than 130 million in 2003, we believe that findings for these two states could offer insights for Nigeria as a whole on the following grounds.[1] First, the states offer some geographic variation—with one located in southwestern Nigeria and the other in central Nigeria—as well as considerable ethnic diversity. Second, the adult HIV prevalence rates in the two states are not too far from the national average of about 5.0%—3.9% for Oyo State, and 6.3% for Plateau State—or roughly about 82,000 HIV-infected adults in Oyo State, and 81,000 in Plateau State.[2]

SAMPLING PROCEDURE, DATA, AND METHODOLOGY

In this section we describe the sampling approach and the methods used to assess the impact of HIV/AIDS among households in Oyo and Plateau states.

Sampling Procedure

Our intention was to sample two categories of households—1,200 "general" households (600 each in the two states) that may or may not have members with HIV and 300 households explicitly identified to have HIV-positive members, about 150 in each state. Moreover, 150 households were to be interviewed in each urban local government area (LGA) and 150 households interviewed in each rural LGA, respectively.

The census data on population (for 1991) and geographic area for each state were obtained from the Nigerian Population Commission website and http://www.nigeriabusinessinfo.com/nigeria-population.htm. Projected population for 2003, owing to the lack of a census since 1991, was obtained from the United Nations website http://esa.un.org/unpp/p2k0data.asp.

HIV prevalence data was obtained from the NACA (National Action Committee on AIDS) website: www.naca.gov.ng. Estimates of adults with HIV in the two states are based on HIV prevalence rates reported by NACA, combined with age-distribution data from the National Population Commission, and projected populations in the two states from the United Nations.

Consider first the "general" household survey. In each state, we chose for sampling purposes four LGAs so as to be representative of both rural and urban areas. In Oyo State, Ibadan and Ogbomoso were the two urban LGAs, and Igboora and Saki were the two rural LGAs. In Plateau, Jos and Pankshin were chosen as the two urban LGAs and Barakin-Ladi and Jos-North were the two rural locations. Jos-North replaced the Shendam LGA, owing to ethnic strife during the period of the field survey.

In choosing the set of sample households, we adopted a stratified random sampling procedure within each chosen LGA. The stratification was based on classification of residential areas by economic status — low, medium, and high. Within each stratum, streets were randomly chosen, followed by a systematic selection of houses on the basis of the number of buildings in each street. Only one household within each identified building was sampled. Where more than one household lived in a building, selection was by ballot. The same procedure was used for sampling rural households, except that stratification of residential areas by living standards was not felt necessary, given the more economically homogeneous nature of the population. This sampling procedure was adopted after our attempt to use the enumeration area maps of the National Population Commission for the national census to guide the sampling process did not work well, because the relevant maps were more than a decade old. The maps are being updated and should enable a better sampling frame for household-level data collection in future years.

The survey was administered to respondents by first introducing the study to the heads of household and obtaining their verbal consent. Only after the consent was given did a trained enumerator proceed to a structured questionnaire that was then filled out by household responses.

For households explicitly identified to have HIV-positive members, a somewhat different strategy was pursued in data collection. Unlike the "general" household sample, households of people living with HIV/AIDS were sampled purposively. The choice of the sampling procedure reflects the inherent limitation of a probability sampling approach in identifying a sufficiently large sample given the unwillingness of infected persons to "self-identify" because of the stigma associated with HIV-positive status.

Specifically, the sample population of households with an HIV-infected member was accessed as follows. The research study was first introduced to hospitals and nongovernmental organizations (NGOs) working with people with HIV and the consent of eligible respondents was initially received verbally through the representatives of these organizations. Only then were trained field workers introduced to people living with HIV/AIDS, at a location convenient to the prospective respondent. At the time of this introduction, the prospective respondents were again introduced to the objectives of the study, and their consent was obtained in writing. Due to limited NGO activities in rural areas, the majority of this population was identified from urban locations. Hospitals were the main entry point for rural locations.

In the end, our sample sizes were close to — but not identical to — the sample sizes that we originally envisaged. Table 9-2 presents some summary statistics showing that a total of 1,495 households were sampled in the end, 1,143 of "general" households, and 352 households that had an adult member explicitly identified with HIV. About 131 households experienced a death of a family member.

Table 9-2. Economic Impact of HIV/AIDS on Households

State	Number of Households	Mean Household Size	Annual PCE (naira in thousands)	Christian (percent)	Muslim (percent)	Female (percent)	Asset Index
Oyo							
With HIV	154	4.3	124.2	52.7	45.7	50.7	0.902
Without HIV	599	5.4	132.5	61.0	38.6	48.7	1.065
All	753	5.2	131.1	59.6	39.9	48.8	1.032
Plateau							
With HIV	198	6.2	111.6	90.4	8.0	63.1	-0.896
Without HIV	544	6.4	99.0	85.3	12.2	49.5	-1.106
All	742	6.4	102.3	86.6	11.1	50.0	-1.050

Abbreviation: PCE: per capita expenditure

Data

The survey collected data on a variety of household- and individual-level variables. This included demographic information on each household member—such as age, sex, marital status, and relationship to head of household—as well as any deaths that occurred in the household in the year preceding the survey.

The data also included information a variety of socioeconomic characteristics of individual members and the households, including years of schooling, literacy status, earnings, occupational status income from sources other than labor earnings, household expenditure, asset holdings, and other indicators of living conditions.

Apart from this socioeconomic and demographic information, the survey collected data on individual health status, illness in the four weeks preceding the survey, hospitalizations in the year preceding the survey, the type of health facility where treatment was sought, out-of-pocket health expenditures, transportation expenses linked to care, funeral expenses (in case of death), the length of time for which an individual was unable to perform normal activities, time spent in caregiving by non-ill members of the household, and the main sources of financing of health spending by the household.

Both sets of respondents (corresponding to households with HIV and without HIV) were also queried about their views and concerns regarding the future of children and orphans of people with HIV, the social stigma associated with HIV, as well the likelihood of smooth inheritance transfers following the death of one or more parents. Individuals with HIV were additionally queried about mental stresses they faced, including any steps they had taken to address the sources of this stress.

To assess households' economic status we used two types of indicators. First we derived an asset index, based on household responses to questions on the assets they owned and their living conditions, based on the "principal component" method. Second, we used an indicator of household consumption expenditures. Because data on expenditures for some of the households were missing, and also because the simplistic nature of the questionnaire did not allow for inclusion of items such as imputed spending on self-owned housing, we adopted the following procedure for imputation: An ordinary least squares regression of household consumer expenditures in the last year on household asset holdings was used to "fit" expenditures for cases in which the observations were missing. The resulting information and other relevant household data are presented in Table 9-2.

Data from Table 9-2 suggest that in the sample population, members of households with HIV and members of households without HIV were broadly comparable in terms of per capita expenditures, religious composition, the proportion of females, and asset holdings. It should be noted, however, that the per capita expenditures in our sample were substantially higher than the estimated per capita GDP at market prices of 70,000 to 75,000 naira, a range that results from different estimates of Nigeria's population.[3] This discrepancy between our sample and Nigeria's per capita GDP can at least be partially explained. First, Nigeria has a substantial black market economy, so one can imagine that some consumer expenditures are likely to go unreported in estimates of national income. Second, Oyo and Plateau states are not among the poorest states in Nigeria and presumably have average incomes (and expenditures) that are somewhat higher than the national average. Finally, with nearly 60% of our sample urban, we can imagine that the gap between the two sets of estimates would be further narrowed if the appropriate share of rural populations could be accounted for. On the other hand, one ought to expect GDP per capita to be substantially higher than household spending from standard national economic accounting principles because these estimates also include savings. With no recent studies of consumer spending available, one can do little to address this discrepancy directly, except to point to this as an area for future research. To the extent that the sample of individuals in our study is relatively rich, one can imagine, based on earlier work for Africa and elsewhere, that any evidence of adverse household impacts of AIDS would be conservative.

Methodology

In assessing the adverse implications of AIDS on households in Oyo and Plateau states, the cross-sectional nature of our data limits the analyses that we can perform and the conclusions that we can derive, especially if we are concerned with changes over time. Nonetheless there are analyses that can offer potentially useful insights.

These include first, assessing whether individuals and households with HIV, or that recently experienced an adult death, used more health care and spent more out of pocket on health than comparable groups that did not have HIV or experience an adult death. Second, information on the way health care is financed and the extent of caregiving provided across different categories of households can yield important insights about the sacrifices households are making and the coping strategies they are adopting. Finally, information on respondent assessments about HIV-related stigma and protection of property following the death of an adult household member will be useful in assessing the severity of impacts.

---

[3]As per statistics reported by the International Monetary Fund, in 2003, Nigeria's GDP at current prices was about 7,545 billion naira. The above finding obtains if we assume that GDP at current prices continues to grow at average annual rates experienced during the preceding two years.

Table 9-3A. Morbidity and Health Expenditures in the Last Month in Oyo and Plateau States, 2004

State	Percentage reporting illness in the past month	Mean days ill person not able to perform normal activities	Days spent per ill person as inpatient of health facility	Average health expenditures per ill person (in naira)	Average outpatient spending per ill person (in naira)	Percentage private facilities (non-public, non-mission)
Oyo						
With HIV	55.8	5.7	2.3	7,757	1,747	53.5
Without HIV	13.6	4.0	1.1	3,754	2,199	59.9
All	15.2	4.2	1.3	4,327	2,134	58.9
Plateau						
With HIV	47.0	7.5	1.5	4,774	2,479	23.1
Without HIV	7.9	4.6	1.1	5,179	1,505	41.7
All	9.5	5.3	1.2	5,097	1,705	37.5

Source: Authors' estimates
Note: "Average health expenditures" (column 5) include both inpatient and outpatient spending on health

Table 9-3B. Morbidity and Health Expenditures in the Last Month in Oyo and Plateau States (Female), 2004

State	Percentage reporting illness in the past month	Mean days ill person not able to perform normal activities	Days spent per ill person as inpatient of health facility	Average health expenditures per ill person (in naira)	Average outpatient spending per ill person (in naira)	Percentage private facilities (non-public, non-mission)
Oyo						
With HIV	59.0	4.8	2.0	7,632	1,971	45.7
Without HIV	13.3	3.9	1.0	2,311	1,005	61.8
All	15.1	4.0	1.1	3,152	1,158	59.0
Plateau						
With HIV	50.4	7.2	1.5	5,867	2,881	19.7
Without HIV	6.9	4.2	1.2	7,241	2,033	37.8
All	9.2	5.1	1.3	6,846	2,277	32.1

Source: Authors' estimates
Note: "Average health expenditures" (column 5) include both inpatient and outpatient spending on health

FINDINGS AND DISCUSSION

Tables 9-3A, 9-3B, and 9-3C describe the pattern of morbidity in the month preceding the survey, indicators of severity of illness, amounts spent on inpatient and outpatient care, and type of facility used by people living with HIV/AIDS (PLWHAs) and those not identified as infected.

The data presented in these tables suggest two conclusions that hold for both Oyo and Plateau states. First, individuals with HIV were considerably more likely to report an illness in the last month. Second,

State	Percentage reporting illness in the past month	Mean days ill person not able to perform normal activities	Days spent per ill person as inpatient of health facility	Average health expenditures per ill person (in naira)	Average outpatient spending per ill person (in naira)	Percentage private facilities (non-public, non-mission)
Oyo						
With HIV	52.6	6.8	2.5	7,900	1,489	62.5
Without HIV	13.9	4.1	1.3	5,068	3,285	58.2
All	15.3	4.4	1.4	5,434	3,053	58.8
Plateau						
With HIV	41.1	8.2	1.7	2,481	1,634	30.0
Without HIV	8.8	4.9	1.0	3,610	1,104	44.7
All	9.8	5.4	1.1	3,466	1,172	42.6

Table 9-3C. Morbidity and Health Expenditures in the Past Month in Oyo and Plateau States (Male), 2004

Source: Authors' estimates;s
Note: "Average health expenditures" (column 5) include both inpatient and outpatient spending on health

they are likely to have a more severe illness as measured in terms of the average numbers of days they are unable to perform their normal activities and the duration of inpatient stays.

The data also suggest some inter-state differences as well. In Oyo State, people with HIV tended to spend substantially greater amounts out-of-pocket relative to people without HIV, mainly because they use more inpatient care, and because they also rely to a much greater extent on the private sector compared to their counterparts in Plateau State. However, because morbidity prevalence among PLWHAs is much greater than for those who are not identified as being infected, it also follows that on a *per capita basis* (all people whether sick or not), health expenditures on HIV-positive persons are much greater than those who do not have HIV in Oyo State. Our conclusions do not change even when we break the data down by gender.

Prima facie then, HIV/AIDS imposes a greater burden of health spending on affected households in Oyo State. Indeed, households that have one or more HIV-positive members reported one-month morbidity rates among their members of 22% and 11% in Oyo and Plateau states respectively, compared to 13.6% and 9.4% among households that did not report HIV-positive members. Moreover, the morbidity data also suggest that HIV potentially imposes income losses on households owing to the greater length of normal activity days lost by sick members. From Tables 9-3B and 9-3C we see that compared to women, sick male HIV-positive members tend to lose a greater number of normal activity days, and this could signal losses in household income if the sick person is the family breadwinner. The lower out-of-pocket spending by HIV-positive individuals in Plateau State revealed by our data suggests that public services there reach HIV-positive individuals more effectively than in Oyo State, and this may be worthy of further investigation.

Our comparisons could potentially be confounded by the fact that the data on HIV-positive individuals derive primarily from urban areas (75% of the sample) and relate to adults, whereas that is not the

Table 9-4A. Hospitalization and Health Expenditures in the Last Year in Oyo and Plateau States, 2004

State	Percentage reporting hospitalization in the past month	Days spent per ill person as inpatient of health facility	Average health expenditures per hospitalized person (naira in thousands)	Percentage private facilities (non-public, non-mission)
Oyo				
With HIV	51.3	9.9	50.4	31.7
Without HIV	4.5	10.7	24.6	35.9
All	6.3	10.5	33.2	34.5
Plateau				
With HIV	20.2	23.2	25.9	20.0
Without HIV	3.9	13.0	18.2	33.9
All	4.5	14.9	19.7	31.3

Source: Authors' estimates

Table 9-4B. Hospitalization and Health Expenditures in Reference Year, By Gender, Oyo and Plateau States, 2004

Gender	Percentage reporting hospitalization in the past month	Days spent per ill person as inpatient of health facility	Average health expenditures per hospitalized person (naira in thousands)	Percentage private facilities (non-public, non-mission)
Male				
With HIV	34.9	14.2	36.7	32.7
Without HIV	4.5	14.4	24.1	32.1
All	5.6	14.4	26.8	32.2
Female				
With HIV	33.0	14.4	46.5	23.9
Without HIV	3.7	8.8	17.8	38.3
All	5.1	10.5	26.9	33.9

Source: Authors' estimates

case for the non-HIV sample. To this end, we redid the analyses in Tables 9-3A, 9-3B, and 9-3C for adults living in urban areas only, although we do not report our results here. None of our conclusions change if we focus only on adults aged 20 to 59 years living in urban areas.[4]

In addition to morbidity, health care utilization, and health spending in the month preceding the survey, we inquired about hospitalization in the one year preceding the survey. The relevant data are reported in Tables 9-4A and 9-4B.[5]

---

[4]The results are available from the authors upon request.
[5]The number of hospitalizations was not sufficiently large to permit us to break the gender data down further by state.

State	Percentage reporting hospitalization in the past month	Mean days ill person not able to perform normal activities	Average hours of caregiving per day per hospitalized case	Whether normal activity given up by caregiver (%)
Table 9-5A. Caregiving for Hospitalized Persons, Plateau and Oyo States, 2004				
Oyo				
With HIV	51.3	43.2	10.1	78.2
Without HIV	4.5	19.8	9.4	75.5
All	6.3	27.3	9.6	76.4
Plateau				
With HIV	20.2	48.9	12.9	90.0
Without HIV	3.9	27.0	12.8	92.0
All	4.5	31.1	12.8	91.6

Source: Authors' estimates

Our main finding is that PLWHAs are at a greater likelihood of being hospitalized, and once hospitalized they are likely to incur greater expenditures on average than people who do not have HIV. As can be seen from the tables, this is true, irrespective of whether we consider the hospitalization data separately by state or gender. Our results remain unchanged if we focus only on comparisons across adults in the age range of 20 to 59 years living in urban areas of Oyo and Plateau states.

It is well known that health expenditures tend to concentrate in the last year of life of an individual. Because our sample of individuals with AIDS was essentially that of individuals who were alive (otherwise they would not have been interviewed), our analysis perhaps did not fully capture the role of adult mortality in influencing health spending among individuals with AIDS. Thus we compared the average health expenditures among households that experienced an adult (aged 20 to 59 years) death in the year preceding the survey with those that did not. Focusing on hospitalization expenditures only, we found that per capita expenditures on hospitalization among households that experienced an adult death in the preceding year—2,591 naira—was nearly double that of households that did not experience an adult death—1,285 naira. Further breakdown by state and gender was not feasible owing to the small number of adult deaths in our sample (there were only 115 reported adult deaths).

Potential Impacts of HIV-Related Health Spending on Income and Consumption

In the absence of longitudinal data it is difficult to draw ready conclusions about the effects of HIV-related morbidity and health expenditures on household income and/or consumption. However, we can generate some circumstantial evidence in the form of time spent away from normal activities by the ill person and time spent by others on caregiving responsibilities. Tables 9-5A and 9-5B offer some information in this respect for hospitalization in the year preceding the survey.

We have already noted that PLWHAs have a greater likelihood of being hospitalized than those who do not have HIV. However, Tables 9-5A and 9-5B also indicate that the length of time away from normal

Gender	Percentage reporting hospitalization in the past month	Mean days ill person not able to perform normal activities	Average hours of caregiving per day per hospitalized case	Whether normal activity given up by caregiver (%)
Male				
With HIV	34.9	42.9	11.4	86.5
Without HIV	4.5	25.5	11.6	87.1
All	5.6	29.3	11.5	87.0
Female				
With HIV	33.0	46.7	10.8	78.8
Without HIV	3.7	20.8	10.6	80.1
All	5.1	28.9	10.6	79.7

Table 9-5B. Caregiving for Hospitalized Persons, Plateau and Oyo States, by Gender, 2004

Source: Authors' estimates

activities for hospitalized PLWHAs is higher than for people without HIV. There do not appear to be significant differences in the average daily level of caregiving and the sacrifice of "normal activities" by caregivers across PLWHAs and those who do not have HIV. When combined with the greater likelihood of hospitalization and length of time away from normal activity, however, this information suggests that the household likely faces declines in earnings from the affected adult household members and possibly declines in schooling if children are drafted into caregiving.

We could also assess the potential impact of HIV on household consumption by examining the share of health spending in total consumption spending and comparing it across households with HIV infected members and those without. Table 9-6 presents this information.

The third column in Table 9-6 shows that among households with hospitalized HIV-infected members, inpatient care spending as a proportion of household per capita expenditure is nearly three times as high as among households with hospitalized but non-HIV–infected members in Oyo State; in Plateau State, it is twice as high. That is, not only is the likelihood of hospitalization greater if a household has an HIV-positive member, but if the HIV-positive member is hospitalized, a greater chunk of expenditures is devoted to inpatient care. Data in column 5 of Table 9-6 bring these two conclusions together and show that annual per capita expenditures on hospitalization are much higher among households that have HIV-positive members than those who do not.

The economic burdens imposed by the health care expenditures of PLWHAs, coupled with a strong suspicion of an income loss caused through increased amounts of caregiving and time away from work activity by the sick person, indicate a decline in non-health consumption among household members. However, without longitudinal data, it is difficult to conclude whether consumption increased among households with HIV-positive members, or fell, following the incurring of these expenditures, compared to the situation before the illness or hospitalization event. For instance, if households that experienced an

		Spending among households as	Inpatient care spending	Percentage of households
State	Percentage reporting hospitalization in the past year	percentage of annual PCE, if HIV-positive member is hospitalized	per capita among all households (in naira)	selling assets to finance inpatient care
Oyo				
With HIV	51.3	45.6	8570	29.9
Without HIV	4.5	16.8	690	3.7
All	6.3	30.8	2025	16.1
Plateau				
With HIV	20.2	27.5	1842	28.4
Without HIV	3.9	14.2	532	22.2
All	4.5	19.3	870	24.5

Table 9-6. Burden of Inpatient Care Spending in Reference Year, Oyo and Plateau States, 2004

Source: Authors' estimates; PCE = Per Capita Expenditure within Households

HIV-related hospitalization also had better access to insurance, then higher health expenditures may not lead to lowered consumption.

The way household health expenditures are financed can offer some clues as to their likely impact on households' current and future consumption possibilities. Table 9-6 shows that among households that experienced hospitalization in the last one year, those with HIV-positive members were much more likely to sell assets to finance inpatient care than those without HIV-positive members. Although we do not possess additional information about the nature of assets sold, if the households did indeed end up selling durable or income-earning assets such as cattle, the implications for their future consumption opportunities are obvious. Further insight into the financing options open to households is provided by Figures 9-1 to 9-4, which describe the main sources of financing for inpatient care among households that had HIV-positive individuals and those that did not.[6]

Note that self-financing and support from relatives and the community are the major sources of inpatient care financing in our sample households. This is true irrespective of whether we are talking about Oyo State or about Plateau State. But there are some inter-state differences. The role of self-financing appears to be more important in Plateau, presumably reflecting the higher average income levels in that state. Residents of Plateau State also have better access to public facilities, which lowers the scale of spending required, whereas the role of community financing is relatively more important in Oyo State. Notice also that community financing is lower and reliance on self-financing sharply higher among households with HIV–positive members, relative to those without, in Oyo State. Given our earlier observation of higher out-of-pocket spending on inpatient care by households with HIV-positive members, this finding suggests limited community ability to offer insurance against health-related financial risks to PLWHAs.

---

[6]Similar findings emerge if we look at the sources of financing for treatment in the month preceding the survey.

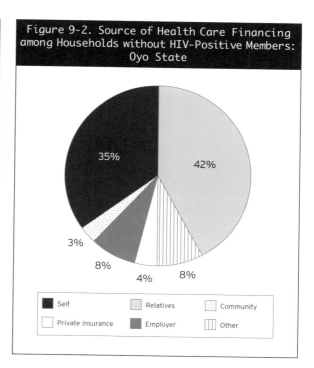

Figure 9-1. Source of Health Care Financing among Households with HIV-Positive Members: Oyo State

62%
33%
1%
0%
3%
1%

Self   Relatives   Community
Private Insurance   Employer   Other

Figure 9-2. Source of Health Care Financing among Households without HIV-Positive Members: Oyo State

35%
42%
3%
8%
4%
8%

Self   Relatives   Community
Private Insurance   Employer   Other

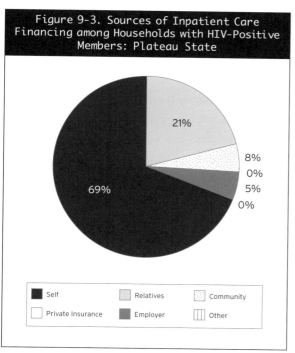

Figure 9-3. Sources of Inpatient Care Financing among Households with HIV-Positive Members: Plateau State

21%
8%
0%
5%
0%
69%

Self   Relatives   Community
Private Insurance   Employer   Other

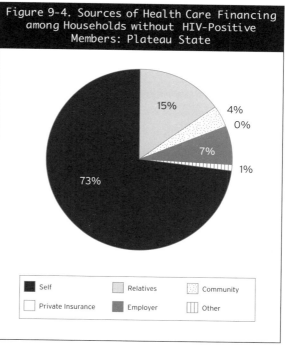

Figure 9-4. Sources of Health Care Financing among Households without HIV-Positive Members: Plateau State

15%
4%
0%
7%
1%
73%

Self   Relatives   Community
Private Insurance   Employer   Other

Table 9-7. Respondents' Perceptions About Well-Being of Children with HIV-Positive Parents and Control of Property upon Death, Oyo and Plateau States, 2004

	People with HIV	People without HIV	Combined
Wills and Property: Perception			
Property disposed as intended	75.5	68.8	71.2
Property grabbed if husband dies	67.2	52.2	55.9
Property grabbed if wife dies	20.7	23.0	22.5
Property grabbed if both parents die	58.1	44.2	47.5
Wills and Property: Experience			
Was property of widow/widower grabbed?	27.0	18.2	21.2
Children/Orphans of HIV-Positive Parents: Assessment of Discrimination and Mistreatment			
Treated differently	40.9	35.3	36.6
Ever neglected or underfed	82.4	69.9	73.2
Ever physically abused	69.4	37.6	46.0
Ever verbally abused	84.0	69.3	73.2

Source: Authors' estimates

There are two other crucial differences between households with HIV-positive members and those without. First, households with HIV-positive members appear to have less access to financial support from employers for health care. Second, in a setting where private health insurance coverage is low in any event, there is no evidence that it provides a source of support for inpatient care expenditures to any of the households that have HIV-positive members. In Oyo State, households not affected by HIV seem to be able to count on some support from private insurance, relative to households that are affected by HIV. In Plateau State, there seems to be no evidence of health coverage by private insurance, irrespective of HIV status.

Taken together, these different bits of evidence suggest that households affected by HIV are likely to incur greater income losses and higher health spending compared to households without HIV-positive members, all else the same. Whether these adverse financial shocks translate into consumption expenditure declines in the short run or the long run depends on the existence of buffers, or insurance, against such shocks. The evidence presented suggests that available insurance mechanisms are limited and that households with HIV-positive members, particularly in Oyo State, are forced to rely on themselves for financing health spending.

Property Losses for Survivors and the Outlook for Children

The adverse implications of HIV for affected households could be considerably more serious if, upon the death of one or both spouses, their property was grabbed by others, so that the financial welfare of their

Table 9-8. The Principal Concerns of People with HIV/AIDS in Oyo and Plateau States

Concerns of People with HIV/AIDS	State	
	Oyo	Plateau
Children: Worries		
Any	71.0	44.7
Inadequate education	57.3	37.3
Unable to survive	47.3	36.7
Lack of guardian	8.4	15.3
No emotional support	29.8	33.3
May be HIV positive	19.8	15.3
Children: Actions to Address Worries		
Any		
Asset purchases	76.3	40.0
Income generation	37.4	32.7
Prepare will	3.1	12.0
Appoint guardian	5.3	14.0
Advise for survival	36.6	32.0
Other Worries		
Illness, physical discomfort	75.3	36.4
Death	48.1	25.2
Declining ability to work	47.4	38.3
Treated badly	18.2	11.2
Perceived badly	27.3	10.3

Source: Authors' estimates

survivors, especially orphans, is seriously threatened. Such circumstances are not uncommon, particularly in developing countries where legal systems are weak, and the survivors are either uninformed, or not strong enough to protect their property rights.

To assess the threat of property loss following the death of one or both parents, we asked respondents about the likelihood of such losses (Table 9-7, top panel). The data reveal a strong perception among respondent households that property is grabbed following the death of adults in the household. It is particularly noteworthy that the perceived risk of property grabbing by others is considerably greater when the husband dies than when the wife dies, regardless of the type of household. Also interesting is that respondents of households with HIV perceive a greater risk of property grabbing upon the death of adult members than households without HIV-positive members.

We also asked respondents who were widows or widowers about their own experience with property grabbing. Although the sample was small, the findings were nevertheless instructive. The proportion reporting actual property grabbing was lower than the proportion perceiving property grabbing, but not insignificant. Fully one-fifth reported some property being grabbed following the death of a spouse, and the share of respondents with HIV reporting property grabbing was greater by 50% than respondents who did not have HIV.

Table 9-7 also highlights concerns regarding respondents' perceptions of the difficulties children of PLWHAs are likely to face upon the death of their parents. In general, a very high proportion of respondents believe that the children or orphans of HIV-infected people are likely to face differential treatment, greater abuse, and neglect, with obvious implications for their future economic and psychological well-being. Once again PLWHAs perceive a greater risk of such discrimination than those not infected.

Further research may well be needed to verify these perceptions and preliminary findings about the financial risks and discrimination that the survivors of HIV-infected people face. However, they do point to an important area for policy action to address some of the negative implications of HIV on households.

Psychic Costs

Economic implications are not the only way in which HIV can influence households; psychological costs may well be rooted in economics and societal responses to the epidemic. We asked HIV-positive respondents about their worries and found a variety of issues of great concern to them. Table 9-8 summarizes some of their responses.

The first panel in Table 9-8 highlights a number of concerns that HIV-positive individuals have about their children, ranging from their future survival to their educational opportunities to their possible lack of emotional support. The middle panel focuses on actions that individuals have taken toward addressing these concerns. The last panel points to additional worries about themselves, ranging from physical discomfort to a lack of ability to work, discrimination, and approaching death.

Table 9-8 highlights some of the respondents' approaches toward addressing their concerns about their children's future, including acquiring additional assets, taking up additional income-generation activities, and training their children for survival. While admirable, their own health care requirements, their inability to work, and the likelihood that their assets will be grabbed by others suggest that these may be inefficient mechanisms for their intended purpose—and thus unlikely to ameliorate the original concerns. Much remains to be done in addressing the psychological well-being and economic concerns of affected households.

CONCLUSION

Like those in other sub-Saharan African countries, HIV-affected households in Nigeria are likely to face both economic and psychological challenges, including the likelihood of substantial income loss within households and an increased burden of caregiving and out-of-pocket health care spending. Our research suggests inadequate community and formal insurance, forcing households to become increasingly self-reliant in meeting their health care expenses and income losses. The likelihood of property loss and discrimination will exacerbate already severe financial burdens on households.

Our study highlights possible directions for policy action. Based on data for Plateau State, it does appear that subsidized access to public sector and mission facilities can ameliorate the financial burden from health care faced by households with HIV-positive members. Increasing public sector access is obviously important, given that other sources of formal insurance, including by employers and third-party insurers, appears to have limited coverage among PLWHAs. Making public services more accessible and subsidizing access to mission facilities offer promising ways to address at least some of the economic difficulties faced by households with HIV. How might these be achieved? Although we did not collect detailed information on public facilities, our study suggests taking a closer look at the experience of Plateau State, given what appears to a more effective performance of health facilities in public and mission sectors there. While robust inference must await future research, we conjecture that some combination of closer proximity, subsidized access to antiretrovirals, and a better system of care and support for PLWHAs is likely to have been crucial. If so, subsidies for public and mission facilities may have to target these very services for improvement.

When a lack of information on the demand side precludes access to public and mission facilities by PLWHAs, the government and the mission sector will have to work with the private sector and civil society organizations to promote such access. As an illustration, increased coordination with traditional health care providers, witch doctors, and others in rural areas that often treat PLWHAs may lead to more referrals to public facilities that can offer better treatment of opportunistic infections and HIV. This will not always be easy because the traditional providers will lose "business" as a result. Thus one element of the strategy might be to provide some medical training or formal recognition by the government, or even involvement of such providers in government health programs, including direct remuneration for referrals.

Other elements of the private sector could also be co-opted. For instance, tax deductions could be provided to firms for expenditures they incurred on treatments for PLWHAs. Because household impacts are sometimes driven by HIV-positive status and discrimination in the workplace, the Nigerian government could work with organizations providing social and private insurance to offer discounted premiums to firms that undertake HIV prevention programs for their employees and do not discriminate against PLWHAs in decisions to hire and fire.

Because income loss owing to the death or loss of a job for the breadwinner is a crucial element in the hardships that households face, a second area for policy intervention would be increasing access of

PLWHAs to income-generation schemes. There is some recent literature that highlights the potential role of microfinancing schemes as a means to promote income generation among PLWHAs in Africa (9). Much can also be learned from the experience of successful microfinance institutions worldwide, particularly the Grameen Bank in Bangladesh, the BancoSol in Bolivia, and institutions in other African countries such as Benin and Ghana that have helped address the financial needs of poor entrepreneurs, including women (21–23). Pilot programs along the lines seen in these other countries may be a useful first step in this direction, initiated perhaps with some combination of federal and state government financial support and civil society operation of microfinance schemes, with regulatory oversight by local bodies and banking authorities.

While access to income generation is useful, protection of existing assets of PLWHAs is obviously important. Thus, another area for policy action is better protection of the property rights of survivors, especially those with HIV-positive parents. Two elements are involved: addressing the generally poor means of protection of property rights (especially land rights) that exists in Nigeria at present, and addressing the special requirements of HIV-infected people and their survivors. We believe a multi-pronged approach is needed here, one that uses both short- and long-term strategies. Some obvious steps include enhancing greater community awareness and participation in defining and respecting property rights, intermediated by civil society organizations, better official record keeping of property ownership, and encouraging individuals, particularly those with HIV, to prepare living wills. The government may also consider giving high priority in civil cases to those involving the property rights of children and widows, perhaps accompanied by subsidized access to lawyers for needy cases. Other longer-term steps may include promoting efforts that reduce discriminatory treatment of HIV-infected people and their survivors, raise women's status in society, and foster judicial reforms directed toward greater transparency and speedy disposal of cases.

Such interventions do require planning and resources, of course, and thus set out a rich agenda for action by the National Planning Commission, the Ministry of Finance, and other government agencies concerned with poverty reduction and HIV in Nigeria. Clearly more resources will be needed for health care, HIV prevention initiatives, and the piloting of income generation and microfinance institutions. Regulatory interventions for microfinance banks as well as judicial reform relating to property rights of children and widows may require additional action by the Ministry of Justice.

Our findings and proposed agenda for action are based on imperfect knowledge. For instance, we believe much could be done to improve upon the data collected for our study. Clearly, the relatively small size of sample households and the fact the sample is somewhat urban-based are sources of concern in assessing whether our findings are truly representative of the population. The focus on only two Nigerian states means that our findings may not readily carry over to other states. Moreover, because the survey was undertaken over a period of just one month, it might not have captured any seasonal biases, if such biases interact with HIV status. Without longitudinal analysis, our conclusions are strongly suggestive rather than conclusive in terms of indicating causal direction. Future research must inevitably focus on addressing these gaps in Nigeria, by extending these analyses to other states, correcting for seasonal biases, and undertaking longitudinal studies.

In addition to the purely methodological aspects of our research, a number of other issues need further exploration. How, for example, are resources on health allocated to different levels of health facilities and who benefits from them? What are the key factors that lead public and mission facilities to effectively serve PLWHAs and reduce the financial impact of AIDS on them? What are the loopholes in the laws and the associated system for their implementation that allows for dispossession of property from their legal owners? How do differences in community organization and norms across Nigeria affect the ways in which individuals with HIV cope with the financial and psychological impacts of HIV? The significant political, geographic, ethnic, and linguistic variation that exists across communities in Nigeria constitutes a fascinating laboratory in which to assess these questions.

ACKNOWLEDGMENTS

We are grateful to a number of individuals and institutions for their encouragement, comments, and material help in undertaking this work. We are especially thankful to Professors Phyllis Kanki and Michael Reich, and Dr. Wole Odutolu at the AIDS Prevention Initiative in Nigeria. Dr. Soji Adeyi provided extremely thoughtful comments that have improved this work. At the Nigerian Institute of Social and Economic Research (NISER) we benefited from the guidance and advice of Dr. D. O. Ajakaiye, Dr. A. Sunmola, Ms. Nancy Nelson-Twakor, Mr. L. N. Chete, and Mr. A. O. Ajala. Dr. A. O. Okesola (Oyo State AIDS Control Programme) and Mr. Bala Mitok Rumtong (Plateau State AIDS Control Programme) provided us with access to data on expenditures on HIV/AIDS. Seminar participants at Harvard and NISER provided several useful comments that benefited this study.

REFERENCES

1. Bolton P, Ndogoni L. Cross-cultural assessment of trauma-related mental illness. Draft report. Baltimore, Maryland: Johns Hopkins University, 2001. Accessed at www.certi.org/publications/policy/ugandafinahreport.htm on July 10, 2005.

2. Germann S. Psychosocial impact of HIV/AIDS on children. *AIDS Bulletin*, 2004;13(2). Accessed at www.mrc.ac.za/aids/june2004/impact.htm on July 10, 2005.

3. Bechu N. The impact of AIDS on the economy of families in Cote d'Ivoire: changes in consumption among AIDS affected households. In: Ainsworth M, Fransen L, Over M, eds. *Confronting AIDS: Evidence from the Developing World*, Washington, DC: World Bank, 1998.

4. Booysen F, van Rensburg D, Bachmann M, Engelbrecht M, Steyn F. The socio-economic impact of HIV/AIDS on households in South Africa. Accessed at www.mrc.ac.za/aids/march2002/economic.htm on July 10, 2005.

5. Over M. Coping with the impact of AIDS. *Finance Dev*, 1998:22–24.

6. Donovan C, Bailey L, Mpyisi E, Weber M. Prime Age Adult Morbidity and Mortality in Rural Rwanda: Effects on Household Income, Agricultural Production and Food Security Strategies. Kigali, Rwanda: Ministry of Agriculture, Livestock and Forestry, 2003.

7. Nampanya-Serpell N. Social and economic risk factors for HIV/AIDS affected families in Zambia. Paper presented at the International AIDS Economics Network's Economics of AIDS Symposium, Durban, South Africa, July 7–8, 2000. Accessed at www.iaen.org/conferences/durpapers/papers.htm on July 10, 2005.

8. Nyamukapa C, Gregson S. Contrasting primary school outcomes of paternal and maternal orphans in Manicaland, Zimbabwe: HIV/AIDS and weaknesses in the extended family system. Draft report. London, United Kingdom: Imperial College Faculty of Medicine, 2004.

9. Mutangandura G. Household welfare impacts of mortality of adult females in Zimbabwe: implications for policy and program development. Draft report. Chapel Hill, North Carolina: University of North Carolina, Carolina Population Center, 2000.

10. Yamano T, Jayne TS. Measuring the impacts of working-age adult mortality on small-scale farm households in Kenya. *World Development*, 2004;32: 91–119.

11. Barnett T, Blaikie P. *AIDS in Africa: Its Present and Future Impact.* New York: The Guilford Press, 1992.

12. Mujinja P, Over M. The impact of AIDS on health care utilization and expenditure by the fatally ill in northwest Tanzania. *IX International Conference on AIDS*, Berlin, Germany, June 6–11, 1993 (abstract WS-D123-1).

13. Bollinger L, Stover J. *The Economic Impact of AIDS in Zambia.* Draft report. Washington, DC: Futures Group International, 1999.

14. Menon R, Wawer MJ, Konde-Lule JK, Sewankambo NK, Li C. The economic impact of adult mortality on households in Rakai district, Uganda. In: Ainsworth M, Fransen L, Over M, eds. *Confronting AIDS: Evidence from the Developing World*, Washington, DC: World Bank, 1998.

15. Over M, Lundberg M, Mujinja P. Source of finance assistance for households suffering an adult death. Working Paper No. 2508. Washington, DC: World Bank, 2000. Accessed at http://econ.worldbank.org/files/1320_wps2508.pdf on July 10, 2005.

16. Memfih N. Assessing the socioeconomic effects of HIV/AIDS at the level of households in Cameroon. Draft report. Buea, Cameroon: Faculty of Social and Management Sciences, Department of Economics and Management, 2005.

17. Ainsworth M, Dayton J. The impact of the AIDS epidemic on the health of the elderly in Tanzania. Draft report. Washington, DC: World Bank, Development Research Group, 2001.

18. Bloom D, Glied S. Who is bearing the burden of the AIDS epidemic in Asia? In: Bloom D, Lyons L, eds. *Economic Implications of AIDS in Asia.* New Delhi: Oxford University Press, 1993

19. Bloom D, Mahal A, Christiansen L, et al. Socio-economic dimensions of AIDS in Sri Lanka. In: Bloom D, Godwin P, eds. *The Economics of HIV and AIDS: The Case of South and Southeast Asia.* New Delhi: Oxford University Press, 1997.

20. Guinness L, Alban A. *The Economic Impact of AIDS in Africa: A Review of the Literature.* UNAIDS background paper for the Africa Development Forum. Geneva: UNAIDS, 2000.

21. Basu A, Blavy R, Yulek M. Microfinance in Africa: experience and lessons from selected African countries. Working paper number WP/04/174. Washington, DC: World Bank, 2004.

22. Gonzalez-Vega C, Schreiner M, Meyer R, Rodriguez-Meza J, Navajas S. BancoSol: the challenge of growth for microfinance institutions. In: Schneider H, ed. *Microfinance for the Poor.* Paris: Organisation for Economic Co-operation and Development, 1997.

23. Schreiner M. *The Performance of Subsidized Microfinance Organizations — BancoSol of Bolivia and the Grameen Bank of Bangladesh.* Lewiston, New York: Edwin Mellen Press, 2003.

10

THE STIGMATIZATION OF PEOPLE LIVING WITH HIV/AIDS

Lawrence Adeokun,* Prosper Okonkwo,†
and Oladapo A. Ladipo*

The HIV/AIDS epidemic is less advanced in Nigeria than in East African and southern African countries, and so the issues relating to stigmatization and discrimination of people living with HIV/AIDS (PLWHAs) have not been as fully explored in Nigeria. Information on the stigma of AIDS in Nigeria has been limited to a number of abstracts published in international HIV/AIDS conference proceedings (1). The themes that emerge most often in those abstracts include victims' perceptions of the stigma (2); battles against workplace discrimination and consequent encounters with judicial prejudice (3); and the reluctance of PLWHAs to share their test results because of the stigma attached to AIDS (4).

Other themes include the role PLWHAs may play in prevention programs as well as the role of counseling in reducing stigma (5). The understanding is that PLWHAs have largely transcended the fear that others have of AIDS and that meeting a PLWHA humanizes the epidemic (6). The theory that training can reduce the stigma of AIDS is explored (7), as is the belief that faith-based organizations are well placed to promote stigma reduction through their repeated contacts with members (8). Health providers' anxiety about their personal safety is also mentioned (4).

In effect, discussions about the stigma of AIDS have primarily focused on the concerns of PLWHAs and only marginally on other actors in the production, perpetuation, and reduction of

*Association for Reproductive and Family Health, Ibadan, Nigeria
†AIDS Prevention Initiative in Nigeria, Ibadan, Nigeria

stigma. Yet for a holistic view of stigma to be gained, these other actors must be included in the framework of analysis. This chapter therefore presents findings from an HIV surveillance survey conducted in four Nigerian markets. This survey explored the impact of behavioral change activities on stigma, discrimination, and related issues. Placing the data and interpretation in proper context, however, requires an elaboration of the various actors and forms of stigma, discrimination, denial, and shame. It is against this background that the significant changes in indices of stigmatization and discrimination over the one-year project period can be fully appreciated.

BASIC DEFINITIONS

Stigma, Discrimination, Denial, and Shame

Stigma is the sign or mark placed on a person or group that sets them apart as different from the rest of society. The stigma attached to individuals can be extended to those who associate with them (9). The stigma that a person carries becomes a liability only when society declares it so. The same label or trait may be considered a deviation from the norm in one culture and may be within the acceptable range of what constitutes the norm in another culture.

The result of carrying a stigma is devaluation by others and discrimination through the withdrawal of rights and privileges to which that individual or group may otherwise be entitled. Discrimination is the societal response to the negative value attached to the stigma an individual may carry.

The stigma is not necessarily prejudicial; it is the adverse reaction of people to the stigma that creates offense. There are, of course, instances in which the stigma is "foreign" to the host community and consequently looked upon as a deviation from the norm. This is the basis for the pity, revulsion, and other reactions that some people have toward those with physical appearances considered odd or distorted.

Stigma may take a tangible form when there are manifestations of the condition of stigma. In Yoruba culture, for example, being albino is an obvious departure from the norm. Despite the frequency of twinning among the Yoruba, twins also are stigmatized. In the instance of HIV/AIDS, the assumption of HIV infection — and thus the stigma — may be false, or the stigma may be based on reliable information, such as when a PLWHA discloses his or her HIV status.

The measurement of stigma can be problematic because stigma takes so many forms. When the form is tangible, the prevalence of stigma can be measured. In the case of an intangible form, however, only the proxies of stigma can be measured. For example, the number of people suffering from a medical condition can only be measured when the diagnosis is readily available. In the same way, the measurement of stigma depends on the form.

In addressing proxy measures, the reaction of people to propositions about stigma can capture the perceptions and attitudes of respondents to the stigmatized condition, tangible or intangible. In the same way, discriminatory attitudes can be measured in responses. The fact that such measurements may be flawed — because of a social desirability bias in the responses people give to discriminatory propositions or scenarios — must be taken into consideration when analyzing the information (10).

For negative attitudes to change, the mindsets of the various stakeholders in what Goffman calls "the mending of the damaged self" must be considered (9). The stigma lies with the "victim," but the resulting discrimination comes from others. Denial and shame are the strategies available to victims in avoiding or bearing the brunt of the discrimination attached to their stigma.

The effects of HIV-related stigma and discrimination are often so severe that most members of society fear them (11,12). Potential victims can prevent or avert stigma and discrimination by going into denial. The denial of a stigmatized condition such as HIV/AIDS may be experienced by those who have not been tested irrespective of their assessment of their vulnerability. Denial is more pronounced in those who have tested HIV positive but fear the stigma attached to their HIV status.

The basis of denial of a trait and the individual's associated shame change constantly in response to shifts in societal values. This is particularly true of traditional societies as they move to modernization and globalization. Changes in the sexual behavior of young people challenge traditional society, as the culture must adapt to the new reality that the ideals of virginity, premarital celibacy, and modest dress codes may be altered by external values.

When denial no longer serves as a protection—either because the confidentiality of the infection has been broken or the symptoms of disease have become apparent—then shame becomes the next logical mechanism available to the infected and affected. This self-imposed sanction reflects the victim's perception of the degree of the physical or moral deviation from the norms of the society. In effect, the more the victim shares the public's view about the stigma, the greater the shame he or she feels.

People who suffer from tuberculosis, weight loss, or certain types of cancer may be rightly or wrongly suspected of being infected with HIV. At this stage the sense of shame and fear of discrimination may lead the victim to withdraw from friends, relatives, and society and even, in some cases, to contemplate suicide. Individuals who have experienced rejection, isolation, and aggression are at high risk of psychiatric symptoms. Psychological stress and fear of AIDS may hamper social and occupational functioning (13), thus enhancing the effects of shame. In a study in Zimbabwe, 9% of respondents stated that they would commit suicide if they found they were HIV positive (14). The victim reciprocates the rejection of society (15).

REASONS FOR THE STIGMA OF AIDS

In 1988, early in the course of the epidemic, AIDS was considered invariably fatal. The predominant impression was that HIV infection was the result of deviant and stigmatized behavior such as homosexual practices, sex work, and drug use (15), as well as sex outside marriage and promiscuity. The identification of already stigmatized groups as "high-risk" increased their vulnerability to stigmatization and discrimination (16). As early prevention programs were being developed, it seemed logical to start with these "high-risk groups." Consequently, prevention messages placed additional distance between PLWHAs and the rest of the community, giving the impression that HIV prevention did not concern the larger community (9).

Another basis of stigma and discrimination in the early stages of the epidemic was the prevailing myth that HIV could be contracted through normal social contact. In Uganda, for example, it was believed that if one person in a family had AIDS, the rest of the family would become infected. Consequently, many community members terminated social relationships when a person's HIV status became known (17).

The blame of women and sex workers for the spread of HIV and other sexually transmitted infections (STIs) has resulted in considerable discrimination against them (18). Criminal sanctions that seek to regulate the sex industry, however, tend to cause sex workers to operate secretly and therefore out of reach of intervention efforts (19).

Men who have sex with men (MSM) had their own concerns about stigma before the HIV epidemic. Early HIV prevalence rates among MSM heightened that sense of insecurity. Because of this anxiety, MSM in Trinidad kept quiet about their sexual orientation and HIV serostatus (20,21). The same association of sexual orientation with HIV infection resulted in the reluctance to share HIV test results in Chile (22).

There is a prevailing notion that PLWHAs are morally irresponsible. This view was observed among some Kenyan medical students, which suggests that medical knowledge of the epidemic does not fully address the fundamental issues of moral sanction and stigma (23). In the general population, in contrast, outright myths about the spread of HIV can fuel considerable stigma. A significant proportion of the population may not know that most HIV-positive people appear and feel well. Many believed that HIV could be transmitted by sharing a public toilet. And as recently as 2003 one in ten respondents surveyed in markets in Oyo State believed mosquitoes could transmit HIV (24).

In the absence of general HIV testing, speculation about the status of individuals can form the basis for stigmatization and discrimination. In high HIV prevalence settings, the death of spouses within a year or two of one another has been taken as rough confirmation that they both died of AIDS (24).

The justifications for stigmatizing PLWHAs vary, as do the patterns of stigma and discrimination they elicit. Those who view HIV as a contagion may reject PLWHAs in forms ranging from the benign to the harsh. Understanding the relationship between the justification and the pattern of stigma is a prerequisite for tailoring stigma-reducing interventions to the social and cultural realities of the situation. The goal of such interventions is to change stigmatizing attitudes and behaviors of members of the target group and thereby reduce or eliminate the negative impacts of stigma. The interventions may include planned activities such as those involved in multimedia-based behavior change communication programs.

SEQUENCE AND FORMS OF STIGMA AND DISCRIMINATION

The advent of voluntary counseling and testing (VCT) prompted the institutional discriminatory treatment of PLWHAs by hospital staff (25). In 1992, a Taiwanese mother who gave birth to an HIV-infected infant went abroad to escape the institutional harassment she received (26). The discriminatory responses from friends and family when they learn of someone's HIV status can be equally devastating. A bisexual man hospitalized for *Pneumocystis carinii* pneumonia in Taiwan committed suicide the night before discharge because his family and landlord were not sure they wanted him home (26).

The economic hardships associated with AIDS also can predominate (27). The intermediate stages of economic deprivation parallel the progression from HIV infection to AIDS-related conditions to the full development of AIDS. That deprivation is hastened when an employer abrogates an HIV-infected employee's rights to employment, insurance, and similar formal support systems.

In one instance, a PLWHA stated that the stigma of AIDS had forced her to resign from her job as a nurse in a private clinic and go into hiding (28). (It is worth speculating that this could have been as much a reaction to the shame she felt as to the sense of stigmatization and discrimination she experienced from colleagues.) Next, at the family level, she was denied inheritance and, although she had two young children, was shut out by her own relatives when she tried to return to her hometown. This is a typical example of the vulnerability of females who relocate from their biological homes to their marital homes. After spending three years homeless, she returned to her relatives in 1994 and forced them to accept her. This can be described as the stage in which those targeted by stigmatization and discrimination fight back in desperation. Later, she joined a group of HIV-positive people called Christian Service Lilongwe, obviously expecting it to be a support group. But the group later rejected her because she decided to go public about her status. Apparently, they feared her revelation would expose them all to stigma. That fear also reflected the sense of shame some members felt about their infection. Similar tales of personal tragedies have emerged over the years (29,30).

A quick review of the stigma associated with smallpox can provide additional insight into the forms of stigma and discrimination. Prior to its eradication in Africa, smallpox was a recurring and deadly annual epidemic and a contagion (31). Despite its ferocity, smallpox—with a 20% to 30% fatality rate—was survivable, even before the advent of vaccination (15). It was neither the deadliness nor its scarring effect on the survivor that formed the basis of the stigma, however. Rather it was the association of the disease with the myth of divine sanction for a spiritual or behavioral infringement that made the disease so stigmatizing. In the Yoruba culture, the disease was named after Sopona, the god of both thunder and retribution. Consequently the avoidance of the victim by outsiders was partly a public health response and partly an instinct to place distance between oneself and something considered evil.

Under these conditions, it comes as no surprise that the attitude of the family in which the infection occurred differed from those of other families. For the index family, secrecy provided the first line of defense against social and moral sanctions. The infected person was kept out of sight and cared for until the disease cleared, leaving behind a telltale sign of infection in the form of pockmarked skin. When the episode resolved, the family may well have discovered that other families from whom they had hidden their relative harbored infected family members of their own.

The immediate family made a distinction between the public health response and the social distance response. They may well have put the infected family member in isolation partly to avoid transmission within the family and partly to keep the infection a secret from the public. Total isolation of the victim was often impracticable, however, particularly in the case of children, who needed family members to provide care.

It is in the eradication of smallpox that the most relevant insight into the reduction of stigma can be found. According to Henderson, in Nigeria, the strategy of surveillance and containment of smallpox was found to be better and more cost effective than other strategies (31). This approach required suspected cases to be quarantined under guard, while all contacts and everyone within a five-mile radius received vaccinations. New stable vaccines and a special needle that protected the vaccine permitted field workers to vaccinate inaccessible populations. Workers used charm, guile, shame, and intimidation to achieve universal cooperation.

The actions of different stakeholders involved in the management of smallpox may offer lessons in reducing the stigma of HIV/AIDS. First, the general view was that smallpox was a visitation on the people. Second, both the infected individuals and their immediate families carried a prevailing sense of shame. Third, the infection was hidden from outsiders. Fourth, the close relatives were prepared, especially in the case of childhood infections, to make an exception to the social avoidance and rejection that could accompany adult infection. Finally, the more severe the outbreak, the less stringent the secrecy attached to infection. Some of these features of the social management of smallpox infection may be applicable to HIV stigma reduction. For example, a study in Uganda found that the higher the level of HIV prevalence, the more open a given population was about HIV infection (17).

CONSEQUENCES OF THE STIGMA OF AIDS ON PREVENTION AND CARE

The consequences of stigma, discrimination, denial, and shame on prevention and care can be viewed from the perspectives of the individual, the society, and the caregivers. In the case of the individual, fear of rejection, discrimination, and even deadly violence can discourage people from taking an HIV test, sharing the results, and complying with treatment even when they learn of the advantages of early detection (29,32). Similarly, the self-imposed sense of shame about HIV infection can affect an individual's ability to take even elementary preventive actions such as condom use (12). For example, a South Pacific woman who knew her husband was having casual sex when away from the family felt too ashamed — presumably of her own helplessness, subordination, and humiliation — to ask him to take precautions against infection (33).

The stigma attached to AIDS not only affects the individual's access to health services and employment, but also their treatment by community, social, and religious groups (34). In Uganda, for example, the earlier notion of AIDS as a terminal condition affected the allocation of resources within the household and the provision of medical treatment (17). The denial of symptoms by a patient or family was common and made resource diversion easier. The fear of stigmatization prevented many HIV-infected rural residents from attending a health center. Instead, they opted for home visits from health workers or care from traditional healers who could be visited at night. An economic consequence of the assumption that AIDS was contagious was a fear of buying produce from a family in which a member was ill. In the political realm, a woman was denied election to a community position because people believed she had AIDS (17).

In response to the fear of stigmatization and social isolation, many PLWHAs avoid becoming involved in community AIDS education even though their involvement would provide a tremendous opportunity for correcting many misconceptions about the virus and its transmission (17). Individuals who belong to an already stigmatized group are less likely to become involved with HIV prevention programs (20).

Entire families share the impact of the infection and the associated stigma. For example, the community may stigmatize children whose parents died of AIDS. Individual family members also endure emotional and physical stress in caring for those infected, especially when they develop full-blown AIDS (35).

AIDS orphans experience major psychosocial effects on the loss of parents, including stigmatization and learning difficulties at school, social ostracism, low levels of social support, discrimination in all areas of life, and economic hardship. In addition, children who lose their parents to AIDS become fearful of losing other people close to them. They also experience desolation, extreme loneliness, a high rate of concealment as to the cause of parental death, and unresolved grief (36).

Society may use stigmatization and discrimination in defense of norms and values, but the public health consequences of driving the HIV/AIDS epidemic underground are devastating to the health, economy, and social life of the society (34). The stigma may lead people to delay being tested, to keep positive test results a secret, and to avoid using condoms with sexual partners for fear of rousing suspicion of HIV infection (14).

When HIV prevalence rates rise, the increased burden of opportunistic infections and diseases such as tuberculosis, diarrhea, and skin cancers places considerable stress on health care systems (38). An equally exponential pressure is placed on home-based caregivers as the economic ability of patients to access formal health services declines.

Some clinicians, intent on avoiding HIV acquisition, employ strategies that turn out to be stigmatizing and discriminatory of PLWHAs. Their fears prompt health providers to take drastic and punitive measures to contain the epidemic, sacrificing, in the process, the principles of informed consent and confidentiality (38). Many fears they harbor about HIV are based on erroneous information, however, such as the notion that AIDS is a contagion (39). When clinicians become more informed about the relative risks of infection from occupational hazards, they tend to adopt rational universal precautions at work. Their families may remain concerned, however, about the risk of caring for PLWHAs (39).

Another concern of health professionals is the dilemma of maintaining confidentiality while weighing the risks of infection for the patient's relatives and lovers as well as for the health care staff if they are not aware of the patient's HIV status. Attempts at resolving the dilemma may give the impression of stigmatization and discrimination in the treatment of HIV-infected patients (39).

SPECIFIC DETERMINANTS OF STIGMA REDUCTION

It is apparent that various stakeholders to the stigma, discrimination, denial, and shame are open to some common and tailored strategies for stigma reduction. Consequently, it is worth identifying the evidence-based determinants of such a reduction. Fear of the unknown entity and ignorance of the actual — as opposed to mythical — impact of that entity are the two negative factors producing stigmatization and discrimination. Conversely, knowledge, information, enlightenment from anti-stigma campaigns, and interventions coupled with the infrastructure for care and support are the positive factors in stigma reduction.

Since the level of fear appears to correlate directly with the level of ignorance about the transmission of HIV, it may be postulated that the higher the level of ignorance, the higher the concomitant fear of the affliction and those affected by it. Deriving from these postulates, the more educated people are about HIV/AIDS, the less stigma they attach to it. In Kenya, a study found that the stigma medical students attached to HIV/AIDS declined with each additional year of education (36).

Within health care systems, the level of knowledge and the inclination of providers determine whether HIV patients receive any kind of counseling. The quality of counseling also depends on the skills available and the commitment of the providers to the process of counseling (40). Improvements in the training of health providers at both the institutional and community levels will lead to a better and more dignified quality of care for HIV-positive patients.

At the same time that fear and ignorance about HIV/AIDS can prompt stigmatizing and discriminatory behavior, there is evidence that competent counseling can reduce fear, encourage openness, and lead to a proactive attitude to prevention and care (41). The content of such counseling includes assurances of the prolonged life possible to PLWHAs if they treat infections, eat well, get enough rest, keep busy to avoid preoccupation with the notion of approaching death, refrain from alcohol and smoking, and exercise regularly (41). To this array of advice can now be added excellent adherence to antiretroviral (ARV) regimens when available.

Assurances given by long-surviving PLWHAs are particularly potent in reducing the stigma attached to HIV/AIDS. PLWHAs can dispel myths, correct inaccuracies, and instill confidence in the process of VCT. Although relatively few individuals in Nigeria are going public with their HIV status, the multiplier effect of their action often converts many more to a rational view of testing and treatment.

In the absence of the testimony of such individuals, behavior change communication (BCC) is a powerful tool for moving individuals from an initial state of indifference or denial to a more proactive state of agreeing to an HIV test and following through with the necessary monitoring and treatment if appropriate. To be effective, the design and implementation of BCC programs must take into account the social and cultural context of the epidemic; the interventions must then be tailored to that context.

THE MARKET PROJECT

To help elucidate the role of stigmatization and discrimination in the HIV/AIDS epidemic in Nigeria, a biomedical and biosocial research team from the Department of Virology at the University College Hospital and the Association for Reproductive and Family Health, also in Ibadan, conducted an HIV surveillance program in two cities in Oyo State. This survey had several objectives:

- To determine the prevalence and, if at all possible, incidence of HIV infection among those under surveillance;
- To give market agents skills in HIV prevention education, counseling, and distribution of barrier methods in their respective markets;

- To encourage peer educators chosen from among the volunteers to carry out a continuous and systematic outreach program in their markets and communities;
- To conduct regular multimedia BCC activities in the markets and neighboring communities; and
- To refer all HIV-positive people for assessment, treatment, and care to the APIN Plus/Harvard PEPFAR clinic site at the University College Hospital in Ibadan while maintaining linkage with the national ARV program.

Methodology

The project recruited more than a thousand volunteer market agents of both sexes in four major markets in Ogbomoso and Ibadan in August 2003. These volunteers participated in four rounds of VCT as part of HIV surveillance, including STI screening and treatment over a two-year period. Apart from monitoring the rate of HIV spread among the volunteers, project staff referred people who tested HIV positive to appropriate institutions for management and support as well as linkage with the national ARV program.

The volunteers also participated in BCC interventions that promoted HIV prevention and risk reduction, including safer sex practices using the dual protection strategy. The program was based on an adaptation of the health belief model to the circumstances of HIV prevention (24). The methods included periodic promotional campaigns, group assemblies, regular review meetings, health talks on various aspects of the epidemic, distribution of educational materials, development of market-based folk theater, and condom distribution.

When BCC activities were combined with biomedical interventions, HIV infection acquired a new meaning, one that was less discrediting than before the onset of the intervention. The myths that dissipated during the period contributed to the reevaluation of the risk of infection and the feasibility of prevention. In effect, the BCC activities targeted so frequently over the two-year period formed the basis of the expectation that stigmatizing attitudes and behaviors of volunteers as well as of other project market traders would be changed, thus reducing or eliminating the negative impacts of stigma on such elements as adherence to periodic HIV testing, and treatment of PLWHAs.

In effect, while the biomedical methods focused on the objective of deriving epidemiologic data, the target of the biosocial methods were sexual risk reduction, adoption of safe sex practices, and the reduction of stigma.

Measurement Problems of Stigmatization

With BCC activities new in the markets and the Yoruba language limited in its ability to convey the subtleties of some sociological concepts, our major challenge was to devise an instrument that captured the main elements of stigma, discrimination, denial, and shame that various stakeholders in the HIV/AIDS epidemic feel. Stigma, discrimination, and predictors of tolerance reported by respondents can be made. They were chosen in the context of the Yoruba perception of the spiritual, moral, and physical basis of disease (42) as well as on their mechanisms for social distance and avoidance.

Table 10-1.
Stigmatizing Statements, Discrimination Questions, and Predictors of Tolerance

STATEMENTS AND QUESTIONS

	Panel 1: Stigmatizing Statements
1	HIV-infected people are promiscuous.
2	HIV/AIDS is a punishment from God.
3	HIV-infected people are responsible for their own problems.
4	HIV-infected people are not useful to anyone.
5	HIV-infected people should not be allowed to mix with uninfected people.

	Panel 2: Discrimination Questions
6	Would you sleep in the same room with someone who has HIV?
7	Would you visit someone with HIV/AIDS in the hospital?
8	Would you help carry someone dying of AIDS to an ambulance?
9	Would you tell others if a relative died of HIV/AIDS after a long illness?

	Panel 3: Predictors of Tolerance
10	Mothers stand by their children.
11	Providers are friendly to HIV-infected people.
12	Some tribes are more tolerant of sick people than others.
13	Better-educated people are more tolerant of those living with HIV/AIDS.
14	Some religious people are better able to look after people living with HIV/AIDS.

The first panel of Table 10-1 shows three moral statements about PLWHAs, one negative assessment, and one punitive prescription for PLWHAs. HIV infection is credited to sexual laxity, divine justice, and self-inflicted misfortune. In addition, PLWHAs are stated as not being useful to society, and the judgment is given that they should not be allowed to mix with those presumed to be uninfected.

The next panel is composed of four questions assessing the degree of social and physical contact that respondents are prepared to make with PLWHAs and the extent to which they would be willing to inform people that a relative had died of AIDS. These items are at the root of the integration of family members into the household. These questions seek to tease out whether the common courtesies accorded family members in traditional society in times of illness would be extended to PLWHAs. Asking whether people would sleep in the same room as a PLWHA is consistent with the prevailing living arrangement in which large families share limited accommodations. Because of the large sizes of bilaterally extended families, the first strains in interpersonal relationships can be manifested in changes in sleeping arrangements. PLWHAs are often hospitalized, especially if they are not on ARV therapy. The AIDS stage is also marked by physical and emotional dependence on others. Access to the basic physical and emotional support from family members is vital to the quality of life of PLWHAs.

Another dimension of stigma is the shame individuals attach to having HIV in the family. Protracted illness is usually associated with HIV infection in high prevalence populations. The respondents' willingness—or lack of willingness—to acknowledge a death from AIDS openly thus becomes a marker for the level of shame attached to AIDS.

In the third panel, five items sought to establish which relationships and institutions were likely to offer support to PLWHAs. Respondents were asked to predict the attitudes of mothers, health providers, ethnic groups, educated people, and religious bodies to PLWHAs.

Data on the benchmark level of prevailing stigma and discrimination attached to HIV/AIDS were collected in August 2003. A general adult population was randomly sampled among traders in the two markets. Each market has an average population of approximately 2,500 people. A total sample of 667 traders was surveyed. The 14-item module required that respondents answer "True," "False," or "Uncertain." Most respondents held strong views and opted for the first two options.

Indices

On each of the first nine items, the percentage responding in the affirmative is a useful index of the extent to which the respondents held stigmatizing and discriminatory attitudes toward PLWHAs. In the last panel, the percentages responding in the affirmative is an indication of the extent of care and support that could be counted upon from the various relationships and institutions.

By comparing the percentages obtained at the baseline and the second survey one year later among two unmatched samples, it is possible to discuss the direction and magnitude of change in the levels of stigmatization and discrimination. This analytical approach is also adopted for testing the impact of three project interventions on stigma reduction.

The possibility of regrouping the items into single indicators was considered but not adopted. The single-item interpretation allowed the elements and basis of stigmatizing and discriminatory attitudes to be easily identified and addressed in anti-stigma BCC activities.

Intervention Procedures

Although this project did not specifically target discrimination as the primary aim, the package of interventions on the HIV surveillance assured that if periodic measurements of stigmatization and discrimination were obtained, they would give an accurate reflection of the extent to which program activities and interventions affected stigma.

The four main project interventions were:

- In-depth training of volunteers on HIV/AIDS with a focus on the role of early detection in the management of infection;
- The implementation of a multimedia BCC intervention that included health talks, risk assessments, and the creation of an amateur drama troupe in each market so the training and learning content could be reinforced in the informal setting of edutainment;
- Biannual participation of volunteers in HIV and syphilis tests based on competent confidential counseling, testing, and notification arrangement and frequent contacts to allow for the discussion of issues arising from those tests; and
- The referral of those testing HIV positive to a reference laboratory for confirmation and linkage with the national ARV program.

Changing Attitudes Toward People Living with HIV/AIDS

As the HIV/AIDS epidemic evolves, two problems emerge in connection with the reactions of the public to those known to be infected. One relates to the prejudices people have about HIV and other STIs in general and the stigma that is consequently attached to HIV infection. The other problem arises from the physical and emotional reactions to PLWHAs as the disease progression makes them more debilitated and dependent on others for their basic needs. Stigma reduction and greater tolerance of PLWHAs are consequently desirable outcomes of interventions aimed at prevention and management of the epidemic. It is evidence that those whose identity has been tarnished can then be redeemed and the stain lifted from them (9).

Survey Results

General Levels of Stigmatization and Discriminatory Attitudes

Table 10-2 shows the baseline and year one levels of stigmatizing and discriminatory attitudes toward PLWHAs in Ogbomoso and Ibadan. In interpreting the responses to the five statements in Panel 1, an affirmative is stigmatizing. Consequently, a decline in percentages over the one-year period is indicative of stigma reduction.

In contrast, an affirmative response to any of the four discrimination questions in Panel 2 is indicative of a non-discriminatory attitude toward PLWHAs. Consequently an increase in the proportion of respondents holding non-discriminatory attitudes is the expected outcome of intervention.

An affirmative response to any of the five statements on the predictors of tolerance in Panel 3 is an indication of the reliance that PLWHAs can place on such relationships and institutions for care and support. Differences at the different surveys are presumed to be related to the experiences of the respondents over the intervening period.

Table 10-2 (Panel 1) shows that for all five statements the affirmative proportions declined significantly (p value between 0.0000 and 0.0003). The fact that HIV is mostly sexually transmitted appears to generate a moralistic attitude toward those who are HIV positive. That attitude toward HIV infection was greater among the Ogbomoso sample than among the Ibadan sample. However, the decline in proportions from 52% to 36% and from 30% to 21% in the respective towns is evidence of the erosion of this moralistic attitude in all project markets. These declines are consistent with the working hypothesis that with greater understanding of the alternative channels of infection, and the unintended impact of sexual networking on "innocent" individuals, HIV infection will lose some of its association with promiscuity. There is a corresponding increase in the awareness in both towns that HIV infection may not be the outcome of an individual's negligence but the outcome of other people's behavior.

Nearly half of the Ogbomoso baseline sample related HIV infection to divine punishment for wrongdoing. The Ibadan proportion was much less at 38%. There was a noticeable softening of this religious hard line toward HIV infection in both towns by the time of the second survey. The religious influence on the formation of prejudices is also implied in the third stigmatizing statement. Much higher proportions in both towns blamed HIV-infected people for their predicament at the baseline. The follow-up survey showed a considerable softening of attitudes. Ibadan respondents held a less prejudicial position, however, as to the culpability of those who are HIV positive in the matter of their transmission.

The Yoruba meaning of "not useful to anyone" is indicative of the assumption of reduced functionality or social and economic relevance of HIV-infected individuals. It is from this meaning that follows the equally

No.	Percentage agreeing that the following statements are true or answering affirmatively to the following questions	Ogbomoso Baseline	Ogbomoso Year 1	Ibadan Baseline	Ibadan Year 1
Panel 1: Stigmatizing Statements					
1	HIV-infected people are promiscuous.	52	36	30	21
2	HIV/AIDS is a punishment from God.	46	34	38	26
3	HIV-infected people are responsible for their own problems.	71	59	55	42
4	HIV-infected people are not useful to anyone.	84	56	60	37
5	HIV-infected people should not be allowed to mix with uninfected people.	80	58	73	50
Panel 2: Discrimination Questions					
6	Would you sleep in the same room with someone who has HIV?	16	45	35	52
7	Would you visit someone with HIV/AIDS in the hospital?	58	67	58	66
8	Would you help carry someone dying of AIDS to an ambulance?	35	53	40	57
9	Would you tell others if a relative died of HIV/AIDS after a long illness?	53	41	37	41
Panel 3: Predictors of Tolerance					
10	Mothers stand by their children.	85	89	79	89
11	Providers are friendly to HIV-infected people.	73	88	74	93
12	Some tribes are more tolerant of sick people than others.	60	61	56	61
13	Better-educated people are more tolerant of those living with HIV/AIDS.	63	65	61	77
14	Some religious people are better able to look after people living with HIV/AIDS.	54	55	55	56

harsh prescription that those infected should not mix with the rest of society. In both cases, there were substantial declines in the number of people holding prejudicial views of PLWHAs.

In Table 10-2, Panel 2, the increases across the board show that the high levels of intolerance of physical and social contacts with PLWHAs in both towns gave way to the preparedness to make such contacts after the one year of project intervention. The changes in this non-discriminatory attitude to the observance of basic social courtesies to PLWHAs were similar in both towns. The only exception was that although more than half of the Ogbomoso respondents were hesitant about informing people about an AIDS death in the family by the end of the year, there was a 12% decline in the proportion holding back such information. It is on this item of reluctance to be open about AIDS in the family that Ibadan did not register any difference.

Table 10-2, Panel 3, shows that mothers received a high endorsement as reliable sources of care and support for PLWHAs. In both towns, there were significant increases in the impression that mothers remain reliable sources of care and support. Mothers are noted for their filial loyalty; it is a matter of experience whether this loyalty will stand in the face of the demands AIDS imposes on their physical, economic, and emotional capacities. Similarly, there is a prevailing view that health providers should be free from the prejudices of the public and thus tolerant of the sick. There was a substantial increase in this expectation by the second survey. Just over nine in every 10 expected health providers to show tolerance toward PLWHAs. Although this expectation may or may not be borne out by fact, it does emphasize the assumption that the health system can cope with the emotional demands of the epidemic.

The potential impact of ethnicity on normative attitudes to PLWHAs was largely unchanged in both cities. It would appear that this is a normative view held by the respondents. Education also showed limited change as a predictor of tolerance in Ogbomoso, where approximately two-thirds believed that being better educated made for greater tolerance of PLWHAs.

Faith-based organizations were often cited as potential sources of care and support for PLWHAs. Over half the sample at each survey remained convinced that religious people are well suited to look after PLWHAs. That level remains unchanged over the project period.

Armed with the predominantly favorable improvement in attitudes to PLWHA recorded at the end of a year, the rest of the chapter will explore the contribution of three project intervention elements to those improvements. The three elements hypothesized as critical to the reduction of stigma and discrimination are: participation in the intensive training of volunteers at the start of the project; participation in the sustained multimedia and phased BCC programs; and participation in the VCT exercises. Data on these determinants are presented in the rest of the chapter to show how their associations with reductions in stigma and discrimination.

Training

Awareness creation about HIV/AIDS usually takes the form of campaigns with or without the distribution of educational materials and condoms. These events are additional to the short and compressed messages that are passed on in the mass media. What such activities achieve is an increase in basic knowledge without giving the target population enough information and understanding upon which to fully initiate and sustain behavior change. On this project, that problem was addressed by conducting a five-day training of volunteers on various aspects of HIV/AIDS transmission, prevention, screening, and management of infection. The training alone was evaluated at the end of the five days and it was apparent that some of the volunteers had initiated some changes during the training. The training addressed the issue of stigma and was expected to succeed in changing the negative attitudes of people toward PLWHAs.

Multimedia Activities

During and after the training, the project activities included the use of multimedia. One of the video clips used during the training turned out to be a persistent reference point for viewers about what changed their indifference to the epidemic. Medically explicit videos of STIs and of people at different stages of AIDS development can be powerful in drawing attention to the hazards of risky sexual behavior. Similarly, the use of multimedia BCC intervention and the regular contacts between project staff and the volunteer market agents over the course of two years were expected to reinforce the positive aspects of training and reduce the negative images of HIV infection and AIDS as incurable and always fatal.

Participation in VCT Exercises

Apart from the training and the BCC interventions, the ultimate goal of HIV surveillance was to recruit volunteers for the four rounds of biannual HIV and syphilis tests. (The project's high ethical standards meant that those who did not benefit from either the training or the BCC interventions could still benefit from the pre- and post-test counseling provided to each volunteer.) These counseling sessions were aimed at helping to reduce the volunteers' stigmatizing and discriminatory attitudes toward PLWHAs.

The Impact of Training on Reducing the Stigma of AIDS

It is often remarked that stigmatization and discrimination are the major barriers to VCT and a culture of openness about HIV status. Project activities increased the understanding and appreciation of the dynamics of the epidemic. Consequently, they should contribute to declines in stigmatizing and discriminatory attitudes in the respective surveys.

Table 10-3 shows the percentages affirming statements or questions at the baseline and follow-up survey cross-tabulated by their respondents' participation or non-participation at the initial training session. Since the interpretation of the direction of change remains the same as for the general level, the following summary statements are adequate for clarifying the findings.

In Table 10-3, Panel 1, those who did not attend the training session were considerably more likely to be moralistic about HIV infection than those who attended. The one exception was that of ascribing the infection to divine justice. There was no significant differences on this item. With reference to the culpability of HIV-infected individuals, training appears to have made people soften their judgmental stances. Similarly, training made people less severe in their assessment of the contributions or involvement of PLWHAs in society. The impact of training on stigma reduction appeared more pronounced in Ibadan than in Ogbomoso.

Table 10-3 (Panel 2) shows that training made a significant difference in the level of non-discriminatory attitudes reported for all items. The only exception was that those who did not receive training in Ogbomoso were more likely to tell others of an AIDS-related death in the family than those who received training. There was no significant difference between the two groups in Ibadan. In both towns, those who took part in the training were slightly more reticent about sharing information about the HIV status of a dead relative. This might be the effect of the greater emphasis that VCT programs place on the ethics surrounding the notification of results. The confidentiality of results may have been extended to the confidentiality of the HIV status of relatives who had died of AIDS.

Table 10-3 (Panel 3) shows that expectations of care and support and tolerance of PLWHAs from some relevant others—such as mothers, health providers, and religious affiliates—are largely normative, as there were no significant differences between those who trained and those who did not. It is

Table 10-3. Percentage of Affirmative Responses to Stigmatizing Statements, Discrimination Questions, and Predictors of Tolerance at Baseline and at Year 1 Surveys by Trainee Status

No.	Percentage agreeing that the following statements are true or answering affirmatively to the following questions	Ogbomoso		Ibadan	
		At training (152)	Not at training (326)	At training (122)	Not at training (377)
Panel 1: Stigmatizing Statements					
1	HIV-infected people are promiscuous.	22	42	15	23
2	HIV/AIDS is a punishment from God.	36	33	25	27
3	HIV-infected people are responsible for their own problems.	39	69	30	45
4	HIV-infected people are not useful to anyone.	41	63	16	43
5	HIV-infected people should not be allowed to mix with uninfected people.	48	63	36	55
Panel 2: Discrimination Questions					
6	Would you sleep in the same room with someone who has HIV?	65	36	80	43
7	Would you visit someone with HIV/AIDS in the hospital?	76	63	90	58
8	Would you help carry someone dying of AIDS to an ambulance?	63	49	85	48
9	Would you tell others if a relative died of HIV/AIDS after a long illness?	34	44	39	41
Panel 3: Predictors of Tolerance					
10	Mothers stand by their children.	93	87	94	88
11	Providers are friendly to HIV-infected people.	90	87	95	93
12	Some tribes are more tolerant of sick people than others.	72	56	59	62
13	Better-educated people are more tolerant of those living with HIV/AIDS.	70	62	78	76
14	Some religious people are better able to look after people living with HIV/AIDS.	64	51	61	55

remarkable that the Yoruba have a perception that some other tribes are less discriminatory of differences in physical appearance or social behavior than other tribes.

The Impact of BCC Participation on Reducing the Stigma of AIDS
Table 10-4 shows the relationship between participation in BCC activities and the levels of stigmatizing and discriminatory attitudes at the follow-up survey in August 2004. Apart from the initial training, the sustained multimedia BCC program served the purpose of encouraging a stage-by-stage management of appreciating and adopting new strategies and lifestyles for prevention and management of HIV infection. The BCC programs builds upon the training by deepening the understanding of participants and offering solutions to problems associated with HIV testing. Consequently, it is no surprise that the pattern of responses to stigmatizing statements in Table 10-4, Panel 1, triangulates with the findings about training. It also reaffirms the correlation between being at the training and being at the BCC activities.

No.	Percentage agreeing that the following statements are true or answering affirmatively to the following questions	Ogbomoso		Ibadan	
		At BCC (185)	Not at BCC (293)	At BCC (164)	Not at BCC (335)
Panel 1: Stigmatizing Statements					
1	HIV-infected people are promiscuous.	20	46	13	25
2	HIV/AIDS is a punishment from God.	33	35	23	27
3	HIV-infected people are responsible for their own problems.	40	72	29	48
4	HIV-infected people are not useful to anyone.	43	64	18	48
5	HIV-infected people should not be allowed to mix with uninfected people.	49	64	35	57
Panel 2: Discrimination Questions					
6	Would you sleep in the same room with someone who has HIV?	61	36	73	42
7	Would you visit someone with HIV/AIDS in the hospital?	75	62	84	57
8	Would you help carry someone dying of AIDS to an ambulance?	61	49	78	46
9	Would you tell others if a relative died of HIV/AIDS after a long illness?	38	42	38	42
Panel 3: Predictors of Tolerance					
10	Mothers stand by their children.	94	86	95	87
11	Providers are friendly to HIV-infected people.	90	87	95	92
12	Some tribes are more tolerant of sick people than others.	67	57	61	62
13	Better-educated people are more tolerant of those living with HIV/AIDS.	68	63	82	74
14	Some religious people are better able to look after people living with HIV/AIDS.	60	53	50	59

Table 10-4. Percentage of Affirmative Responses to Stigmatizing Statements, Discrimination Questions, and Predictors of Tolerance at Baseline and Year 1 Surveys by BCC Participation Status

Abbreviation: BCC: behavior change communication

Table 10-4 lends credence also to the differentiation between those who took part in project activities and those who did not.

In Table 10-4, Panel 1, it is also clear that those who were exposed to project activities and to the BCC activities in particular gained some insight into the morally neutral circumstances in which people can be infected with HIV and the possibilities for people to live with the infection for years while pursuing their normal economic and social activities. The one domain in which both groups in both towns were less likely to yield ground to superior argument was the religious one. About the same proportion of both groups believed that HIV/AIDS is a punishment from God. The Ibadan groups, however, were less dogmatic about this belief.

For Table 10-4, Panel 2, too, participation in BCC activities proved as effective as training or reinforced the benefits of training in reducing discriminatory attitudes. The reticence about telling outsiders if a family member had died of HIV/AIDS was retained by those who participated in the BCC activities. In effect, it is worth noting that for those who did not participate in the training, the sustained BCC activities offered a viable alternative to stigma reduction.

Table 10-4 (Panel 3) shows that another benefit of participation in BCC activities is the enhancement of the norms surrounding the notion that mothers, health providers, and educated people make reliable sources for providing PLWHAs with care and support.

The Impact of Participation in VCT on Reducing the Stigma of AIDS

The last determinant of stigma reduction investigated was the impact of participating in the VCT exercises. The decision to take the HIV test once, and especially two to four times in the course of the two-year study, was taken as a major behavior change modification and recognition of the role that VCT plays in HIV prevention and management. It was also expected that those who took the HIV test would have a more tolerant view of people who turn out to be infected.

Panels 1 to 3 of Table 10-5 show the differences in responses by the participation or non-participation of the respondents in the two rounds of VCT carried out during the project year. A comparison of the impact of training with that of VCT participation — Table 10-3, Panel 1, and Table 10-5, Panel 1 — shows that in Ogbomoso no significant difference appeared in the pattern of responses between those who trained and those who took part in the HIV tests with regards to stigma statement. However, those who took the HIV tests showed a greater readiness to help carry someone dying of AIDS than those who trained.

In Ibadan, on the other hand, those who trained were significantly more likely to become involved in the care of PLWHAs (Table 10-5, Panel 2) than those who had only been tested for HIV. A confounding factor in this analysis is that the proportion of those who tested without participating in the training was not higher in Ibadan than in Ogbomoso. In effect, an explanation must be sought in the more cosmopolitan trends observed in Ibadan than in Ogbomoso.

When it came to estimating the position of some tribes, social classes, and religious groups about tolerance of PLWHAs, the absence of large differences between groups remained the dominant feature of participation or non-participation in VCT exercises and stigma reduction.

CONCLUSION

When social scientists explore strategies for reducing the stigma of AIDS, they tend to focus on the choice of actors, such as faith-based organizations; the quality of counseling (43); and the human rights of already stigmatized groups (38). Such recommendations, however, are often not evidence based. Other suggestions focus on the choice of methodology, such as the suitability of message content and the encouragement of support groups (9).

In this chapter we used the evidence-based approach to establish some components of project intervention that may individually or collectively contribute to stigma reduction. In addition to demonstrating that training, BCC programs, and HIV surveillance can help reduce the stigma of AIDS, we

Table 10-5. Percentage of Affirmative Responses to Stigmatizing Statements, Discrimination Questions, and Predictors of Tolerance at Baseline and Year 1 Surveys by VCT Participation Status

No.	Percentage agreeing that the following statements are true or answering affirmatively to the following questions	Ogbomoso		Ibadan	
		Those tested (201)	Those not tested (277)	Those tested (171)	Those not tested (328)
Panel 1: Stigmatizing Statements					
1	HIV-infected people are promiscuous.	23	44	13	25
2	HIV/AIDS is a punishment from God.	37	33	23	28
3	HIV-infected people are responsible for their own problems.	41	70	35	45
4	HIV-infected people are not useful to anyone.	34	69	19	45
5	HIV-infected people should not be allowed to mix with uninfected people.	40	69	41	55
Panel 2: Discrimination Questions					
6	Would you sleep in the same room with someone who has HIV?	67	66	68	68
7	Would you visit someone with HIV/AIDS in the hospital?	77	61	81	58
8	Would you help carry someone dying of AIDS to an ambulance?	70	43	73	48
9	Would you tell others if a relative died of HIV/AIDS after a long illness?	37	43	42	40
Panel 3: Predictors of Tolerance					
10	Mothers stand by their children.	92	87	94	87
11	Providers are friendly to HIV-infected people.	88	88	96	92
12	Some tribes are more tolerant of sick people than others.	60	62	60	63
13	Better-educated people are more tolerant of those living with HIV/AIDS.	60	68	79	76
14	Some religious people are better able to look after people living with HIV/AIDS.	56	55	56	56

Abbreviations: VCT: volunteer counseling and testing

identified some of the expectations of the public about where PLWHAs should receive their care and support. In this connection, the faith in health providers as a source of care and solace for PLWHAs will require that clinicians be prepared for this responsibility through training and appropriate logistical support in coping with the physical and emotional demands of the epidemic.

The major outcome of the analysis is the validation of the hypothesis that improved understanding of an epidemic leads to reductions in the stigma of AIDS. The corollary is that detailed training within HIV surveillance provides more understanding than the basics of HIV/AIDS available in the mass media and has more impact on stigma reduction.

Although the evidence is conclusive as to the impact of training, participation in BCC activities, and HIV testing on reducing stigmatizing attitudes, some ambiguity remains about the relationship between each of the three elements of intervention and non-discrimination. The reporting of non-discriminatory attitudes as if they were norms may have been the result of the desire of the respondents to be socially correct. While pronouncing judgment on the morals of an HIV-infected person may be consistent with their understanding of the epidemic, it is another matter to refuse to help a PLWHA. People may have an intellectual inconsistency in their positions, but this is the dilemma of investigating phenomena that are subject to a social desirability bias.

REFERENCES

1. Nigerian Institute of Medical Research. *Nigeria's Contribution to Regional and Global Meetings on HIV/AIDS/STIs: 1986–2005.* 2nd ed. Lagos: Nigerian Institute of Medical Research, 2005.

2. Okonkwo A. *Attitudes of Journalists Towards People Living with HIV/AIDS in Nigeria: A Personal Experience.* Lagos: Nigerian Institute of Medical Research, 2005:115–116.

3. Ahamefule G. *Human Rights Violation: My Experience as a Person Living with HIV.* Lagos: Nigerian Institute of Medical Research, 2005;118.

4. Ugo U. Non-disclosure of sero-status due to high stigmatization in communities. Lagos: Nigerian Institute of Medical Research, 2005;224.

5. Opara O. The need to make HIV carriers acceptable in the society through HIV counseling. *XIV International AIDS Conference,* Barcelona, Spain, July 7–12, 2002 (abstract TuPeG5557).

6. Sabatier R. Crossing the threshold of fear. *AIDS Watch,* 1988;(3):2–3.

7. Obishai A. *Reducing Stigma and Preventing HIV Transmission in Nigerian Health Facilities.* Lagos: Nigerian Institute of Medical Research, 2005;177.

8. Okoli Rev., Omeogu CO, Onumonu C. *Faith Based Organizations' Use of Sermons as a Tool for HIV Awareness Creation.* Lagos: Nigerian Institute of Medical Research, 2005;190–191.

9. Goffman E. *Stigma: Notes on the Management of a Spoiled Identity.* Englewood Cliffs: Prentice Hall, Inc., 1963.

10. Guest G, Bunce A, Johnson L, Akumatey B, Adeokun L. Fear, hope and social desirability bias among women at high risk for HIV in West Africa. *J Fam Plann Reprod Health Care,* 2005;31(4):285–287.

11. Anonymous. Standing up to stigma. *AIDS Action,* 2000;47:2.

12. Aggleton P. *HIV and AIDS-Related Stigmatization, Discrimination and Denial: Forms, Contexts and Determinants. Research Studies from Uganda and India.* Geneva: UNAIDS, 2000.

13. Modesto Meza J, Aguilera A, Avery AE. Psychiatric and social aspects of AIDS: report of 4 cases. *Acta Psiquiatr Psicol Am Lat,* 1994;40(2):146–150.

14. Moyo I, Low A, Ray CS, Katsumbe TM, Chisvo D, Mbengeranwa OL, Gumbo N. Knowledge and attitudes on AIDS relevant for the establishment of community care in the city of Harare. *Cent Afr J Med,* 1993;39(3):45–49.

15. Koop CE. Individual freedom and the public interest. In: Fleming AF, Carballo M, FitzSimons DW, Bailey MR, Mann J, eds. *The Global Impact of AIDS.* New York: Alan R. Liss, Inc., 1988:307–311.

16. Lara y Mateos RM. Stigmatizing diseases: the case of HIV/AIDS. [Enfermedades estigmatizadoras: el caso del VIH/SIDA.] *Investigacion en Salud,* 2000;2(1):13–20.

17. Muyinda H, Seeley J, Pickering H, Barton T. Social aspects of AIDS-related stigma in rural Uganda. *Health Place,* 1997;3(3):143–147.

18. Maduna-Butshe AC. Women sex workers and the HIV pandemic: stigma and blame in context. *S Af AIDS News,* 1997;5(1):8–11.

19. Gasu J. Legal and ethical aspects of sexual health and living with HIV/AIDS. In: *Summary of Proceedings of the 1st African Youth Conference on Sexual Health,* Accra, Ghana, September 30–October 6, 1996. Accra, Ghana: Ghana United Nations Students and Youth (GUNSA), 1996:25–27.

20. Sealey G. We are our own worst enemies. In: Reid E, ed. *HIV and AIDS: The Global Inter-Connection.* West Hartford, Connecticut: Kumarian Press, 1995:108–119.

21. Nack A. Damaged goods: women managing the stigma of STDs. *Deviant Behav,* 2000;21(2):95–121.

22. Astorga Munoz MA. AIDS: the patient's perspective. In: Fuenzalida-Puelma H, Linares Parada AM, Serrano Laertu D, eds. *Ethics and Law in the Study of AIDS*. Washington, DC: Pan American Health Organization, 1992;(530):253–257.

23. Baguma PK. AIDS-related stigma, personal risks and career objectives among Makerere medical students. *J Community Appl Soc Psychol*, 1992;2(2):105–112.

24. Adeokun LA, Ladipo OA, Odutolu O, et al. Bridging the knowledge-behavior gap through HIV/AIDS surveillance in four markets in Ogbomoso and Ibadan, Nigeria. *Arch Ibadan Med*, 2004;5:59–65.

25. Brown L. Facing stigma and discrimination. *Global AIDSLink*, 1999;(57):17,23.

26. Chang PY, Lin KC, Chuang CY, et al. Status and trend of HIV-1 infection and AIDS in Taiwan, December, 1991. *Asian Pac J Allergy Immunol*, 1992;10(1):65–68.

27. Dying villagers appeal for help. *AIDS Asia*, 2001;3 (3–4):12.

28. Chinula T. Catherine's story. *Pac AIDS Alert Bull*, 2001;(23):14–15.

29. Wright K. The stigma of AIDS. *WIPHN News*, 2000;25:6–7.

30. Baggaley R. Zambia: a church where brothers are not brothers. *AIDS Anal Afr*, 1994;4(3):5–6.

31. Henderson DA. Smallpox: epitaph for a killer? *Natl Geogr Mag*, 1978;154(6):796–805.

32. Anonymous. Stigma, poor health infrastructure blamed for increasing HIV/AIDS cases in Nigeria. *AIDS Wkly*, 2001;16:18.

33. Anonymous. Women living with HIV/AIDS: personal histories. Personal statement by a woman living with HIV in the South Pacific. In: Berer M. *Women and HIV/AIDS: An International Resource Book*. London: Pandora Press, 1993:248–249.

34. Anonymous. Challenging stigma and discrimination. *AIDS Action*, 2000;(47):1.

35. Junaid A. AIDS: young people talk about how AIDS affects family life. Developing Countries Farm Radio Network Package 59, script 5. *Voices*, 2001;(59 Suppl):5.

36. Devine S, Graham D. How having HIV positive parents affects the lives of orphans. *AIDSNET Newsl*, 1999;1(3):38–45.

37. Raviglione MC, Luelmo F. Update on the global epidemiology of tuberculosis. *Curr Issues Public Health*, 1996;2(4):192–197.

38. Hamblin J. *People Living with HIV: The Law, Ethics and Discrimination*. New York: United Nations Development Programme, 1993.

39. Delph Y. AIDS: the doctor's perspective. In: Fuenzalida-Puelma H, Linares Parada AM, Serrano Laertu D, eds. *Ethics and Law in the Study of AIDS*. Washington, DC: Pan American Health Organization, 1992:258–263.

40. Calderon S. Testing positive in El Salvador: HIV stigma continues, but counseling improves. *Impact HIV*, 1999;1(2):25,27.

41. Serunkuuma R. Living with HIV/AIDS: a personal testimony. *AIDS Health Promot Exch*, 1994;(3):7.

42. Odebiyi AI. Food taboos in maternal and child health: the views of traditional healers in Ile-Ife, Nigeria. *Soc Sci Med*, 1989;28(9):985–996.

43. Miller D, Jeffries DJ, Green J, Harris JR, Pinching AJ. HTLV-III: should testing ever be routine? *Br Med J (Clin Res Ed)*, 1986;292(6525):941–943.

II

CONTROLLING HIV/AIDS IN NIGERIA

On the
Waterfront

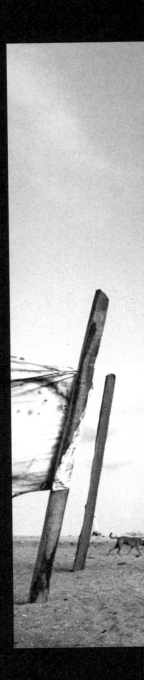

THE BAR BEACH IN LAGOS USED TO BE NOTORIOUS
as the site where criminals were executed.
Now a popular recreation spot known for its
long stretch of sand and refreshing breezes,
it features some of the most expensive hotels
in Africa; a standard room can cost US$320
a night. Not far away, just across a lagoon
that laps the shores of Victoria Island, is
Kuramo Beach, a string of squatter villages
where that same US$320 would represent
more than a year's wage for most residents.

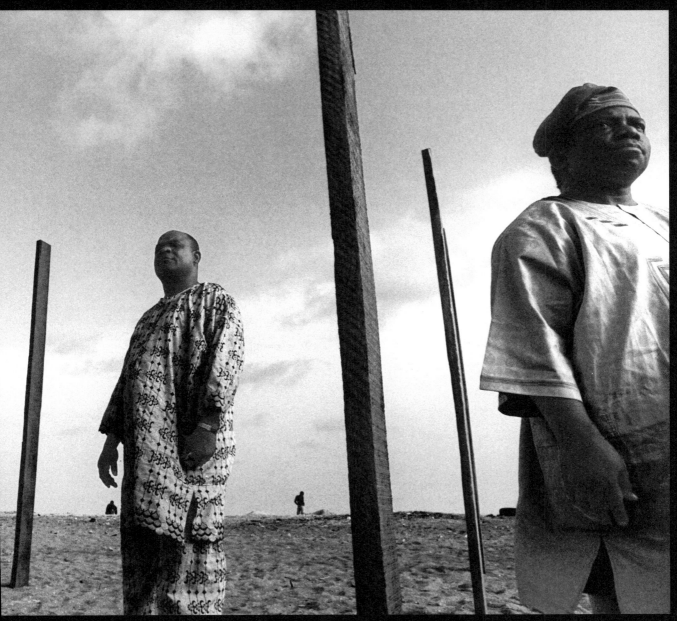

Professors David Olaleye (left) and Isaac Adewole, both experts on HIV/AIDS in Nigeria, stand at the construction site for the new AIDS clinic at Kuramo Beach.

More than 15,000 villagers live in shanties along the long, narrow strip of Kuramo Beach. Nearly a dozen people share each shanty. Most of these shelters have sand floors, thatched roofs, and walls patched together from shipping cartons; those who can afford better materials use wooden planks for the walls and corrugated iron for the roofs. The villages lack running water and proper sanitation. Electricity becomes available only when someone manages to tap into the city grid illegally.

Kuramo residents struggle for basic survival. Some eke out a living selling fish caught in the nearby polluted waters, while others operate makeshift bars or run small businesses out of their homes. But most women find themselves selling their bodies to earn enough money for food. Even young girls join the sex trade, servicing men old enough to be their grandfathers. Here poverty and desperation have fueled the HIV epidemic. And here the AIDS Prevention Initiative in Nigeria (APIN) has pitched its tent.

APIN became involved in Kuramo Beach after Dr. Folasade Ogunsola, a physician and microbiologist, expressed interest in reaching out to a community of female sex workers at high risk of HIV infection. She teamed up with another physician, Dr. Job Ailuogwemhe, and the two met with a local pastor who had started an elementary school in Kuramo as a first step toward empowering residents and giving them economic options.

"When we started," Dr. Ogunsola says, "we realized we should create a family clinic because Kuramo community members desperately needed access to health care. So we began by meeting with the village chiefs, or *Baale*, to gain their acceptance and approval for the clinic. We also held weekly rallies to educate the villagers about HIV and to build community trust in the program."

APIN has since built the clinic, whose materials are a combination of concrete for strength and wood to help it blend with other community structures. The clinic is equipped with electricity and running water, enabling the two full-time nurses and several part-time physicians to provide services to dozens of villagers each day.

Children receive vaccinations, often for the first time in their lives. Adults gain access to routine medical care, services for HIV disease, and AIDS education.

"We're interested in teaching Kuramo Beach residents how to protect themselves against HIV and other sexually transmitted infections," Dr. Ogunsola says. "Clinic staff now offer voluntary counseling and testing services at the same time they're developing a profile of the HIV epidemic in Kuramo." That profile is already alarming, with high rates of HIV infection among the sex workers.

In 2005, the Kuramo Clinic became a satellite for the Harvard PEPFAR program. Patients found to be infected with HIV are driven to Lagos University Teaching Hospital, where they receive further medical evaluation to determine their eligibility for antiretroviral therapy. Already several dozen villagers are receiving free, lifesaving antiretrovirals.

"It's my dream," Dr. Ogunsola says, "that the clinic will survive the harsh and volatile environment of Kuramo Beach and one day provide HIV treatment and care to all the villagers in need. I'm also hoping to set up a community association so the people themselves can eventually take over the clinic."

"This program has affected so many villagers' lives already," Dr. Ailuogwemhe adds. "Many of these people have never believed that anyone cared about them. It has been a tremendous boost for them to have a free clinic in their midst—and to know they will be cared for if they turn out to be infected with HIV. They have felt encouraged to come forward. Condom use has increased dramatically, and many women have felt empowered to leave sex work altogether."

THE NATIONAL RESPONSE TO HIV/AIDS

Oluwole Odutolu,* Babatunde A. Ahonsi,†
Michael Gboun,‡ and Oluwatoyin M. Jolayemi*

Nigeria has set for itself the goals of reversing the trend of its HIV epidemic by 25% in 2009 and subsequently eradicating the epidemic (1). Yet meeting these goals will require a tremendous, unprecedented national response.

NATIONAL MODELS OF SUCCESS

Historically, the response to HIV/AIDS has run a parallel course from one country to another. The association of HIV/AIDS with sex, disease, and death triggered initial reactions of denial and fear and bred stigmatization and discrimination (2). AIDS was then tagged the disease of sex workers and homosexuals, making it less attractive for support. Similarly, early biomedical successes were tempered by the lack of a vaccine and curative drugs, and bringing in the human rights dimension to a public health problem compromised the "John Snow approach" of finding and dealing with the source of infection. National programs also grappled with the epidemic as a behavioral issue that could be "fixed" by promoting safer sex. Governments underestimated the roles that migration,

*AIDS Prevention Initiative in Nigeria, Abuja, Nigeria
†Ford Foundation (West Africa), Lagos, Nigeria
‡UNAIDS Inter-Country Team for East and Southern Africa, Pretoria, South Africa

poverty, gender inequality, war, and conflict play in the spread of HIV. They restricted their thinking and approach to HIV/AIDS as solely a health problem and realized only relatively late the full devastating impact of the epidemic.

Each national program has passed through several stages in response to the changing realities of the epidemic. National public health policies have differed in their approaches and results, though, and some countries seem to have successfully tackled the crisis. For example, although both Senegal and Nigeria recorded their first AIDS case in 1986, Nigeria has not mounted the same level of response as Senegal. Senegal has consistently maintained a prevalence of less than 2% (3), while several years ago Nigeria found itself on the threshold of a 6% national prevalence rate (4). Although one cannot pinpoint the one factor that led to the pattern, Senegal responded by rapidly setting up a national AIDS program and had a strong political support (5). The religious organizations played a great role, and the country's long-established public health policy of registering sex workers and tracking and treating their sexually transmitted infections (STIs) helped significantly in controlling the epidemic. The Philippines had a similar experience (5).

Despite financial constraints, Uganda has been able to reverse the course of its epidemic through strong political leadership and openness about HIV/AIDS. Since 1986, Ugandans have developed personal behavioral change strategies that have dramatically reduced HIV prevalence. Personal communication networks that transmitted information about AIDS drove these changes. A second important feature of the Ugandan response was leadership. President Yoweri Museveni not only championed open and frank talks about AIDS, but he also made sure that the epidemic was placed on the political agenda at all levels (6). Uganda also started the multisectoral approach to create greater involvement of all sectors and communities. Their research has led Moore and Hogg to suggest that "decreasing HIV prevalence in Uganda is not due to the natural course of the epidemic but reflects real success in terms of HIV control policies" (7).

Similarly, Thailand has, through its policy of 100% condom use among sex workers, recorded a significant reduction in the country's HIV prevalence (8), and Brazil has been a trailblazer in providing people living with HIV/AIDS (PLWHAs) in that country with universal access to antiretroviral (ARV) therapy (9).

In its 2004 report on the global AIDS epidemic, UNAIDS issued a positive scorecard on the global AIDS response with the claim that national responses are improving but still fall short of what is needed (10). The report notes in particular improvements in national leadership and a marked increase in resources. The report also records significant progress in strategies, policies, legislation, action, faith-based leadership, and civil society and community mobilization. International resources have increased through the World Bank Multi-Country AIDS Program; the Global Fund on AIDS, Tuberculosis and Malaria; and the U.S. President's Emergency Plan for AIDS Relief (PEPFAR). Widespread partnerships are resulting in broadening national ownership and increasing transparency. Private sector engagement is resulting in workplace programs, leadership and advocacy for AIDS work, and partnerships with the community and government for a strengthened response to the epidemic. The multisectoral approach is said to be paying off; AIDS has been mainstreamed into institutional activities while districts and communities have been empowered as decentralization takes root. Lastly, strategic information continues to guide policy and programs. (See Table 11-1.)

Evidence has been accruing that we are beginning to understand the epidemic and what works (11). Drawing from this body of evidence, we know that a number of factors—including national leadership and political commitment at all levels; a multisectoral approach; a strong STI program; a single, consistent

---

Table 11-1. Progress Update on the Global Response to the AIDS Epidemic, 2004

National responses are improving but still fall short of what is needed.

- Nearly one-third of countries lack policies that ensure women's equal access to critical prevention and care services.
- Most countries have ratified international conventions on human rights, but effective implementation of these agreements is weak. Only 40% of countries have legal measures in place to prohibit discrimination against people living with HIV/AIDS.
- Three-quarters of countries report that national activity and progress monitoring and evaluation remain major challenges. Only 43% of countries have a national monitoring and evaluation plan and only 24% have a national monitoring and evaluation budget.
- Only 20% of transnational companies have adopted comprehensive workplace policies addressing HIV/AIDS. At the country level, implementation of workplace policies is inadequate.
- Many senior political leaders from countries where HIV prevalence is low and the epidemic is concentrated in key populations at higher risk remain detached from the response to HIV/AIDS.

Source: UNAIDS. *2004 Report on the Global AIDS Epidemic.* Geneva: UNAIDS, 2004

---

behavior change message; and the institution of treatment—all work together to reduce HIV prevalence rates and to mitigate the impact of HIV/AIDS.

FRAMING THE DISCOURSE

Although up-to-date, Nigeria has not yet determined the right mix of policies and programmatic approaches for tackling the HIV/AIDS crisis; the country has been muddling through by basically following the trend in approaches recommended or dictated by United Nations agencies—such as the World Health Organization (WHO) and UNAIDS—and other international organizations that have been at the forefront of responding to the epidemic. Approaches have ranged from primarily a biomedical one to the promotion of behavior change, essentially switching from a health sector response to a multisectoral approach.

The country and its citizens also painfully passed through a period of long denial. Official denial meant neither the federal government nor the state governments committed the needed human and financial resources to prevention and control of HIV infection. The worst period was 1994 through 1999. But throughout this period, some international organizations and emerging Nigerian civil society organizations (CSOs) were able to mount responses to the epidemic, particularly in the areas of information, education, and communication; community mobilization; and capacity building for programming.

The HIV situation in Nigeria midway into the first decade of the twenty-first century is serious enough given that about one in twenty adult Nigerians may be living with the virus (12). Yet the situation could have been much worse but for the early and progressively intensive and extensive efforts by

CSOs to galvanize popular and official responses around HIV prevention, vulnerability reduction, and impact mitigation at individual, community, and national levels. Indeed, one could argue that the official development and implementation of a multisectoral national response to HIV/AIDS—starting in 2001 with the formulation of a three-year HIV/AIDS Emergency Action Plan (HEAP) (1)—could have happened later and at a slower pace. Such a worse scenario was probably avoided because of the momentum generated by the earlier response efforts of CSOs beginning in the late 1980s and the push from their more recent HIV prevention interventions, research efforts, demonstration service delivery projects, and sustained policy advocacy activities since the mid-1990s.

This chapter will examine the responses of both the public sector and the civil society sector to the HIV epidemic between 1986 and 2005. (The commercial sector is excluded because, setting aside its traditional engagement in health products marketing and health service delivery for profit, its engagement as part of the national response came much later and has been of a limited, sector-specific nature.) Both the public sector and the civil society sector have their own strengths; each is more adept at engaging with particular aspects of the national response and, therefore, each contributes in different but complementary ways. For example, relative to CSOs, national governments in many parts of the world tend to, for reasons of political expediency, prevaricate around issues of providing sexual health information and clinical services to adolescents and young adults in deference to religious and cultural sensitivities and associated interest groups (13). On the other hand, though, the mass delivery of sexual health education to adolescents through the school system almost always entails a heavy reliance on the policy directives and administrative structures of the public sector.

Nonetheless, a key motivation for our analysis is the fact that although many sound and progressive policies, action plans, and protocols pertaining to health and other development issues have always been instituted by the Nigerian government, they have usually not been adequately implemented or sustained (14,15). Often implicated are such factors as cognitive, communication, and operational gaps between the three tiers and relevant units of government; poor coordination and collaboration between the public, private, and civil society sectors; human and financial resource shortfalls; discontinuities of policy and policy instruments; misapplications of efforts and resources; infrastructural challenges; and leadership deficits (13,16). The national response to the HIV epidemic has also suffered from this syndrome (15,17,18). This has to be a key consideration in any serious assessment of the relative roles of the civil society and public sectors in the national efforts at curtailing HIV spread and mitigating its impact.

According to Barnett and Whiteside, the national response should take guidance from six conceptual phases: timing and targeting; information, observation, or instruction; advocacy and ownership; process versus product; scaling up and sustainability; and the myth of coping (2). Timing and targeting are captured in Table 11-2, which shows the six stages, the epidemiologic features and appropriate prevention strategies of each stage, and the expected impact and response.

Stage	Epidemiology and Prevention	Impact and Response
Stage 1: No one with AIDS is identified, some HIV infections	HIV prevalence > 0.5% in high-risk groups, targeted prevention	Planning only required
Stage 2: A few cases of AIDS are seen by medical services, more people are infected with HIV	HIV < 5% in high-risk groups, targeted prevention	Impact on medical demand and use facilities; need to plan for this
Stage 3: Medical services see many with AIDS; some policy makers are aware of HIV/AIDS; the incidence of reported tuberculosis cases increases	Prevalence > 5% in high-risk populations. Targeted prevention but general information	Impact still mainly medical but need to begin human resources planning and targeted mitigation especially for the most vulnerable groups, institutions, and sectors
Stage 4: AIDS cases threaten to overwhelm health services; widespread general population awareness of HIV/AIDS	Prevalence > 5% in women attending antenatal clinics. Information available to all, continuing targeting of high-risk groups	Impact now broader; need to start looking at the education sector and all government activities. Private sector plans for impact
Stage 5: Unusual levels of severe illness and death in the 15-to-50 age group produce coping problems, a large number of orphans, and the loss of key household and community members; tuberculosis becomes a major killer	Prevalence > 20% in women attending antenatal clinics and has been so for five years. Full battery of prevention according to resources	Impact at all levels. Resources need to be equally diverse. They may include targeted relief or targeted antiretroviral treatment
Stage 6: Loss of human resources in specialized roles in production and economic and social activities; reproduction decreases the ability of the households, communities, enterprises, and districts to govern, manage, and provision themselves effectively. Responses range from creative and innovative ways of coping to failure of social and economic entities	Prevalence > 15% in the 15-to-49 age group and has been so for five years. Most now need to be focused on key groups and interventions. Efforts to reach those below the age of 15 and those above 15; emphasis on voluntary counseling and testing	This impact requires massive intervention at all levels. One emphasis should be on children in crisis, including orphans. Local programs need to be scaled up and made acceptable, perhaps with donor funds

Table 11-2. The Evolution of the HIV/AIDS Epidemic and Its Consequences

THE PUBLIC SECTOR RESPONSE

In terms of structures, the public sector's response to the HIV epidemic began shortly after the official recognition of the presence of HIV in Nigeria with the establishment in 1987 of the National Experts Advisory Committee on AIDS to advise the federal government on how best to respond to the problem (14). The Federal Ministry of Health (FMOH) took responsibility for coordinating the national response from 1986 to 1999. The health sector HIV/AIDS strategy was within the framework of the Department of Disease Control and by design the approach was biomedical, although laced with health education and policy formulation. Table 11-3 details the core components of the response: prevention and health promotion; treatment; health standards and health systems; and informed policy and strategic development. The National AIDS and STD Control Program (NASCP) in the FMOH coordinated the response. This period showed significant progress in some major areas, but much of the progress was through CSOs. The public

Table 11-3. Core Components of the Health Sector Response from 1988 to 2004

Core Components	Strategic Approaches
Prevention and health promotion	• Providing support for the development of broad-based programs to educate the general population about HIV/AIDS • Promoting safer and responsible sexual behavior and practices • Targeting interventions to high-risk groups • Promoting harm reduction
Treatment	• Increasing access to services to diagnose and manage STIs • Strengthening tuberculosis services • Providing a continuum of care from home to health facility
Health standards and health systems	• Ensuring the safety of blood and blood products • Promoting universal safety precautions • Setting and promoting national standards for the public, private, and community-based delivery of HIV/AIDS prevention, health promotion, and treatment and care • Building capacity and strengthening health systems
Informed policy and strategic development	• Establishing or/and strengthening epidemiologic and behavioral surveillance for HIV and other STIs • Elaborating plans to generate resources • Strengthening accountability and monitoring systems for both human and financial resources • Countering the stigmatization and discrimination of PLWHAs • Reviewing policies, laws, and regulations • Mobilizing communities, NGOs, PLWHAs, vulnerable groups, and the business sector

Abbreviations: NGO: nongovernmental organization; PLWHA: person living with HIV/AIDS; STI: sexually transmitted infection

sector was able to institute structures to ensure the safety of blood and blood products, establish and strengthen epidemiological surveillance for HIV and other STIs, and promote syndromic management of STIs.

Blood Safety

Partly because of the limited data then available to policy makers and the early recognition that the most efficient route of HIV transmission was through blood and blood products, the Nigerian government especially at the federal level focused much of its response efforts in the pre-1999 era on blood safety; in fact, more than 10% of the 20-page 1997 national AIDS policy document focused on this issue (18). The development of a national blood safety program received much of its impetus from the technical support of the World Health Organization and the funding support of Britain's Department for International Development (DFID) (14). The program, which started with 21 screening centers in 1988–1989, had by 1995 grown to include nearly 120 centers. Guidelines were issued, service protocols developed and disseminated, testing equipment purchased and distributed, and many laboratory technologists trained across the country.

By the early 1990s, however, Nigeria had acquired a pariah state status among donor countries because of widespread violation of citizens' human rights, and little governmental funding of the AIDS control program was forthcoming to compensate for the rapid reduction in donor funds. The quality of the program began to drop drastically. Indeed, according to the acting national AIDS program coordinator at that time, a 1995 survey of the program's equipment, service delivery, and technical know-how situation showed that 75% of the equipment across the country was not in use, a range of disparate practices prevailed, and no mechanisms were in place for ongoing monitoring, evaluation, and technical support (14). Some of the consequences of this suboptimal situation were long delays—sometimes as long as a month—in getting test results in some parts of the country and a fairly high frequency of false positives from testing blood samples for HIV antibodies. It is no surprise therefore that the 2003 national AIDS policy seeks to foster stronger partnerships between the federal and state ministries of health in the standardization, accreditation, and quality control of blood transfusion services across the country (12).

Epidemiologic Surveillance for HIV/AIDS and STIs

The strongest component of Nigeria's public sector response to HIV/AIDS has perhaps been its epidemiologic surveillance. The FMOH—in collaboration with UN agencies, the U.S. Centers for Disease Control and Prevention (CDC), DFID, Family Health International (FHI), the POLICY Project, and the state ministries of health—has over the years monitored the epidemic and developed information to inform the review of policies and the strategic direction of the national response.

Nigeria's first-generation HIV/AIDS surveillance system started in 1986, when all public health facilities were mandated to report any diagnosed AIDS case in the country to the FMOH. HIV/AIDS was a reportable disease until 1994. From 1986 to 1996, HIV/AIDS/STI data focused on reported AIDS cases, blood screening data, and HIV sentinel surveillance seroprevalence among specific groups, such as sex workers, long-distance truck drivers, tuberculosis patients, STI patients, and pregnant women attending antenatal clinics.

Since 1996 the FMOH, in collaboration with development partners, has strengthened and implemented all the components of the second-generation surveillance guidelines of WHO/UNAIDS. The country's second-generation HIV/AIDS surveillance system includes AIDS case reporting, STI surveillance, HIV surveillance, behavior surveillance, coordination of research, and effective use of surveillance data. The first national HIV/AIDS–related behavioral surveillance household study in selected centers was conducted by the FMOH in collaboration with DFID, the Society for Family Health, and the AIDS Prevention Initiative in Nigeria (APIN) in 2002.

An evaluation of the Medium-Term Plan II (MTP II) (19), implemented between 1993 and 1998, was later contracted to a multidisciplinary committee on an ad-hoc basis. The situation and response analysis included a desk review, interviews, collection and analysis of service records, facility inspection, and surveys. The evaluation report, a narrative of findings from the six geopolitical zones, looked at the outcome of some preventive interventions conducted during the period, including the promotion of safer sex behavior, the diagnosis and treatment of STIs, blood safety measures, the reduction of HIV transmission through injections and other skin-piercing instruments, and the increased accessibility of health care to people with HIV. Others efforts included the establishment of voluntary counseling and testing (VCT) centers, local production of condoms, and advocacy to policy makers.

The report appraised the contributions of the government, development partners, professional associations, and other CSOs toward the implementation of the plan. Apart from the ministry of health, other sectors were adjudged to have elicited a negative response (unaware), no response (indifference), or a weak response. In fact, the health sector response was considered weak because the government did not fund the plan and donor participation was limited because it fell within the period of Nigeria's autocratic military rule, for which the country was under sanctions. Although NASCP was charged with coordinating the plan, it was hindered not only by a lack of funds but also by logistical problems, poor political commitment, inadequate staffing, and incomplete participation by the states. The report concluded that the MTP II was poorly implemented; the report's findings fed into the design of HEAP (20).

Multisectoral National HIV/AIDS Response Under HEAP: 2000–2004

Following the restoration of civilian democratic rule in the country in 1999, the federal response to HIV/AIDS changed dramatically. The national response was guided by HEAP and coordinated through the National Action Committee on AIDS (NACA), which was formally established in 2001. The critical shift in the response to HIV prevention and control was in the more coordinated involvement of line ministries, CSOs, and international organizations. There was—and still is—political commitment from the president, who established the Presidential Committee on AIDS, composed of ministers of the line ministries and technical experts. NACA was established to coordinate the response at the national level; at the state and local government levels are state action committees on AIDS (SACAs) and local action committees on AIDS (LACAs). Other components include the United Nations Expanded Theme Group, the Partnership Forum, the Youth Forum, and the Interfaith Forum.

The new national strategic plan, HEAP, was designed to have nationwide coverage and was planned for implementation at the national, state, and local government levels. The critical factors considered to influence the success of HEAP were political commitment, resource availability, and skills development. Detailed activity schedules were prepared for each of the components outlining the strategies, timeframe, and indices of output indicators and implementing agencies. Roles and responsibilities at the national, state, and local government levels were also clearly delineated.

HEAP also identified priority interventions, including:

- **Preventive interventions targeted at high-risk groups.** These groups include sex workers and their clients, long-distance transport workers, school and university students, street children, the military, the police, prisoners, and PLWHAs.
- **Preventive interventions for the general population.** These interventions included improvement of blood safety, implementation of sexual education and lifestyle education in schools and through non-formal educational channels, expansion of services for STIs and reproductive tract infections, and increased availability of low-cost condoms and VCT.

- **Care and support for people infected with and affected by HIV.** Public sector hospitals and community networks were expected to provide this care and support, including prevention of mother-to-child transmission of HIV (PMTCT), management of the HIV/tuberculosis co-infection, and treatment of opportunistic infections.

The implementation of HEAP showed increased HIV-related activities in the country, with networks formed for CSOs, PLWHAs, and HIV/AIDS researchers. Nigeria was able to attract funding from the World Bank, USAID, DFID, the Bill & Melinda Gates Foundation, and the Ford Foundation. Several projects were implemented across the length and breadth of the country. The estimated direct HIV/AIDS related budget of the government through HEAP was US$236 million, with a national government contribution of US$40 million over a three-to-five-year period. This figure does not reflect all the indirect cost related to the HIV/AIDS epidemic, however.

The national response received the largest resource base in its history between 2001 and 2004. For the first time, Nigeria began direct services to mitigate the impact of HIV on the infected and affected, including PMTCT, provision of ARVs to treat PLWHAs, care and support in the communities, and care of orphans and other vulnerable children.

Although HEAP has not been fully evaluated, stakeholders collaborated on a review in December 2004. Although many gaps were identified, the framework has helped to harness resources and galvanize actions toward a more effective national response to the HIV epidemic. Some of the notable adverse comments were that states were not effectively mobilized to action, coordination was weak at the center, and access to such services as PMTCT and antiretroviral treatment (ART) was limited. A newer plan, the National HIV/AIDS Strategic Framework, has been developed for 2005–2009.

The post-1999 period also witnessed the review of the 1997 national HIV/AIDS policy and the development of the 2003 National Policy on HIV/AIDS, which is more comprehensive and wider in scope than the previous one. The new policy addressed more pressing issues relating to stigmatization, discrimination, impact mitigation, and monitoring and evaluation, and it detailed achievement targets for 2005–2009. The implementation was encapsulated in the principle of multisectoralism. In addition to the new policy, NACA, in collaboration with partners, developed the National HIV/AIDS Behavior Change Communication Strategy. In April 2004, NACA launched the Nigerian National Response Information Management System for HIV/AIDS (NNRIMS) (21), designed to tackle the major challenges in monitoring, evaluating, and reporting on HIV/AIDS initiatives and their impact nationally. Some of the strategic initiatives, actions, and programs that the public sector has developed, especially since 1999, follow.

Development of National Policies and Program Frameworks

The development of national policies is one area in which the leadership of the public sector has been unmistakably strong. In fact, since 2000, Nigeria, under the leadership of NACA, has witnessed a deluge of policy documents that articulate sound strategies, clear targets, and strong action plans for reducing HIV spread and mitigating its impact (13,16,22). In terms of an operational framework, NACA is responsible for coordinating the HIV/AIDS response in Nigeria. As such it acts as a liaison between the government and the private sector and non-profit sectors, coordinating initiatives, steering policies, framing the important issues, and helping organizations develop capacity. NACA is also expected to serve as the clearinghouse for HIV-related information, material, and databases. Implementation of these strategies, however, rests with the many organizations, both local and international, whose mandate is to address HIV/AIDS.

At the policy level, the post-1999 product list includes the National Policy on HIV/AIDS, the National Health Policy and Strategy, the National Reproductive Health Policy, the National Youth Development Policy, the National Policy on Population for Sustainable Development, the National Policy on Women, the National Policy on HIV/AIDS in the Workplace, and the National Curriculum on Sexuality Education. At the action plan and framework level, the list includes HEAP, the National HIV/AIDS Strategic Framework, the National Health Sector Strategic Plan, NNRIMS, and the National HIV/AIDS Behavior Change Communication Strategy. Sector-specific policies have also been developed since 2003 for the education, labor, and internal affairs (which includes the Prisons Service) sectors by the respective line ministries, although the associated strategic and annual implementation plans for translating them into programs and services have yet to be instituted.

It is notable, from the acknowledgments and preface sections of all these documents, that external donor agencies and their implementing partners have played a dominant role in funding and facilitating the processes that led to the writing of these policies and action plans.

On the positive side, the drive for a truly multisectoral response to the HIV epidemic has informed the development of many of these policies and frameworks, and most have been developed out of a fairly broad-based participatory process (1,16). Typically, the process included the production of several drafts that were then critically reviewed at different stages by all the invited stakeholders, including ten key line ministries at different levels of government (health, education, defense, internal affairs, information, women and youth, labor, agriculture and rural development, police affairs, and culture and tourism); the organized private sector; nongovernmental organizations (NGOs); community-based organizations (CBOs); donor agencies; the academic community; faith-based organizations; and women's and youth organizations (16).

But questions continue to be raised about how representative the involved stakeholders are and how well they provide feedback to their constituencies given the continuing poor familiarity with and adoption of the key tenets and recommendations of these policies at the community level (1,15,22). Even more worrying is the issue of ineffective communication of policies from the federal to the lower tiers of government and their units, which are supposed to implement these policies (15,16,22). For example, few of the SACAs and LACAs that are charged with translating the multisectoral approach to HIV prevention and impact mitigation into reality on the ground are so engaged. Finally, the myriad problems alluded to earlier that lie behind the legendary policy-reality gaps in Nigeria continue to characterize ongoing efforts at implementing these laudable policies. One manifestation of this malaise is the as-yet limited implementation of the presidential directive given in 2003 that each line ministry at the federal level should include a line item for HIV/AIDS in its budget. Nevertheless, to buttress the general point about the clarity and soundness of policy strategies and frameworks developed through the leadership of NACA, we elaborate below on two recently released strategic plans.

National HIV/AIDS Behavior Change Communication Strategy

In 2004, NACA launched the National HIV/AIDS Behavior Change Communication Strategy for 2004–2008 (22). The five-year document was developed through a highly collaborative process coordinated by NACA and supported by USAID, with the Center for Communication Programs of Johns Hopkins University and FHI as the immediate technical partners. The development process was undertaken between 2003 and 2004. The vision behind the development of the strategy was to help attain the national goal of reducing the rate of spread of HIV infection by 25% from the current rate of 5.0% to 4.4% by 2008. The goal of the strategy is to attain a coordinated national response for HIV-related behavior change communication (BCC) programming that ensures coherent, uniform, evidence-based, community-oriented, and theory-driven interventions from all stakeholders and that produces a measurable impact within the shortest possible time.

The strategy document seeks to provide a practical and useful strategic instrument for addressing HIV-related BCC issues in Nigeria. It also seeks to empower all stakeholders and to coordinate a comprehensive, audience-responsive, and culturally appropriate BCC program for the control and mitigation of HIV/AIDS in Nigeria. The document identifies:

- The key issues related to HIV-related BCC in Nigeria;
- The conceptual framework and analysis of most effective strategies to help ensure verifiable impact;
- The five-year vision, goal, and target indicators that need to be met to achieve that vision in all priority areas;
- The priority audiences, relevant strategies, and key interventions that should be addressed; and
- Practical timelines for rolling out the overall strategy to maximize impact.

The strategy identifies five priority audiences based on their overall role in HIV transmission in Nigeria and in line with research findings and the provisions of the National Policy on HIV/AIDS: men and women of reproductive age (15 to 49 years old); young people; health care providers; people who engage in high-risk behavior or most-at-risk people; and PLWHAs. Each priority audience has been further segmented to identify subgroups with clearly different desired behavioral outcomes or situations. Objectives, strategic approaches, activities, related research needs, potential partners, implementing agencies, and gatekeepers were developed for each priority audience. The strategy focuses principally around prevention, but also addresses care, support, treatment, and capacity building.

The Nigeria National Response Information Management System for HIV/AIDS

As mentioned earlier, NNRIMS was designed to address some of the major challenges facing the national response to HIV/AIDS related to monitoring, evaluating, and reporting on HIV/AIDS activities and their impact. The NNRIMS is intended to provide decision makers and program implementers with accurate, updated information on the status of Nigeria's response to the epidemic and its outcomes. It will support decision-making, improve accountability, and ensure the documentation of lessons learned. NNRIMS will also provide guidelines for monitoring the implementation of the national HIV/AIDS plans, evaluating the effectiveness of the HIV/AIDS response and various specific interventions, and building the capacity for monitoring the response at all levels. It is hoped that the document will be operationalized and the indicators validated shortly while baseline information on the national response can be quickly obtained to serve as a standardized benchmark for tracking the epidemic.

Providing Program Norms and Standards and Service Guidelines and Protocols

The fecundity of the public sector in developing policies for tackling the epidemic has been matched over the years by an associated growth in the production of norms and standards, technical guidelines, and protocols for delivering programs and services. Documents have been disseminated on such topics as blood safety, ARV treatment, VCT, tuberculosis treatment, PMTCT, and management of STIs (12,13,16,17).

But while most public sector organizations are aware of these guidelines and protocols and follow some of them, service managers often do not have access to these documents. The agencies also usually do not have the requisite technical guidance and support for establishing and maintaining high-quality care, especially at the primary and secondary levels of the health care delivery system. Moreover, few formal links exist between private and public sector programs and services.

Coordination of Development Partners

Nigeria has received extensive support from development partners, including the UN agencies, the CDC, APIN, DFID, and the United States Agency for International Development (USAID). An Expanded Theme Group for HIV/AIDS, in addition to the UN Theme Group, has become fully operational, with all development partners incorporated by 2001.

Over the years, the United Nations System Response has facilitated the development of important and strategic instruments to curb the devastating impact of HIV/AIDS in the country. Noteworthy is the World Health Organization's singular technical and programmatic support to the national response during the early years of the country's epidemic, especially during the days of the Global Programme on AIDS. The commitment to the national response is well articulated in the UN Development Assistance Framework.

The UN's HIV/AIDS response is coordinated through the HIV/AIDS Theme Group. The UN has jointly developed a country support strategic framework. The major highlights of the framework include:

- Active social and participatory involvement of relevant stakeholders in assessment, planning, program implementation, and monitoring and evaluation.
- A stakeholder-driven, multi-track communication and advocacy system designed to promote communication between stakeholder groups.

- Provision of clear linkages between HIV/AIDS, poverty, social governance, and sustainable livelihood.
- Development of institutional partnerships and capacity enhancement for the provision of drugs and transfer of appropriate health technologies to enhance community, household, and individual actions.
- Development of PMTCT capacity.

Research Coordination

To use all the available data generated on HIV/AIDS to make meaningful decisions, the FMOH, in collaboration with NACA and other development partners, inaugurated the National HIV/AIDS/STI/ORID Research Network in 2001. The members include representatives from the public and private sectors, development partners, universities, state governments, PLWHA organizations, and CSOs. This fully operational network facilitated the implementation of the Fourth National Conference on HIV/AIDS in Nigeria, held in 2004.

Prevention of Mother-to-Child Transmission

Nigeria began its PMTCT program in July 2002 with the goals of generating information for the formulation of a national policy and implementation guidelines for a comprehensive PMTCT intervention in Nigeria and providing effective PMTCT services for women of reproductive age in selected health facilities in Nigeria. The coordination of the program rests with the FMOH, while the task team and the core partners' forum provide technical and financial support to the program. The task team is composed of site principal investigators and professionals in obstetrics and gynecology, pediatrics, nursing, and nutrition, as well as officials from the ministry and development partners. The core partners' forum includes UNICEF, APIN, the CDC, USAID, and USAID–implementing partners, particularly Pathfinder International, FHI, and the POLICY Project. This program was pilot tested in eleven teaching hospitals on the basis of two centers in each geopolitical zone. The program has one of the most efficient monitoring and evaluation systems, which resulted from the collaboration of the task team, NASCP, and the core partners' forum members, especially the CDC. The program has similarly contributed positively to increasing access to VCT, universal precautions, infant feeding counseling, and improved laboratory infrastructure.

While early results showed that the nevirapine prophylaxis worked in reducing transmission (24), evidence suggests that in a universally breastfeeding population, the ARV regimen has to be reconsidered, and a task team committee has recommended the use of triple therapy—zidovudine, stavudine, and nevirapine—or another combination of full highly active antiretroviral therapy, or HAART, for HIV-positive women. Nevirapine, as one of three drugs provided under the national ARV program, runs the risk of resistance development, which is a sign of virologic failure in HIV-infected women who may move from PMTCT to PMTCT Plus. This calls for a more inclusive approach to the management of care of HIV-infected women, their infants, and their entire families.

Access to PMTCT is also a critical issue as the program currently reaches less than 1% of women of childbearing age who need it either for VCT alone or the entire PMTCT. Similarly, the PMTCT program did not cover some high-prevalence states, such as Akwa Ibom, Cross River, and Benue, thus raising the question of equity in terms of targeting services to places they are most needed. The centers were recently increased to 67, however, with all ARV centers becoming PMTCT sites. APIN in particular is experimenting on statewide coverage in Plateau and Oyo States with a target of 50% coverage in 2005. The national program, however, is being evaluated.

If Nigeria is to meet its national PMTCT goal of providing services for 20% of women who need the service by 2005 and 50% by 2010, then it must significantly scale up the program by decentralizing it to secondary and primary health care delivery levels. Nigeria has grants from the Global Fund for HIV/AIDS, Tuberculosis and Malaria and support from UNICEF, APIN, and PEPFAR through the CDC and USAID to expand the service rapidly. The country only requires the political will, commitment, and enhancement of its human and institutional capacity to achieve the scale up.

Access to Antiretrovirals

One of the most significant developments in the national response since the re-establishment of civilian democratic rule in 1999 has been the institution of a national AIDS treatment program geared toward expanding poor PLWHAs' access to antiretroviral drugs (13,16). It was announced in April 2001 as "Africa's largest antiretroviral treatment program," with the annual allocation of approximately $3.7 million for the procurement of ARVs from India that will be used to treat 10,000 adults and 5,000 children (16,17). The decision was followed by studies on the safety and efficacy of a combination of stavudine, lamivudine, and nevirapine. The findings showed that two nucleoside reverse transcriptase inhibitors, when combined with nevirapine, reduced viral loads to below-detectable levels (25). This was again followed by two multi-center studies and clinical trials on several ARV combinations. A national ARV protocol and guideline has since been implemented.

Twenty-five centers were created around the country, mainly in federal institutions. Although the number varies from one institution to another, the program has been able to provide treatment to more than 13,684 adults using generic drugs from CIPLA and Ranbaxy; the pediatric guideline has yet to be completed. The national ARV Access program is highly subsidized, with PLWHAs paying 1,000 naira (US$8) per month for the drugs. In December 2004, a total of 11,435 people were reported to be on the initiative while about 2,249 were on other protocols in which the facilities provide unsubsidized ARV to patients.

The program does not, however, cover the cost of laboratory diagnostics for hematology, chemistry, CD4+ counts, or viral load. These tests can cost as much as 15,000 naira to 20,000 naira (US$100 to US$120). PLWHAs must be tested before being recruited to the program and agree to present themselves every three months for monitoring. The cost of the tests has served to deter some PLWHAs from entering the program. The inclusion criteria into the scheme include a CD4+ count of less than 200 without symptoms, a CD4+ count of less than 350 with symptoms, or a confirmed AIDS diagnosis. The government also has made provision for second-line drugs, which include zidovudine, didanosine, and indinavir.

The Nigerian program is bold and ambitious, and it has contributed to a drastic reduction in ARV prices globally. ARV procurement has been financed solely by the federal government, which spent an estimated US$7.6 million on ARVs from 2001 to 2003; US$11.4 million was budgeted for 2004. At present the country is grappling with the issue of scale up as access is curtailed by the locations of the sites and the unavailability of drugs for many PLWHAs in the existing centers; almost every site is afflicted with the "waiting list syndrome." The WHO, through its 3-by-5 Initiative, projected that 400,000 Nigerians should have been on ARVs by the end of 2005. Fortunately, Nigeria is benefiting from PEPFAR, which is expected to place a total of 20,000 new cases on ARV in 2005–2006 and an additional 100,000 PLWHAs in the following five years. In addition, Nigeria still has an outstanding grant with the Global Fund for scaling up access to ARVs.

Recent assessments of the program implementation indicate, however, a significantly slower than planned progress in scale up and a number of persisting challenges that threaten its ongoing effectiveness and long-term sustainability (16,17). These challenges include budgetary shortfalls and discontinuous release of funds, inventory control and distribution problems, inadequate laboratory backstopping, human resource scarcity and training deficiencies, health-care infrastructure deficits, inadequate involvement of PLWHAs and related community groups, and poor technical guidance, support, and coordination for all treatment centers—both within and outside of the public sector program—to forge a comprehensive ART program.

The situation may improve with time as many of these challenges could just be teething problems that come with the rapid establishment of any enormous national program in a developing country like Nigeria. Nearly four years into the program, however, several problems—such as the lack of equipment to assess drug resistance, the nine-hour waits to be seen that PLWHAs have experienced on clinic days in some centers, and a pediatric component that has yet to gather steam—are calls for concern (16). Nonetheless, it stands to reason that despite these problems and the relatively small number of people currently being treated, the institution of the national ART program and its continuing scale up must be helping to reverse the strong fatalism and stigma with which HIV has been associated in Nigeria (26,27).

This assessment of the public sector's role in the national response to HIV between 1986 and 2004 is less then flattering. But it also indicates that the situation has been improving since 1999. Even so, certain unwholesome trends persist, including poor communication and a lack of trust between tiers of the sector, weak intersectoral coordination, inadequate and irregular financing, an increasing dependence on donors, and enormous human capacity deficits. NACA has championed ongoing efforts to address some of these problems through the HIV program development project funded by the World Bank. It has also strengthened partnerships among the civil society and private sectors around HIV prevention, care, and support, partly funded out of a Global Fund grant. NACA's role since 2002 is also noteworthy as—with the support of donor agencies and such international CSOs as ActionAid (15,24)—it has strengthened networking among HIV-focused CSOs through the Civil Society Consultative Group on HIV/AIDS in Nigeria (CISCGHAN) and the Network of People Living with HIV/AIDS in Nigeria (NEPWHAN) and between the CSOs and the public and private sectors. Ensuring the sustainability of these efforts must be a major priority in the years to come if Nigeria is to make significant progress in stemming the spread of HIV and mitigating its impact.

THE CIVIL SOCIETY RESPONSE

Nigerian CSOs have been active in an organized and informed way in the HIV response since the mid-1980s. In 1985, for example, the Society for Family Health (SFH), a national CSO based in Abuja, took the first steps in what is now an internationally acclaimed nationwide HIV prevention program focused primarily on the social marketing of condoms (28,29). Similarly, following early research findings about the groups most at risk of HIV infection, STOPAIDS, a Lagos-based CSO, launched an HIV prevention education and counseling intervention among long-distance truck drivers that later covered motor parks in different regions of the country (Onitsha in the southeast, Lagos in the southwest, Port Harcourt in the Niger Delta, and Kano and Hadejia in the north-central zone) (30). Most CSOs active in the HIV field in Nigeria are not the intermediary, change- and development-oriented types like SFH and STOPAIDS, however. Instead, they tend to be community-based and faith-based organizations preoccupied mainly with small-scale care and welfare services (15,23). Table 11-4 shows the seven broad areas of CSOs' relative dominance within the national response.

Exploratory and Basic Behavioral Research

An often-ignored fact about the knowledge-production landscape in Nigeria is its increasing diversification since the economic crisis of the 1980s to include CSOs. In no field has this been more obvious than in reproductive health, as suggested by the 2003–2004 assessment of 138 academic journals in Nigeria by the National Universities Commission, which ranked as first a CSO-published journal, the *African Journal of Reproductive Health* (31). Indeed, Nigerian CSOs working on HIV issues have been active in conducting pioneering, though often small-scale and formative, research on important behavioral topics, especially since the late 1990s. But these efforts have not greatly affected the research, practitioner, and policy communities because they have usually been neither published nor widely disseminated. Two CSO-led research efforts around brothel sex work and public attitudes toward PLWHAs help illustrate this point.

To the best of our knowledge, the first attempts to systematically inquire into HIV stigmatization among cross-sections of the general Nigerian public, beyond health workers or trainees, were conducted during 1998–99 by two health and development CSOs — Pathfinder International working in Benue State, and the Social and Economic Rights Action Center (SERAC), a Lagos-based human rights CSO, which surveyed seven locations across Nigeria (29,32–34). While we have yet to see the published version of the SERAC study, the Pathfinder study was only publicly disseminated through an international journal in 2002 (35). Nonetheless, the utility of these studies can be gauged by the fact that the SERAC study, for example, which revealed widespread violations of the rights of PLWHAs, informed its development of programs to legally advocate for the rights of PLWHAs. In 2001 this resulted in the first court case in Nigeria's history that sought to defend the human rights of a PLWHA by prosecuting

Table 11-4. Areas of Sectoral Predominance within the National Response, 1987–2004

Public Sector	Civil Society
Blood safety	Condom use promotion
Expansion of antiretroviral access	Youth-focused interventions
Prevention of mother-to-child transmission of HIV	PLWHA care and support, including organizing for self-help and advocacy
Development of policies and program frameworks	Exploratory and basic behavioral research
Provision of program norms and standards and service guidelines and protocols	HIV prevention and VCT among high-risk groups
Sentinel and behavioral surveillance	Mass media engagement, training, and mobilization
	Legal reform advocacy and legal aid for PLWHAs

Source: Authors' analysis
Abbreviations: PLWHA: person living with HIV/AIDS; VCT: voluntary counseling and testing

a private hospital in Lagos for its wrongful dismissal of a nurse living with HIV (14). Other CSOs such as the Center for the Right to Health have since sprung up to expand efforts at promoting and defending the rights of PLWHAs (35). Similarly, the research efforts of SFH have contributed greatly to a better understanding of the socioeconomic correlates and regional differentials in condom use and other sexual-health–seeking behaviors of sex workers and their clients in Nigeria (36,37).

HIV Prevention and VCT among High-Risk Groups

As mentioned earlier, CSOs have led the way in HIV prevention interventions targeting high-risk groups since the late 1980s, with the notable example of the work among transport workers and motor park communities dating back to 1987. Another example of national CSO leadership can be found in the work of the Nigerian chapter of the Society for Women and AIDS in Africa (SWAAN), which has since 1990 provided prevention education, voluntary HIV counseling, and community-based HIV care services among low-income women across Nigeria, including sex workers (38,39).

Founded in 1989, SWAAN is a national volunteer organization of professional and community women that has seen its membership grow from 40 in 1990 to 2,500 by 2002, with branches in 22 states (40). With funding from a diversified base of external donor agencies and international NGOs, it has relied heavily on culturally sensitive information materials, community outreach, and participatory training activities to:

- mobilize nearly 3,500 peer health educators for HIV prevention education in schools spread across Nigeria between 1996 and 2000;
- provide income and safer sex negotiation skills training to more than 500 sex workers between 1996 and 2001; and
- provide, since the mid-1990s, home visits, care, and psychosocial support to PLWHAs in nine states through more than 90 members and more than 200 community health workers it trained for this purpose.

Given the sensitive nature of the complex issues surrounding HIV prevention in Nigeria, it is likely that the demonstration and diffusion effects of the efforts of SWAAN and similarly focused CSOs would be creating an impact far beyond what is implied by the number of people they have trained and the number they have directly reached with their services.

Similarly, the only sustained, multi-site efforts at preventing HIV spread and mitigating its impact among prison inmates and prison barrack communities across Nigeria have been led since 1994 by Life Link Organization, a Lagos-based CSO (14,40). It has worked, largely with funding from the Ford Foundation and Family Health International, among these especially hard-to-reach and grossly underserved communities. Its formative research — which had shown the high prevalence of behaviors and attitudes conducive to HIV spread among prison inmates and residents of prison barracks — led to its working with prison inmates, wardens, guards, administrators, prison training colleges, and the spouses and children of prison staff in more than 20 prison communities in eight states across Nigeria (Lagos, Edo, Kano, Akwa Ibom, Kaduna, Oyo, Enugu, and Ogun) and the Federal Capital Territory.

Life Link's prisons work has entailed the development and dissemination of locally appropriate HIV information and communication materials, training and motivation of peer educators, HIV counseling, confidential testing and referral services, and care and support services. Beginning around 2000, these activities have directly reached more than 11,000 prisoners annually. In addition, Life Link's advocacy and outreach efforts with the prison service authorities and their supervising ministry, the Federal Ministry of Internal Affairs, led to the formulation of a national AIDS policy for the national prison service in 2004. Life Link remains the only CSO in Nigeria that is working nationally on HIV prevention and care in prisons and surrounding barrack communities.

Condom Use Promotion

CSO-led efforts to promote condom use and to ensure easier access to free or affordable condoms by sexually active Nigerians seem to have escalated in response to the growing HIV epidemic. Indeed, the number of CSOs working in the AIDS and reproductive health fields has increased exponentially in Nigeria, which since the early 1990s has increasingly employed a strategy of promoting condom use. A 2001 study, for example, identified 61 women's NGOs and NGO networks spread across Nigeria, of which more than 90% were involved in reproductive health promotion activities, such as STI/HIV prevention education, counseling, and referrals, as well as birth spacing counseling and referrals (36,41). During numerous working visits to these organizations in different parts of Nigeria, we have also observed that they all dispense — sometimes surreptitiously — condoms for free, or at heavily subsidized prices, to the requesting members of their target populations.

YOUTH-FOCUSED INTERVENTIONS

The leadership of Nigerian health and development CSOs in promoting HIV prevention initiatives among adolescents and young adults in Nigeria has been well documented since the late 1980s. Some of the leading CSOs highlighted in this literature are Action Health Incorporated (AHI), a Lagos-based youth-serving CSO founded in 1989 (14,42–46), and Adolescent Health Information Project (AHIP), a Kano-based youth-focused CSO founded in 1989 (41,44). Other youth-serving CSOs include the Association for Family and Reproductive Health (ARFH), based in Ibadan since 1989 (38,47); the Calabar-headquartered Girls' Power Initiative (GPI), which has been active since 1994 (41,44,48); and the Community Life Project, which has worked out of Lagos since 1992 (14,49). The literature about their efforts reveals the following:

- CSOs provide most of the available youth-friendly reproductive health clinic services, including HIV counseling, referrals, and syndromic management of STIs for in-school and unmarried out-of-school adolescents in Nigeria (38,39,44,46,49).
- An increasing number of CSOs spread across Nigeria are providing peer-to-peer HIV education to thousands of young people in and out of school and are disseminating youth-focused HIV prevention messages to the larger population through distribution of information materials, community outreach, and the mass media (38,43,44,48–50).
- Some CSOs have successfully advocated policy and legislative changes that support HIV prevention efforts among youth; examples include GPI's central role in convincing the Cross River State legislature to pass a bill in 2000 prohibiting forced and early marriage for girls (49) and the Edo State legislature in 2002 to enact legislation prohibiting female genital cutting (41). Similarly, AHI played a leading role in the official institution of the National Family Life and HIV Education Curriculum, which has resulted in the gradual integration of HIV education into secondary school curricula in a number of states (45), while in the late 1990s the Ibadan-based Association for Reproductive and Family Health successfully promoted the official adoption of a sex education curriculum in Oyo State and its implementation in public secondary schools throughout the state in collaboration with the state government (41).
- Many youth-serving CSOs are also conducting interventions that reach thousands of young people and that have the potential to reduce youth vulnerability to HIV infection through such vehicles as career guidance, employment skills training, gender consciousness raising, and leadership development (44,47,49).
- Most of the leading youth-serving CSOs have provided mentorship to younger CSOs with similar missions and have inspired the establishment of a growing number of youth-led, youth-serving organizations focusing on HIV prevention (38,43,48).

These CSOs are concentrated in urban areas, mostly in the south and middle belt of Nigeria, and depend heavily on external funding agencies (15,41). It cannot be a coincidence that the revised National

Policy on HIV/AIDS (1) and the National HIV/AIDS Strategic Framework (51) both give prominent attention to many of these youth-focused interventions.

There remains, however, the challenge of unevenness in the quality and content of HIV-related information, counseling, and clinic services provided by the growing number of youth-serving CSOs spread across Nigeria. This unevenness calls for more systematic evaluations of these programs. But the only published peer-reviewed paper we know that is relevant to this issue shows that when carefully planned and implemented, peer education–centered approaches do significantly improve the sexual health knowledge, such as modes of HIV transmission, and attitudes, such as support for greater access to contraceptive information. Peer education–centered approaches also moderately help to delay sexual debut and increase condom use among Nigerian adolescents and young adults (38).

Mass Media Engagement, Training, and Mobilization

Only since 2001 has the Nigerian mass media begun a strong positive engagement with the country's struggles to control HIV spread and deal with stigma. Prior to this, it engaged in sensationalistic and fear-engendering coverage of HIV-related stories and issues in ways that did not help the civil society and public sector efforts to prevent the spread of HIV and destigmatize AIDS (14). This situation seems to have changed only when CSO-led initiatives shifted their approach from working through the media to working with the media. The work of Journalists Against AIDS (JAAIDS), a Lagos-based media CSO, provides one of the best illustrations of the more effective approach.

Formed in late 1997, JAAIDS seeks to contribute to the prevention, care, and control of HIV in Nigeria by educating and building the skills of media professionals reporting on AIDS and by pursuing media-based advocacy for more effective national HIV policies and programs. Drawing its support from a number of external multilateral, private, and internal governmental funding agencies, as well as partnerships with several international NGOs (14,26,50), JAAIDS has been particularly active since 2001. That year JAAIDS began to organize training seminars for media practitioners around the country, facilitate regular access to updated and accurate HIV information for journalists, motivate stronger media and community responses to HIV with an annual awards program, and provide a widely used Web-based discussion forum on HIV (the Nigeria AIDS e-Forum).

The more recent advocacy campaigns of JAAIDS have focused on issues of access to HIV treatment, media activism, and community participation in stigma reduction. A 2004 independent participatory assessment of the impact of JAAIDs' large-scale media mobilization efforts revealed that, across all the geopolitical zones of the country, many Nigerian media practitioners, reporters, and editors have become more knowledgeable about HIV; have reduced sensationalized, stigmatizing, and inaccurate reporting of AIDS issues; and have begun in-house capacity building around HIV prevention, care, and support (26).

PLWHA Care and Support Through Organizing for Self-Help and Policy Advocacy

At the Paris AIDS Summit in December 1994, the global community endorsed the principle of greater involvement of PLWHAs in policy making and program development and implementation (52), as did

Nigeria in 1996, going by statements in the 1997 national policy on AIDS (53). Yet Nigerians living with HIV remained invisible in the country's response to HIV for much of the first 15 years of the Nigerian epidemic, although since the mid-1990s some PLWHA support groups had been meeting regularly under the aegis of various health care institutions and CSOs such as STOPAIDS and the Nigerian Network on Ethics, Law and HIV/AIDS (15,22,31).

Few informed observers would argue with the assertion that the autonomous and activist self-organizing, mobilization, and national level policy advocacy by Nigerian PLWHAs around issues of access to care and stigma reduction only began in 2000 following the formation of AIDS Alliance in Nigeria (AAN), the first CSO to be exclusively founded for and by PLWHAs, in Lagos in December 1999 (54). Prior to this, the umbrella organization for PLWHAs in Nigeria — NEPWHAN, which had been formed more than a year earlier with encouragement from donor agencies, the FMOH, and some health and development CSOs — remained dormant. One of the authors witnessed the beginnings of PLWHA activism in Nigeria and can confirm that a key reason for NEPWHAN's dormancy in its first three years of existence was the failure of the National AIDS and STDs Control Program to fulfill its promise, made during NEPWHAN's inauguration in mid-1998, to provide an office and meeting space for the organization and to facilitate its institutionalization. It is important to note that AAN's establishment was facilitated by the technical support that its founders received from other CSOs, especially the Lagos-based Center for the Right to Health and Health Matters Incorporated.

Nonetheless, the rapid emergence of Nigerian PLWHAs out of invisibility and passivity since 2000 has been remarkable. The process was triggered by AAN, which also housed NEPWHAN until late 2001, largely with funding support from the Ford Foundation and Family Health International (14,55). AAN led an aggressive media campaign to combat the discriminatory treatment that PLWHAs faced in Nigeria and demand for more effective and stronger official responses to PLWHA concerns and needs through advocacy visits to the president, state governors, legislators, and numerous donor agencies and national and international CSOs (56). AAN also helped facilitate the formation of support groups of PLWHAs across Nigeria and participated in relevant national and international conferences such as the epoch-making African Summit on HIV/AIDS, Tuberculosis and Other Related Infectious Diseases held in Abuja in April 2001.

Among the approaches that AAN pioneered between 2000 and 2002 were the PLWHA-managed, telephone-based HIV counseling and referral services; weekly radio and national television programs on HIV issues run by and focused on PLWHAs; and regular national media appearances, which included strong critiques of publicized cure claimants, through press interviews and the convening of international and national press briefings (55,56). In addition, AAN has been active in disseminating HIV prevention information and awareness creation through music concerts, radio and television programs, and the distribution of such materials as educational leaflets, handbills, and face caps. The organization has also engaged in care and support activities through referrals of PLWHAs to designated public health facilities for the treatment of HIV and opportunistic infections.

AAN's national visibility and efforts helped to revive NEPWHAN and partly account for the rapid proliferation of PLWHA support groups since 2001, as indicated by a 2004 mapping exercise (23). More importantly, AAN has helped to give a human face to the Nigerian epidemic, assisted in the gradual de-stigmatization and normalization of HIV, promoted HIV prevention education efforts, and helped facilitate the ongoing expansion of access to care and treatment for poor PLWHAs. Significant internal conflicts persist, however, and the organized PLWHA community has been plagued by various management and technical capacity problems. This situation is not uncommon of PLWHA and other identity-based groups across the developing world (56). It is a challenge that demands a coordinated response from all relevant stakeholders, and it is encouraging that NACA and a number of donor agencies have recently taken up that challenge (23).

Legal Reform Advocacy and Legal Aid for PLWHAs

As acknowledged in the revised National Policy on HIV/AIDS (1), some of Nigeria's laws must be reformed to create a more enabling environment for combating HIV-related stigmatization and discrimination in Nigeria. To the best of our knowledge, sustained interventions geared to achieving this goal have originated from CSOs and only since 1999. We had earlier alluded to the pioneering legal activism effort of SERAC to test Nigerian laws for how well they protect the rights of PLWHAs. This early case revealed how poorly informed about HIV many members of the legal profession in Nigeria were (14). It is therefore significant that a Lagos-based CSO, the Center for the Right to Health (CRH), which was founded by a former staff member of SERAC, has emerged on the national stage as an intermediary for HIV-focused legal reform advocacy and capacity building on issues related to the law, human rights, and ethics, as may be gauged from some of its publications (36,57,58).

Since 1999, CRH has, with multiple external donor–sourced funding, worked with the judiciary, other CSOs, PLWHA groups, and health care delivery services to promote respect for ethics and human rights in health-care policies and practices that affect Nigerians living with HIV. CRH's main strategies have been research and information dissemination; training and sensitization of health care providers, members of the judiciary, and CSO staff; VCT provision; and legal counseling and litigation for PLWHAs. CRH also provides technical support to other CSOs, including CBOs working on issues related to HIV and the law. Most of the organization's training and information activities draw or target beneficiaries from across Nigeria, while the reach of its VCT and legal counseling services has been expanded since 2003 with the establishment of offices and centers in Owerri in the southeast and in Abuja in the country's center. CRH's work represents some of the newer developments that have helped the national response to HIV in Nigeria become more truly multisectoral and multidisciplinary since 2000.

The Ongoing Contributions of CSOs

The initiatives of health- and development-related CSOs have been more varied and have proliferated more rapidly than those of the public sector, although some remain small in scale and narrow in reach.

These CSO-led initiatives have also focused more on issues that relate to the underlying drivers of HIV transmission in Nigeria—such as the lack of access to sexual health information and services by youth and the particular social and economic vulnerabilities of women—than on the more biomedical response issues. But like those of the public sector, most CSO-driven interventions have been sustained more by funding from external than internal sources. This raises questions about local ownership and sustainability of the national response should a sudden loss of interest in HIV or in Nigeria by foreign donor agencies occur in the near future. The increasing collaboration among the CSOs and between them and public sector agencies do, however, offer hope about the long-term robustness of the national response should the external environment deteriorate.

TWO CASE STUDIES OF CSO CONTRIBUTIONS

The current National Policy on HIV/AIDS emphasizes the importance of preventing HIV spread among young people and breaking the silence around sexual behavior and health issues if the epidemic is to be curbed sooner rather than later (1). The policy also clearly recognizes the urgency of curtailing HIV transmission through increased condom use within high risk and highly vulnerable groups such as sex workers and their clients, long-distance truck drivers, and migrant laborers. Given the limited nature of public sector responses on these issues until around 2001, it is useful to examine what sort of planned social and policy change strategies by key CSOs enabled the evolution of national-level interventions around them. The efforts of AHI and SFH since the late 1980s provide good case studies for identifying and illustrating the utility of these strategies.

Action Health Incorporated and the National Family Life and HIV Education Curriculum

The leadership of AHI in the development, institution, and gradual implementation of Nigeria's National Family Life and HIV Education Curriculum for secondary schools is well documented in the reproductive health literature (44,45,59) and in publications by the organization itself (43,47,60). Table 11-5 briefly summarizes the curriculum's history and AHI's role in it.

Since 1989 AHI has worked to improve the sexual and reproductive health of adolescents in Nigeria. With funding from a range of external donor agencies and financial and technical support from several international NGOs, AHI has implemented model projects and outreach activities in Lagos State and, more recently, nationally through partner CSOs, among secondary school students, out-of-school youth, parent groups, CBOs, opinion and religious leaders, and policy makers at local, state, and federal levels to expand the access of Nigerian adolescents to youth-friendly reproductive health information, counseling, and clinic services (43,45,47,60). Particularly significant, however, has been AHI's sustained efforts for more than a decade to promote the development, institution, and implementation of school-based sexuality education in Nigeria. This process unfolded gradually since 1992.

First, following strong evidence from studies conducted in the late 1980s and early 1990s that young Nigerians bore a disproportionate share of the country's reproductive ill-health burden, AHI and a

Table 11-5. Chronology of the Development and Institution of the National Family Life and HIV Education Curriculum, 1995–2005

1995–96	Convening by Action Health Incorporated of a multisectoral coalition of more than 80 youth-health-interested NGO representatives, public agency officials, health professionals, civil servants, and researchers and its adoption of the Guidelines for Comprehensive Sexuality Education in Nigeria.
1999	First National Conference on Adolescent Reproductive Health and Development, which endorsed the institution of sexuality education in Nigerian schools from the upper primary to the tertiary level.
2000	Finalization of the draft of the National Sexuality Education Curriculum under the aegis of the Nigerian Educational Research and Development Council with technical support from Action Health Incorporated.
2001	Approval by the National Council on Education on the sexuality education curriculum for implementation in schools throughout Nigeria.
2003	Revision and breaking into two of the national sexuality education curriculum as FLHE.
2004	Commencement of classroom teaching of the FLHE throughout junior secondary schools in Lagos State with technical backstopping by Action Health Incorporated.
2005	Pre-implementation activities by ministries of education in collaboration with local CSOs in a number of states, including Enugu, Cross River, and Plateau.

Source: Authors' analysis
Abbreviations: CSO: civil society organization; FLHE: Family Life and HIV Education Curriculum; NGO: nongovernmental organization

number of similar organizations began to see the breaking of the culture of silence around youth sexual health issues and the expansion of youth access to accurate and relevant sexuality and reproductive health information as potentially effective responses. This led AHI, in 1992, to establish a technical and collaborative relationship with the Sexuality Information and Education Council of the United States and to convene, in 1995, a coalition of more than 80 youth-serving CSOs, health professionals, public servants, relevant federal ministries, professional associations, and donor agencies from around the country. This coalition evolved quickly into a national task force that helped to draw up and issue in 1996 the *Guidelines for Comprehensive Sexuality Education in Nigeria*. The document set out the framework for providing Nigerian youth with age-appropriate, medically accurate information on a broad set of topics related to human development, reproductive health, gender roles, relationships and intimacy, abstinence, HIV and other STIs, and contraception.

Following its release, some CSO members of the task force—including AHIP in northern Nigeria, GPI with centers in southeast and midwest Nigeria, SWAAN with more than 20 state chapters across Nigeria, the Association for Reproductive and Family Health in southwest Nigeria, and AHI itself—immediately began to adopt the guidelines in carrying out model youth sexuality education in schools and youth centers in their states of operation. These CSOs also continued to advocate for the development and adoption of a national sexuality education curriculum by the federal government for implementation in schools throughout Nigeria. Subsequently, AHI facilitated a process that culminated in 1999 in the first federal-government–convened, donor-backed, multisectoral, and broadly participatory national conference on adolescent reproductive health (61). This conference, in which more than a hundred youths participated from across Nigeria, was historic as it endorsed the call by Nigerian youth-serving and other health and development CSOs for the federal government to develop and adopt a national comprehensive sexuality education curriculum. Led by AHI, these groups continued their advocacy in the intervening period, resulting in 2001 in the policy statement by the National Council on Education, the country's highest policy-making body on education, which endorsed the step that such a curriculum be instituted nationally across the three tiers of the educational system in Nigeria.

From the second half of 2002, however, following increased media attention to the curriculum, opposition to its implementation at the state level from some religious organizations and political interest groups began to gather steam (43,61). In response, the federal government began revising the curriculum in 2003. The government changed the title of the curriculum to the "more acceptable" National Family Life and HIV Education Curriculum; divided it into a junior level and a secondary school level; excised the treatment of such sensitive topics as masturbation, sexual orientation, and sexual dysfunction, especially from the junior-level curriculum; and directed that its implementation be adapted to suit local circumstances by state governments.

Much of the curriculum's content, however, remained intact and strong enough to give young people a sound sexual health education. AHI followed the release of the new curriculum with technical and operational partnerships that enabled the Lagos State Ministry of Education in 2004 to commence the classroom implementation of the curriculum in more than 300 public junior secondary schools throughout the state with an estimated student population of nearly 150,000. Other CSOs have begun to work with their state governments to replicate the Lagos model in a number of states across southern and middle Nigeria (43,45). Implementation of the curriculum has also been given a prominent place in the 2005 National HIV/AIDS Strategic Framework (51).

SFH and the Expansion of Condom Availability, Accessibility, and Use

SFH has earned global recognition for its research-informed social marketing of condoms and sexual health BCC programs, which have resulted in a steady growth in condom use and other protective sexual practices among sexually active populations in Nigeria, especially in the urban areas (30,62). SFH recently emerged as the first Nigerian CSO to receive direct funding from the U.S. Agency for International Development. With 17 offices and more than 150 field-based health communicators (who double as salespeople) spread across Nigeria, SFH now supplies approximately 80% of the condoms sold annually within the country (63).

Founded in 1985 by such eminent Nigerians as the one-time federal minister of health, the late Olikoye Ransome-Kuti, Justice Ifeyinwa Nzeako, and the Emir of Dass, in collaboration with the Washington, DC–based Population Services International, SFH relies on an integrated set of multiple strategies for its HIV prevention education and condom use promotion programs, which became national in scope in 1993. SFH now conducts sexual health communication activities among vulnerable populations throughout Nigeria in such settings as motor parks, brothels, markets, worksites, schools, and vocational institutions using peer education, drama, and the production and distribution of customized informational materials (62–64). These programs, primarily funded by the DFID, tend to reach large numbers of Nigerians; the nearly 1,000 junction-town dramas it conducted with HIV and family planning–related storylines in 2002 reached approximately 1.7 million Nigerians (65).

To encourage sexual health behavior change in the general population, SFH relies heavily on mass media campaigns, touring street theater troupes, the marketing of contraceptive products, and VCT services. Its radio drama series and condom advertisement blitz over the Nigerian airwaves and on billboards have remained prominent since the mid-1990s. SFH also maintains an active research and evaluation unit, which usually furnishes its program managers with the evidence base for the careful planning and execution of numerous interventions. This unit has become an important source of behavioral data relevant to Nigeria's HIV prevention efforts as evidenced by its brothel-based sex work research (65) and its Nigerbus National Multi-Round Surveys (NNMS) of 15- to 50-year-old Nigerians (63,65), which have since 1998 generated data that are useful for monitoring trends in the adoption of protective sexual practices.

The NNMS is a bimonthly, multistage sample survey of 2,500 male and 2,500 female Nigerians aged 15 to 50 years selected proportionately from across all 36 states and the Federal Capital Territory (65). The survey — which is fairly urban-biased despite being equally spread between rural and urban areas — collects information on the social, economic, and demographic characteristics of respondents, as well as their knowledge, attitudes, and practices regarding past and recent sexual activities, sexual health-seeking behaviors, and other HIV-prevention–related behaviors. In summarizing some of the data generated by the NNMS since 1998, Table 11-6 gives a rough sense of the impact of SFH programs on the spread of HIV preventive practices among Nigerians, especially condom use.

The figures suggest a steady rise in condom sales in Nigeria, which translates into a tripling of the annual number of condoms marketed by SFH from 50 million in 1998 to 150 million in 2004. This trend is thought to be partly the result of the condoms' relative cheapness and ease of availability through pharmacies across Nigeria, as well as the aggressive marketing of condoms backed by strong sexual BCC activities (63,65). It is also noteworthy that the condom sales trends are broadly in the same direction as the adoption of protective sexual practices. Consistent condom use in commercial and casual sex, for example, appears to have risen steadily between 1998 and 2002 as the number of condoms distributed by SFH nationwide has risen steadily, despite continuing reports of embarrassment at buying condoms by more than half of the respondents throughout the period.

While not all of the observed increases in the adoption of HIV prevention practices by Nigerians indicated in Table 11-6 can be attributed to SFH's social marketing of condoms and sexual BCC programs, a definitive explanation of these trends is unlikely to be complete without giving some prominence to them. As with most of the other health and development CSOs discussed in this chapter, however, SFH's programs and associated costs have been mainly covered, over the years, by funding from bilateral external donor agencies, especially USAID and DFID.

Key Insights into Change-Inducing Strategies

The two case studies offer a number of lessons about strategies that CSOs should be encouraged to adopt for maximizing the impact of their programs on major health and development challenges

Table 11-6. Trends in Condom Sales (Annual Totals) by the Society for Family Health[1] and Percentage Adopting HIV Prevention-Related Practices (Mid-Year Estimates)[2], 1998–2003

Index	1998	1999	2000	2001	2002	2003
Number of condoms sold (in millions)	50.0	58.1	75.1	116.3	132.3	136.1
% who consistently used condoms (last two months) in non-spousal sex	29.6	26.0	32.9	37.0	55.9	--
% who used condoms consistently in commercial or casual sex	56.4	63.5	70.0	72.7	86.3	--
% who are embarrassed to buy condoms	59.9	57.6	58.0	54.0	56.3	--
% of 15- to 17-year-olds who have never had sex	64.0	68.6	73.0	81.5	81.1	--

[1]Refers to condoms sold by the Society for Family Health, which is estimated to be about 80% of all condoms sold in Nigeria.
[2]Respondents are 15- to 50-year-olds selected systematically from across Nigeria, with an urban bias in the sampling.

Sources: Society for Family Health: Annual Report of 2004 Activities; the Nigerbus National Multi-round Surveys; and activity records supplied in September 2004 by Zacch Akinyemi, general manager of social marketing at the Society for Family Health, Abuja.

fronting countries like Nigeria. First, while SFH has used mass-scale strategies entailing wide presence in the field, AHI has relied more on catalytic and networking strategies. Both broad strategies have produced significant impacts that have helped to strengthen the national response. Second, although both organizations have in recent years become increasingly involved in a wider range of interventions, they have retained a strong focus on a single core issue since they began operating more than 15 years ago. The lesson here is that without carving a niche for itself, a CSO in a country like Nigeria may find it difficult to command the kind of convening or mobilizing influence for fielding initiatives that seek to have national-level impact and the kind of local and international reputation that facilitates successful fundraising. Finally, the two case studies clearly suggest that Nigeria now has intermediary-type CSOs, at least in the reproductive health field, that can serve as nodes for efforts to address the observed weaknesses within the civil society sector as a whole.

Current Challenges and Opportunities in CSO Engagement

Our analysis thus far suggests that health and development CSOs have provided Nigeria with many of the building blocks required for waging a strong national response to the HIV epidemic. CSOs seem better equipped to work at the community level with the most vulnerable groups and on issues that relate more to the root causes of the escalation of HIV spread in Nigeria, such as ignorance and gender inequality, than on the more proximate issues, such as blood contamination and high STI burdens, which have attracted more of a public sector response. CSOs have shown — as with SWAAN and SFH among sex workers and Life Link Organization among prison inmates and barracks communities — how to effectively plan and deliver HIV prevention and care services to hard-to-reach, needy, and underserved populations. But given how few CSOs of this type there are and how limited their access to resources is (2,15), what can the government, donor agencies, and CSOs do to increase the number of CSOs and enhance their contribution to HIV prevention and impact mitigation?

First, the best practices that these CSOs have developed should receive greater government recognition and donor support. Second, the CSOs themselves must become more adept at documenting and disseminating their success stories. Third, given the comparative strength of CSOs at getting HIV programs to underserved or hard-to-reach populations, every level of government should forge more healthy two-way partnerships with CSOs, and donors should be more willing to support these efforts.

At present, CSOs find it easier to work with and are more accepted by local communities and council governments than state and federal government agencies, which sometimes treat them with suspicion and cynicism (15,41,50). This reluctance is probably a legacy of the long years of military dictatorship during the 1980s and 1990s. But in the face of a health and development emergency like the HIV epidemic, Nigeria can ill afford this response. The official AIDS programs at the three levels of governments need to work more actively with local and national CSOs in the design, implementation, and monitoring of programs. This seems not to be happening yet, especially at the state level (15). The public sector must be more willing to share financial and technical resources with CSOs to support them in delivering services in areas and communities and on issues that CSOs are better suited to tackle. In return, the CSOs should become more open to sharing information with the government about their work, funding, and structure.

NACA's recent efforts to forge stronger partnerships with CSOs as a way of mainstreaming them within the national response are commendable. But the approach of working almost exclusively with two umbrella CSO networks, CISCGHAN and NEPWHAN, needs to be expanded and refined. The HIV epidemic is such an enormous, multidimensional problem that it may not always be effective to work through such multi-issue, multi-constituency loose networks. We have found that CSOs working collectively have been better able to form successful partnerships and joint actions with government at state and federal levels when the issues are narrow and well defined. The development and institution of the National Family Life and HIV Education curriculum provides a good illustration of this approach. Perhaps a nodal strategy of public sector–civil society partnerships around specific components of the national response would be more productive. There could be capacity strengthening for the public sector in identified areas of weakness. NACA could identify leading CSOs that have earned a reputation for solid work over a sustained period around each component issue to spearhead the development of partnerships with the relevant units of government.

It must be stated, however, that two large threats to CSOs' continued contribution to the strengthening of the national response to HIV remain poorly addressed. These are the twin issues of donor dependency and significant human and institutional capacity deficits (15,18,41). On the latter, many Nigerian health and development NGOs lack research and advocacy skills (15,41), and when they are available, those skills tend to be concentrated at the top of the organization in a general context of widespread lack of professionalism (2). This is partly a reflection of the relative youth of this sector, the technical and complex nature of some of the issues around HIV, Nigeria's generally low level of development, and the reluctance of donor agencies to fund the rather hard, long, and dirty work of building the technical and managerial capacities of CSOs.

The problem of donor dependency also extends to the public sector HIV programs and is therefore doubly worrisome. Leaders in the HIV field in both the civil society and public sectors must strengthen their advocacy campaigns for better governmental and private sector funding of HIV programs in Nigeria. Legislators and members of the executive arm of government need to be more aggressively sensitized on the dangers that AIDS pose to national development and security and the great need for the country to rely less on external funding in responding to it. This is a task that requires the combativeness and persistence of activist CSOs in the health and development field. The CSOs themselves must also, in the interim, begin to diversify their sources of funding to include internally generated revenues and long-term investment initiatives that can enable them build up their autonomous asset base.

OTHER MAJOR INITIATIVES SINCE 1999

One of the benefits of the restoration of civilian democratic rule in Nigeria and the recent increase in international support for HIV prevention and treatment in Africa has been the huge increase in funding for AIDS programs in Nigeria by bilateral and multilateral development assistance agencies since 2000. The main elements of four major initiatives fielded between 2000 and 2005 follow.

The World Bank–Supported HIV/AIDS Program Development Project

The World Bank–supported HIV/AIDS Program Development Project was conceived to form part of the framework of the HIV/AIDS Emergency Action Plan (HEAP) for 2001–2004. The overall objective of the project has been to help Nigeria reduce the spread and mitigate the impact of HIV infection by strengthening its multisectoral response to the epidemic through the implementation of a comprehensive program. The program was planned to build the capacity of such institutions as NACA, the line ministries, the SACAs, the state line ministries, and CSOs, including support groups of PLWHAs; expand public sector response; and establish the HIV/AIDS Funds for competitive disbursement to organizations to implement projects. The total credit from the World Bank is US$90.3 million to be shared among the federal government, 18 states, and the Federal Capital Territory (66). But it has since been extended to all 36 states. Implementation was slow initially, but the project has benefited from continuous reviews leading to involvement of more states and greater fund disbursement to the project.

Global Fund–Supported Programs

The sole purpose of the Global Fund for AIDS, Tuberculosis and Malaria is to channel large sums of money to programs fighting AIDS, tuberculosis, and malaria in a bid to reverse the course of the epidemics and to stem their devastation, especially in developing countries (67). The Global Fund has committed US$66.46 million to Nigeria for HIV-related projects (68). This fund is intended to expand the country's antiretroviral program, to develop six centers of excellence for PMTCT, and to promote the effective participation of CSOs in the national response to HIV/AIDS. The Country Coordinating Mechanism manages the fund, while the principal recipients are NACA and the Yakubu Gowon Centre (69).

NACA has received approximately US$11.8 million to expand the ART program in Nigeria; the funds are being used to supplement the government supply of both first-line and second-line drugs to the ART centers, upgrade facilities and strengthen capacity at 25 treatment centers, scale up access to many more centers, enhance quality of care by providing additional training to health care workers, and improve coordination between the public and private sectors.

The PMTCT grant will support the development of six centers of excellence to provide VCT services for 18,000 women, to offer ART to 1,000 HIV-infected women, and to train health care workers.

The civil society grant is intended to help improve the coordination of HIV/AIDS interventions by CSOs and to document and disseminate some of the key lessons learned in the response to the Nigerian epidemic. Some of the funds will also be used to establish resource centers in 12 states.

NACA has also provided four-wheel-drive cars to enhance operations at the PMTCT sites, strengthened VCT services, and supported NASCP in building its human and institutional capacity. Judging from the fact that these grants were given during the first round and signed in 2003, implementation has been slow. NACA and NASCP need to move more quickly to access the remaining funds for critical areas of the response and correct the misconception that the absorptive capacity is poor.

DFID-Supported Programs

DFID has major commitments to two HIV/AIDS programs in Nigeria: Promoting Sexual and Reproductive Health for HIV/AIDS Reduction (PSRHH) and Strengthening the National Response to HIV/AIDS (SNR). The PSRHH program is a seven-year, £52 million national BCC and condom social marketing program that began in January 2002 (69). The program's goal is to improve sexual and reproductive health among poor and vulnerable populations in Nigeria by building on the lessons learned in the development and management of Nigeria's Contraceptive Social Marketing Programme, which the British government supported. Population Services International, SFH, and ActionAid-Nigeria are the implementing agencies for the PSRHH program.

SNR is a five-year, £25 million program that began in 2004 (69). FHI is the lead implementing agency with ActionAid-Nigeria and Voluntary Services Overseas as collaborating partners. The program is being implemented in six high prevalence states with the goal of reducing "the impact of HIV/AIDS on the lives and livelihoods of poor people in Nigeria." The purpose is the continued development and implementation of a multisectoral, human rights–based Nigerian response to the epidemic, focusing on selected, high-priority locations where DFID's inputs can make a difference. The program aims to build the capacity of the SACAs to effectively coordinate the state-level responses; increase access in selected high-impact locations to effective, community-level services for people vulnerable to HIV/AIDS; reduce HIV-related stigmatization; promote the rights of vulnerable people; and strengthen local leadership to mobilize and sustain a multisectoral response at community levels.

Other DFID activities include institutional support to NACA and technical assistance for the development of the HIV/AIDS Health Sector Strategic Plan.

AIDS Prevention Initiative in Nigeria

APIN is a project of the Harvard School of Public Health with US$25 million funding from the Bill & Melinda Gates Foundation (70). The project seeks to develop and support an effective, knowledge-based HIV prevention program for Nigeria in collaboration with Nigerian academics, professionals, policy makers, researchers, and health workers at the national, state, and community levels. The overall goal of the project is to reduce the rate of growth of the HIV epidemic and ultimately reverse its course. The project has contributed substantially to human and institutional capacity building, with improved laboratory structures leading to five reference HIV laboratories in the country. It has also led to the implementation of a PMTCT program and has instituted and generated information on surveillance in some subpopulations. The project has been operational since 2000 in four states and at the national level.

In 2004, Harvard also won a grant to implement PEPFAR in Nigeria. It has since initiated an ARV treatment program in six sites in the country. The PEPFAR is a US$15 billion initiative of the U.S. government for the treatment and care of PLWHAs in 14 countries, including Nigeria. The Nigerian program proposes to provide ARV treatment for 200,000 Nigerians within a five-year period (2005–2009).

CRITICAL ISSUES FOR CONSIDERATION

Given the discussion thus far, a number of issues arise that require closer and more systematic attention if the national response is to fulfill its potential for significantly reducing HIV spread and effectively mitigating its impact at all levels of the Nigerian society and economy.

The Three Ones

The United Nations agencies working on HIV/AIDS and other stakeholders have agreed to a new set of guiding principles called the "Three Ones": one agreed-upon AIDS action framework that provides the basis for coordinating the work of all partners; one national AIDS coordinating body with a broad-based multisectoral mandate; and one agreed-upon country-level monitoring and evaluation system (71). The national response must reflect and promote the Three Ones. Nigeria already has one coordinating body (NACA); the National HIV/AIDS Strategic Framework, which will be the agreed-upon action framework until 2009; and a monitoring and evaluation system (NNRIMS). It is hoped that with technical assistance from UNAIDS and other development partners, NACA's coordination role will be enhanced.

Harmonization and Coordination

At the national level, all stakeholders need to accept that an effective AIDS response can only be achieved if countries own and drive it within their own borders. International assistance is important, but it only works if it is embedded within a national response. NACA, in the driver's seat, should be more proactive about coordination and with the international partners ensure harmonization and alignment.

Promoting Evidence-Based Interventions

NNRIMS set in motion the systematic gathering of data about the epidemic. As more evidence accrues about what works in response to the epidemic, such information should be used to inform policy and practice. Unfortunately, political interference and sectional interest sometimes obstruct the use of scientific evidence in developing consensus on effective approaches. NACA's monitoring and evaluation capacity should be strengthened to effectively coordinate state and local government data collection and analysis.

Meeting International Obligations

Nigeria is a signatory to the Millennium Development Goals (MDG), adopted at the Millennium Summit in September 2000, which calls for expanded efforts to halt and reverse the spread of HIV by 2015. Another important document to which Nigeria is a signatory is the Declaration of Commitment on HIV/AIDS adopted by the United Nations General Assembly Special Session on HIV/AIDS (UNGASS) in June 2001, which commits member states and the global community to taking strong and immediate action to address the HIV/AIDS crisis (72). UNGASS calls for achieving a number of specific goals, such as reducing HIV prevalence among young men and women, expanding care and support, and protecting human rights.

The UNGASS declaration reflects the critical importance of accurate information. By making concrete, time-bound targets in the declaration and requiring that efforts be undertaken to measure global success in reaching these targets, the member states envisioned that the declaration would promote greater urgency and solidarity in the campaign against the epidemic. They also affirmed the need to make such information widely available to all interested individuals and stakeholders.

A number of indicators were formulated to measure the attempts of the various nations in reaching these goals. To monitor progress toward the actualization of the targets, countries were requested to make biennial reports on their national response and the epidemic using these indicators. Countries therefore had to develop methods to ensure regularity in reporting. Nigeria was among the nations that submitted the first report, in 2003 (73); subsequent reports are expected biennially. To be able to access resources when the need arises, Nigeria must continue to report on the state of its epidemic.

Capacity Building at the State and Local Government Levels

As mentioned earlier, national response has been dominated in the public sector by federal institutions. A recent survey on the state action committees on AIDS and their local government counterparts showed that they lack both managerial and project management skills. This has hampered the implementation of the World Bank–assisted project in nearly all the states, except Lagos, Plateau, and Oyo. NACA, SNR, Support to International Partnership Against AIDS in Africa, APIN, and other partners have set a national program for capacity building for the SACAs. A critical mass of people must be trained in project management, and these groups, in collaboration with other partners who may be implementing projects in particular states, must continuously monitor those skills.

Scaling Up Interventions

Nigeria must scale up its HIV/AIDS interventions massively in the next five years if will ever achieve the goal it set for itself in the 2003 national policy and meet international obligations under the UNGASS and the MDG. Program leaders must consider the following:

- Scaling up interventions to young people aged 15 to 24 years who seem to be driving the epidemic is critical, as the prevalence rate in this group is higher than the national median average and they constitute nearly 20% of the population.
- Scaling up interventions to core transmitters (high-risk groups) and the bridge populations remains a viable strategy for controlling the epidemic. Efforts should be intensified and more resources should be directed to making this happen.
- Promoting VCT is necessary for deepening and broadening prevention and as a gateway to providing care and support and reducing stigmatization and discrimination.
- Scaling up PMTCT from the present 11 sites in teaching hospitals to the secondary level health institutions quickly would likely help stem the epidemic and mitigate its impact at the household level.
- The national ART program must be expanded and the implementation of a plan to produce ARVs in Nigeria itself must be fast-tracked. The latter may be critical to ensuring the program's long-term sustainability.
- Some unanswered questions remain about the impact of the epidemic on Nigeria. More in-depth studies are needed on the socioeconomic impacts of HIV/AIDS and their implications for national development, allowing a sharper focus for efforts to mitigate the impact of the epidemic.

Upstream Interventions

Responses must take the determinants of the epidemic into account in order to address them. Although some of the factors that drive the epidemic are structural and environmental in nature, policy makers and program experts often pay attention only to biomedical and behavioral interventions. According to Piot, "poverty, ignorance, unemployment and inequality are the handmaidens of the epidemic. They help spread HIV, and AIDS, in turn, undermines development" (74). Poverty and gender inequality contribute to women's decisions to become involved in transactional sex and their inability to negotiate for condom use. The plight of such vulnerable groups as sex workers and economically disadvantaged housewives contribute to the epidemic in Nigeria (75). As a result, "upstream" interventions are needed, with the goal of empowering people to make decisions that reduce their risk of infection and to adhere to behavior that protects them from transmission. Such interventions should include poverty reduction, enhancing the status of women, and appropriate educational programs for displaced persons. Nigeria can accommodate these interventions under the National Economic Empowerment and Development Strategy (NEEDS) (76) and the states' equivalent (SEEDS).

THE RIGHT MIX OF TREATMENT AND PREVENTION

Nigeria has received major funds for treatment, but it has also experienced a relative reduction in resources for prevention. To be successful in stemming the spread of HIV, the country must achieve the right mix of treatment and prevention.

Stover et al. opines that the widespread availability of treatment can enable the full impact of prevention efforts to be attained (77). Salomon et al. forecast different scenarios looking at four types of responses to the HIV epidemic: a baseline, which maintains the status quo of ineffective prevention (as observed in Nigeria up to the mid-1990s) and treatment; a treatment-centered response; a prevention-centered response; and a combined response (78).

A baseline projection for sub-Saharan Africa shows that the annual number of new adult infections will rise from 2.4 to 3.7 million between 2004 and 2020 and the AIDS mortality will rise from 1.8 million to 2.6 million. But if the treatment-centered approach were taken, the HIV infection rate would decrease by 6% compared to the baseline by 2020 and the mortality rate would decline initially by 33% but converge to baseline values by 2020. A prevention-centered response would have a greater impact on new infections, with a 50% reduction in annual incidence by 2020; the mortality trend in the prevention-centered response is more favorable than the treatment-centered response because of reduced incidence (an annual incidence of 34% to 64% and a reduction in annual mortality of 20% to 42% by 2020). The combined-treatment-and-effective-prevention response would have salutary effects, in which both infections and deaths averted could be substantially higher (the annual number of new infections would be 74% lower and the annual mortality rate would be 47% lower by 2020) (78).

The implication of these scenarios is that with an estimated four to six million Nigerians already infected, Nigeria runs the risk of a 50% increase by 2020 if the present prevention efforts are ineffective despite increased access to treatment. The rising rates of infection would also have devastating implications for the already fragile health system and the elevated mortality rates from AIDS. At the same time, Nigeria could turn the tide by creating a combined response to the epidemic.

Integration of HIV Prevention and Treatment

Nigeria must scale up its HIV interventions massively in the next five years if will ever be able to achieve the goal it set for itself in the 2003 national policy and meet international obligations under the UNGASS and the MDG. Interventions to high-risk groups such as sex workers and long-distance drivers should receive top priority. The second priority area should be the prevention of HIV infection among young people. Investment in prevention efforts targeting this enormous and vulnerable group will yield a high dividend. Large-scale school behavior change programs and modified curricula will also go a long way toward achieving the desired result. PMTCT should be a third area of priority, with care of orphans and vulnerable children a fourth area. Closely linked with this would be care and support for women and children infected and affected by HIV/AIDS. Prioritizing these strategies is important for two reasons: resources are limited, and money should be spent where it will give the highest yield in terms of number of new cases prevented.

Integration of prevention efforts with treatment efforts is also vital. The Global HIV Prevention Working Group (79) identified five strategies:

- **Expand access to HIV testing:** Because VCT is a critical entry point for both prevention and ART services, testing programs should be significantly expanded and aggressively promoted. Wherever ART is available, VCT should be universally offered, provided that individuals retain the right to opt out of testing. This approach not only identifies people who will need treatment but also provides prevention education for those who are HIV negative.
- **Incorporate HIV prevention in health care settings:** All health care workers should be trained to provide HIV prevention counseling, access to condoms and other prevention tools, and screening for STIs. Risk reduction strategies should also be integrated into initiatives that promote ARV adherence. Prevention and treatment services should be tailored to meet the specific needs of women, recognizing the multiple social, legal, and economic disadvantages they confront. Special efforts will similarly be needed to make integrated prevention and treatment a reality for young people, who often do not enter the care system until they are adults.
- **Promote ART in prevention services:** Prevention outreach programs should promote HIV testing, educate communities about HIV treatments, and facilitate linkages to care.
- **Reassess donor and government priorities:** Donors and national programs should prioritize integration of prevention in ART settings.
- **Add research, monitoring, and evaluation components:** Efforts on research, monitoring, and evaluation should be strengthened and expanded to identify the most effective strategies for integrating HIV prevention and treatment.

Resource Implications

The simultaneous scale up of prevention and treatment will require an enormous amount of resources. On the global level, the UNAIDS recommends that spending from all sources increase from US$10.5 billion in 2005 to US$15 billion in 2007. The implication for Nigeria is that given the currently available funds from all sources, the government and donors should increase funding for HIV programs by around 300% between 2005 and 2009. The Global Fund, the World Bank Multi-Country AIDS Program, DFID, and PEPFAR already have funds allocated to Nigeria, and the country can seek more funds from other multilateral and bilateral organizations. Nigeria must also eliminate any obstructive low absorptive capacity—associated partly with administrative choke points—to enable funds to be quickly applied to scale up efforts, in order to reap a meaningful impact from such interventions.

Funds should be committed to short- and long-term strategies to build sustainable capacity in Nigeria, allowing the country to deliver essential services, to expand and improve its health care infrastructure, and to expand training programs for health care personnel.

CONCLUSION

Despite a substantial initial delay in tackling the epidemic, the Nigerian national response is well situated to respond positively in the next few years, judging by its present structure; its political and international organizational support; the laid-down brickwork of policies, frameworks, and guidelines; the recorded successes in programs and services; the increased funding; the ever-developing human and institutional capacity; and NACA's improved coordination and harmonization of roles. Promoting ownership and the scaling up of prevention interventions and promoting access to treatment and care will be essential factors in the country's success.

While the Nigerian national response to the HIV epidemic is on the right track, it still must increase the implementation rate and make interventions more evidence-based. Capacity building for the state and local government implementers is critical, and CSOs should be encouraged to continue their interventions while ensuring they are properly funded. Impact mitigation is crucial as the country has begun to see many children orphaned by AIDS and many homes lose their breadwinners to the disease. The response should remain proactive in every sector if Nigeria is to the meet its goal of reducing the HIV prevalence rate by 25% by the year 2009.

Evidence-based decision-making on promoting abstinence, delaying sexual debut, reducing the number of sexual partners, and encouraging condom use will be essential for bringing the epidemic under control. The national response should continue to build the country's capacity to track the epidemic and analyze trends, follow changes in behavior patterns and respond appropriately, measure the social and economic impact, monitor program indicators, evaluate progress, and conduct operations research.

Finally, achieving a sustainable integration of prevention interventions with ART will be critical to success. Nigeria's national response cannot hinge on either prevention or treatment alone but should include a massive scale-up of prevention strategies as access to ART is expanded. Nigeria must tap the potential for treatment to enhance prevention, as only effective prevention will make treatment affordable in the long run.

REFERENCES

1. Federal Government of Nigeria. *National Policy on HIV/AIDS*. Abuja: Federal Government of Nigeria, 2003.

2. Barnett T, Whiteside A. *AIDS in the Twenty-First Century: Disease and Globalization*. New York: Palgrave Macmillan, 2002.

3. UNAIDS. UNAIDS report for 2003: most deaths and new infections ever; some good news. *AIDS Treatment News*, 2003;396:2.

4. Federal Ministry of Health. *National HIV Sero-prevalence Sentinel Survey, 2001*. Abuja: Federal Ministry of Health, 2001.

5. UNAIDS. *Acting Early to Prevent AIDS: The Case of Senegal*. UNAIDS Best Practice Collection (June). Geneva: UNAIDS, 1999.

6. Kaleeba N, Kadowe JN, Lalinaki D, Williams G. *Open Secret: People Facing up to HIV and AIDS in Uganda*. Strategies of Hope Series No. 15 (July). London: ActionAid, 2000.

7. Moore DM, Hogg RS. Trends in antenatal human immunodeficiency virus prevalence in western Kenya and eastern Uganda: evidence of differences in health policies? *Int J Epidemiol*, 2004;33:542–548.

8. Viravaidya M. AIDS in South and Southeast Asia. HIV/AIDS: perspective Thailand. *AIDS Patient Care STDs*, 2001;15(8):437–438.

9. Loo VS, Diaz T, Gadelha AM, Campos DP, Pilloto JH. Managing HIV-infected patients on antiretroviral therapy in Rio de Janeiro, Brazil: do providers follow national guidelines? *AIDS Care*, 2004;16(7): 834–840.

10. UNAIDS. *2004 Report on the Global AIDS Epidemic*. Geneva: UNAIDS, 2004.

11. World Bank. *Can Africa Claim the 21st Century?* Washington, DC: World Bank, 2000.

12. Federal Ministry of Health. *2003 National HIV Sero-prevalence Sentinel Survey*. Abuja: Federal Ministry of Health, 2004.

13. Abantu for Development. *Empowering Youth Through Comprehensive Reproductive Health Programs*. London/Accra: Abantu for Development, 2004.

14. Peterson J, Obileye O. *Access to Drugs for HIV/AIDS and Related Opportunistic Infections in Nigeria*. Abuja: POLICY Project/Nigeria, 2002.

15. Ahanihu E. *Closing Ranks: An Account of Nigeria's Response to HIV/AIDS, 1986–2003*. Ibadan: Spectrum Books, 2005.

16. Action Aid/Nigeria. *Mapping Civil Society's Involvement in HIV/AIDS Programmes in Nigeria*. Abuja: Action Aid, 2001.

17. Falobi O, Akanni O, eds. *Slow Progress: An Analysis of Implementation of Policies and Action on HIV/AIDS Care and Treatment in Nigeria*. Lagos: Journalists Against AIDS, 2004.

18. Partners for Health, Deliver, and POLICY Project. *Nigeria: Rapid assessment of HIV/AIDS Care in the Public and Private Sectors*. Bethesda, Maryland: The Partners for Health Reform*plus* Project and Abt Associates Inc., 2004.

19. Federal Ministry of Health. *Report of the National Evaluation Committee on HIV/AIDS on the National Response to the Medium Term Plan II (1993–1997)*. Abuja: Federal Ministry of Health, 2000.

20. Federal Ministry of Health. *HIV/AIDS Emergency Action Plan: 2001–2004*. Abuja: Federal Ministry of Health, 2001.

21. Federal Ministry of Health. *Nigeria National Response Information Management System (NNRIMS) Guidelines and Indicators*. Abuja: Federal Ministry of Health, 2004.

22. National Action Committee on AIDS. *National HIV/AIDS Behavior Change Communication Strategy (2004–2008)*. Abuja: National Action Committee on AIDS, 2004.

23. Touray KS. *Mapping of Support Groups for People Living with HIV/AIDS (PLWHAs) in Nigeria: National Report*. Abuja: National Action Committee on AIDS, 2005.

24. Odutolu O, Davies A, Fatusi A, Okonkwo P, Ejembi C. Policy options for the Nigerian PMTCT program. *XV International AIDS Conference*, Bangkok, Thailand, July 11–16, 2004 (abstract ThPeE7988).

25. Idigbe EO, Adewole TA, Eisen G, et al. Management of HIV-1 infection with a combination of nevirapine, stavudine and lamivudine: a preliminary report on the Nigeria antiretroviral program. *J Acquir Immune Def Syndr*, 2005;40(1):65–69.

26. Falobi O, ed. *Beyond the Shadow: Unmasking HIV/AIDS-related Stigma and Discrimination in Nigeria*. Lagos: Journalists Against AIDS, 2004.

27. Reis C, Heisler M, Amowitz LL, et al. Discriminatory attitudes and practices of health workers toward patients with HIV/AIDS in Nigeria. *PLoS Med*, 2005;2:1–10.

28. Society for Family Health. *SFH News*, January–June 1997.

29. Population Services International. SFH: first Nigerian NGO to get direct U.S. funding. *Profile: Social Marketing and Communications for Health*, June 2005.

30. Nwabuko B. STOPAIDS organization: 10 years on the road. *STOPAIDS News*, 1997;1:4–5.

31. Editorial opinion. The quality of academic journals. *The Guardian* (Nigeria), July 11, 2005.

32. Morka F. Living the HIV+ life. *Access Magazine*, 1999; 1:1–3.

33. Pathfinder International-Nigeria. *Report of Qualitative Research on Acceptance of PLWHA*. Lagos: Pathfinder International, 1999.

34. Alubo O, Zwandor A, Jolayemi T, et al. Acceptance and stigmatization of PLWHA in Nigeria. *AIDS Care*, 2002;14:117–125.

35. Center for the Right to Health. *Human Rights and HIV/AIDS: Experiences of People Living with HIV/AIDS in Nigeria*. Lagos: Center for the Right to Health, 2001. Accessed at *www.crhonline.org/pubdetail.php/pubid=2* on July 1, 2005.

36. NGO Networks for Health. *Women's NGO Networks in Nigeria: Providing Reproductive Health Information and Services and Promoting Reproductive Rights*. Washington, DC: NGO Networks for Health, 2001.

37. Development Research and Projects Centre. *Women's NGOs and NGO Networks in Nigeria: A Profile*. Kano: Development Research and Projects Centre, 2001.

38. Mba ND. *Youth-for-Youth Health, Gender and Development NGOs: Report of a Mapping Exercise Prepared for the Ford Foundation*. Lagos: Ford Foundation, 2004.

39. Society for Women and AIDS in Africa Nigeria. *SWAAN Profile*. Lagos: SWAAN, 2003.

40. Life Link Organization (Nigeria). *LLO Newsletter* (10th anniversary issue), 2004;1:1–3.

41. Development Research and Projects Centre. *Women's NGOs and NGO Networks in Nigeria: A Profile*. Kano: Development Research and Projects Centre, 2001.

42. Action Health Incorporated. *Enabling Access: a Report of the Sexuality Education/Family Life Implementation Forum*. Lagos: Action Health Incorporated, 2004.

43. Bryant E. Lessons for living: Nigerian youth are fighting AIDS by tackling a new curriculum and teaching each other. *Ford Foundation Report*, 2004;35: 8–15.

44. Brocato V. *Establishing National Guidelines for Comprehensive Sexuality Education: Lessons and Inspiration from Nigeria*. New York: SIECUS, 2005.

45. Action Health Incorporated. *Providing Youth-Friendly Health Services: The AHI Youth Clinic*. Lagos: Action Health Incorporated, 2002.

46. Action Health Incorporated. *The AHI Story (1989–2001)*. Lagos: Action Health Incorporated, 2002.

47. Brieger WR, Delano GE, Lane C, et al. West African Youth Initiative: outcome of a reproductive health program. *J Adolesc Health*, 2001;29:436–446.

48. Madunagu B, Osakue G. *GPI at Ten: A Decade of Roses, Thorns and Change*. Calabar: Girls' Power Initiative, 2004.

49. Iwere N, Kohl RD. Applying the MSI scaling up framework: scaling up the Community Life Project in Nigeria. Prepared for the Annual Meeting and Exposition of the American Public Health Association, New Orleans, Louisiana, November 5–9, 2005.

50. Journalists Against AIDS. *Evaluation Report: Mobilizing the Media towards HIV/AIDS Prevention, Care and Support in Nigeria*. Lagos: Journalists Against AIDS, 2004.

51. National Action Committee on AIDS. *National HIV/AIDS Strategic Framework: 2005–2009*. Abuja: National Action Committee on AIDS, 2005.

52. UNAIDS. *UNAIDS and Nongovernmental Organizations*. Geneva: UNAIDS, 1999.

53. Federal Ministry of Health. *National Policy on HIV/AIDS/STIs Control*. Abuja: Federal Ministry of Health, 1997.

54. AIDS Alliance in Nigeria. *Positive News*. Lagos: AIDS Alliance in Nigeria, 2001;1:1–17.

55. AIDS Alliance in Nigeria. *Positive News*. Lagos: AIDS Alliance in Nigeria, 2003;2:1–3.

56. Center for African Family Studies. *Positive Action*. Nairobi: Center for African Family Studies, 2001; 1–4.

57. Center for the Right to Health. *HIV/AIDS and Human Rights: Your Rights in Clinical Trials*. Lagos: Center for the Right to Health, 2002.

58. Center for the Right to Health. *HIV/AIDS and Human Rights: Role of the Judiciary*. Lagos: Center for the Right to Health, 2001.

59. Esiet AO, Whitaker C. Coming to terms with politics and gender: the evolution of an adolescent reproductive health program in Nigeria. In: Haberland N, Measham D, eds. *Responding to Cairo: Case Studies of Changing Practice in Reproductive Health and Family Planning*. New York: Population Council, 2002:149–167.

60. Action Health Incorporated. *A Unique Partnership for Adolescents' Well-being in Nigeria*. Lagos: Action Health Incorporated, 2002.

61. Adepoju A. Sexuality education in Nigeria: evolution, challenges and prospects. *Understanding Human Sexuality Seminar Series*, 2005;3:1–18.

62. Society for Family Health. *Annual Report for Year 2004 Activities*. Abuja: Society for Family Health, 2004.

63. Society for Family Health. *PSRHH HIV/AIDS Prevention and Impact Mitigation Strategic Framework*. Abuja: Society for Family Health, 2004.

64. Akinyemi Z. Personal communication (with the general manager of social marketing at the Society for Family Health between September 2004 and August 2005).

65. Ankomah A, Anyanti J, Omoregie G, et al. *National Behavioural Survey 2: Brothel Based Sex Work in Nigeria*. Abuja: Society for Family Health, 2004.

66. World Bank. *Nigeria: HIV/AIDS Program Development Project*. Project Appraisal Document, P070291. Washington, DC: World Bank, 2001.

67. Global Fund for AIDS, Tuberculosis and Malaria. *A Force for Change: The Global Fund at 30 Months*. Geneva: Global Fund for AIDS, Tuberculosis and Malaria, 2004.

68. Global Fund for AIDS, Tuberculosis and Malaria. *Portfolio of Grants in Nigeria*. Accessed at www. theglobalfund.org/search/portfolio.aspx?lang= en&countryID=NGA on July 1, 2005.

69. Department for International Development. *DFID Programmes in Nigeria*. London: Department for International Development, May 2005;14.

70. AIDS Prevention Initiative in Nigeria. Accessed at www.apin.harvard.edu on July 1, 2005.

71. UNAIDS. *"Three Ones" Key Principles: Coordination of National Responses to HIV/AIDS*. Geneva: UNAIDS, 2004.

72. United Nations. *Declaration of Commitment on HIV/AIDS: United Nations General Assembly Special Session on HIV/AIDS, 25–27 June 2001*. Geneva: United Nations, 2001.

73. United Nations. *A Report on the UNGASS Indicators in Nigeria: A Follow-Up to the Declaration of Commitment on HIV/AIDS, Reporting Period: January–December, 2002*. Geneva: United Nations, 2004.

74. Piot P. *AIDS: The Need for an Exceptional Response to an Unprecedented Crisis*. A Presidential Fellows Lecture. World Bank/UNAIDS, 2003.

75. Omoridion FI. Sexual networking among market women in Benin City, Bendel State, Nigeria. *Health Transit Rev*, 1993;3:159–169.

76. Federal Government of Nigeria. *National Economic Empowerment and Development Strategy (NEEDS)*. Abuja: Federal Government of Nigeria, 2004.

77. Stover J, Walker N, Garnett GP, et al. Can we reverse the HIV/AIDS pandemic with an expanded response? *Lancet*, 2002;360:73–77.

78. Salomon JA, Hogan DR, Stover J, et al. Integrating HIV prevention and treatment: from slogan to impact. *PLoS Med*, 2005;2(1).

79. Global HIV Prevention Working Group. *HIV Prevention in the Era of Expanded Treatment Access. Report 2004*. Geneva: Global HIV Prevention Working Group, 2004.

12

BUILDING EFFECTIVE INFRASTRUCTURES
FOR HIV/AIDS CONTROL

Job Ailuogwemhe* and Jean-Louis Sankalé*

Nigeria, like many African nations affected by HIV/AIDS, faces the daunting task of responding to an unprecedented health emergency at the same time it needs to rebuild a dilapidated health infrastructure. An estimated 20% of the four to six million Nigerians already living with HIV/AIDS may need antiretroviral therapy (ART). In 2001, the Nigerian government launched what was then one of the world's most ambitious ART programs, aimed at providing provide ART to 10,000 individuals through 25 treatment centers. This program has since entered a phase of rapid expansion, which raises two crucial questions: Can the country's current infrastructure accommodate such an expansion, and is the concomitant development of an adequate infrastructure possible?

The lack of an adequate infrastructure and limitations in human resources have been cited as major limiting factors in the ART expansion in such countries as Botswana (1,2). How will Nigeria fare, especially given the fact that, in 2000, the World Health Organization ranked Nigeria's health care system as one of the worst in the world (3)?

Through our work with the AIDS Prevention Initiative in Nigeria (APIN) since 2001 and the President's Emergency Plan for AIDS Relief (PEPFAR) grant based at Harvard since 2004, we have contributed to the upgrading of several health facilities across Nigeria and evaluated many others.

*Department of Immunology and Infectious Diseases, Harvard School of Public Health, and AIDS Prevention Initiative in Nigeria, Boston, Massachusetts, USA

Based on our firsthand observations and available documents, we will describe and critique the infrastructures for HIV/AIDS control in Nigeria, particularly the biomedical infrastructures. We will examine the constraints on those infrastructures and the ability of existing infrastructures to meet current and future needs. We will also analyze the Nigerian experience in the context of the current ART expansion and try to chart the way forward.

HIV AND THE NIGERIAN HEALTH CARE SYSTEM

Nigeria, like many countries, initially regarded the HIV/AIDS epidemic as a health issue. In 1987, a year after the first AIDS case was reported in Nigeria, the National AIDS/STDs Control Program (NASCP) was created under the auspices of the Federal Ministry of Health (FMOH). At the time, though, the country was suffering from a lack of democracy, accountability, and transparency. During the political and social instability, most health infrastructures were neglected. Scant resources and the lack of political will—compounded by the international community's political and economic ostracism of Nigeria—limited the potential impact any program could have on HIV/AIDS control.

Nigeria's return to a democratically elected government in 1999 brought the country's first signs of a coordinated national response to the growing epidemic. In April 2001, President Olusegun Obasanjo put his political weight behind the fight against AIDS in Africa by inviting African heads of state to attend the African Summit on HIV/AIDS, Tuberculosis, and Other Related Infectious Diseases, the first of its kind in Africa. The implications of this political statement were enormous, and Nigeria has since made significant strides toward the development of adequate infrastructures and institutions for controlling the epidemic.

The FMOH takes primary responsibility for responding to health issues in the country. The HIV/AIDS efforts of the FMOH are conducted through NASCP, working in line with the state ministries of health, HIV and other sexually transmitted infection (STI) programs, and local government authority AIDS action managers. NASCP coordinates national programs that are implemented by federal and parastatal institutions across the country or by institutions at the state or local government level.

In the public sector, treatment and care for HIV rely primarily on the public health delivery system. Nigeria has a three-tiered health care delivery system: primary health care; secondary health care; and tertiary health care. The tertiary health care centers, which consist of the university teaching hospitals and the federal medical centers, are evenly distributed across all the 36 states and the Federal Capital Territory. The general hospitals and state hospitals make up the secondary tier, with each state having at least one hospital, along with one or more branches spread across the state. The primary health care centers, which are the first line of access to health care delivery, are located in local government areas.

The three-tiered system of health care is sometimes a mixed blessing, as different political and administrative structures have authority and control over each tier of the system. The failings of institutions at one tier can place undue strain on the other tiers without the possibility for these levels of government to remediate the failings of the troubled institution. Instances of duplication and even competition between institutions at different tiers have also been noted.

Other governmental institutions that do not belong to the general health care delivery system remain integral parts of the HIV/AIDS care and treatment delivery. These FMOH-affiliated parastatal institutions include the Nigerian Institute of Medical Research, the Nigerian Institute of Pharmaceutical Research and Development, and public and government hospitals. These hospitals include all military hospitals, police hospitals, and hospitals owned by such government agencies as the Nigerian National Petroleum Corporation, the Nigerian Railways, the Nigerian Ports Authority, the Central Bank of Nigeria, and the Nigerian Prison Services.

Complementing the government health institutions are private-sector hospitals and clinics, including for-profit clinics, which tend to be smaller operations in larger cities. Nigeria's private-health sector is not well regulated, and few data are available on the extent to which private practitioners are involved in HIV care and treatment (4). A number of large firms, such as the major oil companies, and missionary groups also run clinics and hospitals (4). Many of these clinics and hospitals work with community-based organizations and faith-based organizations to conduct AIDS support services in communities across the country.

Governmental agencies at the federal, state, and local levels tend to suffer significantly from inadequate resources. Despite a formal organizational structure of the various health infrastructures in Nigeria, the health referral system is simply non-operational. Many disparities exist between structures at the same levels. Federal institutions, for example, vary widely in their ability to provide comprehensive HIV services. At the primary health care level, HIV services, when available, are often limited to HIV testing and, in few pilot sites, prevention of mother-to-child transmission services. Most HIV-related services are performed at secondary state hospitals or even only in tertiary centers, such as teaching hospitals and federal medical centers. With the recent paradigm shift resulting from the introduction of ART, the medical aspects of HIV have been addressed after many years of neglect and hopelessness. When the federal government's ambitious ART program effectively started in 2002, it reached its goals rapidly given the immense latent need for ART. The federal government is spearheading the current rapid expansion with funding from bilateral and multilateral cooperation, including the PEPFAR program, and implementation by Nigerian institutions, both public and private, in cooperation with external implementation partners.

THE INFRASTRUCTURE FOR HIV CARE AND TREATMENT

In the current context of ART provision, HIV/AIDS is viewed as a chronic disease, and most people receive treatment in clinics on an outpatient basis. This is not to suggest that AIDS is not burdening admissions facilities; in some instances, people living with HIV/AIDS account for the majority of admitted patients in some wards.

The Clinical Setting

Although outpatient HIV clinics follow several modalities, most HIV-infected patients attend clinics in which physicians and nurses who specialize in HIV/AIDS treat HIV-infected patients exclusively. The two most common modalities consist of the HIV clinic with a devoted building, such as at University College Hospital in Ibadan and Jos University Teaching Hospital, and an HIV clinic in a more general outpatient facility with devoted time for HIV patients as seen at the University of Maiduguri Teaching Hospital and Lagos University Teaching Hospital.

In the institutions we have visited, facilities dedicated to HIV/AIDS care—often with an attached pharmacy, record office, and laboratories—seem to be better at delivering appropriate care and ensuring patient retention than facilities with no particular specialty. The specialized facilities also have the advantage of not taking away consulting slots from other hospital departments. The main drawbacks are the costs associated with creating a specialized structure, the stigma attached to a building or part of a building devoted entirely to HIV care, and, in the long run, the non-integration of HIV services into the routine services provided by the facility at large.

APIN and more recently the Harvard PEPFAR program in Nigeria have helped several institutions organize and equip their outpatient service facilities for HIV care and treatment. These institutions tend to favor specialized structures for HIV care in an effort to allow a significant expansion of the services provided.

Pharmacies

Pharmacies in federal hospitals are generally large facilities with much more space than the existing stocks require. These pharmacies are staffed by several pharmacists with adequate general training but often limited knowledge of the issues relating to ART. A system of stock management is operated with the use of bin cards. When computers exist, they are usually not used for record keeping and stock maintenance. Refrigeration and a stable supply of electricity continue to be critical issues. In the six sites where the Harvard PEPFAR program is operational—University College Hospital, Jos University Teaching Hospital, Lagos University Teaching Hospital, the University of Maiduguri Teaching Hospital, the Nigerian Institute of Medical Research, and the 68 Nigerian Army Reference Hospital—the pharmacies have been significantly upgraded with the provision of dedicated emergency power generators, operational computerized information systems, refrigerators, and increased security to prevent break-ins.

Laboratories

The laboratory infrastructure is the most expensive and specialized part of any institutional framework for HIV/AIDS care (5,6). In Nigeria, policymakers and decision makers have tended to view laboratories in the narrow context of HIV screening. Over the years, many laboratories across the country were equipped with necessary HIV screening tools, such as equipment for performing ELISA assays. Once rapid tests requiring no specialized instruments were adopted, though, the perceived needs of infrastructure development contracted even further. Until recently, this development tended to be limited to training sessions for personnel conducting rapid tests in nearly empty, dilapidated laboratories.

At the onset of the ART program no laboratory in the country had the full capacity needed to monitor treatment response and toxicity properly. Only a handful of institutions had the capacity to perform CD4+ counts, a necessary test for decision-making in HIV therapy. The federal government program provided the training and technical capacity for CD4+ tests to be performed in the 25 treatment centers using a manual microscopic technique. This technology is labor intensive, and one laboratory technician cannot reliably perform more than 10 tests a day. This pace cannot accommodate the expansion of ART in these centers and in other centers that would rely on them for laboratory support.

Through a generous donation from MTN Nigeria, a telecommunications company, APIN was able to equip two federal treatment centers—at University College Hospital and Jos University Teaching Hospital—with flow-cytometry–based instruments (7), which allow technicians to process more than 100 CD4+ tests daily. The instruments cut the cost of the tests four- to fivefold. All Harvard PEPFAR program sites are now equipped with these instruments. Many other programs in Nigeria, particularly the other PEPFAR programs, have opted for that investment as well.

Similarly, when the ART program started in Nigeria, only one center had the capacity to perform viral load tests routinely; these tests are used to measure the virus level in the blood of infected individuals and thereby allow clinicians to assess treatment efficacy. This center, the Nigerian Institute of Medical Research, had been upgraded and equipped by a grant from the Ford Foundation.

APIN, a project based at the Harvard School of Public Health (HSPH) and sponsored by the Bill & Melinda Gates Foundation, has significantly affected the level of infrastructures available in its four target states of Borno, Lagos, Oyo, and Plateau. All APIN sites now routinely perform HIV viral load tests with technical assistance and/or equipment provided by HSPH.

When HSPH became a PEPFAR implementation partner, it further expanded the capacity of its collaborating centers. HSPH has provided training and retraining of health professional and laboratory personnel and helped upgrade or establish six laboratories for HIV and STI services. To our knowledge these sites—University College Hospital, Jos University Teaching Hospital, University of Maiduguri Teaching Hospital, Lagos University Teaching Hospital, Nigerian Institute of Medical Research, and 68 Nigerian Army Reference Hospital—are the only public institutions in the country to provide a complete laboratory monitoring of ART response and toxicity by providing serodiagnosis with Western-blot confirmation, hematology, chemical pathology, flow-cytometry–based CD4+ determination, and viral load on a routine basis for nearly all their patients.

In addition, five of these centers are Nigeria's only facilities to perform infant diagnostics using polymerase chain reaction (PCR), the only technique capable of diagnosing HIV infection in infants. In addition, most sites have been involved in projects in collaboration with HSPH to conduct surveillance studies of the HIV strains circulating in Nigeria and of the drug resistance levels in various patient populations.

Additional efforts by the federal government, some state governments, HSPH, other PEPFAR implementation partners, and several international development partners are rapidly changing the face of

Nigeria's biomedical infrastructures. Laboratories that support prevention and treatment efforts are being upgraded and developed in various parts of the country. Flow-cytometry–based CD4+ determination is becoming more and more available, enabling more accurate and less expensive CD4+ counts. Despite all this progress, the pace of laboratory development cannot keep up with the pace of the increased demand for HIV care and treatment.

One remaining criterion for being able to provide the best quality care available to Nigerians living with HIV/AIDS is the capacity to perform drug-resistance testing. At the programmatic level this testing is desirable to enable periodic assessments of resistance levels, to establish patterns of resistance development in strains circulating in Nigeria, and to provide a tool for evaluating adherence (8–10). These activities are now conducted in partnership with HSPH for sites participating in APIN or the Harvard PEPFAR program.

CONSTRAINTS ON INFRASTRUCTURES FOR HIV/AIDS CONTROL IN NIGERIA

The biomedical infrastructure for HIV/AIDS control in Nigeria faces many major problems. Among the most pressing are an inadequate definition of needs, a lack of sustained commitment and insufficient funds from the government, a lowest-common-denominator effect, inadequate manpower, a weak commitment from development partners, equipment maintenance requirements, the need for quality management and accreditation, and the high costs of treatment-response and toxicity monitoring in ART.

An Inadequate Definition of Needs

The burden of HIV on the Nigerian health care system is generally inferred from surveillance data conducted in various patients groups during biennial national serosurveys and local studies and from the attendance at HIV clinics. The country has no systematic information system, however, that would allow an exact picture of the situation to emerge. Unfortunately, most Nigerian hospitals have a paper-based and often obsolete patient record system. Such systems can be rudimentary, particularly at the state hospital and primary health center levels. In that context, it is not always possible to establish reliable health statistics on HIV. The problem is usually compounded by the lack of proper diagnostics and investigational facilities. The system, as it exists, does not allow a full assessment of the burden that HIV/AIDS poses on the health system. Monitoring of HIV/AIDS–related activity is usually performed in a vertical manner within the boundaries of specific programs such as the government ART program, or through such periodic surveys as the biennial seroprevalence survey.

The lack of reliable systematic data leads to an underestimate of the strain that HIV places on the heath system. More importantly, the care and treatment requirements can only be guessed at based on imperfect data and general estimates. As an illustration, we can cite the case of an HIV clinic in a

Nigerian teaching hospital that started with visits in physicians' offices and has since moved to three different locations in four years, each time more than doubling its capacity. The clinic increased its frequency to become daily only to find itself overwhelmed within months of each move. In this particular case, we did not witness an explosion of AIDS cases in the city but rather a latent need that the previous facilities and services had not met. The existence of adequate data to predict the needs and plan for the appropriate infrastructures would have prevented the costly exercise of refurbishing new facilities and moving to clinics that would prove too small too fast.

A Lack of Sustained Commitment and Insufficient Funds from the Government

Nigeria's political history has been characterized by instability, with the attendant consequence of a lack of continuity in government policies and programs. A direct result was a lack of sustainable development in the country's health care delivery system. By the time Nigeria's first AIDS case was reported in 1986, the quality of the existing health care delivery infrastructure and institutions had already declined. The democratic institutions in place since 1999, however, have been able to reverse that trend. Unfortunately, despite the commitment of the government, the extent of the decay is such that the pace of rehabilitation of the health infrastructure is not fast enough for tackling the HIV/AIDS crisis. Fund allocation is also an issue, with each component of the health sector jostling for its share of limited resources. The Nigerian government has begun renovating eight teaching hospitals; to date, two of these hospitals have been renovated and commissioned (11).

A Lowest-Common-Denominator Effect

Nigeria is a large federal country, yet it is still traditionally divided along various geographic, religious, and sociocultural fracture lines. The central government is truly at the center of power as it exerts control over resources and most aspects of policy. In most of its administrative and political decisions, the federal government pays obsessive attention to issues of fairness and balance between states and regions of the country. This has the unintended consequence of stymieing progress, as some infrastructure developments may be regarded negatively if concentrated in a region or a state. Government officials have frowned on some infrastructure upgrades because the upgrades were possible only in few centers, creating the perception of inequality or injustice. This regard for equity risks spreading the limited resources so thin to the point of irrelevance.

Inadequate Manpower

Nigeria is probably the African country that has provided the largest number of physicians and other health professionals to nations in Europe and North America, as well as to other countries that, if not more developed, have at least better wages or living conditions than Nigeria. According to the Association of Nigerian Physicians in the Americas, for example, more than 2,500 physicians born or trained in Nigeria are now working in North America. Despite this brain drain, Nigeria still abounds in well-trained health professionals, many of whom are underemployed because of the lack of openings in public institutions. Yet another major constraint on infrastructures for HIV/AIDS control in Nigeria, therefore, is inadequate manpower.

The chronic shortage of health care delivery personnel in Nigerian hospitals is especially evident in the AIDS field. The most highly trained HIV/AIDS experts are always in constant demand and working on multiple projects. The Nigerian government, with the assistance of APIN, has developed a basic training curriculum that has been used to educate a large number of health professionals across the country. Yet with the advent of ART, HIV medicine and laboratory sciences have become fields of high specialization that require advance training that is currently only available through apprenticeship. No Nigerian university has established HIV/AIDS as a field of study. It will be difficult to develop good infrastructural capacities for HIV/AIDS control and upgrade existing ones if there are insufficient numbers of well-trained personnel to run these facilities.

Most of the infrastructures for HIV/AIDS control in Nigeria are plagued with a shortage of competent professionals, and institutions that are well staffed usually find it difficult to retain their staff. Similarly, institutions have not established strategies and policies for retaining personnel with specialized HIV training. For instance, nurses and counselors who received HIV-specific training are sometimes redeployed in another position, often within the same institution, where their recently acquired skills are not applied.

A Weak Commitment from Development Partners

The policies of many international development partners play an unintended role in the problem of inadequate manpower in Nigeria. Most agencies involved in HIV/AIDS prevention and control efforts in Nigeria are goal driven, and an enormous pressure is placed on them to show results within a specific timeframe. Instead of training new personnel or building new infrastructures, many of these agencies engage the services of a few highly skilled professionals, while others rely on the expertise of experienced personnel from abroad. This has in no small measure contributed to the shortfall in the development of infrastructures for HIV/AIDS control.

Furthermore, donor agencies usually fund projects on a two-to-five-year basis to meet short-term goals; such a timeframe often is not enough to build a sustainable infrastructural capacity — nor is that capacity ordinarily part of the funder's indicators of success. In addition, many international partners tend to circumvent paralyzing government bureaucracies by administering programs themselves in an effort to save time and be more efficient. The net effect is the tendency toward multiple, semi-autonomous, overlapping projects clustered in some regions of the country. Local expertise is often diverted onto the projects, creating vacancies in other areas. Once a project has been completed, however, personnel and equipment are often dispersed, creating no lasting impact on infrastructural development.

Equipment Maintenance Requirements

Modern laboratories charged with the follow-up of ART patients—such as the ones developed by APIN and the Harvard PEPFAR program—represent significant investments in equipment. The average cost of equipping a complete laboratory—one that can perform high-volume hematology, chemical pathology, flow-cytometry–based CD4+ determination, viral load, and DNA PCR—approaches US$300,000. Such an investment needs to be protected by having in place plans that allow preventive maintenance and timely emergency repairs. As often as possible, equipment and automated systems provided by companies that offer techinical support and maintain a representative in Nigeria should be selected. Given the poor quality of the power supply, surge protectors must be installed on all expensive or crucial pieces of equipment. Unfortunately, for many instruments the technical competence for maintenance and repair is not available in the country. As the infrastructure system develops the need for training will grow even more urgent.

Quality Management and Accreditation

Nigeria has no functioning laboratory accreditation system. Quality assurance and quality control were foreign concepts to most of the laboratories we visited, and not a single laboratory had a quality-management plan. No segment of the health system, in fact, seems to have a quality-management plan. There is a need for laboratory system specialists trained in quality management. The Standards Organisation of Nigeria, a member of the International Organisation for Standardisation, does not have health-related industries or institutions certified, with the exception of three pharmaceutical manufacturers and distributors. APIN has instituted a limited system of quality assurance and control for the laboratories affiliated with the project, and a significant strengthening of this system is under way through the Harvard PEPFAR program.

Costs of Treatment Response and Toxicity Monitoring in ART

In recent years there has been a growing advocacy effort around the globe for access to ART in resource-constrained countries (12). This has led to significantly reduced prices for drugs and the development of many generic versions and new formulations. Unfortunately, the global community at large did not show the same level of effort for advocacy for laboratory monitoring of the treatment (5,6). This is not to say that prices have not dropped. In recent years we have witnessed a more than threefold decrease in the price of reagents for viral load for most resource-constrained countries. Prices of CD4+ assays have also fallen, and less expensive alternatives have been developed. Yet laboratory monitoring—including the cost of reagents and the associated cost of supplies, personnel, and infrastructure buildup and maintenance—accounts for a sizable portion of the cost of maintaining an individual on ART.

For instance, the government of Nigeria has been subsidizing drugs for ART without a similar effort toward treatment monitoring, resulting in a situation in which most patients were being treated without proper monitoring. It has been estimated that treatment monitoring would account for 23% of the total cost of treatment and one-half to two-thirds of patients' out-of-pocket expenses (13). The establishment of the Harvard PEPFAR program has helped alleviate this problem in areas in which the program is operating, but the problem remains acute in other areas.

CONCLUSION: THE WAY FORWARD

Nigeria, whose population represents 20% to 25% of those living in Africa, faces enormous challenges with the HIV/AIDS epidemic. Although no other African nation has had an experience directly applicable to Nigeria as a whole, two countries—Botswana and Senegal—offer relevant lessons from their experience with building ART programs (2,14).

Botswana, a sparsely populated country on a large landmass, has high prevalence rates of HIV infection. The country's ART program started in the capital, Gaborone, and rapidly expanded to most areas of the country without the development of sophisticated infrastructures. The program operated with referral of blood samples for monitoring tests to a central laboratory in Gaborone. Later, a second laboratory opened in the second largest city. The main emphasis in rolling out the ART program has been on training; Botswana has developed an exemplary training curriculum for health care workers, which has since served as a model for many countries, including Nigeria (2). Serious concerns have arisen, however, about the ability of the central laboratory to cope with the volume of test requests and the ability of the program to be monitored and evaluated properly. The Harvard PEPFAR program in Botswana is helping the Botswana government in bolstering its monitoring and evaluation capacities.

Senegal, in contrast, is a smaller country with a larger population and a low HIV prevalence rate. The government ART program, one of the first in Africa, began in the capital, Dakar, and was later rolled out to the various regional capitals of the country only when the adequate infrastructures were in place. Although the delay in the roll out dampened the success of the initial start of the program, it ensured that patients were provided adequate care and that the program was monitored properly.

In Nigeria, the ART program was started without addressing most of the country's infrastructure issues. The recent involvement of such projects as APIN and such programs such as the Harvard PEPFAR has been changing the picture significantly. Infrastructures are being developed in many cities around the country. Several key elements still need to be addressed, however, to prevent future problems:

- Government decision makers, the donor community, and implementing partners must demonstrate a strong and sustained commitment to infrastructure rehabilitation in particular laboratories.
- The country has an urgent need to improve not only its health and HIV data collection and analysis, but also its epidemiologic research to be able to properly define the needs of each town, city, state, and region of the country. The development of appropriate infrastructures is contingent on the definition of the needs in matters of care and treatment of HIV.
- Training of more HIV specialists must take priority. The government is conducting training programs to update health professionals, but the pace must be accelerated. Universities should not only reinforce HIV in curriculums, but also develop an HIV specialization in all aspects of social and biomedical sciences as well as medicine.

- Health institutions involved in HIV care and treatment must develop flexible and efficient horizontal networking to be able to address the needs of patients. The agility of such a system requires that the networks be organized on objectively defined and practical parameters that would not impede their functioning.
- Vertical networking must also be reestablished to allow the secondary and primary health care systems to fulfill their roles and alleviate the burden on the tertiary institutions. At present, ART centers are not only treating patients who need ART, but are also monitoring thousands of otherwise healthy individuals infected with HIV and patients on ART who are stable. The system could become more efficient if this monitoring role could be devolved to the lower tiers of the health system. It would be unrealistic to wait for the full repair of the Nigerian health care system, but it can be conceived of a system in which tertiary centers would partner with secondary or primary health centers. Some centers would refer patients to other centers for follow-up and in exchange provide training and other technical support.
- Several reference centers that would operate with the most modern techniques are required, not only to serve as referral points for difficult cases but also to conduct clinical and operational research in treatment and care of HIV. Continuous research is necessary to develop evidence-based solutions to the problems that need to be tackled. A lack of commitment to research is a serious impediment to developing appropriate solutions to the various problems the ART programs face in many African countries. Often the emergency of the situation requires that solutions be found in the experience of another country. In general, though, the balance must be struck between reinventing the wheel and taking a one-size-fits-all approach. These centers would be ideal sites for developing quality control systems for other laboratories.
- Nigerian institutions and their implementing partners should harmonize their various technical platforms for four reasons: to ensure that results are comparable from one center to another; to facilitate the contracting of any maintenance needs outside of Nigeria; to be able to buy reagents and other consumables from a single manufacturer in bulk, thereby reducing costs and increasing the likelihood of sustainability; and to facilitate the implementation of quality assurance and control measures.

To contain its HIV/AIDS epidemic effectively, Nigeria must pay much more attention to developing its infrastructural capacity by strengthening institutions and enhancing the training of health care delivery personnel in the area of HIV. Although the best way to approach these goals has been the subject of much debate, experts seem to agree that decision makers in Nigeria must significantly increase their commitment toward building new infrastructures and upgrading or maintaining existing ones. Nigerian institutions have tended to rely on the help of international development partners. Yet to attract the necessary funding and technical expertise, they should first demonstrate a strong commitment and a clear expression of infrastructural development needs.

Overcoming the constraints will not be easy. In recent years, though, one of the best approaches for Nigerian tertiary institutions has been to establish collaborations with international institutions and organizations in all areas relevant to HIV control. The need to strengthen Nigerian biomedical institutions is critical, and collaboration with international institutions, if built on a well-defined intervention and research agenda, can help strengthen capacity significantly by offering long-term partnerships. Large multilateral and bilateral efforts at the government level are rarely amenable to the in-depth partnership required to uplift existing institutions. They are, however, necessary for the establishment of new large institutions. We are already witnessing positive developments in the direction of institutional partnerships. Since 2001 HSPH has forged collaborations with six Nigerian institutions through APIN and more recently the Harvard PEPFAR program. Other public and private institutions—including the University of Maryland, Johns Hopkins University, Family Health International, and the U.S. Centers for Disease Control and Prevention—are involved in various direct collaborations with different Nigerian institutions as well.

The federal government of Nigeria must provide an enabling environment that will encourage international developmental agencies to embark on long-term projects that incorporate funding for local infrastructural development. There is also a need for greater cooperation between policy makers and researchers to increase the indigenous capacity to conduct research and promote the use of research results in formulating policies. Research is needed to define the monitoring strategies that afford the greatest attainable care to patients with HIV while taking into account the limitations of the resource-poor setting. Research results—when incorporated into the policy and strategies design and health programs implementation at all levels of the country's health system—will go a long way toward helping planners and policy makers develop effective long-term infrastructural development objectives.

REFERENCES

1. Ogundipe S. HIV and AIDS: lessons from Botswana. *Vanguard*, December 26, 2005.

2. Wester CW, Bussmann H, Avalos A, et al. Establishment of a public antiretroviral treatment clinic for adults in urban Botswana: lessons learned. *Clin Infect Dis*, 2005;40(7):1041–1044.

3. World Health Organization. *World Health Report.* Geneva: World Health Organization, 2000.

4. Partners for Health Reformplus, DELIVER, and POLICY Project. *Nigeria: Rapid Assessment of HIV/AIDS Care in the Public and Private Sectors.* Bethesda, Maryland: The Partners for Health Reformplus Project, Abt Associates Inc., 2004.

5. Stephenson J. Cheaper HIV drugs for poor nations bring a new challenge: monitoring treatment. *JAMA*, 2002;288(2):151–153.

6. Tucker T, Yeats J. Laboratory monitoring of HIV—after access to antiretroviral drugs, the next challenge for the developing world. *S Afr Med J*, 2001; 91(8):615.

7. Imade GE, Badung B, Pam S, et al. Comparison of a new, affordable flow cytometric method and the manual magnetic bead technique for CD4 T-lymphocyte counting in a northern Nigerian setting. *Clin Diagn Lab Immunol*, 2005;12(1):224–227.

8. Lazzari S, de Felici A, Sobel H, et al. HIV drug resistance surveillance: summary of an April 2003 WHO consultation. *AIDS*, 2004;18(Suppl 3):S49–S53.

9. Moatti JP, Spire B, Kazatchkine M. Drug resistance and adherence to HIV/AIDS antiretroviral treatment: against a double standard between the north and the south. *AIDS*, 2004;18(Suppl 3):S55–S61.

10. World Health Organization. *Report on Inventory of Laboratories in Africa Involved in Genotypic and Phenotypic HIV-1 Antiretroviral Drug-Resistance Testing.* Brazzaville: Regional Office for Africa, World Health Organization, 2001.

11. Address by His Excellency, President Olusegun Obasanjo, GCFR, at the Commissioning of the Federal Government/Vamed Project, University College Hospital, Ibadan, November 5, 2005. Accessed at www.nigeriafirst.org/article_5196.shtml on January 24, 2006.

12. Kallings LO, Vella S. Access to HIV/AIDS care and treatment in the south of the world. *AIDS*, 2001; 15(7):IAS1–3.

13. Kombe G, Galaty G, Nwagbara C. *Scaling Up Antiretroviral Treatment in the Public Sector in Nigeria: A Comprehensive Analysis of Resource Requirements.* Bethesda, Maryland: The Partners for Health Reformplus Project, Abt Associates Inc., 2004.

14. Desclaux A, Ciss M, Taverne B, et al. Access to antiretroviral drugs and AIDS management in Senegal. *AIDS*, 2003;17(Suppl 3):S95–S101.

AIDS IN NIGERIA - *A Portfolio by Photojournalist Dominic Chavez*

WHEN DOMINIC CHAVEZ VISITED NIGERIA IN APRIL 2004 to photograph a nation on the threshold of an explosive HIV epidemic, he witnessed the full spectrum of life, from an HIV-infected mother giving birth, to a father awaiting treatment in a clinic with his children, to a young woman dying from an AIDS-related opportunistic infection.

Chavez captured on film a former soldier who now champions the rights of people living with HIV/AIDS, a toddler orphaned by AIDS, and sex workers who struggle to protect themselves from the virus at the same time they struggle to make a living. He photographed outreach workers giving condom demonstrations, technicians learning the latest laboratory protocols, and high-level government officials holding cabinet meetings on HIV prevention strategies.

For ten days Chavez visited three cities: Abuja, the capital; Jos, in the center of the country; and Lagos, in the southwest. He took his camera into an antiretroviral treatment clinic, a classroom in which sex workers receive AIDS education, a state-of-the-art HIV laboratory, a labor and delivery room, and a prevention-of-mother-to-child-transmission-of-HIV clinic. In all those places he sought to capture the vulnerability of people whose lives have been forever altered by an insidious virus, the determination of a cadre of scientists and outreach workers tackling the epidemic, and the courage and resilience of a nation facing what may prove to be the gravest threat in its history.

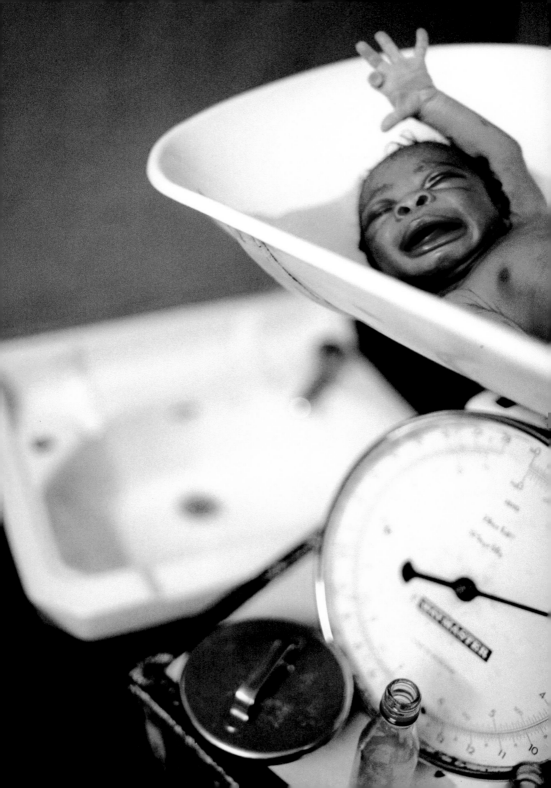

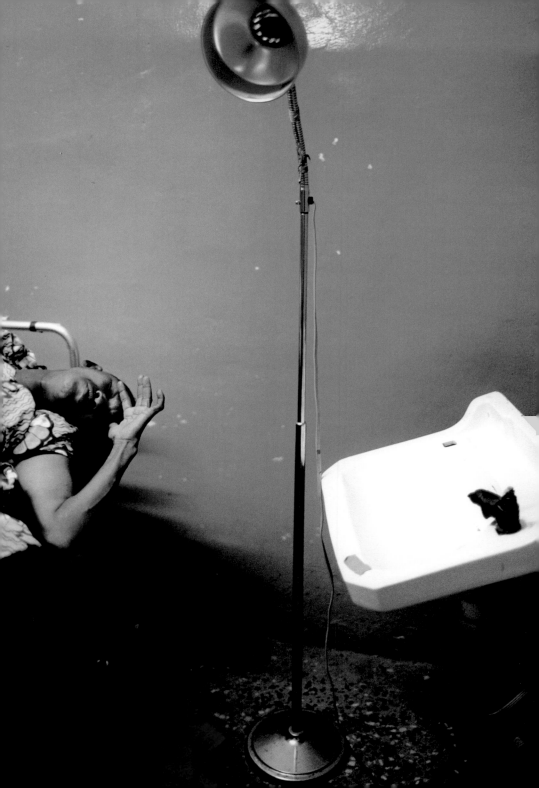

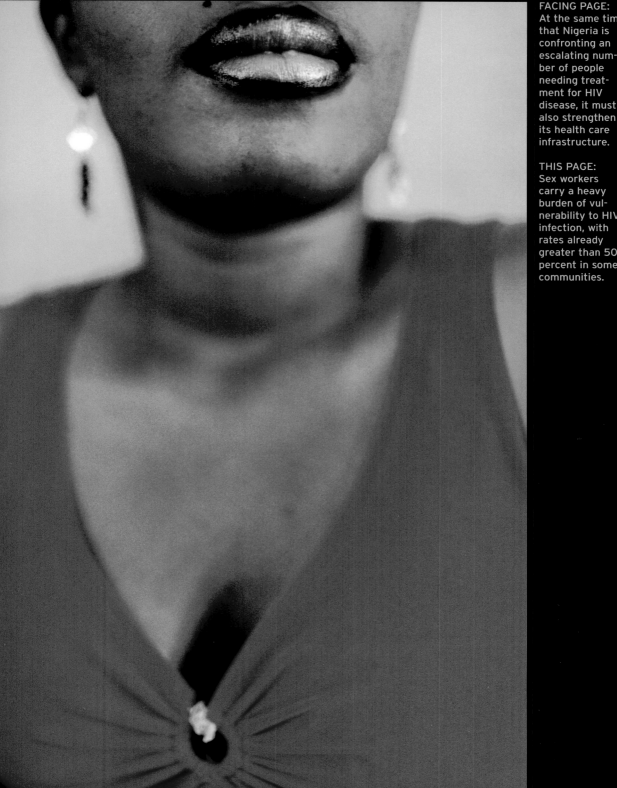

FACING PAGE:
At the same tim
that Nigeria is
confronting an
escalating num-
ber of people
needing treat-
ment for HIV
disease, it must
also strengthen
its health care
infrastructure.

THIS PAGE:
Sex workers
carry a heavy
burden of vul-
nerability to HIV
infection, with
rates already
greater than 50
percent in some
communities.

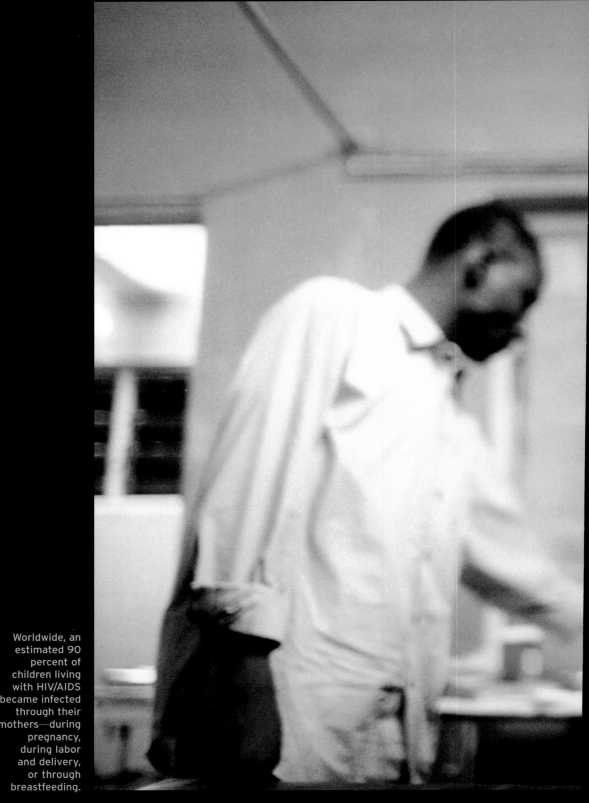

Worldwide, an
estimated 90
percent of
children living
with HIV/AIDS
became infected
through their
mothers—during
pregnancy,
during labor
and delivery,
or through
breastfeeding.

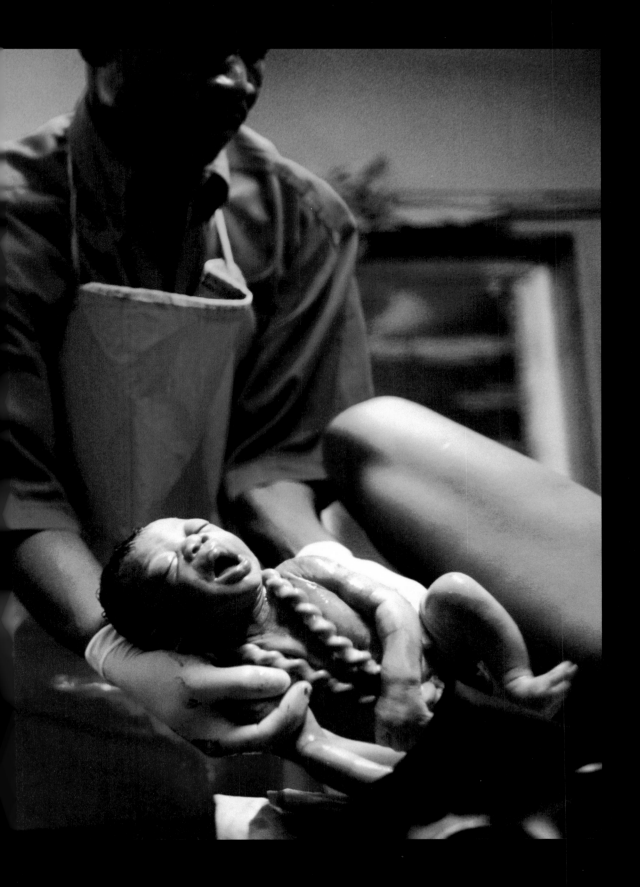

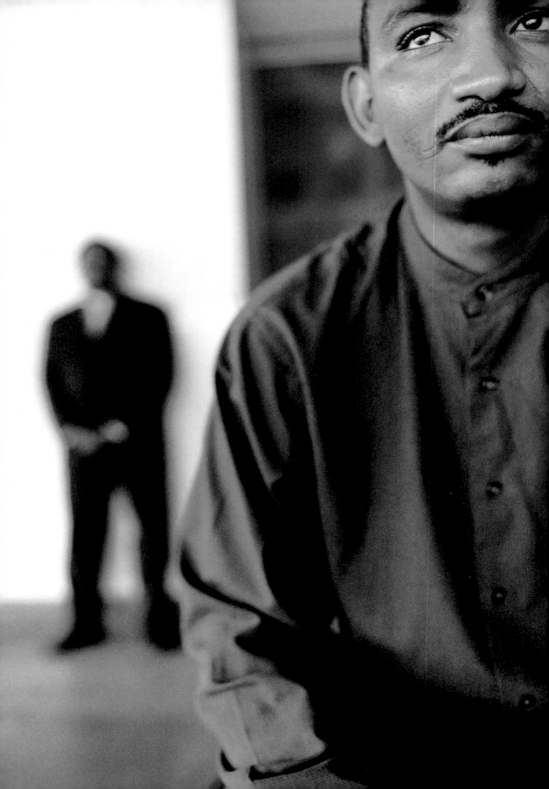

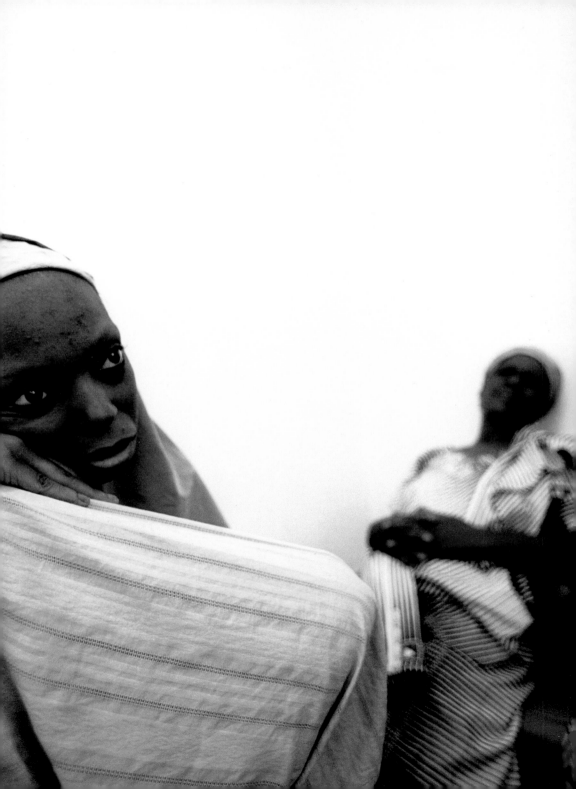

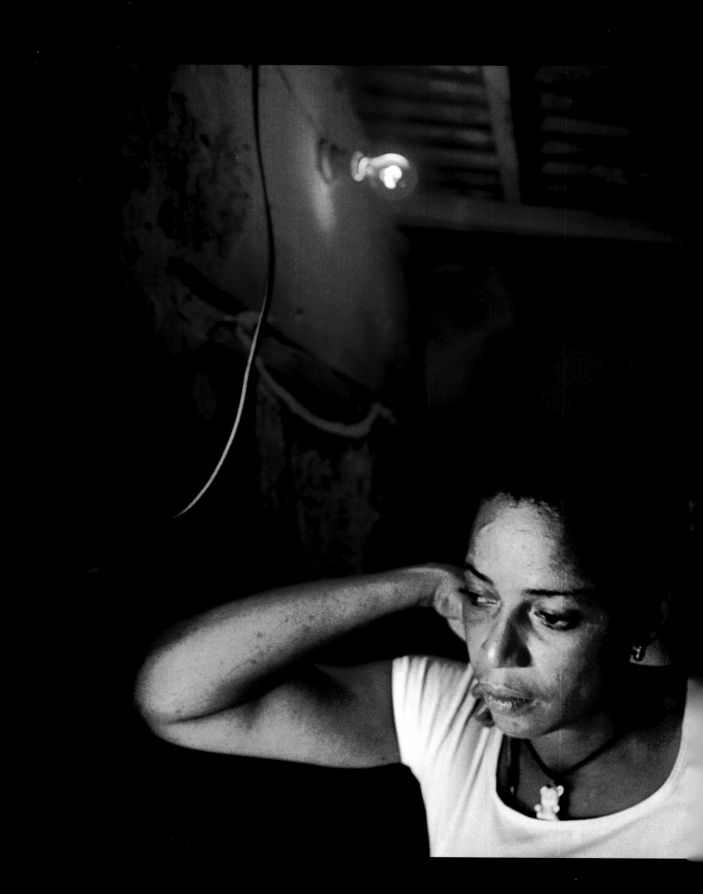

With leadership
from a number
of innovative
civil society
organizations,
peer educators
are playing
critical roles in
teaching society's
most vulnerable
people about
the risks of
HIV infection.

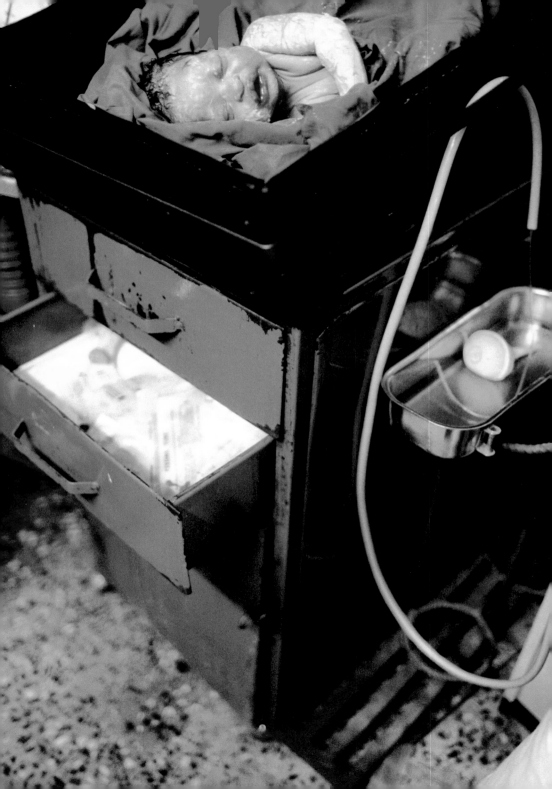

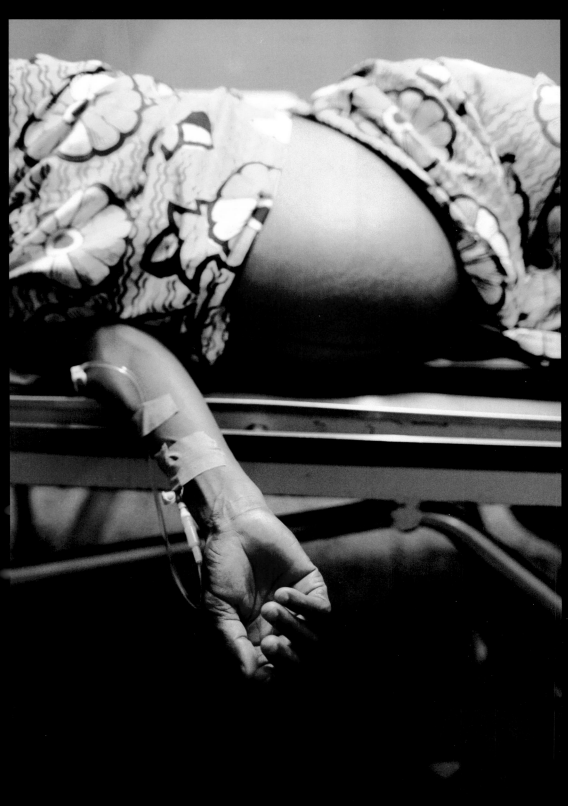

FACING PAGE:
The rates of
mother-to-child
transmission
of HIV have
plummeted
in developed
countries. Sub-
Saharan Africa
now accounts
for more than
90 percent of
the world's HIV-
infected babies.

THIS PAGE:
Like this woman
in labor, as many
as six million
Nigerians are
already infected
with HIV. Some
experts fear that
number could
climb to as
high as fifteen
million by 2015.

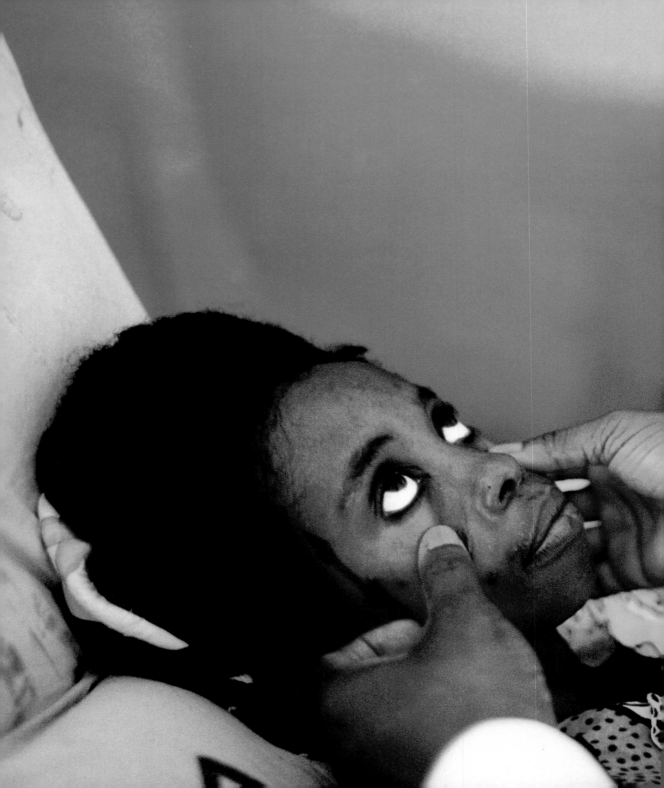

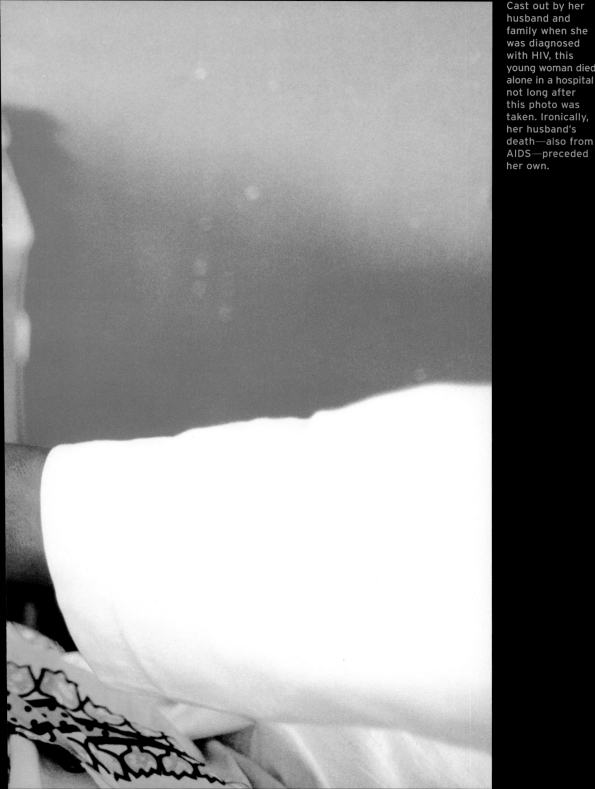

Cast out by her husband and family when she was diagnosed with HIV, this young woman died alone in a hospital not long after this photo was taken. Ironically, her husband's death—also from AIDS—preceded her own.

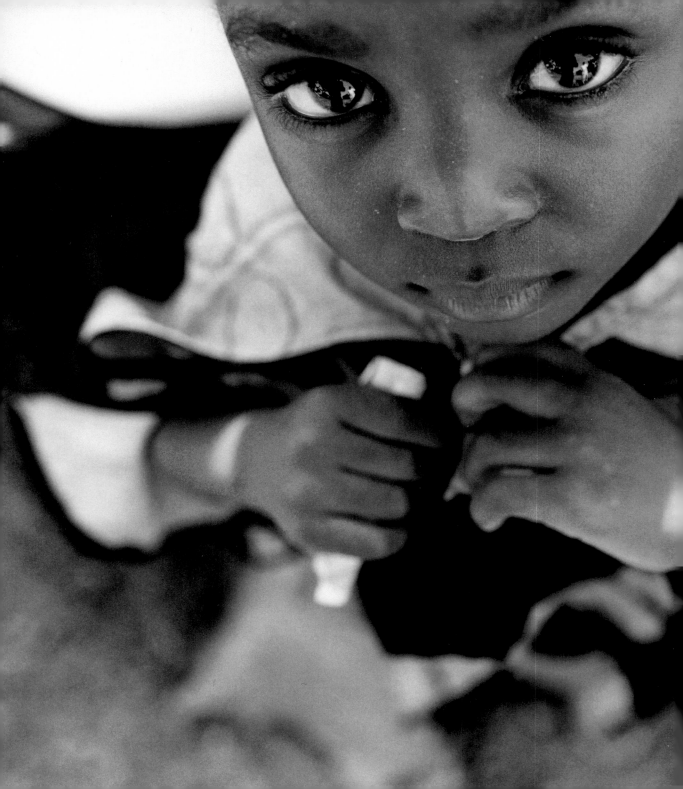

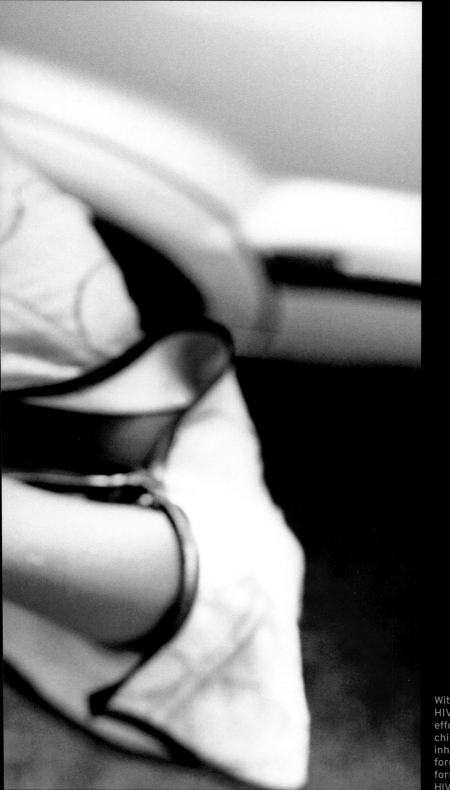

Without concerted
HIV prevention
efforts, Nigerian
children may
inherit a world
forever trans-
formed by the
HIV/AIDS epidemic.

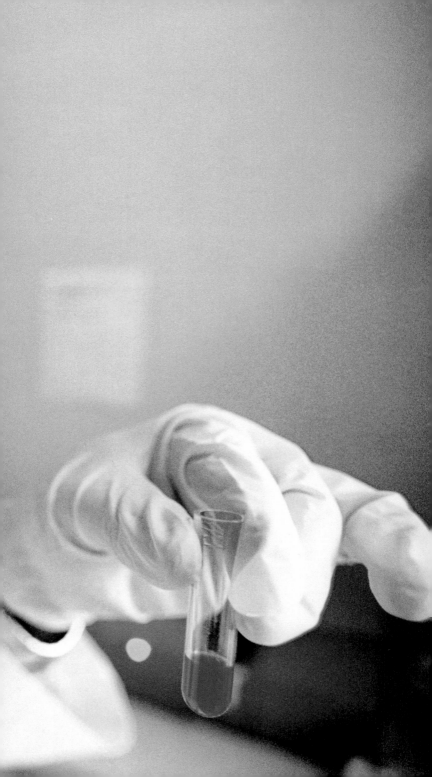

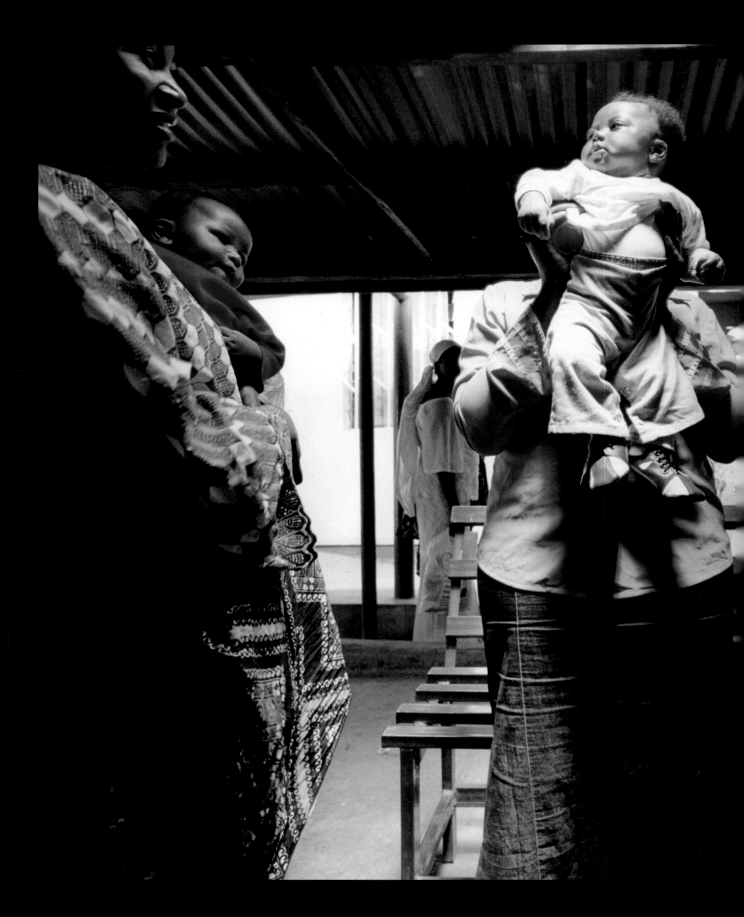

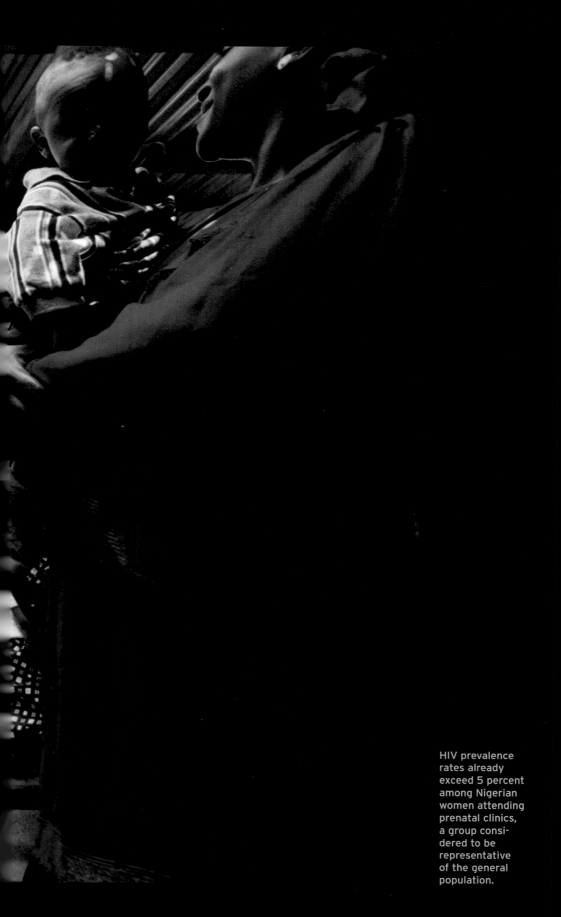

HIV prevalence
rates already
exceed 5 percent
among Nigerian
women attending
prenatal clinics,
a group consi-
dered to be
representative
of the general
population.

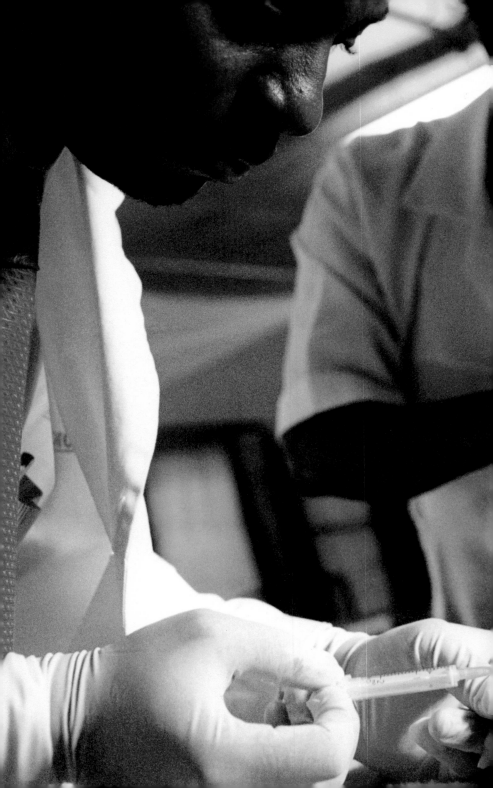

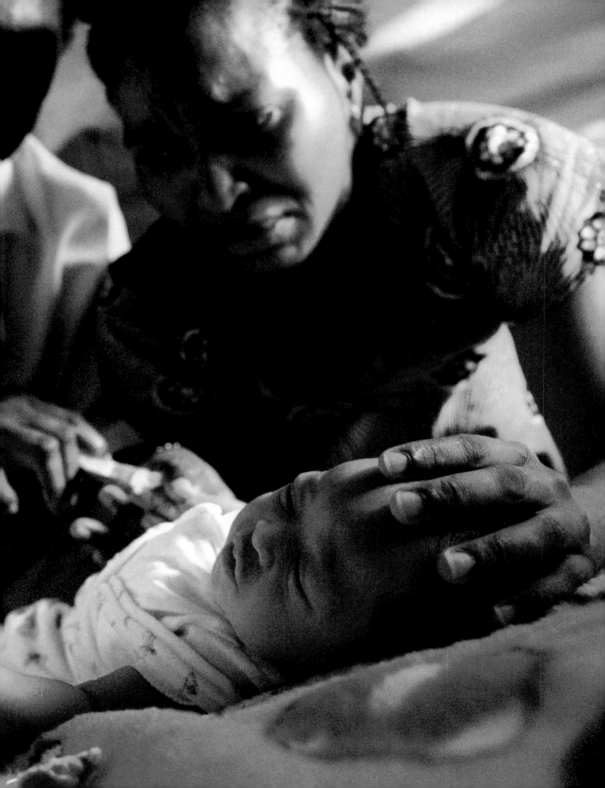

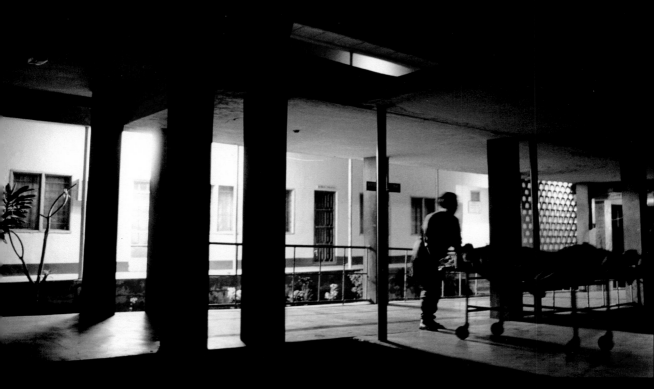

n early morning
ight, an HIV-
nfected woman
s transported to
he labor ward at
Jos University
Teaching Hospital.
She and her
physicians are
hoping to avoid
transmission
of the virus to
her baby.

13

THE ROLE OF CIVIL SOCIETY ORGANIZATIONS IN HIV/AIDS CONTROL

Irene Ogbogu* and Omokhudu Idogho†

The concept of civil society, one of the most popular paradigms of the twentieth century, conveys different meanings to different people. To the poor in Nigeria, for example, civil society may represent the only access to the few services available. To others, though, it may represent the voice of Nigeria Labor Congress, which has become synonymous with fighting for pro-poor policies from the government.

In his book on civil society, Michael Edwards draws from earlier work by such civil society thinkers as Thomas Hobbes and Alexis de Tocqueville to present three theoretical frameworks for viewing civil society: as an association of people with similar goals; as a "good" society or utopia that defines development; or as a "public sphere" in which the right and appropriate interplay of all the actors in the tri-sector model leads to development action (1).

In this chapter we use the term "civil society organization," or CSO, to refer to all associations and networks between the family and the state in which membership and activities are voluntary (2). This definition encompasses such organizations as local and international nongovernmental organizations, community-based organizations, faith-based organizations, community development associations, support groups for people living with HIV/AIDS (PLWHAs), professional associations, and trade unions.

---

*Women's Health, Education and Development, Abuja, Nigeria
†ActionAid International Nigeria, Abuja, Nigeria

Other categories include such networks and coalitions as the Civil Society Consultative Group on HIV/AIDS in Nigeria, the Network of People Living with HIV/AIDS, the National Network on Reproductive Health, the Nigerian Network of Sex Work Projects, the National Union of Road Transport Workers, and the Christian Health Association of Nigeria. While these examples suggest the range of groups included in the term "civil society organization," a great deal of ambiguity remains in the statutory and general understanding among practitioners in the field (3), especially in Nigeria.

In furtherance of humanity's search for the right recipe for development, CSOs have taken center stage. The HIV epidemic is one area on which they have made their mark during the past two decades. This trend has translated to the now-recognized best practice of creating multisectoral and multidisciplinary partnerships at national and international levels to respond to an epidemic that may prove to be humanity's biggest challenge ever.

THE COMPARATIVE COMPETENCIES OF CSOS

HIV is intimately linked to sex and sexuality, areas that norms and taboos moderate in Nigeria. Community leadership and structures in turn tend to regulate these norms and taboos. While government policies may create environments that enable change, the reality is that the obstacles to such change lie outside the control of formal policies and processes and more within the domain of community's socialization processes and upbringing—the informal policy arena (4). The unique strength of CSOs is their ability to provide platforms to challenge some of these informal policies, particularly if they are indigenous to that locality and well accepted in the communities. Their use of more participatory approaches and integration with communities place them at a vantage point to be able to tackle the social and cultural determinants driving the epidemic in a way that the public sector struggles to do.

One such area is outreach to female sex workers. The illegality of commercial sex work hampers government efforts to promote safer sex among this critical segment of society. As a result, CSOs must step in to fill this gap. CSOs are particularly adept at uniting the underprivileged and marginalized fringes of society, building their capacities, giving them "voices," and promoting their social inclusion. The pioneering efforts of such organizations as The AIDS Support Organization (TASO) in Uganda are oft-cited examples of the contribution CSOs can make to HIV/AIDS prevention, care, and support. Uganda's success in reducing its rate of HIV infection has been attributed to the highly politicized and energized civil society at the forefront of the country's response (3).

THE EVOLUTION OF NIGERIAN CSOS AND HIV-RELATED ACTIVITIES

Nigeria is blessed with a flourishing CSO sector, especially in traditional institutions, such as community development associations and women's groups. From time immemorial these groups have served as a source of vital social capital across many Nigerian communities and in the Diasporas.

By contrast, more formal nongovernmental organizations (NGOs) are a recent phenomenon, with roots in the years of the country's military dictatorship. NGOs were the main organizations with which Nigeria's international development partners were willing to cooperate. Some of the earlier organizations were formed by civil servants who, privy to donor policies, were quick to set up shop. Donor requirements of formal registration disenfranchised most indigenous groups in favor of these newer creations, a trend that continues.

In the earlier phase of Nigeria's response to the epidemic, before 1999, the predominant role of local CSOs was program implementation (3), with some limited attempt by a few international NGOs to mediate in the policy formulation process. The CSO response was fragmented, limited in scope (5), and even incoherent. Their funding was mainly limited to implementing interventions; few donors were willing to invest in strengthening local organization until the Department for International Development (DFID) funded its Capacity Building for Decentralized Development Project. Relationships among CSOs were marked by mistrust, competition, and limited collaboration.

Some NGOs did make their marks, however; examples include STOPAIDS, the Association for Reproductive and Family Health, Action Health Incorporated, the Society for Family Health, and Planned Parenthood Federation of Nigeria. After the advent of democracy in 1999 and the development of the HIV/AIDS Emergency Action Plan (HEAP) the following year, all stakeholders recognized the need for CSOs to broaden their roles beyond program implementation.

With DFID support, ActionAid International Nigeria and Family Health International facilitated a national forum of CSOs of all shades, which gave birth to the Civil Society Consultative Group on HIV/AIDS in Nigeria (CISCGHAN). Initially composed of 75 members, the coalition now has more than 350 members spread across the country (6). A facilitating committee of 16 members from all the geopolitical zones manages the coalition, whose initial operation was based on the concept of a "virtual secretariat." This concept has since evolved with the establishment of a fully functional office and enhanced capacity to manage programs, including a grant from the Global Fund on AIDS, Tuberculosis and Malaria to strengthen the civil society response across the country.

The Network of People Living with HIV/AIDS (NEPWHAN) originated in 1998 under the auspices of PLWHA-friendly NGOs and some faith-based organizations. Its poor funding base precluded tangible activities or projects, however, until 2000, when the Federal Ministry of Health, working through its National AIDS and STD Control Program (NASCP) along with a number of NGOs and faith-based organizations, brought together PLWHAs from all over the country again in a bid to re-establish and invigorate the network. The meeting succeeded in reviving the network. The network opened a permanent office in 2003 and has managed to catalyze the emergence of PLWHA support groups across the country. It has also been able to engage the national response in a coordinated way despite limited funding.

POLICY FORMULATION, IMPLEMENTATION, AND EVALUATION FOR CSOS

Medium-Term Plans I and II

The involvement of CSOs with Nigeria's Medium-Term Plans (MTEPs) I and II was limited to the implementation of a few interventions. Donors funded most of these interventions, and CSOs tended to design such programs outside the parameters of the plans. The formal partnership that CSOs formed with the government were ad hoc; personal recognition was the key criterion for being able to take a seat at the table. Competition was intense among CSOs, and little collaboration was discernible. The CSOs also lacked a systematic framework for influencing the policy formulation processes. Each organization seemed more preoccupied with scrounging resources for their own initiatives than building a common voice on issues. Most donors supported the cost of the program interventions of such CSOs; little was spent in the institutional development of CSOs. The situational analysis that preceded the development of HEAP described the CSO contribution as receiving little government recognition (5).

HIV/AIDS Emergency Action Plan

The emergence of CISCGHAN in 2000 provided the first opportunity for local CSOs to provide coherent input to Nigeria's HIV/AIDS policy formulation process. The inaugural meeting of CISCGHAN provided its members with a forum to articulate, based on their years of experience in program implementation at the community level, what they considered to be important for the CSO input in the national response. The result of this policy research and analysis session became known as "CISCGHAN core position statements." These 16 statements provided the framework in which CISCGHAN engaged other actors in shaping the HEAP document and the emerging institutional arrangements of the National Action Committee on AIDS (NACA). With its motto "the voice of CSOs working on HIV/AIDS in Nigeria" (7), CISCGHAN maintained four representatives in NACA before NACA became reconstituted in 2003. With the following words, CISCGHAN summarizes its bold mission: "CISCGHAN exists to coordinate, facilitate and advocate and to ensure the needs and issues of CSOs working on HIV/AIDS are addressed and to provide a coordinated and coherent input into the national response to the HIV/AIDS epidemic."

The "arena" in which CISCGHAN and other CSOs had to operate differed markedly as the government, through NACA, displayed a better understanding of the role of CSOs in policy development. They were thus able to maximize the input of CSOs into the process. The CSOs, for their part, soon realized that their understanding of policy formulation processes was limited. While they had gained a seat at the table, many still struggled to ensure a bidirectional flow of information between CISCGHAN and the wider CSO constituencies. Some CSO practitioners in Nigeria even believed that the government had more or less co-opted CISCGHAN, and the network would thus find it difficult to take any principled position if it disagreed with what NACA wanted.

International NGOS also were actively involved in developing HEAP. They provided a broad perspective by drawing on experiences with the best practices in parts of the world where programs were more mature. Several were involved in building the capacity of local organizations to understand the policy process, especially policy research and analysis; drawing from their field experience and capacity for networking (as distinct from networks); and developing platforms to push their policy agendas. Others, however, maintained a narrower interest, as they were keen to gain mileage for their organizations, especially from the government. Collaboration among the international NGOs also was weak, as everyone had made it to the policy table yet few had any distinct positions to argue. The media, with the exception of specialized media NGOs, rarely were represented at the table, unlike other countries where the media are known to set the policy agenda; public interest news and coverage were limited at that time. A handful of media representatives, however, attended some of the sessions held during the development of HEAP.

The World Bank Multi-Country AIDS Program

CISCGHAN also engaged in the consultation process of the World Bank Multi-Country AIDS Program (MAP) to ensure that the the program implementation manual for the World Bank HIV/AIDS Fund (HAF) reflected the needs of CSOs. The then moderator of CISCGHAN worked closely with the World Bank and NACA to determine how the HIV/AIDS Fund and the implementing organ for the project would operate, especially with regards to the revision of conditions that CSOs have to meet in order to access the HAF, such as the issue of counterpart funding and the years of existence. MAP has earmarked 33% of its funds for CSOs and community interventions.

State Action Committees on AIDS and Local Action Committees on AIDS

While CISCGHAN as a vehicle clearly succeeded in formalizing CSO involvement in policy formulation, the situation differed at the state level, as CSOs could not organize. Participation in the emerging SACAs and LACAs became arbitrary, as the SACAs invited NGOs they were comfortable with to the table. Some states — such as Lagos, Plateau, and Akwa Ibom — had a fair amount of CSO representation. Yet most CSO members of SACAs rarely fed back to other CSOs, and they lacked a coordinated process for collating issues from their constituencies and feeding the information back to the SACAs. The limited capacity and weak funding base of most SACAs resulted in few activities in their states. Their inability to strengthen the capacity of their CSOs became one outcome of this coordination challenge.

Contributions of Faith-Based Organizations

Although faith-based organizations wield considerable influence in defining "informal policies" — some of which hinder efforts to promote safer sex and positive living, their involvement in the formulation of the HEAP document was minimal. Since the development of HEAP, however, NACA has made a concerted effort to bring faith-based organizations on board in a structured way. This is important in view of the fact that the creation of an enabling environment is one key strategy articulated in HEAP (8).

Network of People with HIV/AIDS in Nigeria

NEPWHAN was formed at a time when PLWHAs were not involved in NGO programs in accordance with the GIPA—or Greater Involvement of People Living with HIV/AIDS—principle. They were viewed as beneficiaries rather than major stakeholders and had input into neither the design nor the development of HIV/AIDS interventions. The network was created to address the absence of rights-focused approaches and abuses of PLWHAs' fundamental human rights. It serves as a coordinating body for PLWHA support groups across the country. Since its formation, NEPWHAN has demonstrated tremendous potential as an advocacy group and a logical entry point as gatekeepers for HIV/AIDS interventions. It has succeeded in creating a defined advocacy and consultative position in all relevant bodies in terms of facilitating activities such as access to care, research, and the creation of a legal and policy framework for HIV/AIDS.

NEPWHAN's major challenge may lie in its decentralization. Currently, its work is confined to the national level, leading to a disconnect with its state PLWHA groups.

CSOS AND PROGRAM INTERVENTION IN NIGERIA

CSOs are now significant actors in HIV/AIDS program implementation in Nigeria. The programs range from prevention to care and support; the country has few impact-mitigation programs.

A review of the major programs shows that international NGOs working with and through local CSOs manage more than 70% of the program interventions (Table 13-1) (9). This scenario is not unexpected, as most donors, upon consideration of the history of corruption in the public service and the bureaucracy involved in getting anything done, would rather give resources to CSOs that can rapidly deploy them. The CSO sector also has contributed to providing the few data sources available, such as the National HIV/AIDS and Reproductive Health Survey and the Nigerian Demographic and Health Survey. This section presents some of the previous and ongoing interventions in which CSOs have been involved.

Prevention

High-Risk Groups

Communities with high-risk behavior—characterized by large numbers of brothel-based sex workers and transactional sex— are common in Nigeria. Working with this group is challenging for two principal reasons: it must deal with the migratory nature of sex workers and long-distance drivers and the illegality of the sex trade means that society views working with sex workers as encouraging the trade. A number of development partners have commended the pioneering work of such organizations as Women's Health, Education and Development (WHED), which works with sex workers in the northern part of the country, and Nka Iban Uko and the Society for Women and AIDS in Africa, Nigeria (SWAAN), which work in the south.

These groups are still active in the sector, with such new entrants as ActionAid Nigeria and the Society for Family Health's Promoting Sexual and Reproductive Health for HIV/AIDS Reduction (PSRHH) project, which seeks to conduct sex worker interventions in more than a hundred communities across Nigeria. These communities deploy a mix of program interventions, such as peer facilitation,

Table 13-1. Major Programs and Implementing Agencies in Nigeria

Program	Description	Agencies	Total Amount
World Bank Multi-Country AIDS Program	Resources both public sector and CSO HIV/AIDS responses	Funded by the World Bank; implemented by the National Program Team (NPT)	US$90.3 million for 2002-2006
Promoting Sexual and Reproductive Health and HIV/AIDS Reduction (PSRHH)	Major prevention program targeting MARPs and young people; provides research capacity for the national response	Funded by DFID and USAID; implemented by Population Services International, ActionAid, and the Society for Family Health	Approximately US$90 million; included in DFID and USAID commitments listed below
Nigeria AIDS Response Fund	Funds CSOs response to HIV/AIDS, with a special focus on gender	Funded by CIDA; implemented by Pathfinder International	Can$4.8 million for 2004-2008
POLICY Project	Public sector policies in reproductive health and HIV/AIDS in Nigeria	Funded by USAID and implemented by the Futures Group's POLICY Project	US$6.155 million for 2000-2004
AIDS Prevention Initiative in Nigeria (APIN)	Provides serosurveillance for HIV and other STIs, scales up prevention interventions among high-risk groups, conducts research, builds laboratory capacities, funds CSO interventions, catalyzes government policy responses	Funded by the Bill & Melinda Gates Foundation and implemented by the Harvard School of Public Health	US$25 million for 2001-2005
DFID Nigeria HIV/AIDS/ reproductive health programs	DFID commitment to HIV/AIDS over seven years, less investment in wider health sector	Multiple implementing organization for programs such as PSRHH, Strengthening Nigeria Response, and Partnership for the Transformation of Health Systems (PATHS)	£81.5 million (US$123 million) for 2001-2008
USAID program	request for proposals were due in the last quarter of 2003	Implementing partners were selected after a bid process	More than US$82 million for 2004-2009 (US$99 million in related sectors, reproductive health, maternal and child health, and enabling environment)
Global Fund for AIDS, Tuberculosis and Malaria	PMTCT program; promotion of CSO participation in the HIV/AIDS response; the national antiretroviral program	National Action Committee on AIDS/Yakubu Gowon Centre	US$28 million for 2004-2005

Abbreviations: CIDA: Canadian International Development Agency; CSO: civil society organization; DFID: Department for International Development; MARPs: most at risk people; PMTCT: prevention of mother-to-child transmission of HIV; STIs: sexually transmitted infections; USAID: United States Agency for International Development

peer education, the provision of services, advocacy work targeted at reducing police harassment, and the promotion of condom use in brothels.

The PSRHH project has also introduced a water-based lubricant in addition to other existing products such as condoms. The water-based lubricant is intended to prevent the frequent condom breakage that sex workers report experiencing when using petroleum-based lubricants.

Youth

Young people are the primary target group in HIV prevention. CSOs continue to implement various programs targeted to this group, ranging from school-based programs to out-of-school programs. Examples include the pioneering work of the Association for Reproductive and Family Health in its expanded life-skills program and the youth-friendly centers of Action Health Incorporated.

Other notable youth CSOs include the Adolescent Health and Information Project in Kano, the Girls Power Initiative in Calabar, Life Vanguards in Osogbo, and the Halt AIDS Group in Jos. Ford Foundation West Africa has supported many of these organizations using the youth development approach to tackle youth sexuality problems, gender issues, and livelihood issues. These programs have demonstrated how better livelihood support reduces the vulnerability of young women to HIV infection. UNICEF Nigeria has also funded a large number of in-school peer education programs.

In addition, CSOs have been instrumental in developing sexuality curricula for schools and contributing to the adolescent sexuality policy of Nigeria.

Care and Support

The involvement of CSOs in home-based care is relatively new (3), with a number of CSOs operating on a small scale scattered across the country. Some of the initial CSO experiences were in Benue State under a DFID-supported project on sexually transmitted infections. PLWHA support groups also have flourished in the past five years with the active support of NEPWHAN.

As the HIV epidemic in Nigeria matures, the need for care and support will grow. Newer programs focus on care and support and include CSOs as program managers and implementers. Some CSOs — such as Mothers Welfare Group in Kaduna, Living Hope Care in Ilesha, and the Family Health and Population Action Committee in Ibadan — have successfully pioneered home-based care of PLWHAs and even sparked many support groups.

CSO involvement in facility care has been limited mostly to work in mission hospitals and clinics providing care to PLWHAs. Some of these institutions have facilities for voluntary counseling and testing and, for those taking antiretrovirals, monitoring capabilities for CD4+ counts and other laboratory tests excluding viral load. Some of these hospitals provide prevention of mother-to-child transmission of HIV services. Several NGOs — such as the Centre for the Right to Health, Treatment Literacy Action, and AIDS Alliance in Nigeria — are involved in treatment literacy and access to antiretroviral treatment programs.

RECENT ACHIEVEMENTS AND ONGOING CHALLENGES

Since 2000 Nigeria has seen a flurry of activities in the HIV/AIDS sector with an increased level of engagement by the international development actors. The new era builds on best practices from around the world and has adopted a multisectoral, multidisciplinary approach. CSOs have been key beneficiaries of this new approach as their roles within the national response to HIV/AIDS have broadened and become more resourceful. In some way international NGOs have responded to this challenge with increased capacity and a more collaborative approach to bidding, designing, implementing, and evaluating their programs. While the international NGO presence in Nigeria has grown tremendously since 2001 to take advantage of the increased in-country funding opportunities, not much can be said for local CSOs capacity building; although there are more funders, CSOs still lack the technical and institutional capacity for an effective response. This is evidenced by the inability of local CSOs to take a significant leadership role in any of the bigger programs that donors have put up for bidding. This section of the chapter critically reviews some of the achievements, lessons, and challenges CSOs have faced since 2000.

Recent Achievements

CSOs have already made a number of strides in Nigeria's HIV/AIDS control efforts. Among their achievements are:

- **A more coordinated approach.** The emergence of CISCGHAN, NEPWHAN, and the Nigeria AIDS Research Network has led to some coordination in terms of the civil society contribution to the national response. This achievement has made representation in NACA and the United Nations' Expanded Theme Group on HIV/AIDS easy and systematic. With more than 400 local CSOs involved in HIV/AIDS programs in Nigeria, the coordination of their input into any national process is important. Such coordination is not the norm at the state level, however; with the exception of five states, CSO input into the SACAs still tends to be sporadic and unsystematic.

- **An increased capacity.** The increased engagement of CSOs in HIV/AIDS interventions has resulted in an increased capacity for fundraising and program work. The CSO capacity for influencing policy and networking has also increased tremendously. The use of bidding options by donor for contracting their implementing partners has resulted in international NGOs scaling up their in-country capacity for program implementation. The process has relegated local CSOs to the background, however, as they have become subgrantees to the larger international NGOs. Most of the programs have provisions for strengthening the institutional capacity of local CSOs to enable them to participate more actively in future bid process as equals.

- **A greater involvement in policy development.** The civil society mapping by ActionAid in 2001 showed that most CSOs were seen only as program implementers. The emergence of CISCGHAN and the development of the HEAP strategy provided the basis for the formal involvement of CSOs in influencing policy in Nigeria. The success in getting the needs of CSOs reflected in HEAP is one such achievement. CSOs have since continued their involvement in policy influencing, including such processes as adolescent sexuality policies and the Nigeria Economic Empowerment and Development Strategy (NEEDS).

- **Better collaboration and networking.** The CSO communities have become more collaborative in seeking funding and implementing programs. Information flow has improved, with the Nigeria e-forum acting as a medium of information flow. Networking has also flourished as other networks at state and zonal levels are emerging. One example is the Northern Coalition of PLWHA Support Groups. Program coordination is still weak, however, as CSOs continue to duplicate efforts, tread paths that others have walked, and relearn lessons already mastered.

- **A greater role in program implementation and research.** Most program interventions in Nigeria are being managed by international NGOs working with local counterparts. Some of the larger programs—such as PSRHH and the AIDS Prevention Initiative in Nigeria—have a national focus. Other CSO-managed programs include the Canadian International Development Agency–funded Nigeria AIDS Responsive Fund project, with Pathfinder International, UNICEF programs, and the POLICY Project of the Futures Group. Most HIV/AIDS research is coordinated in partnership with government and other actors such as the Society for Family Health. The Global Fund grant to CISCGHAN is a clear testimony of the growing role of the coalition in program implementation in the country.

- **A broadened participation beyond NGOs.** The range of organizations involved in HIV/AIDS work has also broadened to include faith-based organizations, community groups, and specialized media groups. The faith-based response at the grassroots level, in fact, kick-started the national response. An example is the Catholic Diocese of Makurdi, which initiated the first home-based care program and information, education, and communication materials development. In 2004, members of the Islamic and Christian communities came together to form the Interfaith Coalition on HIV/AIDS. Private sector initiatives for HIV/AIDS prevention and control include HIV/AIDS hotlines supported by Coca-Cola and Vmobile Nigeria. MTN also has a Partnership Against AIDS in Communities program in six states. Cadbury, Unilever, and Nigerian Brewery are examples of private sector organizations that have instituted HIV/AIDS workplace policies.

- **Stronger partnerships with government agencies and the private sector.** Partnerships have deepened between CSOs and government agencies and between CSOs and the private sector. The government and private sector now recognize the competence of CSOs and value their contribution to the national response. For their part, CSOs now recognize the role of government in policy design and evaluation. In 2003 alone, these enhanced collaborations led to the development of such subsidiary strategies as the behavior change communication strategy of Nigeria, the monitoring and evaluation framework, and the rural access strategy.

Ongoing Challenges

Tapping the Power of Indigenous CSOs

CSOs that are indigenous to a community have been shown to better than nonindigenous organizations at driving HIV/AIDS program interventions that achieve a genuine impact on that community. This notion is stated clearly in the Panos Institute report *Missing the Message:* "What works is when the energy, anger and mobilization of civil society have been at the forefront of the response to HIV and AIDS" (9). This publication attributes the success of the Uganda civil society sector primarily to the fact that its response was internally driven rather than built on external resources. Community-based organizations in Uganda had to adapt their normal functioning to the reality of AIDS when little external money was available. They were thus already fully politicized on the issue. When external funds arrived, the organizations were able to build on this energy, and success was quick in coming.

In Nigeria, external money has driven most of the HIV/AIDS response. For CSOs, the focus has been on program and project implementation, and most local CSOs have lacked a deep understanding of sexual and reproductive health and HIV/AIDS issues beyond that implementation. *Missing the Message* recognizes this gap and emphasizes the need "within civil society, to increase emphasis on advocacy" (9). Programming must focus on bridging the skills gaps, dealing with the inappropriate motivations of some CSO actors, and deepening the understanding of networking and collaborative programming.

The Need to Build Institutional Capacity

While the CSO capacity for implementing programs is generally good, most of those skills lie within the narrow confines of prevention efforts that focus on sensitization and information, education, and communication (10). Few CSOs have the skills and capacity to run a care and support program; indeed, few PLWHA support groups can fully define the parameters of positive living. Fewer still are working on treatment literacy and wider health sector reform issues. The capacity for policy analysis and influencing needs significant strengthening.

International NGOs that focus on the capacity building of local CSOs tend to focus on building technical capacity rather than institutional capacity. The result is that the institutional capacity of decades-old organizations lags behind that of their programs. This weak capacity translates to an inability to engage fully in policy development and a dependence on the government for assistance in being involved in this process. CSOs' scope of input is thus already limited because reliance on government support compromises their independence. Donors should be willing, therefore, to support the holistic development of local CSOs, including their institutional capacity.

The Challenges Inherent in Networks

The evolution of CISCGHAN and NEPWHAN as institutions highlights the challenge of running structures that promote networking as distinct from a network NGO. This distinction is important, as network NGOs tend to compete in the same market as their members, a trend that eventually leads to conflicts of interest.

At inception CISCGHAN viewed its role primarily as articulating the CSO position on HIV/AIDS issues and strengthening members' capacity through training by other members. Several years down the line, however, the coalition has found itself pressured to broker funds for members. Other members have become disenchanted by what they perceive as the coalition's failure to meet members' expectations, which were primarily for CISCGHAN to raise funds for its members. The understanding of members, most of whom joined the organization after its inception, thus differs from the initial ideal that led to the birth of the coalition. The Global Fund project remains a key test of whether CISCGHAN will survive where others have failed in combining networking with being a network NGO.

A Diversity of Motivations

The motivations of CSOs are as varied as the kinds of organizations the sector represents. Coalitions and networks such as CISCGHAN seek to increase resources for their members' interventions, broaden the CSO participation in the national response, and ensure the judicious use of available resources. NEPWHAN and a host of support groups work to enhance the quality of life for PLWHAs, increase access to public-sector antiretroviral programs, and ensure greater involvement of PLWHAs. The over-riding interest of faith-based organizations is to ensure the non-pollution of their doctrine. They seek to reduce the "Westernizing influence" of secular NGOs while remaining committed to service delivery; they are also concerned about reducing that Westernizing influence on their own doctrine. Other CSOs' greatest concerns are securing funds for their programs and gaining recognition in their communities

In response to such varied motivations, NACA must create a functional coordination framework that attempts to balance the different interests within the sector, and the different organizations need to reflect always on their comparative competence and work toward synergizing their programs.

The Need for Documentation

A lack of documentation tends to be a weakness of CSOs in Nigeria; they rarely capture programming lessons, experiences, or successes. The project mentality of donors has contributed to this state of affairs as most CSOs' only recourse to documentation is writing up the donor report. The lack of such vital program information leads to reinvented wheels and a waste of scarce resources. Skills for documentation are weak, and the lack of an effective monitoring system further limits projects, as there is no frame-work to capture change.

The Difficulty of Resource Mobilization

CSOs have found it increasingly difficult to secure funds for their activities because the dwindling resources cannot meet their growing needs. Several other factors are exacerbating the situation: a colos-sal increase in the number of CSOs, a lack of government investment in CSOs, and the changing political agendas of the donors from which the CSOs derive much of their funding. These agenda changes have resulted in the shifting of resources from one thematic area to another.

Learning to Navigate Donor Politics

Donors have diverse motives for working in any country, and those motives determine their actions in that particular country. Their motives may encompass different developmental ideals, for example, which they may not necessarily impose but they may propagate as much as possible while serving as a vehicle for driving political interest.

In addition, most donors have favored groups that are aligned with their political interests. These groups benefit from the funding for as long as they help achieve the donors' goals. Thematic priorities and geographic considerations play important roles in donor politics as donors often dispense most of their resources on a particular thematic or geographic region for reasons best known to them; unfortu-nately, this tendency deprives other resource-poor areas of assistance.

Perhaps the most obvious example of donor politics is the issue of adopting donor-driven programs to ensure funding for CSOs. This scenario allows donors to determine which programs are conducted with their resources with little or no consideration paid to the communities' needs; such a practice creates a sustainability predicament.

CONCLUSION

The role that CSOs have played in Nigeria's national response to the HIV/AIDS epidemic has enlarged significantly since 2000, with better results and enhanced capacity. The multisectoral approach adopted by the Nigerian government in its HIV/AIDS program has improved the operating space for CSOs' intervention in the sector. Limited capacities and a weak collaboration especially among local CSOs have reduced their ability, however, to fully occupy the space that has been made available to them.

Specific recommendations include:

- **Decentralize the responses and roles of CSOs.** Seen as implementers, CSOs have broadened their roles to include participation in policy formulation, monitoring and evaluation, advocacy, and influencing, especially in the context of the multisectoral approach at the national level. This has not been true at the state level, however. International development partners therefore need to intermediate in this process as the response continues to devolve to the state level. Financial support to enable active CSOs participation in the policy process should be provided. This is important so that CSOs participation can occur without being compromised by government funding. This recommendation is needed especially in the implementation of HEAP's successor, the National HIV/AIDS Strategic Framework.

- **Broaden CSOs beyond NGOs.** The CSO sector continues to be largely limited to more formal NGOs. The untapped potential and the less formal community structure of community-based groups must be leveraged in the scaling up of the national response. Their deeper link with the poor will ensure that the voice of poor people has a directly influence on policy formulation process rather than the existing scenario, in which NGOs act as intermediaries to the people. Broadening CSOs beyond NGOs will require donors to rethink their funding criteria and their engagement in direct capacity building of this local structure but the benefit in the long run will exert an impact beyond the HIV/AIDS sector on wider governance issues in Nigeria.

- **Build the capacity of CSOs.** To be able to progress, CSOs need capacity building. They need skill development in such areas as program design beyond prevention, policy research and advocacy, and TRIPS issues and medicines. International development partners and NACA must prioritize the capacity building of CSOs in a structured way. SACAs, because of their proximity to CSOs in their states, are in a better position to build the capacity of CSOs but they need support from NACA. The larger programs should develop models that the smaller CSOs can adapt for effective nationwide scale-up.

- **Introduce participatory approaches.** A high level of skill in participatory — or "bottom-up" — approaches is one area that makes CSOs distinctive and enables them to work on complex cultural issues on a context-by-context basis. In Nigeria, though, most CSOs lack skills in participatory program design and implementation. Most intervention continues to be didactic and does not reflect the principles of adult learning. The capacity of CSOs must be built for incorporating participatory approaches in their work and exploring options to domesticate participatory methodologies, just as Reflect and Stepping Stones—first developed in Uganda in 1995—incorporate participatory approaches to HIV, sexual health, and gender.

- **Support CSO networking and collaborations.** Collaborations can deepen the skills of CSOs while ensuring optimal program delivery. State and local governments need to support the networking of CSOs. Some donors have already set good examples by compelling CSOs to form consortia to bid for their funding (3); implementing international NGOs need to adopt this same strategy in funding local CSOs.

CSOs have a unique role to play in helping to stem the HIV epidemic in Nigeria and to provide care for those affected by AIDS. With the capacity-building support of governmental agencies and international donors, CSOs can play an even broader and more effective role.

REFERENCES

1. Edwards M. *Civil Society*. Cambridge: Polity Press, 2004;vii.

2. Ibid, 20.

3. ActionAid Nigeria. *Mapping Civil Society Involvement in HIV/AIDS Programs in Nigeria: A Report of Findings in Seven States.* Abuja: ActionAid Nigeria, 2001;26.

4. Idogho O, Kinyanjui C, Ogundipe A. *Reproductive Health/HIV/AIDS Policy Environment in Nigeria: Challenges and Opportunities.* Abuja: ActionAid Nigeria; 2004.

5. National Action Committee on AIDS. *Situation Analysis Report on STD/HIV/AIDS in Nigeria.* Abuja: National Action Committee on AIDS, 2000.

6. Civil Society Consultative Group on HIV/AIDS in Nigeria. Membership List. Abuja: Civil Society Consultative Group on HIV/AIDS in Nigeria, 2003.

7. Civil Society Consultative Group on HIV/AIDS in Nigeria. Core Position Statements on the National Response to HIV/AIDS in Nigeria. Abuja: Civil Society Consultative Group on HIV/AIDS in Nigeria, 2000.

8. National Action Committee on AIDS. HIV/AIDS Emergency Action Plan. Abuja: National Action Committee on AIDS, 2001.

9. The Panos Institute. *Missing the Message: 20 Years of Learning from HIV/AIDS.* London: The Panos Institute, 2003.

10. Odutolu O, Adedimeji A, Odutolu O, Baruwa O, Olatidoye F. Economic empowerment and reproductive health behaviour of young women in Osun State, Nigeria. *Afr J Reprod Health*, 2003;7(3):88–96.

14

REACHING VULNERABLE AND HIGH-RISK GROUPS IN NIGERIA

Viola Adaku Onwuliri* and Oluwatoyin M. Jolayemi†

The worldwide HIV/AIDS epidemic disproportionately affects sub-Saharan Africa, where nearly two-thirds of the world's HIV-infected people live. As of December 2005, women accounted for nearly half of all adults living with HIV worldwide and for 57% in sub-Saharan Africa (1). An estimated 3.2 million Africans became infected in 2005 alone, with people aged 15 to 24 accounting for half of new infections worldwide.

Since the first AIDS case was reported in Nigeria in 1986, the HIV prevalence has grown exponentially from 1.8% in 1991 to 5.8% a decade later. The most recent survey, in 2003, showed a slight but uncertain dip to about 5.0%. HIV is most widespread among adults aged 20 to 24 years, with an average national prevalence of approximately 5.6% in 2003 (2). The significance of these high rates at lower age groups is that people are becoming increasingly exposed to HIV at much younger ages. The surveillance data also reveal that marriage is a risk factor, with 96.6% of HIV-positive women in Nigeria married.

The HIV epidemic in Nigeria has moved from the nascent stage, in which prevalence is less than 5% in all subpopulations, through the concentrated stage, in which prevalence is more than 5% in high-risk populations, to the generalized stage, in which prevalence is greater than 5% among women attending antenatal clinics. Even though HIV is now widespread in Nigeria, evidence strongly suggests

*Department of Biochemistry, Faculty of Medical Sciences, University of Jos, Jos, Nigeria
†AIDS Prevention Initiative in Nigeria, Abuja, Nigeria

that regardless of the stage of the epidemic, the most efficient method to reduce the spread of HIV in the general population is to reduce its transmission among high-risk groups. It is therefore crucial to continue strong HIV interventions targeted at high-risk and bridge populations. The increasing prevalence of HIV among sex workers in Nigeria has been well documented, as evidenced in the national prevalence of HIV among female sex workers (FSWs), which rose from 17.5% in 1991 to 22.5% in 1993 to 36.5% in 1995 (3,4).

The major mode of transmission of HIV in Nigeria is through unsafe sexual intercourse — mainly heterosexual, though anecdotal evidence suggests that the homosexual route is increasing — and, to a lesser extent, through unsafe blood transfusions, unsafe injections, and mother-to-child transmission. The epidemic is being driven by ignorance, fear, stigma, poverty, the low status of women, and sociocultural practices that include high-risk sexual behavior. In developing interventions, policy makers and program designers must take into account the deep-seated, complex factors that fuel the epidemic in terms of what makes people vulnerable and places them at higher risk for contracting HIV.

VULNERABILITY AND RISK

Program designers need to understand such terms as "susceptibility," "vulnerability, and "risk" when developing interventions for vulnerable and high-risk groups.

Susceptibility

"Susceptibility" includes those features of a society that make it more or less likely that an infectious disease will attain epidemic proportions (5). Within the context of HIV/AIDS, women have a biologic vulnerability that makes them more susceptible to contracting HIV than men.

Vulnerability

"Vulnerability" describes those features of a society, social or economic institution, or process that affect the likelihood that excess morbidity and mortality associated with disease will have a negative impact (5). These are beyond the natural factors associated with susceptibility. Poverty, fragmented social issues, and gender inequality all exacerbate vulnerability. These deep-rooted factors weaken people's ability to cope with the impact of AIDS. Addressing vulnerabilities therefore requires long-term, sustainable strategic solutions linked to the development process.

In the context of HIV/AIDS, vulnerability means having little or no control over one's risk of acquiring HIV infection or — for those already infected with or affected by HIV — little or no access to appropriate care and support. Vulnerability has been identified as a major determinant of the spread of HIV (6). Women, children, adolescents, and young adults are considered more vulnerable to HIV/AIDS than older men.

Risk

"Risk" refers to the probability of contracting HIV; it is not a moral judgment on behavior. People at highest risk of transmitting or becoming infected with the virus are known as "high-risk core transmitters" (7).

While HIV epidemics follow diverse courses in different countries, they share common threads with regard to the principal transmission modes and distribution patterns, which help account for the rapid spread of the virus globally since the early 1980s (8). Population subgroups with similar behavior patterns should be exposed to similar risk. But because the socioeconomic context, underlying vulnerabilities, policy, and legal frameworks differ, "high-risk groups" vary from one geographic area to the other. In Nigeria, high-risk groups include FSWs, long-distance truck drivers, commercial motorcyclists, military personnel, police officers, migrant and mobile populations, prisoners, men who have sex with men, and injection drug users. It is important to note, too, that high-risk groups transmit the virus to the general population through their interaction with other population subgroups, known as bridge populations, which in Nigeria include the clients of sex workers and the sexual partners of people in high-risk groups.

High-risk groups engage in risky behaviors such as unsafe sex, commercial sex, injection drug use with contaminated needles, and substance abuse, which beclouds judgment about unprotected sex. For interventions to be effective, their designers much clearly understand the factors that drive people to risky behaviors.

FACTORS CONTRIBUTING TO HIV/AIDS SUSCEPTIBILITY, VULNERABILITY, AND RISK

Many complex and interrelated factors influence people's susceptibility, vulnerability, and risk to HIV. These factors can be classified as biological, sociocultural, gender based, and economic.

Biological Factors

Women are likely more susceptible than men to contract HIV in any given heterosexual encounter because of several naturally occurring biologic factors: the greater area of mucous membrane exposed during sex in women than in men; the greater quantity of fluids transferred from men to women; the higher viral content of male sexual fluids; and the micro tears that can occur in vaginal or rectal tissue from sexual penetration. Young women may be especially susceptible to infection (9). Other cofactors—including the presence of sexually transmitted infections (STIs), especially ulcerative ones such as chancroid, syphilis, and herpes— increase women's vulnerability. While it is relatively easy to diagnose and treat STIs in men, most STIs are asymptomatic in women, and the women may not realize they need treatment. This situation impedes early detection and timely treatment of STIs in women, thus increasing their chances of contracting HIV.

Sociocultural Factors

Sociocultural practices, which differ in many parts of the country, influence behavior and affect access to information, education, counseling, and treatment. In addition, some cultural norms relegate women to a lower social status, thus limiting their access to education, information, employment, training, resources, and the freedom to make choices about their own sexuality. Women, particularly young women, are constrained by prevalent norms that allow them minimal opportunity to negotiate for consensual and safe sex. This lack of control over their own sexuality heightens their risk of HIV infection. They tend to have difficulty introducing condoms into a relationship, particularly with their husbands, for fear of evoking displeasure or anger. Other cultural practices that expose women to HIV include wife inheritance, traditional wife sharing, polygamy, and multiple sex partnering by their men. Early and forced marriages of young girls and intergenerational sex similarly put women at greater risk of contracting HIV. Some of these practices are changing, though.

Many societies, including those in Nigeria, maintain a culture of silence around sexual matters. These sociocultural norms prevent parents from discussing sexually related issues with their children. Furthermore, schools are constrained on the grounds of morals, culture, and religion. Yet studies have found that many young people in Nigeria are sexually active from the age of 13.8 years; in urban areas 32% of women and 57% of men aged 12 to 24 who are sexually active have had two or more partners. The 1992 National Demographic and Health Survey showed that nationally 63% of young people have engaged in unprotected sex by age 19. Reducing HIV infection rates in Nigeria will require a deeper understanding of how these sociocultural practices facilitate HIV transmission and affect prevention efforts (10).

Gender-Based Factors

The gender dimensions of HIV/AIDS have become all too obvious. Gender roles and relations have a significant influence on the course and impact of the HIV/AIDS epidemic throughout the world, especially Africa. Women are particularly vulnerable to HIV infection because of the interrelationships among complex biological, cultural, and socioeconomic factors. The gender imbalance of infections appears greatest among Africa's young women, as those between the ages of 15 and 24 are at least three times more likely to be infected than young men (11). A number of studies have found that male-to-female transmission during sex is about twice as likely to occur as female-to-male transmission, if no other sexually transmitted infections are present (11).

Several reasons are responsible for the feminization of the epidemic. First, as the UNAIDS 2004 report shows, marriage and other long-term monogamous relationships do not protect women from HIV (11). In fact, marriage seems to increases women's risk, as married females have higher HIV infection levels than non-married sexually active females of the same age. Studies in Cambodia have found that 13% of urban and 10% of rural men reported having sex with both sex workers and their wives or steady girlfriends (11). Yet only 1% of married women used condoms during their last sexual intercourse with their husbands.

Second, according to a World Health Organization report in 2002, one in five women report sexual violence by an intimate partner. The abrasion caused by forced vaginal or anal penetration increases the risk of HIV transmission (12).

Third, women shoulder a disproportionate burden of care for the family. While women and girls are expected to provide care and support, men are not required to conform to such behavior. In some instances, young girls are more likely than young boys to withdraw from school to care for ill relatives. This increases their vulnerability to HIV. When people become ill, women and girls may face gender-related issues of access and entitlement to health care and support. Ultimately, when partners die, women may be left without any assets or prevented from using their property. The denial of these basic human rights increases women's and girls' vulnerability to sexual exploitation and abuse—and consequently to HIV.

Women's low socioeconomic status—marked by low income levels, poverty, limited education, and subordination, especially in sexual decision-making—exposes them to a greater risk of HIV infection. The situation is compounded by unhealthy traditional practices such as wife inheritance and wife cleansing, which increase the risk of HIV transmission. Women are frequently blamed for the spread of HIV. They may be barred from inheriting property, dispossessed, and stigmatized.

Economic Factors

It is well established that poverty helps drives the HIV epidemic. Poverty also affects access to good preventive services, care, and treatment. HIV/AIDS sustains the vicious cycle, as the epidemic continues to reverse the gains of productivity and development, widens the gap between the rich and the poor, and undermines economic security.

The poor economic backgrounds of women heighten their vulnerability. Poor people are more prone to transactional sex and are more likely to become involved or be coerced into unprotected intercourse. Children, especially girls, may be removed from school to reduce expenses and increase the household labor capacity. Widowed and deserted women may have to resort to providing sexual favors to survive.

WHO ARE NIGERIA'S VULNERABLE AND HIGH-RISK GROUPS?

Vulnerable and high-risk populations vary from place to place and depend on the prevalent behavior patterns and sociocultural context. In Nigeria, vulnerable groups include women, youth, and orphans. High-risk groups include sex workers, truck drivers, military personnel, prisoners, migrant workers and other mobile people, men who have sex with men, and injection drug users. Other subgroups, of course, could emerge and be classified as high risk. Each subpopulation has its own epidemiology, context, issues relating to vulnerability and risks, and challenges in terms of being reached with interventions.

Women

The number of women living with HIV/AIDS has been increasing steadily worldwide, and Nigeria is no exception. Women should not, of course, be treated as a homogeneous group. They may be poor or rich, young or old, educated or uneducated, in purdah or not—and each group has different needs requiring specific targeted interventions. Both the low status of women and the other gender issues that place them at risk complicate the picture. Thus, more women-specific and comprehensive interventions are needed to respond to the causes of women's vulnerabilities and risk. Components to address include sexuality, family, culture, empowerment, self-esteem, negotiating skills, violence, and interventions in various community settings.

The burden of caring for AIDS orphans usually falls on women, creating extra demands on their time and resources, especially in poor families. Efforts to alleviate these consequences especially for women are also necessary.

Young People

Half of all people newly infected with HIV worldwide are young people, with more than 10 million 15- to 24-year-olds now living with HIV/AIDS (11). In sub-Saharan Africa, more than 60% of all new infections are among youth. Young people are not a homogenous group, of course, and they can be categorized in many ways, such as by gender, school status, and marital status. Such classifications help us understand what makes them vulnerable, why they engage in high-risk behaviors, and what kinds of interventions are appropriate.

In-school youth include those in primary, secondary, and tertiary schools. They are usually literate, and because they attend school, they tend to be easier to reach with prevention interventions, including integration of HIV/AIDS into school curricula. The prevention programs of most schools focus on abstinence even though some students are already sexually active. Program designers face difficulty in including condoms in their prevention initiatives as a result of religious and parental pressures.

Out-of-school youth include street children and hawkers, unemployed youths, artisans, and unskilled laborers. They are often engaged in some economic activity that provides them with access to disposable income, which in turn allows them to engage in risky behaviors such as unsafe sex. Nongovernmental organizations (NGOs) sometimes find it challenging to reach these youth and must develop innovative ways to reach them.

As young people become sexually active, many lack the necessary information and skills needed to protect themselves from contracting HIV. In addition, economic issues make many—especially girls—engage in transactional sex; others are pressured into sex in exchange for good grades or money for fees or clothes.

Female Sex Workers

In many societies, sex work is illegal, resulting in clandestine practices. Nigeria is no exception, with a constitution that is silent on sex work. As a result, sex workers, brothel operators, implementing partners, and even policy makers are uncertain of the legal status of sex work. Nigeria is guided by two legal frameworks: the Penal Code, which operates in northern Nigeria, and the Criminal Code, which operates in southern Nigeria. Both codes criminalize sex work and therefore hinder advocacy efforts on behalf of sex workers' rights. The recent adoption of the Moslem Sharia law in some northern parts of the country has resulted in sex work going underground or relocating to other, more conducive environments, making it more difficult to reach FSWs with interventions.

FSWs in Nigeria are characteristically poor, marginalized, and stigmatized. They lack both formal education and empowerment. Frequency of sex with multiple partners and a high burden of STIs place them at high risk of HIV infection. They often engage in unprotected sex and other risky behaviors, such as substance abuse.

Surveys have consistently shown a high and rising HIV prevalence among sex workers, who are said to be the major reservoir of HIV infection. In some states, such as Lagos, the rates have increased from 2% in 1988–1989 to 12% in 1990–1991 to a whopping 70% by 1995–1996 (13). In Jos, a 52% infection rate has been recorded among brothel-based FSWs (14). A behavioral surveillance survey conducted in 2000 reported that knowledge of HIV prevention methods was low among FSWs, and consistent condom use varied from 24% in Jigawa to 89% in Lagos. FSWs also had a low uptake of HIV testing; only 24% reported having had an HIV test and learning the result (15).

The low economic status of FSWs heightens their vulnerability as they engage in unprotected sex. At other times they may be raped or coerced into violent sex; dry sex, with its consequent abrasion and bleeding, increases their risk of contracting HIV. They are disadvantaged by a lack of self-esteem and adequate negotiation skills, which compromises their ability to manage the situation and to seek legal action (16–21). In addition, FSWs face constant sexual harassment and abuse from law enforcement agents such as police officers. They may be forced to have sex without condoms, sometimes at gunpoint, and their money and valuables may be seized. Their impoverishment makes quitting sex work difficult.

FSWs have clients from all walks of life, from artisans, to motorcyclists, military personnel, businessmen, civil servants, and politicians. These clients may contract HIV from commercial sex, then transmit the virus to their partners in the general population. FSWs also have "boyfriends" with whom they may feel obliged to have sexual intercourse without condoms. These factors militate against HIV/AIDS control. The illegality of sex work makes legal protection of sex workers impracticable and HIV interventions for them difficult. The daunting challenges contribute to the vulnerability, risk, and rising trend of infection among FSWs. Yet targeting interventions to FSWs remains an effective way to reduce the spread of HIV.

Long-Distance Truck Drivers and Commercial Motorcyclists

Long-distance truck drivers in Africa, India, and Thailand have been found to participate in vigorous sexual cultures at roadside settlements and border crossings whose transient residents include poor, often young, women from rural areas. Many of these truckers have multiple sexual partners, and they spread HIV widely through the rural byways. Although long-distance truck drivers have long been implicated in the spread of HIV, the number of published reports on their sexual practices is limited (22). A behavioral surveillance survey conducted in Nigeria in 2000 reported that only 23.6% had knowledge of HIV prevention methods, only 26% consistently used condoms with non-regular partners, and only 13% had ever been tested for HIV (15). Commercial motorcyclists, who tend to be much younger, have access to disposable income, which they often use to engage in high-risk sexual behavior.

Military Personnel and Police Officers

Several aspects of the military environment contribute to their high risk of HIV infection, such as their age group (15 to 24 years old); a professional ethos that excuses risk-taking; and lengthy periods away from home, which can result in their purchasing sex to relieve loneliness (23). In concert, these factors place military and police personnel at high risk for contracting STIs, including HIV. In particular, police have been reported to engage in unsafe sexual behaviors with sex workers or casual contacts. This high-risk subgroup is easier to reach with interventions than others because of the military tradition of discipline.

A knowledge, attitudes, and sexual behavior survey conducted among the Nigerian Armed Forces in 2002 showed Nigerian military personnel are more aware of HIV/AIDS than the general population (24). At the same time, however, many of those same personnel have a poor understanding of HIV and other STIs, underestimate their own risk of contracting HIV, and find themselves in professional and personal situations that lead to behavior that places them at risk of contracting STIs, including HIV. Almost half of the respondents who participated in the various peacekeeping operations admitted having sexual partners during the period away. Furthermore, only half the respondents claimed to use condoms regularly with their non-regular partners. And only 40% of the respondents had been tested for HIV. The fact that military personnel live with and interact freely with the civilian population suggests that they may serve as a potential core transmission group of HIV to the larger population.

Prisoners

Prisoners are at exceptional risk for infection with HIV because of both the connection between injection drug use and incarceration and the not-uncommon practice of unprotected intercourse, both consensual and forced, between male inmates. Other high-risk behaviors during incarceration include the sharing of needles and shaving appliances.

Prisoners are difficult to reach with critical health information, which exacerbates their vulnerability to HIV. There are several controversial issues about prison inmates and HIV/AIDS. Policy does not allow condom distribution to inmates. A recent survey showed that inmates tend to have a poor knowledge of HIV/AIDS, to engage in high-risk behavior, and to have a low uptake of voluntary counseling and testing (VCT) services. The survey further revealed a seroprevalence of 8.82% among prison inmates (25).

Migrant and Mobile Populations

Seasonal workers, including rural farmers, are often away from home for long periods of time, and the social disruption and loneliness resulting from their migration is associated with a higher incidence of casual sexual partners. While away from home, loneliness and stress drive many of these migratory laborers to frequent FSWs. Sexual contact between migrant men and FSWs has helped spread the virus, which advances over an even wider geographic area when the migrants return home to visit their families. Conversely, women whose partners are migratory workers may resort to commercial sex work for economic survival while their partners are absent.

Migration of other workers—including civil servants, business executives, bankers, salesmen, and politicians—both within and between states also poses a major risk factor, as they often engage in unprotected sex away from home. At the same time, the workplace provides an ideal organized setting to reach these workers with behavior change communication programs.

Men Who Have Sex With Men

Homosexuality is not prominent in Nigeria, possibly because male-to-male sex is highly stigmatized; in some cultures it is either a taboo or legally prohibited. Same-sex contacts are becoming increasingly practiced, however, and those who engage in them are becoming more open about it.

HIV transmission results from high-risk factors such as unprotected sex, STIs, and non-condom use during anal sex with a non-regular partner. The use of alcohol and illicit drugs continues to be prevalent among some men who have sex with men (MSM) and is linked to risk for HIV and other STIs. The stigma associated with homosexuality makes reaching MSM difficult. It is therefore important that efforts be made to break all barriers so they can be offered AIDS education, preventive services, and HIV care.

Injection Drug Users

Using or sharing unsterile needles when injecting heroin, cocaine, or other drugs leaves people vulnerable to contracting or transmitting HIV. Another way people may be at risk for contracting HIV is simply by using drugs of abuse, as research has shown that drug and alcohol use can impair judgment and increase the likelihood of engaging in unplanned and unprotected sex (26). Although research has been scanty on the HIV prevalence among drug users in Nigeria, anecdotal data suggest that it is on the rise as more Nigerians are involved in drug use, including alcohol (27,28).

HIV/AIDS POLICIES AND INTERVENTIONS TARGETED AT VULNERABLE AND HIGH-RISK GROUPS

Policies

On the whole, the policy environment for HIV control activities in Nigeria is positive, with a high political commitment by President Olusegun Obasanjo. The implementation of HIV/AIDS control measures in Nigeria is guided by a number of instruments, including the HIV/AIDS Emergency Action Plan (HEAP) (29), the National Policy on HIV/AIDS (3), and the National HIV/AIDS Strategic Framework, launched in 2005 (30). These frameworks all recognize the need to prioritize targeted interventions for vulnerable and high-risk groups. One stated objective of HEAP is "to promote behavior change in both low and high-risk populations." Among its behavior change communication (BCC) strategies, the National HIV/AIDS Strategic Framework recommends that advocacy to brothel owners be increased, long-distance truck drivers be engaged in BCC, and mobile communication units be used at hotspots, in junction towns, and among military personnel.

Interventions

The National Action Committee on AIDS was established to coordinate the country's multisectoral response to HIV/AIDS. Interventions targeted at vulnerable and high-risk groups are therefore implemented by government agencies in collaboration with development partners, civil society organizations, and people living with HIV/AIDS. Even though several interventions are ongoing, the response is still inadequate. A 2005 World Bank report states that the failure to reach people with the highest risk behaviors has likely reduced the efficiency and impact of assistance (31). The government, international donors agencies, and development partners have supported numerous programs whose strategies for working with vulnerable and high-risk groups include prevention, care, support, treatment, and impact mitigation.

Prevention

As UNAIDS pointed out in its 2004 report, prevention is the mainstay of the response to AIDS (11). Interventions targeting vulnerable and high-risk groups resemble those targeting the general population:

- Efforts to raise awareness, which includes sensitization and mobilization of the subgroups through outreach activities and rallies;
- The development and distribution of information, education, and communication (IEC) materials, such as leaflets, posters, and face caps;
- The use of mass media through print and broadcast outlets;
- The employment of BCC strategies, including use of peer educators and condom distribution;
- VCT at the community level, with people referred to testing centers or mobile units; and
- The use of peer educators.

Unfortunately, prevention efforts have been neither comprehensive enough nor implemented at a scale large enough to make a meaningful impact. Condom use has not gained widespread acceptance and VCT is not used enough.

Care, Support, and Treatment

Some programs integrate care and support into prevention efforts or make referrals. This has been largely inadequate, however, as the fact that treatments help to improve uptake of prevention efforts is not maximized.

Impact Mitigation

The links between poverty and HIV/AIDS are well known, with poverty contributing to the increasing vulnerability of certain individuals, especially women and girls. The Nigerian government has launched initiatives aimed at alleviating poverty in the general population. These efforts include the National Poverty Alleviation Program, the National Economic Empowerment and Development Strategy, and the New Partnership for African Development. The Federal Ministry for Women's Affairs and Social Development also has a program for orphans and vulnerable children that is part of the federal government's impact mitigation strategies.

NGOs have supported vocational skills acquisition for vulnerable and high-risk groups. These are inadequate, however, as the lack of economic empowerment could further increase the vulnerability of the groups. Despite the merits of the poverty reduction strategies, linkages with HIV interventions remain weak and require strengthening.

Specific programs include:

- **School-based programs.** These programs serve in-school and out-of-school youth in secondary and tertiary institutions. They focus on such areas as HIV/AIDS education and prevention, use of peer educators, integration of HIV/AIDS into the curriculum, training in life skills, and formation of anti-AIDS youth clubs.

- **Motor park projects.** Through peer educators, these programs provide HIV/AIDS education, BCC strategies, condom distribution, STI prevention, and VCT at various motor parks.
- **Junction town projects.** These projects target long-distance truck drivers, the FSWs they patronize, and vulnerable street hawkers at junction towns with HIV education, condom promotion, and VCT.
- **Sex work projects.** These programs — both brothel and non-brothel based — include interventions targeted at FSWs, their partners and clients, and brothel managers. Among the initiatives are HIV/AIDS education and prevention programs, condom marketing, the training of peer educators, and the empowerment of sex workers through vocational training.
- **The Armed Forces Program on AIDS Control.** AFPAC has been at the forefront of the national battle against HIV/AIDS with expanded prevention and education programs, condom promotion and distribution, provision of VCT services, and widespread training for its personnel. In addition, AFPAC has begun providing treatment to personnel.
- **The Prison Program.** This program, in collaboration with a local NGO — the Life Link Organization (LLO) — focuses on four main target groups: prison personnel, prison inmates, members of the prison officers' wives association, and young people within the prison barracks. The prevention strategy includes HIV/AIDS education; seminars and workshops on HIV/AIDS; and IEC materials, such as posters, handbills, booklets, flip charts, stickers, T-shirts, and face caps. In addition, LLO provides prison inmates with palliative drugs, needles, syringes, shaving instruments, and food supplements. HIV testing services are limited, however, and almost no provision has been made for the care, support, and treatment of infected people. A support group of people living with HIV/AIDS has also been established within the sector.

SUCCESS STORIES

A number of NGOs have achieved remarkable results. Two in particular — the Society of Women Against AIDS in Africa, Nigeria (SWAAN) and the Society of Family Health — merit showcasing.

Society of Women Against AIDS in Africa, Nigeria

With support from the AIDS Prevention Initiative in Nigeria (APIN) and the Bill & Melinda Gates Foundation, SWAAN implemented a project whose goal was to reduce HIV transmission by promoting safer sexual practices among FSWs. The project also targeted clients and brothel owners and managers. The project employed a broad range of strategies, including prevention, care and support, and impact mitigation. Specific prevention activities included provision of basic information and education on HIV/AIDS. The behavior change strategies included development and distribution of IEC materials, condom promotion, and social marketing of condoms. The emphasis on building capacity by training peer educators resulted in increased knowledge and consistent condom use among sex workers. Sex workers were also counseled and referred to the APIN center in the Jos University Teaching Hospital for HIV testing and STI management. The project also included an advocacy component targeted at the police with an aim to reducing harassment of FSWs.

The empowerment program includes vocational training, as FSWs acquire various skills in hairdressing, catering, computer applications, tailoring, fashion design, knitting, tie-dye arts, and baking (32). The challenge was to provide funds for the sex workers to set up their own trade.

The Society for Family Health

The Society for Family Health is implementing the MARC (most-at-risk-community) Programme, a community-level, quasi-experimental demonstration involving 26 communities spread across Nigeria's six health zones. The program consists of six core interventions: edutainment for community residents; participatory interpersonal communication for young persons and most-at-risk males; parent-child communication initiatives for young people; peer activities for both young persons and FSWs; a massive youth awareness program for young people; and access to services for all community residents. Implementation took place at the same pace in all intervention communities from January 2003 to June 2004. MARCs were identifiable by a combination of poverty and high levels of transactional sex, including multiple sexual partnering far higher than the national average.

LESSONS LEARNED

Those working in the HIV/AIDS field have learned a number of valuable lessons in working with vulnerable and high-risk groups:

- Political commitment and leadership at all levels are important ingredients for successful HIV interventions.
- The root causes of poverty must be tackled. Linkages with poverty alleviation programs must be strengthened, as HIV/AIDS interventions alone cannot address vulnerability issues adequately.
- Interventions targeted at vulnerable and high-risk groups must include prevention, care, support, and treatment. Linkages should be encouraged when individual programs cannot provide services.
- The difficulty of reaching some high-risk groups calls for innovative approaches to programming. Programs tailored and responsive to the needs of the groups are more effective than general programs.
- The size and diversity of the Nigerian population have led to a fragmentation of efforts. Coordination and additional resources will be required to scale up efforts and to make any meaningful impact.
- Experience from the field has shown that faith plays a role in sex workers quitting the trade; sex workers who leave or express an intention to leave tend to be those with strong religious backgrounds.

CONCLUSION

Nigeria still faces a number of constraints and challenges in tackling the range of interventions needed to help prevent HIV among vulnerable and high-risk groups:

- The legislation guiding sex work remains unclear, thereby constraining interventions targeted at sex workers.
- The legal environment needs to be made to respond to the rights of vulnerable and high-risk groups. This dilemma has grave implications for the control of HIV among these groups. For instance, stigma-reduction strategies are ongoing, but their pace is slow. Policies to better promote and support gender equality relating to HIV/AIDS issues have still not been addressed.
- FSWs have a high attrition rate, which makes it difficult to follow through and sustain initiatives.
- The cost of services is often prohibitive. Many of the high-risk and vulnerable groups cannot afford prevention services such as HIV testing or condoms.
- Access to treatment for high-risk groups is limited, which could negatively affect other services.

Despite these challenges, targeting high-risk groups remains an effective way to reduce the spread of HIV regardless of the stage of the epidemic. Designing appropriate targeted interventions requires an in-depth understanding of the risk and vulnerabilities associated with various subgroups. HIV interventions need an enabling environment to be successful, and efforts such as reducing stigmatization should be devoted to providing such a conducive environment. To date targeted interventions have mainly focused on prevention, yet for those interventions to work, treatment and poverty reduction strategies also need attention.

ACKNOWLEDGMENTS

Dr. Onwuliri wishes to acknowledge the authorities at the University of Jos for their constant support and encouragement, the members of SWAAN in Plateau State for their enthusiastic support, and the leaders of the AIDS Prevention Initiative in Nigeria for their sponsorship of SWAAN's Sex Workers HIV/AIDS Education Project in Plateau State.

REFERENCES

1. UNAIDS/WHO. *AIDS Epidemic Update: December 2005.* Geneva: UNAIDS, 2005.

2. Federal Ministry of Health. *National HIV Sero-prevalence Sentinel Survey, 2003.* Abuja: Federal Ministry of Health, 2003.

3. National Action Committee on AIDS. *National Policy on HIV/AIDS.* Abuja: National Action Committee on AIDS, 2003.

4. Society for Family Health. *National Behavioural Survey 1: Brothel Based Sex Work in Nigeria.* Abuja: Society for Family Health, 2001.

5. Barnett T, Whiteside A. *AIDS in the Twenty-First Century: Disease and Globalization.* New York: Palgrave Macmillan, 2002.

6. UNAIDS. *Report on the Global HIV/AIDS Epidemic.* Geneva: UNAIDS, 2002a.

7. World Bank. *Averting AIDS Crises in Eastern Europe and Central Asia.* Washington, DC: World Bank, 2003.

8. Tallis V. *Gender and HIV/AIDS: Overview Report.* Brighton, United Kingdom: Bridge/Institute of Development Studies, 2002.

9. World Health Organization. *Gender and HIV/AIDS.* Geneva: World Health Organization, 2006.

10. Federal Office of Statistics. *1992 Nigeria Demographic and Health Survey.* Lagos: Federal Office of Statistics, 1992.

11. UNAIDS. *2004 Report on the Global AIDS Epidemic.* Geneva: UNAIDS, 2004.

12. World Health Organization. *World Report on Violence and Health.* Geneva: World Health Organization, 2002.

13. USAID. *HIV/AIDS in Nigeria: A USAID Brief.* Washington, DC: USAID, 2002.

14. Egah DZ, Sagay AS, Imade G, Pam S. Trends of HIV among SWs in Jos Nigeria: a seven-year review. *XIII International Conference on AIDS and STDs in Africa,* Nairobi, Kenya, September 21–26, 2003 (abstract 954413).

15. Family Health International. *Behavioral Surveillance Survey.* Arlington, Virginia: Family Health International, 2000.

16. Onwuliri VA, Kanki P, Umeh MN, et al. Female sex workers and female condom use in Plateau State, Nigeria. *XIII International Conference on AIDS and STDs in Africa,* Nairobi, Kenya, September 21–26, 2003 (abstract 960067).

17. Onwuliri VA, Kanki P, Umeh MN, Awari H. Educating sex workers in Nigeria. In: *Nigeria's Contributions to Regional and Global Meetings on HIV/ AIDS/STIs (1986–2003).* Lagos: Nigerian Institute of Medical Research, 2003.

18. Lamptey P, Wigley M, Carr D. Facing the HIV/AIDS pandemic. *Popul Bull,* 2002;57(3):1–37.

19. EUROPAP/TAMPEP. *Hustling for Health. Developing Services for Sex Workers in Europe.* Amsterdam: European Network for HIV/STD Prevention in Prostitution EUROPAP/TAMPEP, 1998.

20. Carrington C, Betts C. Risk and violence in different scenarios of commercial sex workers in Panama City. *Research for Sex Work,* 2001;4:29–31.

21. Metzenrath S. In touch with the needs of sex workers. *Research for Sex Work,* 1998;11.

22. Marck J. Long-distance truck drivers' sexual cultures and attempts to reduce HIV risk behaviour amongst them: a review of the African and Asian literature. In: Caldwell J, Caldwell P, Anarfi J, et al., eds. *Resistance to Behavioural Change to Reduce HIV/AIDS Infection.* Canberra, Australia: Health Transition Centre, National Centre for Epidemiology and Population Health, Australian National University, 1999:91–100.

23. UNAIDS. Engaging Uniformed Services in the Fight Against HIV/AIDS. Geneva: UNAIDS, 2003.

24. Adebajo SB, Mafeni J, Moreland S, et al. *Knowledge, Attitudes, and Sexual Behaviour Among the Nigerian Military Concerning HIV/AIDS and STDs: Final Technical Report.* Abuja: POLICY Project, 2002.

25. Labo HS. *Knowledge, Attitudes, Behaviour and Sero-Prevalence Survey in the Nigerian Para-Military.*

26. National Institute on Drug Abuse. *Drug Abuse and AIDS Fact Sheet.* Rockville, Maryland: National Institute on Drug Abuse, 2004.

27. Madubuike N, Onwuliri VA, Effa-Chukwuma J. *A Baseline Assessment of Women Drug Abuse and HIV/AIDS Issues in Nigeria.* Lagos: United Nations Office on Drugs and Crime/National Drug Law Enforcement Agency, 2003.

28. United Nations Office on Drugs and Crime/National Drug Law Enforcement Agency. *Rapid Situation Assessment of Drug Problems in Nigeria.* Lagos: United Nations Office on Drugs and Crime/National Drug Law Enforcement Agency, 1999.

29. National Action Committee on AIDS. *HIV/AIDS Emergency Action Plan: 2001–2004.* Abuja: National Action Committee on AIDS, 2001.

30. National Action Committee on AIDS. *National HIV/ AIDS Strategic Framework.* Abuja: National Action Committee on AIDS, 2005.

31. World Bank. *Committing to Results: Improving the Effectiveness of HIV/AIDS Assistance.* Washington, DC: World Bank, 2005.

32. Onwuliri VA, Kanki P, Umeh MN. The impact of vocational skills acquisition (VSA) on FSW in Plateau State, Nigeria. *Fourth National AIDS Conference,* Abuja, Nigeria, May 2–5, 2004 (abstract A 550).

15

THE ROLES OF BEHAVIOR CHANGE COMMUNICATION AND MASS MEDIA

Adesegun O. Fatusi* and Akin Jimoh†

Nigeria faces a high burden of AIDS, with more than three million people already infected with HIV (1). Other than a slight decrease from 5.8% in 2001 to 5.0% in 2003, the country's HIV sero-prevalence rate has increased progressively since the first case was officially disclosed in 1986 (2,3). The epidemiologic pattern of HIV infection — with sexual behavior, use of contaminated skin-piercing instruments, and mother-to-child transmission as the principal modes of transmission — clearly indicates that behavior modification is central to HIV prevention. The current absence of curative immunological, pharmacological, and related medical interventions against HIV/AIDS makes behavioral interventions more critical than for many other diseases of public health importance. To ensure maximum impact, behavioral interventions must be examined critically and avenues for strengthening them within national programs and community initiatives must be continuously sought.

Evidence from the successful experience of Uganda indicates that appropriate sexual behavior modification can produce a positive impact equivalent to that of a vaccine, with an effectiveness of 80% (4,5). Following their review of the decline of HIV in Thailand, Zambia, and the gay community

*Department of Community Health, College of Health Sciences, Obafemi Awolowo University, Ile-Ife, Nigeria
†Development Communications Network, Lagos, Nigeria

in the United States, Stoneburner and Low-Beer argued that Uganda is not unique and that successful experiences share several basic elements—"the continuum of communication, behavior change, and care" (6). These success stories stimulate interest in ensuring that HIV-related communication programs are sound in concept and produce the desired behavior changes that will halt the spread of HIV and eventually reverse its impact at the population level.

THE NEED FOR BEHAVIOR CHANGE COMMUNICATION

Since HIV/AIDS first emerged globally, the role of behavior change has been recognized as critical to the control of the pandemic. The phrase "education is the only vaccine against AIDS" was commonly aired during the early years to control the epidemic (7). Against this background, considerable efforts and energy were devoted to implementing communication programs to educate people about HIV transmission modes and prevention strategies. The underlying assumption of these early activities was that improving people's knowledge about the infection and disease would lead to avoidance of risky behaviors. According to the information, education, and communication (IEC) model, "clear information presented in an appropriate format and language would persuade those at risk to protect themselves from the virus" (8). Despite over two decades of communication efforts, however, HIV rates have continued to rise globally. It has become increasingly clear that improved knowledge and education do not always lead to positive behavioral changes.

Human behavior is complex, and behavior change, under any circumstance, can be difficult to achieve and maintain. Prochaska and DiClemente have proposed a behavior change model with five distinct stages; this model emphasizes that behavior change is a process rather than a single event, with relapse possible at any point in that process (9). The nature of HIV infection particularly makes behavior change a great challenge. On the one hand, the risky behaviors associated with HIV transmission largely involve sexual acts—and often people's deepest, most intimate feelings. On the other hand, the actions sought by HIV/AIDS control efforts are mainly in the realm of primary prevention and while high-risk behaviors can increase the chances of transmission, they do not always lead to infection. The long incubation period of the virus, with symptoms often appearing many years after initial infection, may also lower the motivation for at-risk individuals to change their behavior. These scenarios present critical challenges in HIV communication and highlight the need for more focused efforts on behavior change, which must go well beyond the basic education and materials dissemination that have been the hallmark of many HIV-related IEC programs.

IEC activities—the first generation of HIV communication interventions—have continuously occupied a central place in HIV prevention efforts (10). With the urgent impulse to "do something and anything" to reduce the ravaging effects of HIV/AIDS, particularly in the first decade of the epidemic, HIV prevention programs pursued such goals as reaching a specified number of people with information and distributing a specific number of condoms, with little attention paid to the ultimate effectiveness of such activities in actually preventing HIV transmission. Scant attention was given to establishing a strong scientific rationale for HIV communication programs and activities. Thus, the use of behavior change models in designing HIV communication programs took some time to evolve and to occur within the context of HIV prevention activities.

Over the years, it has become clear that while IEC programs have resulted in improved knowledge about HIV/AIDS, they have often failed to produce behavior change. As the U.S. Centers for Disease Control and Prevention has noted, "IEC campaigns are often better at imparting knowledge and information than they are at inspiring behavior change" (11). In sub-Saharan Africa, for example, the level of AIDS awareness has increased significantly over the years, with more than 90% of people in the worst affected countries reporting awareness of the virus (8,12). There is little evidence to suggest, however, a concomitant decrease in HIV-related risk behaviors in most countries on the subcontinent. The awareness achieved is usually shallow and includes neither accurate knowledge nor the development of the skills needed to protect individuals from infection. In 2003 the National Demographic and Health Survey (NDHS) showed wide gaps between awareness and correct knowledge of HIV transmission and the appropriate methods of prevention (13).

The results of similar surveys across many African countries have revealed that awareness and knowledge of HIV/AIDS "correlate only loosely with behavior or perception of risk" (12). This realization has increasingly led to the conclusion that awareness, while an essential prerequisite for changing behavior, is insufficient. Thus, the emphasis in HIV/AIDS communication efforts, globally, is increasingly shifting from IEC to behavior change communication (BCC), which has been described as a second-generation HIV communication intervention (10). This programmatic evolution parallels the general development in the health communication field, with the current period noted to be the "era of strategic behavior change communication, founded on behavioral science models" (14).

Some confusion may exist about how BCC differs from IEC. Whereas IEC largely focuses on improved awareness and knowledge, the primary goal of BCC is sustained behavior change. In practice, IEC has often resulted in the production and dissemination of communication materials, while BCC has been used to establish communication that is strategic and integrated into entire programs (15). BCC also has the advantage of being rooted in behavior change models developed in the field of social psychology. BCC has been defined as, "an interactive process with communities (as integrated with an overall program) to develop messages and approaches using a variety of communication channels to develop positive behaviors; promote and sustain individual, community and societal behaviors change; and maintain appropriate behavior" (15).

In the context of HIV/AIDS prevention and control, BCC entails the use of communication approaches and tools to foster positive change in behavior as well as improve knowledge and attitudes about HIV and other sexually transmitted infections. BCC aims to empower individuals and communities to make informed choices about their health and well-being and to act on them. Behavior change approaches recognize that presenting facts alone does not ensure behavior change and that change may take some time to occur. Behavior change interventions are, thus, designed to accommodate the stage of behavior adoption of an individual or group and to cultivate the skills needed to enable and sustain change.

In the context of HIV prevention, BCC programs aim to (15,16):
- increase knowledge about HIV/AIDS and raise awareness of personal risk factors;
- teach vulnerable individuals the skills needed to reduce risky behaviors;
- motivate individuals to adopt and continue safer behaviors;
- increase the use of appropriate HIV prevention and care services by both infected and uninfected persons;
- reduce the fear and stigmatization often associated with HIV/AIDS;
- increase acceptance and ownership of HIV/AIDS programs by the community; and
- advocate to mobilize and increase resources for HIV/AIDS prevention and care programs at community and government levels.

Behavior change models vary widely. Few of these, however, were developed specifically for HIV prevention. One of the best known is the AIDS risk reduction model, which draws its principal constructs from a number of older theories, including the health belief model, the social cognitive theory, and the diffusion of innovation theory (17). A 2005 Nigerian study has proposed an integrated model for addressing HIV/AIDS in sub-Saharan Africa (18). Within the social context of Africa, the model was based on the convergence of three existing theories—social learning, diffusion of innovation, and social networks.

Regardless of whether they were specifically developed for HIV/AIDS, such theories can play valuable roles as frameworks for studying and understanding human behavior as it relates to the epidemic. While each type of behavior is unique, only a limited number of theoretical variables serve as the determinant of any given behavior (19). Appropriate use of existing behavior change theories enable us to understand these variables and their roles in behavior prediction, and thus to identify the determinants of specific behaviors. In so doing, the theories provide us with valuable tools for effective behavior change and become pivotal in the design, implementation, and evaluation of HIV-related BCC activities. Because discussions on individual theories are beyond the scope of this chapter, Table 15-1 presents several common behavior change theories with examples of their applications in the HIV/AIDS field.

Some experts have argued that the current theories and models may not provide an adequate foundation on which to develop interventions (8,20,21) and may be particularly unsuitable in sub-Saharan Africa and the developing world (22). Others have argued that the existing theories are adequate and no new theories are needed; rather, what is needed "is for investigators and interventionists to better understand and correctly utilize existing empirically supported behavioral theories in developing and evaluating behavior change interventions" (19). Overall, there is consensus that well-designed and targeted theory-based behavior change interventions can succeed in achieving desired health-related goals (23), and evidence is growing that these interventions are effective in the area of HIV/AIDS prevention and control (19,24).

Table 15-1. Overview of Most Frequently Used Theories of Human Behavior

Level	Theory of Model	Behavioral Determinants	Examples of Program Application
Individual	Health Belief Model	• Perceived susceptibility • Perceived severity • Perceived benefits and barriers • Cues to action	• Increase level of risk perception • Influence beliefs of severity • Assess and influence beliefs about the benefits of behavior change and the barriers to that change
	Theory of Reasoned Action*	• Attitudes • Subjective norms • Behavioral Intentions	• Assess and influence attitudes • Assess and influence norms in the social group • Assess and influence behavioral intentions
	Social Cognitive Theory Social Learning Theory	• Outcome expectancies • Self-efficacy	• Sexual communication, need for social support to reinforce behavior change • Modeling of safer behavior
	Stages of Change	• Pre-contemplative • Contemplative • Preparation • Action • Maintenance	• Assess and influence outcome expectations and norms, as well as perceived risk • Assess and influence self-efficacy and intentions • Assess and influence self-efficacy, intentions, and outcome expectations • Assess and influence outcome expectations and norms • Assess and influence norms and self-efficacy
	AIDS Risk Reduction Model	• Labeling • Commitment • Enactment and maintenance	• Assess and influence risk perception, aversive emotions, and knowledge • Assess and influence perceptions of enjoyment, self-efficacy, and risk reduction • Assess and influence communication, informal networking, formal help-seeking
Social and Community	Diffusion of Innovation	• Change agent • Communication channels • Context	• Determine who the influential people are in the community • Determine the most effective means to spread information, including community leaders • Assess the types of social networks in the community
	Social Influences	• Context of social interactions • Social norms • Social rewards and punishments	• Equip young people with social skills, including peer pressure resistance skills • Assess and influence social norms
	Social Network Theory	• Social networks • Social support	• Assess the composition of social networks • Assess and develop social supports
	Theory of Gender and Power	• Social sexual norms and power dynamics	• Address the social structure of gender relations
	Empowerment	• Community organization • Community building	• Assess community priorities • Assess key activities of the community and facilitate alliance building
	Social Ecological Model for Health Promotion	• Intra-personal (knowledge, attitudes, risk perception) • Social, organizational, and cultural (social networks) • Political factors (regulation)	• Increase knowledge and skills development and influence risk perception • Community organizing mass media • Advocacy
	Socioeconomic and Environmental Factors	• Policy • Resources and living conditions • Access to prevention	• Advocacy and community organizing • Social services • Increase access to prevention tools, such as condoms

*A more recent theory of planned behavior is an update of the theory of reasoned action. It was developed by one of the authors of the theory of reasoned action to account for behaviors that are subject to forces beyond the individual's control.

Source: King R. Sexual Behaviour Change for HIV: Where Have Theories Taken Us? UNAIDS/99.27E. Geneva: UNAIDS, 1999.

MAKING BCC COUNT IN HIV/AIDS PREVENTION

Behavior change is a complex process motivated by multiple factors, including an awareness of the need to change, an understanding of the benefits of such change, a belief in one's ability to put the required skills into practice in different settings, and confidence in one's ability to maintain new behavior in light of changing circumstances. To be successful, BCC must move people from awareness to action by instilling the belief that desired outcomes will be obtained by changing behavior and by increasing individuals' sense of control over their own behavior. BCC must go beyond an informational or purely cognitive approach to one that combines both informational and emotional appeals. In this regard, the following elements have been identified as being crucial to the success of HIV-related BCC messages and activities (7):

- **The rational element, based on knowledge:** People need to know the basic facts about transmission—how the virus is and is not transmitted, how likely they are to become infected, and what they can do to avoid infection.
- **The emotional element, based on the intensity of attitudes or feelings:** Individuals need to feel an intense and personal vulnerability to the virus in order to develop an emotional commitment to the behaviors needed to avoid it.
- **The practical element, based on personal skills in the new behavior:** People need to be competent in practicing the new behavior and be confident in their ability to do so. They need a sense of self-efficacy to adopt new, health-protective behaviors.
- **The interpersonal element, or social networks:** People need to associate with and be supported by their significant others (such as family members and peer groups) whose knowledge, emotions, and skills can reinforce healthy changes.
- **The structural element, or the social, economic, legal, and technological context in which behavior takes place:** People need to have access to necessary supplies and services (such as condoms and voluntary counseling and testing facilities), and to live in an environment where safer behaviors are accepted and promoted while risky behaviors are discouraged.

Based on its analysis of the techniques employed by successful BCC activities, the U.S. Centers for Disease Control and Prevention has identified best practices in mounting innovative behavior change interventions (11). Successful interventions tend to:

- **Be personalized:** Individually targeted action works best, and in the case of successful large-scale public health projects, the public messages are reinforced interpersonally and in concert with other services and sectors.
- **Be emotionally compelling:** Successful programs go beyond simply providing information to also creating an emotional stake that motivates individuals and people to act positively.
- **Make extensive use of role models:** Role models motivate individuals to change their behaviors by providing concrete examples of behaviors that can be emulated, increasing their confidence in

their ability to change their behaviors, persuading them of the positive benefits of change, and showing them how to change;

- **Demonstrate sensitivity to social and cultural norms and expectations:** To make sense and be useful to target populations, information must be easily integrated into the target audience's social expectations, norms, and values, as well as their political and economic circumstances. The information must also be applicable to their daily lives.
- **Recognize the environment's unique impediments and facilitating factors:** Successful BCC activities recognize the environmental variables that can impede or facilitate the desired behavior change.

Entertainment-Education Strategies

The entertainment-education—also known as "enter-educate" or "edutainment"—approach has been identified as one that most effectively combines these "best practices" elements by disseminating information through the media in a combination of entertainment and education (11). These approaches can be adopted by various entertainment modalities, ranging from professional to amateur street theater, from cartoons and comics to professional acting and drama performances, and from film and popular music to radio and television soap operas.

Entertainment-education is both popular and effective as it focuses on emotional as well as cognitive factors that influence behavior, and is closely aligned with the customs, norms, and narrative forms that the target audiences find familiar. This approach uses role models extensively in line with the social learning theory (25); creates "good" models, "bad" models, and models that transit from bad behaviors and values to good behaviors and values; and shows the consequences of various choices and actions. As indicated in the literature, modeling is often the best way to teach complex behavior (26). Entertainment-education strategies are also based on the idea that self-efficacy will lead to expected results.

The approach fits well in the "entertainment for education" purpose of storytelling, songs, and other community-based activities that are indigenous to Africa. The approach has been used successfully in many reproductive health programs in sub-Saharan Africa as evidenced from evaluation studies. Several notable examples include the "Soul City" television serial in South Africa (8), the *"Twende Na Wakati"* radio drama program in Tanzania (11), and "Choices," a song about sexual responsibility performed by Nigerian music stars King Sunny Ade and Onyeka Onwenu (27). The entertainment-education approach has also been shown to be cost-effective, with an enduring effect (28). Piotrow and colleagues have summarized the strength of the entertainment-education approach in their "nine Ps of enter-educate"—pervasive, popular, personal, participatory, passionate, persuasive, practical, profitable, and proven effective (28). The slogan "sing and the world sings with you; lecture and you lecture alone" aptly summarizes the essence of the entertainment-education approach (28).

The Power of the Mass Media

The mass media—consisting of print outlets, such as newspapers and magazines, and broadcast outlets, such as radio and television—have important roles to play in BCC. While some controversy has arisen about the effectiveness of mass media in public health campaigns aimed at producing healthier behavior (29), the mass media clearly have the capacity to inform and educate people. At the very least, they can provide the foundation for possible behavior change. They can also affect people's perception of social norms, which in turn support people's efforts to change behavior. The media can also play a powerful advocacy role for policies that support sustainable behavior change at the population level. Furthermore, radio and television are important channels for enter-educate approaches such as soap opera and drama series, which are powerful catalysts for behavior change.

The positive impact of the mass media on risk perception, self-efficacy, and other behavioral predictors as well as HIV/AIDS risk behavior has been documented (29,30). As Rogers noted with regard to the growing use of mass communication strategies in health information dissemination, new communication technologies facilitate health information exchange and optimize decision-making (31). The trend in the HIV/AIDS communication field, globally and nationally, is toward the increasing involvement of the media in control efforts.

Findings from the NDHS attest to the importance of the mass media in the Nigerian HIV/AIDS field. The 1999 survey found that the most frequently quoted source of AIDS information was the radio (72.1% of men and 45.6% of women), followed by television (39.8% of men and 46.6% of women), and newspapers (25.4% of men and 9.3% of women).

The National HIV/AIDS and Reproductive Health Survey, conducted in 2003, showed that most Nigerians consider all forms of mass media acceptable for reaching the populace with information about HIV/AIDS and family planning (32). Radio was the most accepted (89.3%), followed by television (82.3%), and the print media (79.8%). The survey also found that most Nigerians listen to the radio regularly, with 50.4% indicating that they listen every day or almost every day; another 18.9% listen at least once a week. Twenty-eight percent watch television every day or almost every day and 12.9% watch television at least once a week.

Thus, the media habits of Nigerians are such that a good proportion can be reached through well-packaged mass media programs, particularly radio programs. The success recorded with the use of mass media techniques in family planning in Nigeria (33–35) lends credence for their use in HIV/AIDS control, as well as for other health and social development activities.

HIV/AIDS COMMUNICATION EFFORTS IN NIGERIA

In general, Nigeria has had a fluctuating experience in its HIV/AIDS response, particularly with regard to communication activities. While the early phase of the epidemic witnessed a predictably slow response, Nigeria was awakened from its state of disbelief about the presence of the virus in the country by the late Olikoye Ransome-Kuti, then the federal health minister, who took many positive steps to encourage a systematic national response. These steps included the public announcement of the death of his brother, Fela Anikulapo-Kuti, a Nigerian musician of considerable national and international fame, as a result of AIDS, and the establishment of a framework for a national HIV/AIDS response from 1986 to 1993. With the change in government in 1993, the nation experienced reductions in the pace and scale of HIV communication activities. Since the country's return to democracy in 1999, the HIV/AIDS response in the country has received a considerable boost and has enjoyed the highest political support in the country. The following section discusses trends in HIV/AIDS communication in Nigeria and associated achievements.

1986–1993

The early epidemic in Nigeria was marked by efforts to establish the institutional framework necessary for prevention efforts and to provide information to the people about HIV/AIDS. While the government initiated the National AIDS Prevention and Control Program (NACP) in 1988, the general attitude of the population and the civil society was one of cynicism and disbelief regarding the disease. In 1989, the federal government set up a multidisciplinary national AIDS committee, which inspired creation by the states of their various AIDS committees. That year also witnessed the development of a three-year Medium-Term Plan (1990–1992) for the prevention and control of HIV/AIDS, which included plans to educate Nigerians about the disease. The government, under the leadership of General Ibrahim Babangida, launched a "National War against HIV/AIDS" in 1991. Financial resources were provided and program efforts received greater impetus as part of this national initiative. In 1992, the NACP and the National Sexually Transmitted Disease Program merged to become the National AIDS and STDs Control Program (NASCP), housed in the Department of Primary Health Care and Disease Control of the Federal Ministry of Health. A second Medium-Term Plan (1993–1997) was developed; it focused on preventing sexual transmission of HIV through behavioral change interventions and the case management of sexually transmitted infections.

Thus, the era witnessed substantial efforts in laying the structural foundations for a national programmatic response to HIV/AIDS, including BCC activities. One of the major achievements of that period in HIV communication was the production of a national documentary on HIV/AIDS titled "Dawn of Reality." The documentary, which featured interviews from many leading national HIV/AIDS experts, also involved people infected with the virus. The scope of distribution of the film for IEC purposes was fairly small, but the airing of the film on national television reached a far larger audience. In general, government-initiated activities dominated the HIV communication landscape in that era with considerable support from the World Health Organization. Unfortunately, no evaluations were conducted to determine the effectiveness and impact of these activities.

1993–1999

The period from 1993 to 1999 was marked by some expansion in the program activity of NASCP, although the government exhibited considerable apathy to large-scale HIV communications, particularly the use of the national television and radio stations. On the other hand, it was an era marked by the strong emergence of the nongovernmental organizations (NGOs) in HIV/AIDS prevention programs, with the majority of them engaged in information sharing and distribution of educational materials. Considerable attention was focused on the most at-risk groups, including long-distance truck drivers, young people, and sex workers. One of the factors that influenced the increased presence and activities of NGOs in HIV/AIDS communication was the rise in available funds from donor agencies, particularly the United States Agency for International Development (USAID).

The U.S. government held sanctions against Nigeria from 1993 to 1999, a period in which the Nigerian government and its agencies were barred from receiving aid from the U.S. government. Therefore, USAID could only work with NGOs during this period. Through the activities of the Joint United Nations Program on HIV/AIDS (UNAIDS), UN agencies, individually and as group, constituted the major sources of donor support to the Nigerian government during this period. The British Department for International Development also supported a number of community-based HIV/AIDS communication initiatives, particularly in Sagamu (Ogun State) and Gboko (Benue State).

During this period, USAID, through the AIDSTECH project (AIDS Technical Support Project) (1988–1992) and AIDSCAP (AIDS Control and Prevention) Project (1992–1997), implemented by Family Health International (FHI), funded NGOs and NGO networks to conduct a range of communication activities (36,37,38). In 1997, musician Fela Anikulapo-Kuti's death from AIDS brought the reality of the disease to bear on the psyche of many Nigerians for the first time. A review of the efforts by FHI showed limited national impact of the programs (38), while analysis of the national response as a whole showed "insufficient nation wide awareness reflected by weak advocacy and information programs toward general populations and specifically at risk groups—youth and women" (39).

1999–2003

Nigeria's HIV/AIDS response witnessed a significant boost with the inception of the civilian administration in 1999. The level of political commitment, the government's presence, and donor activities and support were unprecedented in the history of the epidemic. The national response broadened from a health-focused approach to a multisectoral one with a coordination structure in place—the National Action Committee on AIDS (NACA) at the federal level, the state action committees on AIDS (SACAs) at the state level, and the local action committees on AIDS (LACAs) at the local level.

The country's first action plan on HIV/AIDS—the HIV/AIDS Emergency Action Plan (HEAP)—was approved in 2001 (40). The plan, which was designed to cover a three-year period, placed a premium on BCC objectives, which included: increasing awareness of the epidemic among the general population and key stakeholders; promoting behavior change in both low- and high-risk populations; empowering communities and individuals to design and initiate community-specific action plans; and ensuring that laws and policies encourage the mitigation of the epidemic.

Both governmental and nongovernmental bodies scaled up the level of educational and communication activities considerably with the implicit aim of facilitating behavioral changes and curbing the epidemic. While most program designers and implementers still operated within the mindset of IEC—with the primary focus being on giving more presentations, organizing more workshops, and distributing more educational materials—there was an increasing awareness of the need to shift toward BCC. The faith-based community and networks of people living with HIV/AIDS (PLWHAs) emerged as important forces during this era. A stronger attention was also paid to networking and coalition building among NGOs. Programs and NGOs with a focus on a particular vulnerable population—such as armed forces personnel or men having sex with men—also emerged.

The National Policy on HIV/AIDS, developed in 2003, has a stronger focus on communication activities—especially BCC—than the earlier policy. The policy explicitly states the government's commitment to "foster behavior change as the main means of controlling the epidemic." Moreover, one of its targets is to "improve the behavior and the practice of the general population and high risk groups related to safe sex by 20% by the year 2005 and 50% by the year 2010 (41). Another goal is to "reduce by 25% the percentage of persons openly expressing negative attitudes about persons living with HIV/AIDS by 2005" (41).

Since 1999, most HIV-related BCC activities have taken place in the context of schools and youth-focused settings, faith communities, workplaces, and health facilities.

School-Based Interventions

School-based BCC interventions have been undertaken largely to address risky sexual behaviors and injection drug use among school-based populations. The country has developed and adopted the National Family Life and HIV Education Curriculum, which covers the primary to tertiary levels of education. Its implementation has been poor, however, with a low proportion of secondary schools implementing the curriculum as a result of lack of skilled teachers and an inadequate attention to the issue by state educational authorities. Implementation at the primary school level has been virtually non-existent, while at the tertiary level, the institutional response to HIV/AIDS has been feeble, and awareness of the provision of the national curriculum poor (42). BCC approaches used in educational institutions revolved considerably around in-class instructional approaches coupled with peer education and counseling, training in life skills, extracurricular interactive sessions with guest experts, and enter-educative methods such as drama.

Other Youth-Focused Interventions

Community- and mass media–based BCC approaches have been implemented in various parts of the country. These initiatives complement the school-based approach for the schooling population and provide opportunities to reach the out-of-school population, which has been poorly reached. Community-based programs have been implemented primarily by civil society organizations, with those focused on adolescents playing a leading role. Major BCC approaches included peer education, behavior modeling, sporting activities, and enter-educative approaches such as musical concerts, video shows, and drama. Mass media approaches richly complemented these methods, particularly through the use of adolescent-focused television drama serials such as "I Need to Know"; radio dramas aimed at improving personal risk perception; customized youth magazines; innovative info-commercials such as "Zip Up," a multimedia campaign on abstinence; and social marketing of condoms.

Faith-Based Initiatives

The faith community grew considerably in its response to the Nigerian epidemic and engaged in a variety of BCC programs directed not only at prevention but also at care and support for PLWHAs and mitigation of the impact on those affected. Many faith communities and congregations — such as the Redeemed Christian Church of God, the Anglican Communion, and the Catholic Church — have developed HIV/AIDS policy and programs, of which BCC constitutes a significant element. The Interfaith Coalition on HIV/AIDS, a network organization of faith communities, was also engaged in HIV communication activities. The range of approaches adopted by faith communities included innovative use of sermons in churches and mosques, peer-led approaches among young people as well as their gatekeepers, modeling, publications, and enter-educative methods.

Workplace-Based Interventions

Workplace-based BCC activities occurred in a number of establishments within the formal sector of the economy, including the oil and gas, beverage production, and banking industries. Such BCC activities often included peer education, dissemination of information through formal and informal networks, and the use of multimedia communication methods. These were initiated as an integral part of holistic workplace HIV/AIDS interventions with a number of complementary components, including formulation of an HIV/AIDS policy, condom promotion and distribution, voluntary counseling and testing, and the provision of care and support for the affected and the infected.

The Armed Forces Program for AIDS Control (AFPAC) can be viewed as a special type of workplace intervention in Nigeria. The program has a rich BCC component, which includes peer education; social mobilization directed at military personnel within the barracks and "mammy markets" (the adjoining shanty civilian trading posts and living facilities that often spring up to service military personnel); condom promotion and distribution; video recording and distribution of drama production targeted at military personnel and their families; and integration of HIV/AIDS education into sporting events. AFPAC also strategically organizes an annual HIV/AIDS week, during which enter-educative approaches are used to promote behavior changes among military personnel across the Army, Air Force, and Navy.

Within the informal sector, BCC approaches have been targeted mainly at the most-at-risk groups such as sex workers and transport workers. Many such activities have often taken place within the vicinity of their operational base such as junction towns, motor parks, and brothels. BCC approaches with these groups have commonly included peer education, condom promotion and distribution, dramatic skits, and road shows.

Health Facility–Based Interventions

A stronger focus on BCC emerged within health care settings, although a considerable degree of improvement is still needed to maximize effectiveness. Messages related to this focus have included promotion of safe environments and safer practices to reduce the potential for transmitting HIV within health facilities, discouragement of discrimination and stigmatization of PLWHAs, and promotion of quality AIDS-related prevention and care services, such as voluntary counseling and testing and prevention of mother-to-child transmission in the management of pregnant PLWHAs. Approaches included innovative and targeted educational material and message design, interactive learning methods, counseling, and orientation activities to facilitate improved patient-provider interaction and communication.

MASS MEDIA TRENDS IN COMMUNICATING ABOUT THE HIV EPIDEMIC IN NIGERIA

At the initial stage of the HIV/AIDS challenge, the occasional news items on the pandemic in Nigerian mass media tended to focus on stories and issues from developed countries with little or no local relevance. Moreover, most HIV/AIDS stories failed to make the front page in print or lead in electronic media, because editors gave them a lower priority than stories on politics, business, sports, or the economy. On the other hand, many media reports on local events relating to the epidemic bordered more on sensationalizing the issues with such headlines as, "Another AIDS victim is dead" (43); "New killer sexual disease discovered" (44); "Who's afraid of the big bad AIDS? — Not Nigerian Men" (45); "11 out of 12 AIDS carriers now dead — Medical Director" (46); and "Call girls spread AIDS" (47).

Numerous media reports also bordered on being inaccurate, false, or denying of the reality of the threat that HIV poses to Nigerian society. At other times, media coverage of HIV/AIDS issues in Nigeria was largely limited to government events and activities as well as the reactions on HIV/AIDS from health-focused NGOs, research institutions, and government agencies. The situation has been changing gradually, however, as a recent analysis of mass media reports and activities found a growing media interest in the epidemic and greater involvement of media practitioners in HIV control efforts, particularly communication activities. The use of alternative media strategies — such as street theater, home videos, documentary films, public service announcements, posters, and music — has also increased use.

Content analysis of 2,156 reproductive health articles published in four national print media between 1986 and 1997 showed a greater attention — 56% — on sexually transmitted infections, including HIV, than other major reproductive health issues. Most of the reports, however, covered workshops, conferences, and government pronouncements rather than in-depth field reports and analysis of the country's HIV epidemic. News items rated as the most common type of HIV/AIDS (72% to 82%) reports in various newspapers (48). In general, the media paid little attention to the science and prevention of HIV/AIDS between 1986 and 1997, a period during which the government's activities and support for HIV prevention were low. Most news coverage on the epidemic in that era related to NGO activities rather than accurate descriptions of HIV/AIDS itself.

Since 2000, mass media in Nigeria have recorded major progress in covering the epidemic. A study of print media from March 2002 to March 2003, for example, indicated increased HIV/AIDS coverage and an improved understanding of key issues involved by journalists. Media reports still overwhelmingly tilt to news, however, while features, editorials, and opinion articles lag behind. An analysis of the publications covered in the study showed that news reports, which generally provide little information on the science and control of HIV/AIDS, constituted 74.5% of media reports, followed by news features (18.1%) and opinion pieces (6.8%); editorials constituted only 0.5% (49). The study also showed that the quality of coverage still left much to be desired; based on objective criteria drawn up by a media NGO, only 3% of articles were considered good, while 85% were rated fair.

Greater participation of the media in HIV/AIDS communication stemmed, perhaps, from the realization that they could exercise considerable influence on the public by increasing people's knowledge, influencing attitudes, and promoting debates on HIV/AIDS through a presentation of factual information about HIV. The recognition that the media could play a central role in creating awareness and understanding of the HIV/AIDS, as well as sensitizing and mobilizing the people against the epidemic, encouraged media practitioners to become more active in the HIV/AIDS communication domain at individual, institutional, and professional levels. The emergence of media-based NGOs in the late 1990s, such as Journalists Against AIDS and Development Communications Network, also added impetus to media-based initiatives against HIV/AIDS in Nigeria.

As mentioned earlier, the death of Fela Anikulapo-Kuti in August 1997 marked a turning point in HIV/AIDS reporting in the country. Fela's death received intense media coverage because it marked the first time a prominent Nigerian was publicly associated with HIV/AIDS, bringing the reality of the epidemic to the doorstep of many Nigerians. Yet, Nigerian mass media failed to fully explore the opportunities offered by Fela's death for educating the population about HIV/AIDS.

Other transient increases in HIV/AIDS reporting followed Fela's death. The most notable were the media coverage of the AIDS "cure" proponents between 2000 and 2001 and the claim of the discovery of an effective treatment by a Nigerian surgeon trained in immunology. In the absence of a coherent response from the authorities, the media were awash with reports that a curative drug had indeed been found in Nigeria. Media outlets in Nigeria continue to feature information about unproven AIDS cures; those marketing "cures" even buy media space regularly to advertise their products.

To improve media coverage and participation in HIV/AIDS control efforts, a number of development partners, including donor agencies and government institutions, have offered or supported training programs for media professionals to improve their HIV/AIDS reporting. Support has also been given for the establishment of media resource centers.

Many organizations have waged media campaigns as a practical way to raise AIDS awareness among people in different regions of Nigeria. Such a campaign differs from an institutionalized approach that is led by media organizations as a core component of media programming. Media-led approaches, which are institutional responses of media organizations themselves, have greater potential than media campaigns to improve features, editorials, opinion pieces, and news reports in the media. Media campaigns, which tend to be sponsored events or commercial adverts, are more expensive and less sustainable than media-led approaches.

Overall, it can be argued that the Nigerian mass media, much like most population subgroups, has moved through the usual stages of denial, sensationalism, and blame but is now responding more constructively to the HIV/AIDS epidemic. This is in line with the pattern found within the media elsewhere in Africa (50).

THE DIFFERENCE BCC HAS MADE IN THE NIGERIAN EPIDEMIC

While the level and scope of BCC activity have increased with time, particularly during 1999 to 2003, a missing dimension in Nigeria's HIV/AIDS programming landscape remains the systematic and scientifically rigorous evaluation of the impact of such programs. As a result, it is difficult to identify which approaches have worked best in different circumstances, locations, and population groups. The general impact of HIV communication programs at the population level can be broadly assessed, however, through the findings of successive national surveys. The NDHS reports for 1999 (51) and 2003 (13) enable an evaluation of the possible impact of the programs at the population level within these time periods.

In general, the reports showed that the proportion of adults who were aware of AIDS increased from 89.5% to 97.0% for males and from 74.4% to 86.3% for females between 1999 and 2003 (13,51). By 2003, even in the zones with the lowest level of awareness, 75.5% of women (for the North-East region) and more than 90% of males (for South-South region) were aware of the disease (13). For males, knowledge of the role of condoms in HIV prevention also increased, from 29.4% in 1999 to 53.4% in 2003; and for females the rates were 13.8% in 1999 (36) and 44.6% in 2003 (13). Despite the high level of AIDS awareness, in 2003 only 59.8% of males and 42.3% of females knew that both condom use and limiting sex to one uninfected partner protect against HIV transmission. In 2003, misinformation was still shown to be high, using UNAIDS criteria, as only 28% of men and 20.8% of women held no incorrect belief about AIDS.

Assessment of knowledge about preventing mother-to-child transmission of HIV showed only 6.2% of males and 5.2% of females understood that HIV could be transmitted through breastfeeding and that HIV-infected women could reduce the rate of HIV transmission to their babies by taking antiretrovirals during pregnancy (13). HIV-related discrimination also was high, again using UNAIDS criteria, with only 6.6% of males and 3.3% of females having accepting attitudes toward PLWHAs. In essence, the plethora of BCC activities and other HIV communication initiatives in the country before 1999 and between 1999 and 2003 have had only a marginal impact on HIV-related knowledge and behaviors in Nigeria.

The data also showed that HIV-related high-risk behavior remains a challenge in Nigeria. Among married individuals, for example, only 32.2% of females and 50.1% of males used condoms during sex with non-marital partners (32). Among singles, 33.7% of females and 48.7% of males used condoms with their sexual partners. Furthermore, only 7.6% of males and 6.0% of females had ever undergone HIV testing. Thus, the available data suggest that HIV communication activities in Nigeria may have been largely ineffective in terms of their overall impact on HIV knowledge and preventive behaviors.

While it may be argued that short-term communication efforts—those whose duration lasts less than five years—may ultimately yield quantifiable improvements in behaviors after long-term implementation, and that change may simply be a matter of time, this is not likely to be a sufficient explanation in the Nigerian scenario. Several potential weaknesses in implementing HIV/AIDS communication programs in Nigeria have been identified, including technical weaknesses in the design and implementation of BCC programs, insufficient coverage of programs across the country, and a lack of coordination and poor collaboration among the organizations involved in HIV-related BCC activities in Nigeria.

- **Technical weakness of the programs:** Few organizations involved in HIV interventions in Nigeria, both governmental and nongovernmental, possess the technical expertise for designing theory-based BCC programs. Materials and messages are designed without the benefit of the scientific foundation that would render them more efficacious, and as most BCC-related activities are not based on any particular behavior change theory, their technical quality tends to be dubious. A field study has found that most civil society organizations lack an understanding of how their communication approaches would conceptually lead to behavior change; they simply "hoped" that change would occur (52). The appropriateness of HIV messages that some organizations disseminate also is doubtful, and sometimes groups disseminate conflicting messages (53). The incorporation of inappropriate methods and languages in messages—including the distribution of English-language materials to non-literate audiences—has been reported (52). A lack of skilled human resources for implementing BCC initiatives has been documented at local, state, and federal government agencies (54). Among others, public sector officers charged with responsibility for health education and health promotion activities were found to lack sufficient knowledge about social mobilization, message design, and the use of health educational materials. Prior to 2003, no government department or institution handling HIV prevention communication activities had ever committed a communication strategy or strategic communication plan to print. This was also true of many development partners involved in HIV prevention and other health-related BCC activities in Nigeria (55).
- **Insufficient coverage of programs:** HIV-related BCC activities have been inequitably distributed across the country. Most have been limited to the urban and peri-urban areas, while the rural areas, where approximately two-thirds of Nigerians live, have been largely neglected. Some states have had a comparative over-concentration of donors' presence, to the disadvantage of other states. There has been no correlation between the number of donor-supported HIV/AIDS projects in any given state and its epidemiologic picture; while some states with low seroprevalence rates have enjoyed a continued influx of donor-supported programs, a number of more affected states lack any such programs.
- **The lack of a coordination framework for BCC activities and a poor level of collaboration among actors:** While increasing efforts have been devoted toward ensuring coordination of

HIV/AIDS responses at the federal level since NACA was created, little BCC coordination was done prior to 2003. At the state and local government levels, the capacity of the SACAs and the LACAs to coordinate effectively remained poor (56). BCC actors and activities had no defined coordination framework and little quality control in terms of disseminated messages. The national oversight of programmatic initiatives was poor, such that many development partners were implementing or supporting various HIV communication activities with little or no consultation with relevant government agencies and no reference to any overall national plan. Little communication and information sharing was taking place between the development partners and actors. Moreover, little attention had been paid to documentation of "best practices." Similarly, little effort was devoted to monitoring and evaluation activities to clearly document the impact of BCC approaches and activities as part of the national response (39).

Thus, the HIV-related BCC landscape in Nigeria before 2003 was characterized by a large number of programs of dubious quality and effectiveness, poor targeting of activities in terms of geographic and population focus, low national spread and coverage, and poor coordination and collaboration of efforts.

THE FIVE-YEAR NATIONAL HIV/AIDS BEHAVIOR CHANGE COMMUNICATION STRATEGY

To improve the effectiveness of BCC for HIV/AIDS control in Nigeria, several weaknesses and challenges must be addressed. This realization provided the rationale for the development of a five-year framework, the National HIV/AIDS Behavior Change Communication Strategy, from 2004 to 2008. The development process, coordinated by NACA, involved various groups of stakeholders, including government institutions, national NGOs, a PLWHA network, and international development organizations.

Activities that took place in the development of the strategic framework included:

- A review of best practices from across Africa in HIV/AIDS prevention, care, and support to identify successful, innovative, and evidence-based approaches;
- A review of existing national data on geographic distribution, knowledge, attitudes, practices, and behaviors around HIV/AIDS, as well as the national monitoring and evaluation indicators;
- A review of past, current, and future HIV/AIDS activity plans and materials collated from diverse stakeholders; and
- Consensus building about the priority audiences and the approaches appropriate to reaching them, priority programs and benchmarks, and the roles and responsibilities of partners.

The framework aims to facilitate the achievement of the national policy goal of reducing the rate of HIV infection by 25%, thereby reducing the national seroprevalence level from 5.0% in 2003 to 4.4% by 2008. The goal is to attain a coordinated national response for BCC programming that ensures coherent, uniform, evidence-based, community-oriented, and theory-driven interventions from all stakeholders, with a measurable impact produced within the shortest possible time (57). The strategy document seeks to provide a practical and useful strategic instrument for addressing HIV-related BCC issues in Nigeria and to empower all stakeholders in HIV/AIDS control and mitigation activities in the context of a coordinated, comprehensive, audience-responsive, and culturally appropriate BCC program.

The strategy document identified: key issues for HIV/AIDS in Nigeria; a relevant conceptual framework and analysis of most effective strategies to help ensure verifiable impact; a five-year vision and target indicators that must be met to achieve that vision; priority audiences, relevant strategies, and critical interventions; and practical timelines for rolling out the overall strategy to maximize impact.

The framework involved the use of two behavioral change theories, selected on the basis of demonstrated effectiveness and relevance to HIV/AIDS interventions in sub-Saharan Africa: the information-motivation-behavioral skills (IMB) model and the extended parallel process model (EPPM). The IMB model facilitates an understanding of the context of behavioral skills, while EPPM provides useful insight in terms of message design and dissemination.

The IMB model has been used as a basis for understanding HIV risk and other reproductive health behaviors across different populations in both developed and developing countries, including young people, university undergraduates, men who have sex with men, and long-distance truck drivers (58–62). Standardized measures of the constructs of the model have been developed and validated for use within a number of diverse populations and for different risk behaviors (63–66). The model holds that HIV prevention information, motivation, and behavioral skills are the fundamental determinants of HIV preventive behaviors (Figure 15-1). The model suggests that well-informed people are not necessarily well motivated to practice prevention and vice versa, but also highlights the existence of a relationship between informational and motivational factors.

The EPPM, on the other hand, focuses on the interplay of "fear" and "efficacy" factors in the context of effectiveness of campaign messages (Figure 15-2). It deals with how fear can be channeled in a positive, protective direction instead of a negative, maladaptive direction (67–69). The EPPM postulates that campaign messages should contain a threat component and an efficacy component. The threat portion makes the audience feel vulnerable, and then the efficacy portion convinces individuals that they can perform the recommended response — that is, achieve self-efficacy — and that the recommended response can effectively avert the threat. The EPPM has been applied successfully to HIV risk and preventive behaviors among people of African descent and in sub-Saharan Africa (70–72).

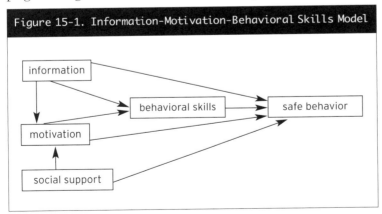

Figure 15-1. Information-Motivation-Behavioral Skills Model

information

behavioral skills

safe behavior

motivation

social support

Source: Fisher JD, Fisher WA. The information-motivation-behavioral skills model. In: DiClemente, R, Crosby R, Kegler M, eds. *Emerging Theories in Health Promotion Practice and Research.* San Francisco, CA: Jossey Bass Publishers, 2002;40-70.

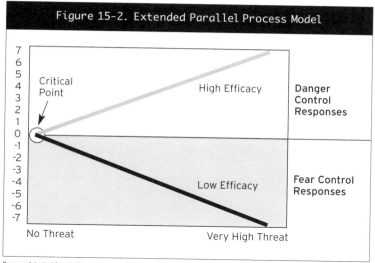

Figure 15-2. Extended Parallel Process Model

Source: Adapted from Witte K, Cameron KA, Lapinski MK, Nzyuko S. A theoretically based evaluation of HIV/AIDS prevention campaigns along the trans-Africa highway in Kenya. *J Health Commun*, 1998;4:345-363.

Audience Segmentation and Strategic Activities

Broadly, the strategy document identified five priority audiences based on their overall role in HIV transmission in Nigeria as documented through past research activities and in line with the focus of the National Policy on HIV/AIDS. These include young people, people with high-risk behavior, health care providers, men and women of reproductive age (15 to 49 years old), and PLWHAs. Each of the priority audiences was further segmented to identify subgroups with clearly different desired behavioral outcomes or situations. Specific objectives, strategic approaches, activities, and related research needs were developed for each priority audience.

While the focus was on primary prevention, in recognition of the importance of the continuum of primary prevention, care, and support to the overall success of HIV prevention efforts, the framework anticipates that 80% of efforts will be devoted to primary prevention, and 20% to other areas (Figure 15-3). The primary prevention activities involved the "ABC" of sexually transmitted infections prevention—Abstinence (delay in sexual initiation); Being faithful (partner reduction); and Condom use (in a correct and consistent manner)—given the proven effectiveness of this approach (73). Other strategic activities indicated in the framework include prevention of mother-to-child transmission; stigma reduction; advocacy among political and community leaders; care, support, and compassion; access to treatment; capacity building; and research, monitoring, and evaluation.

While the framework clearly recognized the differences among the desired behaviors for each priority audience, it also aimed to achieve a holistic approach by recognizing the complementary nature of various strategic activities. For example, as Figure 15-3 shows, for young and single people, abstinence is the major strategic focus, with partner reduction, condom use, and voluntary counseling and referral as complementary approaches. For most-at-risk people, condom use is the main approach, with partner reduction, management of sexually transmitted infections, and voluntary counseling and referral as other strategies. And for men and women of reproductive age, the emphasis is on partner reduction, with voluntary counseling and the reduction of stigmatization as secondary approaches.

The national BCC strategy seeks to use an integrated, multi-channel approach as derived from best practices to provide information, motivation, and behavioral skills building for the various target groups

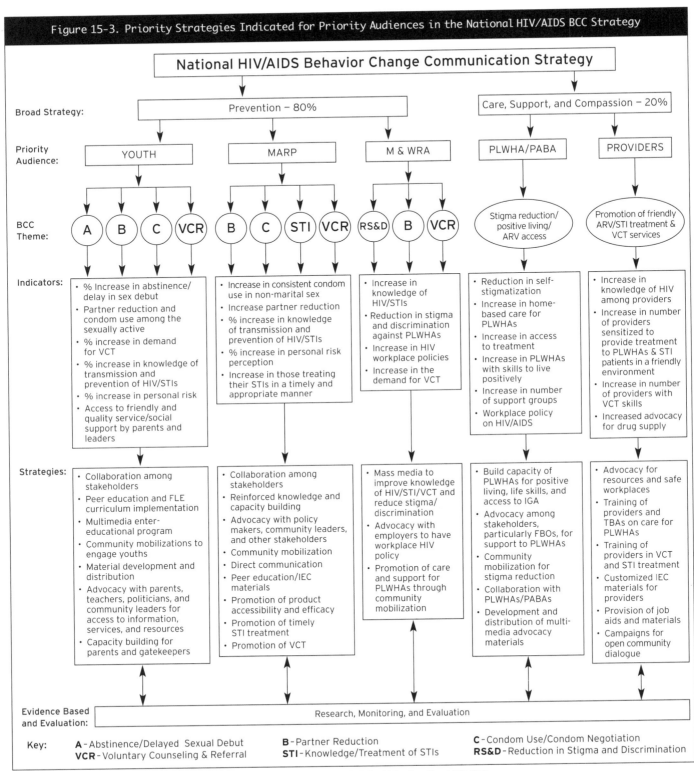

Figure 15-3. Priority Strategies Indicated for Priority Audiences in the National HIV/AIDS BCC Strategy

National HIV/AIDS Behavior Change Communication Strategy

Broad Strategy:
- Prevention – 80%
- Care, Support, and Compassion – 20%

Priority Audience:
- YOUTH
- MARP
- M & WRA
- PLWHA/PABA
- PROVIDERS

BCC Theme:
- YOUTH: A, B, C, VCR
- MARP: B, C, STI, VCR
- M & WRA: RS&D, B, VCR
- PLWHA/PABA: Stigma reduction/ positive living/ ARV access
- PROVIDERS: Promotion of friendly ARV/STI treatment & VCT services

Indicators:

YOUTH:
- % Increase in abstinence/ delay in sex debut
- Partner reduction and condom use among the sexually active
- % increase in demand for VCT
- % increase in knowledge of transmission and prevention of HIV/STIs
- % increase in personal risk
- Access to friendly and quality service/social support by parents and leaders

MARP:
- Increase in consistent condom use in non-marital sex
- Increase partner reduction
- % increase in knowledge of transmission and prevention of HIV/STIs
- % increase in personal risk perception
- Increase in those treating their STIs in a timely and appropriate manner

M & WRA:
- Increase in knowledge of HIV/STIs
- Reduction in stigma and discrimination against PLWHAs
- Increase in HIV workplace policies
- Increase in the demand for VCT

PLWHA/PABA:
- Reduction in self-stigmatization
- Increase in home-based care for PLWHAs
- Increase in access to treatment
- Increase in PLWHAs with skills to live positively
- Increase in number of support groups
- Workplace policy on HIV/AIDS

PROVIDERS:
- Increase in knowledge of HIV among providers
- Increase in number of providers sensitized to provide treatment to PLWHAs & STI patients in a friendly environment
- Increase in number of providers with VCT skills
- Increased advocacy for drug supply

Strategies:

YOUTH:
- Collaboration among stakeholders
- Peer education and FLE curriculum implementation
- Multimedia enter-educational program
- Community mobilizations to engage youths
- Material development and distribution
- Advocacy with parents, teachers, politicians, and community leaders for access to information, services, and resources
- Capacity building for parents and gatekeepers

MARP:
- Collaboration among stakeholders
- Reinforced knowledge and capacity building
- Advocacy with policy makers, community leaders, and other stakeholders
- Community mobilization
- Direct communication
- Peer education/IEC materials
- Promotion of product accessibility and efficacy
- Promotion of timely STI treatment
- Promotion of VCT

M & WRA:
- Mass media to improve knowledge of HIV/STI/VCT and reduce stigma/ discrimination
- Advocacy with employers to have workplace HIV policy
- Promotion of care and support for PLWHAs through community mobilization

PLWHA/PABA:
- Build capacity of PLWHAs for positive living, life skills, and access to IGA
- Advocacy among stakeholders, particularly FBOs, for support to PLWHAs
- Community mobilization for stigma reduction
- Collaboration with PLWHAs/PABAs
- Development and distribution of multi-media advocacy materials

PROVIDERS:
- Advocacy for resources and safe workplaces
- Training of providers and TBAs on care for PLWHAs
- Training of providers in VCT and STI treatment
- Customized IEC materials for providers
- Provision of job aids and materials
- Campaigns for open community dialogue

Evidence Based and Evaluation: Research, Monitoring, and Evaluation

Key:
- **A** - Abstinence/Delayed Sexual Debut
- **B** - Partner Reduction
- **C** - Condom Use/Condom Negotiation
- **VCR** - Voluntary Counseling & Referral
- **STI** - Knowledge/Treatment of STIs
- **RS&D** - Reduction in Stigma and Discrimination

Source: National Action Committee on AIDS. *National HIV/AIDS Behavior Change Communication Strategy.* Abuja: National Action Committee on AIDS, 2004.
Abbreviations: ARV: antiretroviral; FBO: faith-based organization; FLE: family life education; IEC: information, education, and communication; IGA: income-generating activities; MARP: most-at-risk population; PABA: people affected by HIV/AIDS; PLWHA: person living with HIV/AIDS; STI: sexually transmitted infection; TBA: traditional birth attendant; VCT: voluntary counseling and testing

identified. The anticipated use and contribution of the various communication media to impact behavior include:

- Mass media (television, radio, billboards, and print): to build awareness, increase knowledge, promote role models, and influence societal norms.
- Enter-educative approaches: to reinforce awareness and knowledge, clarify misconceptions, desensitize behaviors, and shape societal norms.
- Interpersonal communications: to personalize information, model and practice behavioral skills, and build self-efficacy through skills and confidence-building strategies. Activities that involve significant time, multiple methods, and recurrent sessions with small groups are more effective than others.
- Community mobilization: to sensitize and advocate for societal responses to the HIV epidemic, and to influence policy change to create an enabling environment for sustained behavioral change.

The proposed operational framework corresponds with the existing structure for HIV/AIDS control activities in Nigeria, which is multisectoral in nature and entrusts NACA, the SACAs, and the LACAs with coordination responsibilities. Implementation of specified strategies and activities will be decentralized, resting with the various organizations mandated to address HIV/AIDS while NACA has the coordinating role in the operationalization of the framework.

Overall, the strategic framework is a laudable development as the country's first national document on BCC. While considerable attention has been given to addressing individuals and groups with specific approaches, however, little or no attention has been made to addressing the larger environment. This weakness is one of the major criticisms about the use of psychosocial theories for interventions in the area of sexuality. Most human behaviors, particular sexual behaviors, do not occur in isolation; rather, contextual factors play significant roles in the patterns exhibited. Many experts have underscored the fact that seeking to influence behavior alone is insufficient if the underlying social factors that shape the particular behavior remain unchallenged (74). Change in an individual's behavior is unlikely to be sustainable without some degree of change in the social environment. Thus, significant attention should be paid to the societal context, which the strategic framework has neglected to do thus far. Issues of poverty, gender inequality and inequity, and other related human development conditions must also be addressed for the BCC approaches to achieve their full impact.

Uganda's experience also testifies to the need to address the larger sociocultural and economic context of the disease. The approach in Uganda embraced "ABC" but went beyond it to "D," or Delayed sexual activity, a message young people found to be more acceptable than abstinence. More importantly, the Ugandan approach also included "E" and "F"—Empowerment of women through Financial independence (75).

"Prevention methods such as the 'ABC' approach—Abstinence, Be faithful, and use Condoms—are good but not enough to protect women where gender inequality is pervasive," the executive director of UNAIDS, Peter Piot, noted in his World AIDS Day address in 2004. "We must ensure that women can choose marriage, to decide when and with whom they have sex, and to successfully negotiate condom use" (76). As UNAIDS, the United Nations Population Fund, and the United Nations Development Fund for Women noted in their joint report, the "triple threat of gender inequality, poverty and HIV/AIDS" must be tackled to achieve reduction in the spread of the epidemic and its devastating consequences (75).

The long-term success of BCC programs also requires community involvement and ownership, which must be integrated into the Nigerian program. The Ugandan experience clearly indicates that community processes and initiatives constitute the major pillars for sustainability and success in the fight against HIV/AIDS (6).

CONCLUSION

Behavior change to ensure HIV prevention remains a critical challenge, and, at the same time, a priority in the current fight against the epidemic. While the complex nature of the human behaviors driving the epidemic is recognized, the examples of African countries such as Uganda, where the epidemic has been successfully stemmed, provide encouragement about the effectiveness of BCC strategies.

The National HIV/AIDS BCC Strategy provides Nigeria with a platform for more effective and coordinated BCC responses to the epidemic and the potential to realize the policy goal of reducing the rate of HIV infection by 25% by 2008. The strategic framework captures the essence of policy pronouncement that, "effective communication includes greater public enlightenment, focusing on the removal of socio-cultural barriers; informational barriers; systemic barriers; the improvement in the general public's base knowledge regarding the HIV and AIDS epidemic; and catalyzing community-based responses of HIV and AIDS" (57). The challenge lies with ensuring good implementation on a continued basis. Thus, the document needs to be widely distributed; the capacities of stakeholders must be developed for effective implementation; and good oversight of the implementation and coordination must be ensured to bring the vision of the document to reality and effectively check the spread of HIV in Nigeria.

The mass media has a valuable role to play in disseminating information about HIV/AIDS and Nigeria's strategic framework to fight this disease. Media practitioners also need to be involved in monitoring and reporting on the implementation of the strategic framework and publicizing "good practices." Thus, building the capacity of media practitioners and organizations to contribute appropriately will be important in the context of improving HIV-related BCC in Nigeria. This should entail, among others, building the institutional capacity of media organizations to initiate media-driven responses that are more strategic in nature and that go beyond the present level of activities.

ACKNOWLEDGMENTS

We highly appreciate the efforts of Drs. Titi Abiona, Sola Akinrinade, Jason Blackard, Olawunmi Fatusi, Oluwole Odutolu, and Olorunda Rotimi in reviewing earlier versions of the manuscript.

REFERENCES

1. United Nations Development Programme. *Human Development Report. Nigeria 2004. HIV and AIDS: A Challenge to Sustainable Human Development.* Abuja: United Nations Development Programme, 2004.

2. Federal Ministry of Health. *2003 National HIV Seroprevalence Sentinel Survey.* Abuja: Federal Ministry of Health, 2004.

3. Federal Ministry of Health. *HIV/AIDS: What It Means for Nigeria (Background, Projection, Impact, Interventions, and Policy).* Abuja: Federal Ministry of Health, 2002.

4. Green E, Nantulya V, Stoneburner R, Stover J. *What happened in Uganda? Declining HIV Prevalence, Behavior Change, and the National Response. Project Lessons Learned. Case Study.* Washington: The Synergy Project, USAID, 2002.

5. Stoneburner RL, Low-Beer D. Population-level HIV decline and behavioral risk avoidance in Uganda. *Science,* 2004;30:714–718.

6. Stoneburner RL, Low-Beer D. Behavior and communication change in reducing HIV. Is Uganda unique? *Afr J AIDS Res,* 2003;2:9–21.

7. Liskin L, Church CA, Piotrow PT, Harris JA. *AIDS Education — A Beginning.* Baltimore: Center for Communication Programs, Johns Hopkins School of Public Health, 1989;XVII:1–18.

8. United Nations Population Fund (UNFPA). *Communication for Development Roundtable Report. Focus on HIV/AIDS Communication and Evaluation.* November 26–28, 2001, Managua, Nicaragua. Organized by UNFPA with the Rockefeller Foundation, UNESCO, and the Panos Institute. New York: UNFPA, 2001.

9. Prochaska JO, Diclemente CC, Norcross JC. In search of how people change: Applications to additive behaviors. *Am Psychol,* 1992;47:1102–1114.

10. Kalichman S, Rompa D, Coley B. Lack of positive outcomes from a cognitive-behavioral HIV and AIDS prevention for inner city men: lessons from a controlled pilot study. *AIDS Educ Prev,* 1997; 9:S299–313.

11. U.S. Centers for Disease Control and Prevention. *Global AIDS Program: Strategies.* 2004. Accessed at www.cdc.gov/nchstp/od/gap on January 10, 2005.

12. Scalway T, Deane J. *Critical Challenges in HIV Communication: A Perspective Paper from the Panos London HIV/AIDS Program.* London: Panos, 2002.

13. National Population Commission and ORC Macro. *Nigeria Demographic Health Survey 2003.* Calverton, Maryland: National Population Commission and ORC Macro, 2004.

14. Piotrow PT, Rimon JG II, Payne Meritt A, Saffitz G. *Advancing Health Communication: The PCS Experience in the Field.* Center Publication 103. Baltimore: Center for Communication Programs, Johns Hopkins Bloomberg School of Public Health, 2003.

15. Family Health International, Institute for HIV/AIDS. *Behavior Change Communication (BCC) for HIV/AIDS: A Strategic Framework.* Arlington, Virginia: Family Health International, 2002.

16. USAID. *Behavior Change Communication Programs,* 2004. Accessed at www.usaid.gov/our_work/global_health/aids on January 10, 2005.

17. Catania J, Kegeles S, Coates T. Toward an understanding of risk behavior: an AIDS risk reduction model (ARRM). *Health Educ Q,* 1990;17:53–72.

18. Odutolu O. Convergence of behaviour change models for AIDS risk reduction in sub-Saharan Africa. *Int J Health Planning Manage,* 2005;20(3):239–252.

19. Fishbein M. The role of theory in HIV prevention. *AIDS Care,* 2000;30:273–278.

20. Figueroa ME, Kincaid DL, Rani M, Lewis G. *Communication for Social Change: An Integrated Model for Measuring the Process and Its Outcomes.* Baltimore, Maryland: Center for Communication Programs, Johns Hopkins Bloomberg School of Public Health, 2002.

21. Kelly K, Parker W, Lewis G. Reconceptualising behavior change in the HIV/AIDS context. In: Stones C, ed. *Socio-political and Psychological Perspectives on South Africa.* London: Nova Science, 2000.

22. *Communications Framework for HIV/AIDS: A New Direction.* Geneva: UNAIDS and University Park, Pennsylvania: Pennsylvania State University, 1999.

23. Glanz K, Rimer B. *Theory at a Glance: A Guide for Health Promotion Practice.* Bethesda, Maryland: National Cancer Institute, National Institutes of Health, 1997.

24. King R. *Sexual Behavior Change for HIV: Where Have Theories Taken Us?* Geneva: UNAIDS, 1999.

25. Bandura A. *Social Learning Theory.* Englewood Cliffs, New Jersey: Prentice-Hall Inc., 1977.

26. Clift E. *Information, Education and Communication: Lessons from the Past; Perspectives for the Future.* Geneva: World Health Organization, 2001.

27. Kincaid DL, Jara JR, Coleman PL, Segura F. *Getting the Message: The Communication for Young People Special Project.* Special Study No. 56. Washington, DC: U.S. Agency for International Development, 1988.

28. Piotrow PT, Kincaid DL, Rimon JG II, Rinehart W. *Health Communication: Lessons from Family Planning and Reproductive Health.* Baltimore, Maryland: Center for Communication Programs, Johns Hopkins School of Public Health, 1997.

29. Agha S. The impact of a mass media campaign on personal risk perception, perceived self-efficacy and on other behavioural predictors. *AIDS Care,* 2003; 15:749–762.

30. De Vroome E, Sandfort T, De Vries K, Paalman M, Tielman R. Evaluation of a safe sex campaign regarding AIDS and other sexually transmitted diseases among the young people in the Netherlands. *Health Educ Res,* 1993;6:317–325.

31. Rogers EM. The field of health communication today: an up-to-date report. *J Health Commun,* 1996; 1:15–23.

32. Federal Ministry of Health. *National HIV/AIDS and Reproductive Health Survey,* 2003. Abuja: Federal Ministry of Health, 2003.

33. Ogundimu F. Nigeria: Problems in Communicating Population Control. Working Paper No. 33. Bloomington, Indiana: Population Institute for Research and Training, Indiana University, 1990.

34. Piotrow PT, Rimon JG II, Winnard K, Kincaid DL, Huntington D, Convisser J. Mass media family planning promotion in three Nigerian Cities. *Stud Fam Plann,* 1990;21:265–274.

35. Bankole A. *The Role of Mass Media in Family Planning Promotion in Nigeria.* DHS Working Paper No. 11. Calverton, Maryland: Macro International Inc., 1994.

36. Network. Preventing HIV transmission in "priority" countries. *Network,* 1993;13:18–21.

37. Family Health International. *AIDS Control and Prevention Project Final Report.* Nigeria and Senegal. Arlington, Virginia: Family Health International, 1997(2).

38. Oke O. FHI/IMPACT comprehensive programming for HIV and AIDS in Nigeria. *Fourth National Conference on HIV/AIDS in Nigeria,* Abuja, Nigeria, May 2–5, 2004;173.

39. National Action Committee on AIDS. *HIV/AIDS Emergency Action Plan (HEAP).* Abuja: National Action Committee on AIDS, 2001.

40. National Action Committee on AIDS. *Analysis of the Response on STD/HIV/AIDS in Nigeria.* Abuja: National Action Committee on AIDS, 2000.

41. Federal Government of Nigeria. *National Policy on HIV/AIDS.* Abuja: Federal Government of Nigeria, 2003.

42. Fatusi AO. *Study of African Universities' Response to HIV/AIDS: The Nigerian Universities.* Report of a study submitted to the Association of African University, Ghana, June 2004.

43. The Guardian Newspapers. *Another AIDS victim is dead.* December 5, 1987;2.

44. The Guardian Newspapers. *New killer sexual disease discovered.* September 13, 1986;3.

45. Vanguard Newspapers. *Who's afraid of the big bad AIDS? — Not Nigerian Men.* November 17, 1987;5.

46. Vanguard Newspapers. *11 out of 12 AIDS carriers now dead — Medical Director.* July 6, 1988; 16.

47. Vanguard Newspapers. *Call girls spread AIDS.* March 10, 1988;2.

48. Development Communications Network. *Mass Media Communication Strategies for Reproductive Health Promotion in Nigeria.* Lagos: Development Communications Network, 2001.

49. Journalists Against AIDS. A Slow Awakening: *The Media and HIV/AIDS Epidemic in Nigeria — A Score Card.* Lagos: Journalists Against AIDS, 2003;7–15.

50. Lear D. AIDS in the African Press. *Int Q Community Health Educ,* 1990;10:253–264.

51. National Population Commission and ORC Macro. *1999 Nigeria Demographic and Health Survey.* Calverton, Maryland: National Population Commission and ORC Macro, 2000.

52. ActionAid Nigeria. *Mapping Civil Society's Involvement in HIV/AIDS Program in Nigeria. A Report of Findings in Seven States.* A study commissioned by the UK Department for International Development (DFID). Abuja: ActionAid Nigeria, 2001.

53. Richie-Adewusi F, Oke O, Lariveee C, Ogundehin D. Participatory development of thematic behavior change communication campaign among target groups: the FHI Nigeria experience. *Fourth National Conference on HIV/AIDS in Nigeria,* Abuja, Nigeria, May 2–5, 2004 (abstract A256-1).

54. Umba MA, Fagbemi B, Dennis-Antwi, J, Aneke QC, Shodeinde T, Yola DS, Tamen F. *Report of an Assessment of the Capacity of the Health Sector for Consumer Education and Community Mobilization in Nigeria.* Consultancy report submitted to PATHS, Abuja. March 31, 2004.

55. Fatusi AO. *Review of the Communication Strategies and Activities of the Communication Forum Member Agencies.* Consultancy report submitted to PATHS/JHUCCP, Abuja. January 2005.

56. Oke EA, Dr. Uwakwe CBU, Aderiokun G, Eloike T, Longe O, Banwat S. *Capacity Review of SACAs and LACAs in Nigeria.* Consultancy report submitted to the National Action Committee on AIDS, Abuja, 2003.

57. National Action Committee on AIDS. *National HIV and AIDS Behavior Change Communication. Five-Year Strategy (2004–2008).* Abuja: National Action Committee on AIDS, 2005.

58. Fisher JD, Fisher WA, Misovich SJ, Kimble DL, Malloy TE. Changing AIDS risk behavior: effects of an intervention emphasizing AIDS risk reduction information, motivation, and behavioral skills in a college student population. *Health Psychol,* 1996; 15:114–123.

59. Bryan AD, Fisher JD, Benziger TJ. Determinants of HIV risk among Indian truck drivers: an information-motivation-behavioral skills approach. *Soc Sci Med,* 2001;53:1413–1426.

60. Fisher JD, Bryan AD. Information-motivation-behavioral skills model–based HIV risk behavior change intervention for inner city high school youth. *Health Psychol,* 2002;21:177–186.

61. Fisher JD, Fisher WA. The information-motivation-behavioral skills model. In: DiClemente, R, Crosby R, Kegler M, eds. *Emerging Theories in Health Promotion Practice and Research.* San Francisco, California: Jossey Bass Publishers, 2002;40–70.

62. Kozal MJ, Amico R, Chiarella J, et al. Antiretroviral resistance and high-risk transmission behavior among HIV-positive patients in clinical care. *AIDS,* 2004;18:2185–2189.

63. Fisher JD, Fisher WA, Malloy TE. Empirical tests of an information-motivation-behavioral skills model of AIDS-preventive behavior with gay men and heterosexual university students. *Health Psychol,* 1994;13:238–250.

64. Fisher JD, Fisher WA. The information-motivation-behavioral skills model of AIDS risk behavior change: empirical support and applications. In: Oskamp S, Thompson S, eds. *Understanding and Preventing HIV Risk Behavior: Safer Sex and Drug Use.* Thousand Oaks, California: Sage, 1996;100–127.

65. Misovich SJ, Fisher, WA, Fisher, JD. Understanding and promoting AIDS preventive behavior: measures of AIDS risk reduction information, motivation, behavioral skills and behavior. In: Davis C, Yarber W, eds. *Sexuality and Related Measures: A Compendium.* Syracuse, NY: Society for the Scientific Study of Sex, 1998.

66. Fisher WA, Williams SS, Fisher JD, Malloy TE. Understanding AIDS risk behavior among sexually active urban adolescents. An empirical test of the information-motivation-behavioral skills model. *AIDS Behav,* 1999;3:13–23.

67. Witte K. Fear control and danger control: an empirical test of the extended parallel process model. *Commun Monogr,* 1994;61:113–134.

68. Witte K. Fear as motivator, fear as inhibitor: using the extended parallel process model to explain fear appeal successes and failures. In: Andersen PA, Guerrero LK, eds. *The Handbook of Communication and Emotion: Research, Theory, Applications, and Contexts.* San Diego, CA: Academic Press, 1998;423–450.

69. Stephenson MT, Witte K. Creating fear in a risky world: generating effective health risk messages. In: Rice R, Atkin CK, eds. *Public Communication Campaigns.* 4th ed. Newbury Park, California: Sage, 2001.

70. Cameron KA, Witte K, Lapinski MK, Nzyuko S. Preventing HIV transmission along the trans-Africa highway in Kenya: using persuasive message theory in formative education. *Int Q Community Health Educ,* 1999;18:331–356.

71. Witte K, Cameron KA, Lapinski MK, Nzyuko S. A theoretically based evaluation of HIV/AIDS prevention campaigns along the trans-Africa highway in Kenya. *J Health Commun,* 1998;4:345–363.

72. Witte K, Murray L, Hubbell AP, Liu WY, Sampson J, Morrison K. Addressing cultural orientation in fear appeals: promoting AIDS-protective behaviors among Hispanic immigrants and African-American adolescents, and American and Taiwanese college students. *J Health Commun,* 2001;6:335–358.

73. United States Agency for International Development (USAID). *The "ABCs" of HIV prevention: report of a USAID technical meeting on behavior change approaches to primary prevention of HIV/AIDS*. Washington, DC: Population, Health and Nutrition Information Project, USAID, 2003. Accessed at www.usaid.gov/our_work/global_health/aids/TechAreas/prevention/abc.pdf on January 10, 2005.

74. Wingood GM, DiClemente RJ. The use of psychosocial models for guiding the design and implementation of HIV prevention interventions: translating theory into practice. In: Gibney L, DiClemente RJ, Vermund SH, eds. *Preventing HIV in Developing Countries: Biomedical and Behavioral Approaches. AIDS Prevention and Mental Health*. New York: Kluwer Academic Publishers, 1999;187–204.

75. Women and HIV/AIDS: *Confronting the Crisis*. A joint report by UNAIDS/UNFPA/UNIFEM. *Accessed at www.unfpa.org/hiv/women/report/index.htm* on January 10, 2005.

76. Piot P. Message on the occasion of World AIDS Day, December 1, 2004. *Accessed at www.unaids.org* on January 10, 2005.

16

PREVENTION OF MOTHER-TO-CHILD TRANSMISSION OF HIV

Isaac F. Adewole,* Oluwole Odutolu,†
and Atiene Solomon Sagay‡

The global HIV epidemic continues to expand, with an estimated five million people becoming infected each year. Over the decades, the epidemic, once dominated by infected males, has become progressively feminized. In sub-Saharan Africa, where about two-thirds of the global disease burden resides, 57% of adults living with HIV are women (1). As more women contract the virus, the number of children infected from their mothers has been growing. Worldwide, an estimated 640,000 children acquired HIV in 2004 alone (1), with more than 90% of the infections occurring through mother-to-child transmission.

MOTHER-TO-CHILD TRANSMISSION OF HIV

Mother-to-child transmission (MTCT) of HIV represents an especially tragic dimension of the burden of HIV/AIDS, particularly in resource-constrained settings, where fragile and poorly funded health care systems hamper care and prevention efforts. The impact of this disease is best captured

*University College Hospital, University of Ibadan, Ibadan, Nigeria
†AIDS Prevention Initiative in Nigeria, Abuja, Nigeria
‡Department of Obstetrics and Gynaecology, University of Jos, Jos, Nigeria

by data suggesting that at least one-third of HIV-infected children in developing countries die within their first year of life (2). MTCT has become a critical children's health problem in Africa, contributing to severe morbidity and significant mortality and undermining the impact of programs that had significantly reduced child mortality in previous decades.

HIV and Pregnancy

Women are particularly susceptible to HIV in developing countries, where the male-to-female ratio is less than one. A complex combination of factors — ranging from the biology of the virus, to the anatomy of the female genital tract, to sociocultural traditions — has increased women's vulnerability (3). In the context of MTCT, the high prevalence of HIV among women of reproductive age in sub-Saharan Africa is compounded by a large population of women of reproductive age, high birth rates, a tradition of prolonged breastfeeding, and a lack of effective interventions aimed at preventing MTCT (4).

The first AIDS case was reported in Nigeria in 1986 (5). Since then, prevalence rates among pregnant women have steadily climbed from 0.25% in 1989 to 5.8% in 2001 (6–8). There was, however, a slight but non-statistically significant drop to 5.0% in 2003 (9). These rates contrast with the much steeper increase in HIV rates in South Africa, where the prevalence among pregnant women rose from 1% in 1990 to 25% in 2000 (4). In urban centers in southern Africa, for example, HIV infection rates of 20% to 30% among pregnant women tested anonymously at antenatal clinics are common. Higher rates — including 43% in Botswana and 59% to 70% in Zimbabwe — have also been recorded (10). In many of these hard-hit countries, HIV is by far the most common complication in pregnancy.

Population-based studies of fertility in women with HIV infection in Africa found that pregnancy rates were lower and pregnancy loss was more common in HIV-infected women. Both HIV-positive and HIV-negative women experience a decline in absolute CD4+ cell counts in pregnancy, thought to be caused by hemodilution, yet the percentage of CD4+ cells remains relatively stable. Therefore, percentage, rather than absolute number, may be a more accurate measure of immune function for HIV-infected pregnant women (12–14). When comparing changes in CD4+ count/percentage over time, no difference exists between HIV-positive pregnant and non-pregnant women (15), suggesting that pregnancy does not accelerate a decline in CD4+ cells. In the absence of treatment, HIV RNA levels — or viral load — remain relatively stable throughout pregnancy (16).

Meta-analysis of seven prospective cohort studies found no overall significant differences in death, HIV disease progression, progression to an AIDS-defining illness, or CD4+ count decreases to below $200/mm^3$ between pregnant and non-pregnant HIV-infected women (17). In a subsequent prospective study of 331 HIV-positive women, those with known dates of seroconversion were followed for a median of 5.5 years; during that time 69 women conceived. No differences in progression were found between those who were and were not pregnant during follow-up (18). Overall, the evidence suggests that pregnancy has little or no effect on HIV progression in asymptomatic women or women with early infection, although it may accelerate HIV progression in women with advanced disease (19).

Data have accumulated that HIV disease, especially when more advanced, may result in increases in certain pregnancy complications, such as intrauterine growth retardation, preterm birth, and low birth weight (20–22). Furthermore, concerns have been raised that antiretroviral therapy (ART) itself may increase some adverse outcomes in pregnancy. A study of 497 HIV-infected pregnant women enrolled in a perinatal clinical trial, however, found that risk factors for adverse pregnancy outcomes — such as intrauterine growth retardation, preterm birth, and low birth weight — in antiretroviral-treated women are similar to those reported for uninfected women (23).

Rates and Timing of Mother-to-Child Transmission of HIV

HIV can be transmitted in utero, intrapartum, and during breast-feeding (24,25). Data from polymerase chain reaction (PCR) studies have confirmed the rarity of MTCT early in pregnancy (26). Clinical studies of children born to HIV-positive mothers present two distinct syndromes of acquired infection in the uterus: a smaller group of severely ill babies, suggesting early intrauterine infection (27), and a larger group of apparently healthy babies who develop features of HIV infection after birth, suggesting later infection in pregnancy and around the time of delivery (28).

One of the important contributors to perinatal HIV transmission is birth-canal exposure of the infant to HIV (29). In untreated mothers, Caesarean delivery is reported to offer MTCT risk reduction of 50% to 81% when compared with vaginal delivery (29). Earlier reports indicating that among twins, the first-born infant was at a twice-greater risk of infection than the second-born infant (30) have been

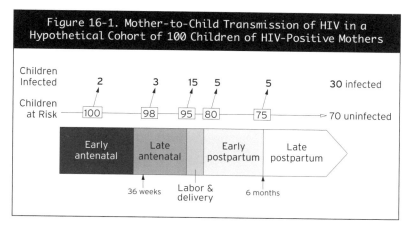

Figure 16-1. Mother-to-Child Transmission of HIV in a Hypothetical Cohort of 100 Children of HIV-Positive Mothers

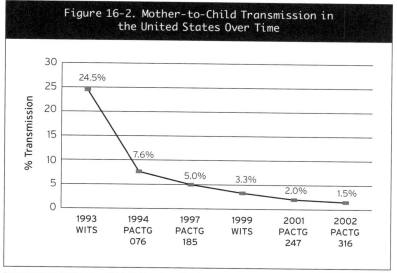

Figure 16-2. Mother-to-Child Transmission in the United States Over Time

Source: Mofenson LM. Overview of Clinical Trials on Prevention of Mother-to-Child HIV Transmission.
Abbreviations: WITS: Women and Infants Transmission Study; PACTG: Pediatric AIDS Clinical Trials Group

challenged by more recent studies that show no such differences (29). HIV transmission through breast milk accounts for up to 20% of infant infections (31). Even when transmission is prevented during pregnancy and delivery by the administration of antiretrovirals, breastfed babies are at ongoing risk of infection.

The rate of MTCT in cohorts of women who have not received any preventive treatment, such as antiretrovirals, is estimated to range from 15% to 25% in industrialized countries to 25% to 45% in developing countries (32). The breakdown according to timing of infection is now thought to be 5% to 10% during pregnancy; 10% to 20% during labor and delivery; and 10% to 20% during breastfeeding (31–33). Figure 16-1 uses a hypothetical cohort of 100 untreated HIV-positive pregnant women to summarize these estimates. The highest rates of MTCT have been found in women in Africa (34–36). MTCT rates in the developed world have fallen to less than 2% in recent years, largely because of the availability and widespread use of effective ART protocols, elective Caesarean delivery, and avoidance of breastfeeding (Figure 16-2) (37–39). Because of high infection rates, high fertility rates, prolonged breastfeeding, and delays in introducing and scaling up prevention of mother-to-child transmission (PMTCT), Africa now accounts for more than 90% of all HIV-infected babies (4).

Bryson, et al. have proposed a working definition to determine the timing of MTCT (28): A child is classified as having been infected during pregnancy (in utero) if the HIV genome is detected within 48 hours of delivery by PCR or viral culture, and during delivery (intrapartum) if those diagnostic tests were negative in a sample taken during the first 48 hours after delivery, but became positive in subsequent samples taken within 7 to 90 days of delivery.

HIV Transmission During Pregnancy

The sperm and the ovum lack the CD4+ receptors and therefore cannot be infected by HIV. This implies that at fertilization, the resulting zygote does not contain the HIV genome. In most HIV-infected women, HIV does *not* cross the placenta from mother to fetus; instead, the placenta acts as a physical barrier that shields the developing fetus from circulating viruses in the mother's blood (40). This protection from the placenta may break down, however, if the mother has a viral, bacterial, or parasitic placental infection during pregnancy; the mother becomes infected with HIV during the pregnancy and hence develops a high level of the virus for a short time; or the mother has a severe immune deficiency associated with AIDS.

Thus, maternal conditions—including untreated placental infections (particularly malaria), recent HIV infection, and advanced HIV disease—have been cited as risk factors for MTCT (41). Similarly, malnutrition during pregnancy may indirectly contribute to MTCT (42); however, one study suggests that vitamin A may increase the risk of vertical transmission (43).

HIV Transmission During Labor and Delivery

Infants of HIV-positive mothers are at great risk of becoming infected with HIV during childbirth. During this single event, 10% to 20% of newborns will acquire HIV infection if no steps are taken to prevent transmission. Most infants who become infected during labor and delivery do so by sucking, imbibing, or aspirating maternal blood or cervical secretions that contain HIV. Several factors—the duration of membrane rupture; acute chorioamnionitis (resulting from untreated infections, including sexually transmitted ones); and invasive delivery techniques that may breach the baby's and/or mother's skin, thus increasing the infant's contact with the mother's blood—have been associated with higher risks of MTCT during labor and delivery (40,41).

HIV Transmission Through Breastfeeding

HIV is present in breast milk, although in viral concentrations significantly lower than those found in blood (44). Studies using animal models suggest that cell-free HIV in breast milk could infect cells of the intestinal mucosa (45,46). M-cells, which are specialized epithelial cells found in the Payer's patches of the intestinal mucosa, may allow infectious agents such as HIV to cross the intact mucosa. M-cells engulf and transport the pathogen and present it to macrophages that indent the serosal surface of the M-cell (47). Results from in vitro studies on rabbit M cells suggest that HIV-1 particles could use M cells to cross the intestinal barrier (48). On average, about 15% of babies born to HIV-positive mothers will become infected through prolonged breastfeeding (24 months or more). This transmission risk is doubled when the mother becomes infected with the virus while breastfeeding (49). Seventy-five percent of infections among breastfed infants occurred before six months of age (50). In a recent study, multivitamin (B, C, and E) supplementation of breastfeeding mothers reduced child mortality and HIV-1 transmission through breastfeeding among immunologically and nutritionally compromised women (43).

Several studies suggest that the risk of MTCT through breastfeeding depends on a number of factors:
- The pattern of breastfeeding (babies who are exclusively breastfed may have a lower risk of becoming infected than those who are also fed with other liquids, milks, or solid foods in the first months of life) (51–53);
- Breast health (mastitis, cracked and bloody nipples, and other indications of breast inflammation are associated with higher risks of transmission);
- Breastfeeding duration;
- Maternal viral load (which is higher with recent infection or advanced disease in the mother);
- Maternal immune status; and
- Maternal nutritional status.

In developed countries, MTCT rates have fallen to as low as 2% of births among HIV-infected mothers with the introduction of HIV counseling and testing, zidovudine prophylaxis, elective Caesarean delivery, and the safe use of infant formula instead of breastfeeding (54). In Africa, however, where these interventions have generally not been available and where prolonged breastfeeding is the norm, about 25% to 35% of HIV-infected mothers pass the virus on to their infants (55). The severity of the MTCT problem in sub-Saharan Africa can be attributed to high rates of HIV infection in women of reproductive age, a large total population of women of reproductive age, high birth rates, and the lack of effective PMTCT interventions.

Table 16-1. Factors Associated with Increased Risk of Mother-to-Child Transmission of HIV		
	Strong Evidence	**Limited Evidence**
Viral	• High viral load • Viral characteristics	• Viral resistance
Maternal	• Advanced disease • Immune deficiency • HIV infection acquired during pregnancy or breastfeeding	• Vitamin A deficiency • Anemia • Chorioamnionitis • Sexually transmitted infections • Frequent unprotected sex • Multiple sexual partners • Smoking • Injection drug use
Obstetric	• Vaginal delivery • Rupture of the membranes for more than four hours	• Invasive or traumatic procedures • Instrumental deliveries • Amniocentesis • Episiotomy • External cephalic version • Intrapartum hemorrhage
Fetal/Neonatal	• Prematurity	• Lesions of the skin and/or mucus membrane (e.g., oral thrush) • Genetic
Breastfeeding	• Prolonged breastfeeding • Mixed feeding • Breast disease (abscess, mastitis, or cracked nipples)	

Determinants of MTCT

A range of factors have been implicated in MTCT. These have been categorized into viral, maternal, obstetric, fetal and neonatal, and breastfeeding factors (Table 16-1).

Viral Factors

Viral load is the most important determinant of MTCT as it correlates significantly with the risk of transmission both in women who have received treatment and those who have not. There is no level of maternal viral load (even when undetectable) below which transmission cannot occur; furthermore, there is no limit of maternal viremia above which MTCT will always occur (56). The risk of vertical transmission is very high when the mother acquires the infection during pregnancy or while breastfeeding. MTCT is also increased if the mother developed full-blown AIDS during pregnancy or breastfeeding.

The selection of drug-resistant mutants, particularly in the setting of zidovudine monotherapy, are independently associated with vertical transmission (57). Emergence of drug-resistant mutants have also been reported with nevirapine monotherapy (58), raising serious concerns about the use of ART monotherapy for perinatal prophylaxis.

A study on MTCT of different HIV-1 subtypes show that subtypes A, C, and intersubtype recombinants are more transmissible than subtype D (59). Among the multiple viral variants that are circulating in the infected mother's blood, in-utero transmission is often associated with the major maternal variant, whereas intrapartum transmission is associated with minor maternal viral variants (60), suggesting that yet unknown selective factors are involved in determining the pattern of viral transmission depending on the timing.

Maternal Factors

The presence of AIDS-defining illnesses or acute HIV disease, which correlates with a high level of viremia and lower CD4+ cell counts, is associated with higher risk of MTCT. In this case, a CD4+ count of around 350 is considered to mark the divide between women who are more or less likely to transmit the virus to their babies (61). A number of studies in tropical Africa have suggested that HIV-infected mothers coinfected with malaria are more likely to transmit HIV to their babies than malaria-negative HIV-infected mothers (62,63). Sexually transmitted infections (STIs) that cause lower genital tract mucosal inflammation increase vaginal shedding of HIV (64), thereby increasing the baby's exposure. Bacterial vaginosis and syphilis have been shown to increase risk of MTCT as well (65,66). Antiretroviral regimens can substantially reduce MTCT of HIV as monotherapy, double therapy, or highly active antiretroviral therapy (HAART) (67,68). Regimens that optimally reduce viral load are more effective in preventing MTCT (68,69), with a transmission rate of 1.1% reported in women receiving HAART (69).

Other maternal factors associated with increased risk of MTCT include unprotected sex with multiple sexual partners, substance abuse, and cigarette smoking (70,71).

Obstetric Factors

Obstetric procedures and conditions that breach the fetal barriers (placenta and amniotic membranes) are associated with increased risk of MTCT. These include abruption placentae, premature rupture of membranes, and chorioamnionitis (72,73). Meta-analysis from 15 prospective cohort studies examined the role of duration of ruptured membranes in perinatal transmission and showed that the likelihood of transmission increased linearly with increasing duration of ruptured membranes, with a 2% increase in risk for each hour increment. Women with clinical AIDS had the most pronounced increase in risk, with a 31% probability of vertical transmission after 24 hours of ruptured membranes (73).

Fetal and Neonatal Factors

Prematurity has been associated with increased risk for perinatal transmission of HIV (74). The cause is unknown but important fetal factors include an immature immune system and genetic susceptibility.

Some babies acquire cellular immunity to HIV before birth. A South African study found that HIV-1–specific T-helper cell responses detected at birth, presumably from in utero exposure, were present in more than one-third of uninfected infants born to HIV-infected mothers (75). These detectable immune responses appeared to provide complete protection against subsequent HIV transmission at delivery and through breastfeeding. The risk of MTCT has been shown to increase when baby and mother are concordant for class 1 human lymphocyte antigen (HLA) genotype, while the risk is low when there is discordance (76). Another genetic factor in the newborn that may confer natural resistance to HIV infection is a homozygous deletion in the CCR-5 receptor gene (77,78).

Breastfeeding-Related Factors

Seroconversion or acute HIV infection occurring in breastfeeding mothers has been reported to double the risk of MTCT to 29% (49), presumably because of the high viral load in the setting. Multivitamin (B, C, and E) supplementation of breastfeeding mothers reduced HIV-1 transmission through breastfeeding among immunologically and nutritionally compromised women (43), indicating that malnutrition may be an important determinant of MTCT. Malnutrition may further increase MTCT risk in resource-constrained settings. Risk of transmission is highest in the earliest months of breastfeeding; however, increased duration of breastfeeding increases risk (79,80). Other potential variables include the presence of cracked nipples or breast abscess, infant oral candidiasis, and the use of exclusive breastfeeding compared with mixed feeding. A randomized clinical trial that compared breastfeeding to formula feeding in Kenya found that formula feeding prevented 44% of infant infections and was associated with a significantly improved HIV-free survival (81).

Pediatric HIV Infection

As mentioned earlier, pediatric HIV infection is fast assuming a serious dimension in developing countries. In addition, the early death of mothers creates a large number of orphans and vulnerable children, many of whom succumb to AIDS or complications of other infections and malnutrition. This trend is eroding gains of child survival efforts of previous decades. For example, the infant mortality rate in Zimbabwe doubled from 30/1,000 to 60/1,000 between 1990 and 1996, while the under-five mortality increased from 8/1,000 to 20/1,000 (82).

Diagnosis of HIV/AIDS in infants can be done by laboratory tests, where available, or by observing AIDS symptoms. The standard HIV test measures HIV antibodies. However, infants born to HIV-infected mothers still carry their mother's antibodies in the blood even if the infants themselves are not infected, for up to 15 months. For this reason, standard HIV antibody tests cannot reliably confirm HIV infection in infants younger than 15 months. The PCR test, which *can* detect HIV much earlier in an infant's life, is prohibitively expensive for widespread use in most African settings. At present only four centers in Nigeria offer DNA PCR testing.

Disease progression in children who acquire HIV infection from their mothers is more rapid in Africa than in developed countries, probably because African children are exposed to early and multiple infections, have high rates of malnutrition and micronutrient deficiencies (83), and have limited access to health care. Recent studies have shown that at least one-third of HIV-infected children in developing countries die within the first year of life (84,85). In a Nigerian teaching hospital, most HIV-infected babies died before their first birthday (86).

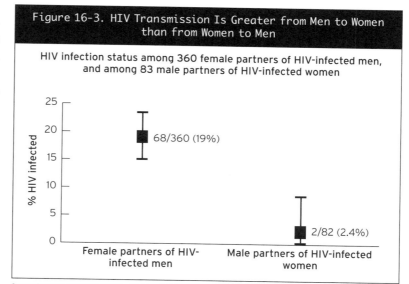

Figure 16-3. HIV Transmission Is Greater from Men to Women than from Women to Men

HIV infection status among 360 female partners of HIV-infected men, and among 83 male partners of HIV-infected women

68/360 (19%)

2/82 (2.4%)

% HIV infected

Female partners of HIV-infected men

Male partners of HIV-infected women

Source: Padian N, Shiboski S, Vittinghoff E, Glass S. Heterosexual transmission of HIV: results from a ten year study. *Am J Epidemiol*, 1997;146:350-357.

Susceptibility of Women

Women are particularly prone to acquiring HIV infection in developing countries because of a multiplicity of factors. For instance, rates of transmission are reported to be two to three times higher for male-to-female transmission than for female-to-male transmission (Figure 16-3) (87–89).

PREVENTION OF MOTHER-TO-CHILD TRANSMISSION OF HIV

In response to the global HIV/AIDS situation, governments, nongovernmental organizations, and international donors, especially the United Nation agencies (90), are now actively involved in the design and implementation of new programs that include essential PMTCT services, such as voluntary counseling and testing (VCT), infant feeding counseling, outreach to communities and families, and antiretroviral therapy. In most cases, the implementation approach has been to incorporate PMTCT into services that already reach pregnant women and women of childbearing age, such as family planning, antenatal care, obstetrical care, and maternal/child health. Many countries in Africa—including Nigeria—are now implementing a range of services to prevent MTCT.

The effectiveness of antiretroviral therapy and the availability of other preventive strategies make PMTCT an effective public health intervention. The outcomes of these interventions are clearly visible in many countries.

Components of a PMTCT Program

On a global scale, prevention of pediatric HIV is now four-pronged: primary prevention of HIV infection among women of childbearing age; prevention of unwanted pregnancies among HIV-infected women; prevention of HIV transmission from infected women to their infants; and care and support of infected women and their infants and families.

Primary Prevention of HIV Infection among Women of Childbearing Age

The best way to prevent HIV infection of children through MTCT, including transmission through breast milk, is to prevent HIV infection of young girls and women of childbearing age. About 70% of the global HIV burden is borne by sub-Saharan Africa, where the principal mode of HIV transmission is heterosexual contact (1). The prevention of HIV transmission among all women of childbearing age, especially adolescent girls, is therefore a major component of a comprehensive PMTCT program. One of the targets set at the United Nations General Assembly Special Session on HIV/AIDS (UNGASS) in 2001 was to ensure that at least 90% of young people should, by 2005, have the information, education, and services they need to defend themselves against HIV infection (91). Educational, behavioral, and cultural interventions should be directed at girls and young women to ensure delay of initiation of sexual activity. It is believed that combining such interventions will result in a significant reduction in heterosexual transmission of HIV, thus limiting the number of prospective women of childbearing age living with HIV.

The promotion of condoms either alone or combined with a more effective method of contraception for dual protection from HIV and other STIs and from unplanned pregnancy is an effective strategy to prevent HIV infection in all sexually active women. Dual protection messages are gradually being integrated into family planning counseling services in Nigeria (92). Other contributory prevention strategies include providing information about sexual health, prevention of STIs, and unwanted pregnancy; tackling livelihood issues; development of negotiation skills; and other life skills that reduce their vulnerability and increase their ability to negotiate safer sex (93,94). Reducing the prevalence and incidence of HIV in this cohort is a critical investment in their adult lives and in the subsequent reduction of pediatric HIV/AIDS.

The Nigerian PMTCT program that is based at the Federal Ministry of Health, unfortunately, has been unable to establish effective linkages with youth programs, which are currently being handled by the Ministry of Education, nongovernmental organizations, and donor agencies, such as the United Nations Population Fund and UNIFEM. Efforts should be made to harmonize PMTCT activities with prevention activities among youths through the National Action Committee on AIDS (NACA) and other implementing ministries and agencies.

Prevention of Unintended Pregnancies among HIV-Infected Women

Every woman has the fundamental right to decide, without coercion, whether to have children. The responsibility of the government and health services is to provide HIV-positive women and their partners with comprehensive information and education about the risks associated with childbearing as part of routine public information about HIV/AIDS, to ensure they have real choices of action, and to respect and support the decisions they reach. This means providing good quality, user-friendly, and easily accessible family planning services so that HIV-positive women can avoid pregnancy if they choose.

Women who choose replacement feeding because of their HIV infection should particularly receive advice on contraception to replace the birth-spacing effect of breastfeeding.

Most HIV-infected women in the developed world use some form of contraception, usually condoms (95). Anecdotal evidence suggests that this is not the case in Nigeria. Women who do not use contraception do not necessarily intend to become pregnant but may lack sufficient power in their sexual relationships, be under pressure from their partners or families to have children, be unaware of their contraceptive options, or believe they cannot become pregnant. They may also have a lifestyle that precludes consistent use of contraception, or simply have decided to take their chances. Unplanned pregnancy also does not necessarily mean unwanted. Some studies show low rates of elective pregnancy termination in HIV-positive women (96), and no significant difference in repeat pregnancy rates between HIV-positive women and HIV-negative ones (97).

The WHO recommends that efforts be made to increase the access of family planning clients to HIV counseling and testing, especially in high-prevalence settings, by integrating HIV counseling or HIV counseling and testing within family planning services or through links with external HIV counseling or testing services (98). This would allow family planning advice and services to be tailored to the specific HIV-risk situation and needs of clients. In this way, providers can best help uninfected women at risk stay uninfected by using dual protection. They can also identify women who are already infected and who require specific care and support services, including counseling on their reproductive choices.

Family planning strategies include:

- **Hormonal contraception.** Hormonal methods of contraception, particularly oral contraceptives, can have significant drug interactions, resulting in either decreased contraceptive effectiveness or increased or decreased concentrations of the co-administered antiretrovirals (ARVs). Use of nelfinavir, ritonavir, amprenavir, lopinavir/ritonavir (Kaletra®), and efavirenz may be associated with decreased effectiveness of oral contraceptives; therefore, an alternative or additional method should be used (99). Concerns have also been raised about a possible increased risk of HIV transmission or acquisition in hormonal contraceptive users. There is evidence that both combined oral contraceptives and progestin-only contraceptives may increase genital tract HIV shedding (64). Given their effectiveness, overall safety, and ease of use, hormonal methods of contraception remain an appropriate option for HIV-infected or at-risk women. Dual protection through consistent condom use should be promoted among these women.

- **Intrauterine contraceptive devices.** The use of intrauterine devices (IUDs) has been linked to increased susceptibility for HIV transmission (100), increased menstrual flow duration, and a foreign body inflammatory reaction, possibly contributing to transmission risk and anemia in HIV-positive women. IUD users are also at increased risk of developing pelvic inflammatory disease and acquiring other STIs and therefore HIV. For these reasons, HIV-infected women should generally avoid the IUD.

- **Spermicides.** Spermicides have in vitro activity against HIV and significant activity against gonorrhea and chlamydia; however, a study of a standard spermicidal dose of nonoxynol-9 (N-9) daily for one week found an increase in irritation, colposcopic and histological evidence of inflammation, and decreased numbers of vaginal lactobacilli in N-9 users, compared with placebo recipients (101). These findings raise concerns that regular use of spermicides may promote HIV transmission. A UNAIDS trial including women in Africa and Thailand found significantly higher HIV seroconversion rates in the N-9 group compared to the placebo group, as well as more frequent occurrence of genital ulcers (102).

- **Condoms.** Consistent condom use provides the best-known protection against sexual transmission of HIV and should be emphasized for all HIV-infected and at-risk women to decrease risk of transmission of HIV and other STIs. During client counseling, it is important to emphasize the dual protection property—prevention of pregnancy and prevention of STIs—of condom use. Condom use should be reinforced for HIV-positive or at-risk women even when prevention of pregnancy is not a concern.

Prevention of HIV Transmission from Infected Mothers to Babies

Specific interventions identified to prevent HIV transmission from an infected mother to her child include ARV use, safer delivery practices, and infant feeding counseling and support. Here too, VCT plays a key role in that HIV-infected women can learn their status as soon as possible to maximize the benefits of subsequent interventions. Among the key strategies are:

- **VCT for HIV in antenatal and labor ward settings.** VCT is a cost-effective intervention for reducing HIV-related risk behavior, particularly when it serves at-risk couples (103). The aim of VCT is to help the woman take necessary action to ensure that she does not become infected with HIV. If she is already infected, however, the aim is to help her protect her own health and the health of her unborn child, her sexual partner, and her other family members (104). PMTCT therefore needs VCT services for identifying women—and families—who may benefit from the interventions. In the absence of VCT services, most women in Africa have no definitive way to learn their HIV status until they themselves fall ill with identifiable symptoms of AIDS, or until they give birth to a baby who is diagnosed with, and dies from, HIV disease. In antenatal and labor ward settings, the Nigerian PMTCT guidelines (105) recommend routine offer of HIV testing, with the opportunity to decline. This is followed by one-on-one post-test counseling and is associated with a high uptake of testing. Availability of rapid testing allows women to be tested and receive their HIV test results at the first prenatal visit. When HIV status is known, mothers can be evaluated for ART eligibility and offered ART treatment and prophylaxis as indicated.

- **Antiretroviral use.** Optimal medical management during pregnancy should include ART to suppress plasma HIV-1 RNA to undetectable levels. A number of short-course ARV regimens—based on zidovudine (106), zidovudine/lamivudine (107), nevirapine (107), zidovudine/nevirapine (108), zidovudine/lamivudine/nevirapine (109), or combinations used in HAART—have been shown to be effective in reducing MTCT (110) in African settings (111). Based on the efficacy and safety of these drug regimens, the recent substantial reduction in cost, and improved availability, new guidelines for the use of ART to prevent MTCT in Nigeria have been formulated. In HIV-infected adults, ART is initiated based on several criteria. When the CD4+ cell count is available, ART is administered for people with WHO Stage IV disease irrespective of CD4+ cell count; WHO Stage III disease with CD4+ cell counts of less than 350/mm³; and WHO Stage I or II disease with CD4+ cell counts less than or equal to 200/mm³. When the CD4+ cell count is unavailable, ART is administered for people with WHO Stage IV disease irrespective of total lymphocyte count; WHO Stage III disease irrespective of total lymphocyte count; and WHO Stage II disease with a total lymphocyte count less than or equal to 1200/mm³. According to the recent Nigerian PMTCT guidelines, pregnancy in HIV-positive women is an indication for prophy-

Table 16-2. Antiretrovirals for Prevention of Mother-to-Child Transmission of HIV

| | HAART available | | | HAART not available | |
	Maternal HAART indicated	Maternal HAART considered[a]	Maternal HAART not yet indicated	Capacity to deliver full range of ARVs for PMTCT exists	Capacity to deliver only minimal range of ARVs for PMTCT exists (e.g., zidovudine not available)
	A	B	C		D
Mother					
Antepartum	HAART	HAART	Zidovudine starting at 28 weeks or as soon as feasible thereafter	–	
Intrapartum	HAART	HAART	Zidovudine + single dose nevirapine[b] Consider:[c] lamivudine	Single-dose nevirapine	
Postpartum	HAART	HAART	Consider:[c] zidovudine + lamivudine for 7 days	–	
Infant	Zidovudine for 7 days[d]	Zidovudine for 7 days[d]	Single dose nevirapine + zidovudine for 7 days[d]	Single-dose nevirapine	

Source: World Health Organization, *Antiretroviral Drugs and the Prevention of Mother-to-Child Transmission of HIV Infection in Resource-Limited Settings.* Accessed at www.who.int/entity/3by5/PMTCTreport_June2005.pdf.

Abbreviations: ARV: antiretroviral; HAART: highly active antiretroviral therapy; PMTCT: prevention of mother-to-child transmission of HIV

[a]**Maternal HAART considered:** the revised World Health Organization adult guidelines recommend HAART be considered for patients with clinical stage I and II with CD4+ cell counts below 350/mm³, particularly if closer to 200-250/mm³. Toxicity to the initiation of long-term nevirapine-containing HAART may be a concern in pregnant women with a CD4+ cell count between 250 and 350/mm³. However, recent data from resource-limited countries among pregnant and postpartum women in Africa and Thailand suggest a low toxicity associated with the use of nevirapine in this context. The expert consultation concluded that nevirapine-containing HAART can be considered in this subgroup, or alternatively a triple-NRTI regimen.

[b]**If the woman receives at least four weeks of zidovudine during pregnancy,** omission of maternal nevirapine dose may be considered.

[c]**If the woman is symptomatic and conditions to deliver the following interventions exist,** a seven-day tail of zidovudine + lamivudine given to the mother after delivery can be considered to reduce the emergence of nevirapine resistance and is advised if HAART is expected to be started soon after delivery.

[d]**If the mother receives less than four weeks of zidovudine or HAART during pregnancy,** infant zidovudine dosing should be extended to four weeks.

lactic ART irrespective of CD4+ count, viral load, or clinical stage of disease (105). Tables 16-2 and 16-3 summarize some of the PMTCT regimens recommended for HIV-positive pregnant women in resource-limited settings.

- **Safer delivery practices.** Labor and delivery management of HIV-infected pregnant women should focus on minimizing the risk for both perinatal transmission of HIV and the potential for maternal and neonatal complications. In non-HAART clinical settings, studies have consistently found that Caesarean delivery performed before onset of labor and rupture of membranes (elective or scheduled) was associated with a significant decrease in perinatal HIV transmission compared with other types of delivery, with reductions ranging from 55% to 80% (112,113). Current opinion recommends elective Caesarean delivery for HIV-infected pregnant women with RNA levels of greater than 1,000 copies/ml near the time of delivery (114). In resource-poor settings, Caesarean section is not accessible to many

Table 16-3. Women Presenting Around Delivery and Having Received no Antiretrovirals for Prevention of Mother-to-Child Transmission of HIV				
	Woman in labor, known to be HIV positive with no prior antiretroviral experience			No maternal ARV PMTCT prophylaxis
	Capacity to deliver full range of ARVs for PMTCT exists		Capacity to deliver only minimal range of ARVs for PMTCT exists (e.g., zidovudine not available)	
	Option 1	Option 2		
Mother				
Intrapartum	Single-dose nevirapine + zidovudine	Zidovudine + lamivudine	Single-dose nevirapine	–
Postpartum		Zidovudine + lamivudine for 7 days	–	–
Infant		Zidovudine + lamivudine for 7 days	Single-dose nevirapine	Single-dose nevirapine + zidovudine for 4 weeks

Source: World Health Organization, *Antiretroviral Drugs and the Prevention of Mother-to-Child Transmission of HIV Infection in Resource-Limited Settings.* Accessed at www.who.int/entity/3by5/PMTCTreport_June2005.pdf.

Abbreviations: ARV: Antiretroviral; PMTCT: prevention of mother-to-child transmission of HIV

Note: In all cases, mothers need to be assessed postpartum for need for therapy.

because of cost, limited availability, and the risk of complications. Invasive obstetrical procedures—such as artificial rupture of membranes, fetal scalp monitoring, and episiotomy—may increase the risk of transmission to the infant. Therefore, their use should be limited to cases of absolute necessity.

- **Infant feeding counseling and support.** All HIV-infected mothers should receive counseling that includes information about the risks and benefits of various infant feeding options and specific guidance in selecting the most suitable option. When replacement feeding is acceptable, feasible, affordable, sustainable, and safe, HIV-infected mothers are advised to avoid breastfeeding. Otherwise, exclusive breastfeeding is recommended during the infant's first months of life. To minimize the risk of HIV transmission, breastfeeding should be discontinued as soon as feasible, taking into account local circumstances, the individual woman's situation, and the risks of replacement feeding. All forms of mixed feeding should be avoided because of associated higher rates of MTCT. Data from the pilot PMTCT centers in Nigeria show that more than 90% of mothers choose breast milk substitutes in sites where the milk is donated.

Provision of Care and Support to HIV-Infected Women, Their Infants, and Their Families

Poverty often compounds the problems of HIV-affected children and families. The impact of AIDS on children may include loss of family and identity, sexual abuse and exploitation, loss of health status, homelessness, exposure to HIV infection, decreased access to and reduced quality of education, increased malnutrition and starvation, and higher rates of infant and under-five mortality.

The impact of AIDS on families and households may include: the emergence of child- or adolescent-headed households; separation of siblings; child abandonment; stress and long-term pathologies; demoralization; poor parental care for children; and female-headed households.

The provision of care and support through PMTCT Plus initiatives has become critical in trying to mitigate these potential impacts of AIDS on children and families. As the prices of ARVs decrease and more resources become available through donor support, PMTCT Plus is expanding rapidly across countries in sub-Saharan Africa. The various elements of care in PMTCT Plus include: health care for adults and children living with HIV/AIDS; early diagnosis of infant HIV-infection status; clinical and immune monitoring; prevention of opportunistic infections; ART; education and counseling; adherence support; social, psychological, and spiritual support; outreach and community linkage; retention in long-term care; and prevention of transmission to others.

In Nigeria, the government's plans to alleviate poverty through skills acquisition and micro-credit schemes are ongoing; however, it is the greater than 90% subsidy on ARVs to support treatment and prevention programs that has the most direct impact on the HIV/AIDS epidemic. Many HIV-infected people are coming out to receive affordable treatment and PMTCT interventions. Access to affordable and effective treatment should gradually transform the perception of HIV/AIDS as a death sentence to that of a treatable chronic disease, with an attendant reduction in stigma.

The Objectives and Strategies of PMTCT

The Nigerian national goal of PMTCT, as stated in the 2003 National Policy on HIV/AIDS, is to reduce MTCT by 50% by 2010 and to increase access to quality confidential counseling and testing services by 50% by that same year (105). Among the specific objectives are:

- To reduce MTCT by 50% by 2010;
- To reduce the prevalence of risky behavior that promotes transmission of HIV among women, their partners, and their children by 30% by 2005;
- To increase demand and uptake for VCT among women of reproductive age by 10% by 2005;
- To prevent unintended pregnancy among HIV-positive women by 50% by 2005;
- To improve access to safe delivery practices for HIV-positive mothers and to ART for HIV-positive mothers and their children;
- To increase support for HIV-positive mothers to practice the infant feeding options of their choice; and
- To improve access of HIV-positive mothers and their families to appropriate care and support.

To achieve these objectives, program administrators are addressing a number of programmatic outputs: administration and coordination of PMTCT; establishment of VCT services in antenatal care settings; community sensitization and support mobilization; provision of a comprehensive care package to pregnant mothers (including infant follow-up); establishment of a system for monitoring and evaluating PMTCT interventions; establishment of a logistics and supplies system; funding; and definitions of the stakeholders' roles. Among the specific activities in support of this work are universal VCT; administration of ARVs to HIV-positive mothers and their infants as stipulated in the PMTCT protocol; infant feeding counseling and support; modification of obstetrical practices; follow-up of babies of HIV-positive mothers; care and support to HIV-positive mothers; and referrals to reproductive health services.

National PMTCT Indicators

Between 2002 and 2004, the Nigerian National PMTCT Task Team, the Federal Ministry of Health (FMOH), and other stakeholders identified a series of indicators to make sound decisions about the status of the national PMTCT program. In addition to identifying specific indicators, several data collection instruments, including several registers and summary forms, were developed and printed for national PMTCT sites. Instruction manuals for completion of the registers and summary forms were developed and made available for distribution with the bound registers. Furthermore, a computerized management information system (MIS) and comprehensive training curriculum for PMTCT data collection and reporting was developed in 2004 in collaboration with the U.S. Centers for Disease Control and Prevention (CDC) and the Institute of Human Virology at the University of Maryland. All 11 first-generation PMTCT centers were provided with computers, the PMTCT-MIS, the training curriculum and manuals, and the national PMTCT program registers and summary forms at a centralized training conducted in Abuja in September 2004. The FMOH maintains the central MIS database and provides technical assistance to the PMTCT sites for continued monitoring of the PMTCT program.

Indicators for the national PMTCT program include the number of pregnant women who receive pretest counseling as well as the number of women who register for antenatal care at the selected program sites, access information on PMTCT/VCT during pregnancy, are tested for HIV during pregnancy or at labor/delivery, return for their HIV test results and receive post-test counseling, test positive for HIV, and receive ART. Other indicators include the number of babies who received prophylactic ART syrup, were fed exclusively from infant formula, were exclusively breastfed, are on mixed feeding, or tested positive for HIV at birth and at 15 months.

CHALLENGES OF PMTCT IN DEVELOPING COUNTRIES

The implementation of a PMTCT project poses special challenges in developing countries with fragile infrastructures and a lack of human and financial resources. The problems are further compounded by a weak political commitment, denial, poverty, sociocultural factors, and illiteracy. The HIV/AIDS epidemic across sub-Saharan Africa remains grave and portends serious social and economic upheaval. In reviewing the situation in South Africa, Bell, et al. cautioned that if nothing is done to combat the HIV/AIDS epidemic, the economy will completely collapse within three generations, as AIDS decimates the workforce, creates large numbers of orphans (who cannot educate themselves), exacerbates poverty and inequality, and puts tremendous pressure on health and social services (115). The most active sector of the Nigerian economy—banking and finance—was found to be hardest hit, as 20% of wives of bankers tested HIV positive in our recent study of risk factors in pregnant women (116), further demonstrating the vulnerability of the economy in a "do-nothing" scenario.

Poor Knowledge of HIV/AIDS

The Behavioral Surveillance Survey conducted in Nigeria showed poor knowledge of HIV/AIDS among pregnant women and health practitioners (117). Many of the pregnant women who exhibited good knowledge about HIV/AIDS had poor knowledge of MTCT. Thirty-two percent (32.6%) of health workers were afraid of people with HIV, while 57.6% suggested that people with HIV/AIDS should be hospitalized. Moreover, there was a clear lack of congruence between the wish of most HIV-positive pregnant women to breastfeed and the formula feeding option currently recommended by health workers. While most patients preferred vaginal births, this was recommended by only 57.7% of health workers. Caesarean section is not readily available in rural areas, where most Nigerians live. The cost of Caesarean birth is prohibitive, and a strong cultural aversion to the procedure persists. Seventy percent of health workers advised HIV-positive pregnant women to avoid subsequent pregnancies. The findings demonstrated an urgent need for training of health care workers and education of women before and during pregnancy.

The Need for Universal Precautions

A major contributing factor to the discriminatory attitude of health care providers is the poor state of the health care system. The services are characterized by chronic shortages of essential protective equipment. PMTCT programs require disposable protective items, facilities for sterilization, and safe handling of body fluids and sharps. There is also a clear need to train health care workers on the essentials of universal precautions. To this end, several tertiary health institutions have developed infection prevention policies through the initiatives of nongovernmental organizations. Recently developed national training curricula for PMTCT, VCT, and ART have sufficiently addressed universal precaution issues. What must now be secured is sustainable funding for the implementation of training plans and provision of the necessary consumables and equipment in health care settings.

The Consequences of Stigmatization

Despite more than 20 years of research and education on HIV/AIDS, there continues to be significant global stigmatization and discrimination against people infected with HIV. Stigmatization and discrimination remain a major fact of life for an estimated 29.4 million people living with HIV in sub-Saharan Africa. As mentioned earlier, women make up the majority of HIV-infected people aged 15 to 49 years old who live in the region — 57%, or 13.5 million (1). Women's vulnerability to HIV is linked to gender issues as well as poverty, lack of economic opportunities, and limited access to education, information, and services. Similarly, stigmatization and discrimination are linked to existing inequities and stereotypes, including racism, poverty, intolerance, and inequality between men and women. As such, the most affected are already the most disadvantaged. There is widespread stigmatization and discrimination toward HIV-infected women in the household, within communities, and in health care institutions.

Nigeria's National Policy on HIV/AIDS recognizes that stigmatization and discrimination facing people infected and affected by HIV/AIDS are significant challenges (118). It prescribes confidential pre- and post-test counseling services and proscribes mandatory testing; however, the policy falls short of issuing sanctions against such acts or providing strategic solutions to the problem. In a similar document, the Swazi national AIDS program (119) developed a strategic framework to guide a broad-based, national response that focuses on three areas: risk reduction (for infection); response management (for care, treatment, and support of those affected); and impact mitigation (to address the far-reaching effects of the epidemic on Swazi society). Under response management, the plan is to address stigmatization and discrimination to create a better environment for people with the virus. The strategies for accomplishing this include passing non-discrimination legislation; developing policies to protect the rights of people with HIV/AIDS; educating communities to support those with the virus; ensuring that those who are affected receive counseling; and training community volunteers to provide care, support, and counseling.

The Need for Voluntary Counseling and Testing

VCT represents the cornerstone of the PMTCT program. In our setting, it is desirable for all pregnant women to receive counseling while testing is made voluntary. This is the basis for the new concept of universal counseling and confidential testing. If ART is to become available, and if a pregnant woman must decide whether she needs it, she must first know and understand the implications of her HIV status. VCT is therefore considered an essential element of services for women in antenatal clinics. In our setting, where men play a key role in the decision-making process, couples counseling is also highly desirable.

Our experiences, as well as reports from other countries, have shown that VCT programs are acceptable to African women in the antenatal setting (120). The movement away from compulsory HIV testing in many facilities thus necessitates immediate, comprehensive training in VCT.

It also must be emphasized that, although women may be seronegative at the time of testing, they may still be vulnerable to subsequent HIV if they do not know the status of their partners or if their partners have other sexual partners. VCT, when properly conducted, has been shown to contribute to an increase in safer sexual behavior at the individual level, and is also likely to reduce the ignorance, fear, and stigma associated with HIV infection in the population at large. HIV counseling and testing in relation to pregnancy and other reproductive health services may prove a valuable entry point for provision of VCT to the wider community of healthy and asymptomatic women and their partners. Certain settings—such as STI clinics, pediatric services, and family planning clinics—may provide an opportunity to offer testing to potential mothers and fathers, while antenatal services allow testing to be offered to women who are already pregnant (121).

Voluntary HIV testing of pregnant women must be confidential and undertaken with informed consent and access to ongoing counseling. Whenever possible, partners should also be counseled and offered VCT. Up to 25% of couples in some developing countries have been found to have serodiscordant HIV results. For these serodiscordant couples, advice about preventing HIV transmission through safer sexual practices has been shown to significantly reduce the rate of transmission to the uninfected partner. In addition, women alone will often be unable to make decisions with financial implications for the family, such as infant feeding decisions. Furthermore, measures to reduce MTCT, especially the avoidance of breastfeeding, make it virtually impossible for HIV-positive women to keep their infection a secret from their families and people in the wider community.

ART in Pregnancy

A breakthrough in the global fight against HIV/AIDS occurred in 1994, when the Pediatric AIDS Clinical Trials Group (PACTG) 076 study in the United States and France demonstrated that zidovudine, an ARV active against HIV, could reduce the risk of MTCT by nearly 70% (67,122). At the International AIDS Conference in Yokohama, Japan, where the announcement was made, a young British HIV-positive woman could not contain her joy. She burst into tears, crying, "You mean I will be able to cuddle my own baby?" Suddenly many HIV-positive couples had hope.

The impressive results of PACTG 076 demonstrated the efficacy of zidovudine in reducing perinatal transmission of HIV. Although conducted in a non-breastfeeding population, it gave hope and stimulated further research into the use of ARVs in preventing mother-to-child transmission. The high cost and the complex dosing regimen also led to the search for cheaper and simpler options and trials of modified zidovudine regimens. These included the modified Thai regimen in which pregnant HIV-positive women were given a four-to-five-week course of zidovudine and provided with safe alternatives to breast milk. The regimen showed that the risk of mother-to-child transmission could be halved, from 18% to 9% (106). Other trials included the CDC-sponsored short-course oral zidovudine trial in Côte d'Ivoire (123) and DITRAME, a short-course oral zidovudine trial in Côte d'Ivoire and Burkina Faso (124). The drawback for these alternative regimens was the absence of a postpartum arm, except for DITRAME, which included an ultra-short postpartum arm of one week. In these breastfeeding populations, the reductions of transmission were 37% and 38%, respectively.

Similarly, the PETRA randomized trial in South Africa, Tanzania, and Uganda used a combination of two ARVs to prevent MTCT. Results showed that when an HIV-positive mother began a combined zidovudine/lamivudine regimen and her newborn also received a postpartum regimen for one week, the chances of the infant becoming infected were reduced 37% (125). As additional studies were conducted (126–128), PMTCT interventions became routine in developed countries, with a short course of combination ART given to the mother, along with enhanced obstetrics practices, short-course postpartum ART for infants, and breast milk substitutes (129).

Subsequently, the HIVNET 012 trial compared peripartum oral zidovudine with nevirapine for mother-infant pairs. Nevirapine had an efficacy of 47% (130,131). The main advantages of nevirapine are its simplicity of dosing and its availability at little or no cost, especially in developing countries with no active donation program. Patients on chronic therapy with nevirapine-containing regimens have been noted to develop non-specific signs and symptoms such as rash, fatigue, malaise, anorexia, nausea, jaundice, and increased transaminases (ALT and AST) (132). The overall risk of hepatic events was 4% (133), while severe or life-threatening rash occurred in approximately 2% of patients receiving nevirapine (134). With single-dose regimens, however, these complications were minimal.

Available data from clinical trials in more than 1,600 mother-infant pairs indicate that single-dose nevirapine prophylaxis to prevent MTCT has had no significant toxicity for either women or their babies. There is grave concern, however, about the development of resistance to nevirapine and other non-nucleoside reverse transcriptase inhibitors (NNRTIs) (135–137). The detection of nevirapine-resistant mutations in women or infected infants exposed to single-dose nevirapine may have clinical significance in terms of response to future NNRTI–containing ART or the potential for transmission of nevirapine-resistant virus to the infant or sexual partners. Concern has also been expressed that transient resistance associated with single-dose nevirapine used for prophylaxis in pregnant women would affect the prevalence of nevirapine resistance in the general population through potential sexual transmission of nevirapine-resistant virus and possibly compromise the efficacy of NNRTI-based regimens on a population basis.

The use of combination ART has not been shown to have adverse effects on pregnancy (138,139). Neurological adverse events were reviewed in infants exposed to zidovudine/lamivudine or placebo in the PETRA study; no increased risk of adverse neurological events was observed in infants exposed to zidovudine/lamivudine compared with placebo (140).

The emerging consensus in the developed world is that pregnant women should receive combination ART for maternal health and well-being and for chemoprophylaxis to reduce mother-to-child transmission of HIV (141). As the costs of ART fall further and national governments become more financially committed, the use of combination ART for treatment should become more feasible in countries across sub-Saharan Africa.

Infant Feeding

Breastfeeding is the norm in Nigeria, despite the inherent danger of transmitting HIV infection. Because breastfeeding is exceedingly common and is socially acceptable, deviation from the practice is not only frowned upon, but it also raises suspicion among in-laws and family members. A woman not breastfeeding her child may suffer significant stigmatization and discrimination.

In Nigeria, the family structure has different layers of decision-making. Sometimes the woman requires the concurrence of her husband or in-laws before she can make such a decision as formula feeding her baby. Our experience suggests that many women who opted to formula feed during prenatal counseling sessions often reneged at the point of implementing their decisions, or they opted to mix feed to please their family members. The cost of breast milk substitutes is another major concern, as many HIV-infected women cannot afford to buy formula.

Formula feeding in the Nigerian setting has its own associated risks. In many areas, there is poor sanitation, a lack of proper energy sources for cooking, and a lack of clean water. Under these conditions, there are significant problems associated with the hygienic preparation of breast milk substitutes. Replacement feeding is often associated with high incidences of diarrhea, respiratory diseases, and malnutrition, all of which are common causes of morbidity and mortality among infants. Thus, apart from the resistance to change from breastfeeding to replacement feeding, there is the additional need to overcome identified risks associated with formula. Activities that support partner disclosure and strengthen breast milk substitute supply and use should substantially bolster ongoing PMTCT programs.

Coutsoudis, et al. have suggested that exclusive breastfeeding in the first three months of life may carry a lower risk of HIV transmission than mixed feeding (51). The WHO recommends that when replacement feeding is acceptable, feasible, affordable, sustainable, and safe, HIV-infected mothers should avoid breast-feeding; otherwise, exclusive breastfeeding is recommended during the infant's first months of life (142). HIV-infected mothers should receive counseling to aid in selecting their option and follow-up counseling, perhaps at the infant welfare clinics, after delivery to help them maintain their decision. Finally, De Cock, et al. have suggested that "perhaps the most feasible strategy for reducing breastfeeding-related transmission in resource-poor settings would be to combine several weeks to months of postnatal ARV prophylaxis of HIV-exposed infants with weaning at about six months" (33). However, this suggestion, along with administration of triple ART to mothers, requires further study.

Cultural Issues

Culture plays an important role in the dynamics of MTCT. In southwestern Nigeria, family members, especially mothers and mothers-in-law, wield substantial powers as to the outcome of serodiscordant relationships (143). HIV infection is a potential source of separation and divorce in these unions. In polygamous settings, one infection in a family can lead to another. The death of a husband often sows the seeds of poverty in a family as the widow may be dispossessed of her husband's property.

THE NIGERIAN PMTCT PROGRAM

Nigeria did not implement PMTCT until July 2002 because, in the face of unstable polity and the quest for democratic reforms, HIV prevention did not become a high priority for the government until 2001, when the national seroprevalence hit 5.8% (8). The projections from the findings of this survey highlighted the grave social and economic consequences of the epidemic in a do-nothing scenario and served as a wake-up call. By starting late, Nigeria stood to learn from the experiences of other countries where UNICEF had implemented PMTCT in collaboration with other UN agencies, the national governments, the U.S. Agency for International Development (USAID), and its implementing partners. UNICEF was one of the few agencies that prompted the implementation of PMTCT in Nigeria. Between conception in 2001 and the final launch in 2002, a joint proposal was developed and partners were recruited alongside the Federal Ministry of Health and UNICEF. Early subscribers to the program included the AIDS Prevention Initiative in Nigeria (APIN), a program of Harvard School of Public Health; the CDC; and other partners including the POLICY Project, Family Health International, the Centre for Development and Population Activities, the United Nations Population Fund, WHO, and Johns Hopkins University.

Although conceived as a pilot project in six tertiary health institutions, eleven such institutions now offer PMTCT services. The goal of the pilot project was to generate information for the formulation of a national policy and implementation guidelines for a comprehensive PMTCT intervention in Nigeria, while the purpose was to provide effective PMTCT services for women of reproductive age in selected reproductive health facilities in Nigeria. UNICEF, APIN, and CDC are providing material and financial resources, technical assistance, capacity building, and site coordination to the project. The National AIDS and STD Control Program of the FMOH coordinates the project. The implementing agencies also form two bodies: the National Task Team on PMTCT and the Core Partners Forum on PMTCT. The National Task Team provides technical know-how, continuous guidance for proper implementation, and advice to the government, while the Core Partners Forum is a platform for project coordination, resource mobilization, and sharing of implementation experiences.

Strategic Options

By the beginning of 2002, Nigeria had begun implementing its HIV/AIDS Emergency Action Plan (HEAP) (144) under a multisectoral approach, with NACA coordinating the national response. This plan states, "NACA and its implementers will focus on developing a strategy to support efforts to prevent HIV transmission between mothers and their children." It fell short of mentioning the use of ARVs as a potential therapeutic strategy and thereby effectively limited itself to primary prevention of HIV among women of childbearing age and the training of health workers. HEAP did, however, reiterate that NACA and its partners would need to address the logistics and procurement issues for ART and medical supplies. Unfortunately, it took NACA and the FMOH some time to identify their respective roles in a multisectoral approach that required the FMOH to loosen its grip on HIV/AIDS prevention interventions, which had hitherto been within its purview alone. The 2003 National Policy on HIV/AIDS (118) clearly filled the gap by declaring that Nigeria would place the highest possible priority on ensuring nationwide access to ARVs for all pregnant women with HIV. This document also identified the policy instrument for achieving its objectives on PMTCT and specifically addressed program details. It also prescribed universal access to VCT for all women of childbearing age in antenatal clinics throughout the country and set a policy target of reducing MTCT 50% by the year 2010. This seems to be in consonance with the UNGASS declaration that established specific goals of reduction of the proportion of infants infected with HIV by 20% by 2005 and by 50% by 2010 (91).

Nigeria was ripe for commencement of a PMTCT program for several reasons. By 2001, the HIV prevalence rate was 5.8% (8), and the country's total fertility rate for 2000–2005 was estimated as 5.4 (118), with only 42% of births attended to by health workers. Among West African countries, Nigeria has the highest number of people living with HIV/AIDS—estimated at four to six million. These conditions could promote unbridled pediatric HIV infection through MTCT in a large population of women of childbearing age. According to the National Population Commission, women of childbearing age constitute 25% of Nigeria's total population.

Many factors hindered initiation of the program, however. The human and institutional capacity to start the program was lacking. Most of the country's public health institutions suffered from gross decay. No government institution offered VCT services, although nongovernmental organizations ran a small number of VCT centers. In terms of resources for implementing the program, an unhealthy rivalry between the FMOH — the oversight ministry under the multisectoral approach — and NACA meant that FMOH was not sure what the source of funding would be. Second, in the timeline for implementing HEAP, PMTCT was to be introduced at a later time than what the FMOH was proposing. The ray of hope for funding the program was, however, the initial support from UNICEF for six centers and the announcement of the first set of grants from the Global Fund for HIV/AIDS, Tuberculosis and Malaria, worth more than US$27 million.

Finally, because of the complexity of the program itself, UNAIDS identified a number of strategic options for countries implementing PMTCT. Among those the planning team considered were the following:

- According to UNAIDS, the seroprevalence of HIV in the country or community will determine the cost of inaction. The advantages of having a PMTCT program in Nigeria outweigh whatever the disadvantages might be. Inaction will probably create a high burden of HIV-infected children with the consequential burden of providing care for them. Unfortunately, high prevalence rates themselves were not used to select the sites for the pilot. Subsequently, the states with the highest burden of HIV infection were not considered in the choice of centers.

- FMOH and its partners made the decision to pilot PMTCT in university teaching hospitals instead of the primary and secondary levels of health care provision in the country (145). This decision was contrary to other UNICEF-assisted centers in Africa. The arguments for the choice are multiple: in Nigeria, all tiers of government are constitutionally required to provide and control health care services concurrently. The federal government has power over university teaching hospitals and federal medical centers, while the state and local governments have authority over state hospitals and primary health centers, respectively. The university teaching hospitals therefore became the centers for implementing PMTCT, as the program was a federal effort. Policy makers at the FMOH level also argue that in terms of human resources, the teaching hospitals have the best mix and types of professionals that can be quickly trained and used later in training at lower levels for the purposes of scaling up PMTCT. The choice of the initial centers and subsequent ones was based on geopolitical considerations, which was unfortunate, as some of the states most affected by HIV/AIDS — such as Cross River, Benue, and Akwa Ibom — still do not have PMTCT services.

- The stigma of AIDS has posed a serious problem for HIV prevention efforts in Nigeria. With the advent of ART, however, HIV infection is becoming considered less a fatal condition than a chronic one, and HIV-positive couples would welcome the introduction of a lifesaving intervention for their children.

- Infant feeding continues to be a difficult issue in Nigeria. In the past few decades, exclusive breastfeeding under the Baby Friendly Hospital Initiative has been heavily promoted among nursing mothers in Africa, and the practice has become entrenched. It was therefore apparent that a pilot project would be needed initially so lessons could be learned about how to make replacement feeding acceptable and safe. The decision whether to breastfeed the infants was to be the exclusive choice of parents after the mother received nutritional counseling.

- Another strategic consideration for the program hinged on resources. The pilot was initially limited to six sites with the hope of expansion when more funds were available. This became reality when APIN and the CDC became partners in the enterprise and more sites began the program.

- Lastly, the choice of ARVs to be used in this pilot program is extremely important. The initial proposal was written with zidovudine as the preferred drug. However, the HIVNET 012 results have suggested that nevirapine might be a better drug for resource-poor settings. Coupled with Boehringer Ingelheim Pharmaceuticals' willingness to donate the drug, the planning team selected nevirapine (130). Nevirapine is an NNRTI with a prolonged half-life that rapidly crosses the placenta and is secreted into breast milk (146,147). The simple regimen consists of a single dose of nevirapine given to the mother at the onset of labor and a treatment suspension to the neonate within 72 hours of delivery.

The program began in July 2002, and all stakeholders did a review of the program after 18 months of implementation. Although logistical problems hindered implementation, the review showed that the program has been well instituted in eight of the eleven institutions, and two were in the top grade. The sites that did not fully implement the program lacked necessary supplies of test kits and consumables. The implementation followed the national guidelines on PMTCT with periodic review performed by the National Task Team and the Core Partners Forum. In all, more than 22,973 women had benefited from the program in terms of health education and group counseling, while about 58% received individual counseling. Forty-four percent of the total number accepted testing, and the HIV prevalence ranged from 3.4% to 11.9%. Nevirapine use among HIV-positive women was less than 60% and delivery in certain hospitals was only 55%. About 40% of the women did not deliver in a hospital, so nevirapine use could not be ascertained. In addition, follow-up of mother-infant pairs was extremely difficult as mothers were uncooperative because of the stigma of AIDS. Most of the infants are still younger than 18 months; however, follow-up in one of the top performing hospitals showed 10 infected children out of 109 — a transmission rate of 9.1%. The prospects are bright, and the coordinating bodies are working assiduously toward the success of the program. However, scaling up requires tremendous efforts in resources, capacity building, and a strong political will in establishing good policies.

RELATING FINDINGS, CONSTRAINTS, AND LESSONS LEARNED TO POLICIES

By design, most of the states currently benefiting from the national PMTCT program are those with a low HIV prevalence. This may have contributed to poor recruitment of infected women in some centers and raises concern regarding the strategic choice of using geopolitical consideration for allocating the centers. For example, the high-prevalence states of Akwa Ibom, Benue, and Cross River, whose prevalence rates range from 7.2% to 12%, have no access to the program and in some cases the nearest center for women who live in those states is hundreds of kilometers away.

Second, the costs of delivery and laboratory services in the teaching hospitals are generally high for the average Nigerian family, coupled with the fact that most people infected with and affected by HIV are of low socioeconomic status. Hence, the group that needs these services most is not being reached. In other instances, women were diagnosed with HIV and received adequate counseling and nevirapine tablets at

34 weeks; however, many did not come back to deliver their babies in the teaching hospitals, because they could not afford the delivery cost. While some returned within the stipulated 72 hours for their babies' nevirapine, a small proportion of the women were lost to follow-up. Therefore, determining the success or failure of the program becomes challenging, as the HIV status of some of the children cannot be determined.

Finally, Nigeria already has an estimated one million HIV-infected women who need PMTCT services. This pilot has provided access to less than 1% of the women who require the services; hence, the need for scale up of services to secondary-level hospitals, mission and private hospitals, and primary health care centers is urgent. To meet the UNGASS and the 2003 National Policy on HIV/AIDS goal of reducing MTCT by 50% by 2010, Nigeria will need a massive scale up of the program.

Scale up should be by decentralization and public-private partnership—both vertical and horizontal. Nigeria has functional decentralization in the health sector from the federal government to the state and local governments, with each tier of government having control over tertiary, secondary, and primary health care services, respectively. Each tier of governance should be encouraged to take up the challenge of implementing PMTCT services. Similarly, it will be necessary for the government to work in partnership with the private health sector, particularly faith-based organizations and other nongovernmental organizations that have expressed interest in starting or have started their own MTCT programs. Government can provide an enabling environment through such means as guidelines, training manuals, and other incentives in terms of training, supervisory visits, and coordination. The FMOH, in a horizontal fashion, should expand services to additional teaching hospitals and the federal medical centers not covered in the ongoing program.

According to UNAIDS, the ability to make PMTCT interventions widely available as quickly as possible depends on political will, the affordability of the interventions, and the strength of existing human resources and infrastructures (148). In Nigeria, human resource requirements can be met only with intensive and purposeful capacity-building using existing training institutions and the critical mass of professionals that were trained during the pilot period. However, there is also a need for a national human resource plan to forecast any human resource needs for the entire HIV/AIDS health sector response.

Most of the 11 centers have been able to establish good VCT services. Importantly, having good VCT services encourages uptake of both VCT and PMTCT, as does the training of physicians, laboratory scientists, and pharmacists. Such training efforts can lead to the development of a critical mass of professionals who can serve as trainers for the next generation of professionals needed as Nigeria continues to scale up its intervention efforts in the next few years. The FMOH is planning to train 2,000 VCT master trainers and 500 PMTCT master trainers using the recently developed national training curricula. These master trainers will be distributed across Nigeria's six geopolitical zones and will help to develop the human resources needed.

Similarly, with regard to the repair and rehabilitation of infrastructures for effective clinical performance, the institutions participating in the PMTCT program have improved infrastructures in order to implement the program. In most cases, laboratories were rehabilitated with the addition of new equipment and technologies, including automated CD4+ estimation machines, facilities for viral load estimation, and PCR facilities. Most labor rooms have been renovated, and equipment has now been supplied, so universal precautions can be taken. Provisions were made for post-exposure prophylaxis (PEP), and in most instances the program stimulated the institutions into having an HIV workplace policy and continuous HIV/AIDS education for health workers. At present, few health institutions—perhaps 5% nationally—offer PEP services.

Affordability is a critical issue for scaling up PMTCT programs nationwide. Can Nigeria truly afford the cost of rapid expansion of PMTCT services? Several factors affect the affordability of PMTCT interventions, including not only the expense of ARVs, but also the costs associated with safe alternatives to breastfeeding, facility upgrading and personnel, HIV tests, personnel training, and monitoring and evaluation efforts. Currently, health care financing is borne by the government at all levels, but a significant proportion is obtained from user fees while health insurance is just kicking off. The government, however, supplements its share of the fund with donor contributions. For the pilot study, most of the funds came from UNICEF, the Bill & Melinda Gates Foundation through APIN, and lately the U.S. government. For the scale up, the federal government already has commitments from the Global Fund and the U.S. President's Emergency Plan for AIDS Relief, or PEPFAR. The user-fee mechanism will also be highly useful when it comes to the cost of delivery; the cost of safe alternatives to breastfeeding (even now it is borne in some cases by the patients); and follow up. Again, a thorough forecast of fund requirements for the scale up of services required by the country will significantly aid in further resource mobilization.

ETHICAL ISSUES IN PMTCT

With particular reference to PMTCT, ethical issues have been raised about the introduction of ART programs for PMTCT in countries where ARVs are not available (149). Some of the concerns are:

- If a mother's access to ARVs is limited to the period of pregnancy and labor, does this amount to treating the mother for the sake of her baby alone?
- Certain PMTCT interventions might encourage the development of drug-resistant strains of HIV.
- In the absence of care and treatment for parents, PMTCT interventions might exacerbate the problem of orphaned children, increasing the burden of care on families and society.
- Is there a place for sterilization of HIV-infected women when we know that they could still infect their partners through unprotected sexual intercourse?
- What reproductive options do serodiscordant couples have?
- The lopsided distribution of PMTCT sites raises serious equity and access issues.

A key principle of health care holds that any measure taken should be in the interests of both the mother and the baby. A useful analogy is the rubella vaccine given to pregnant women to protect their offspring from the ill effects of maternal infection. Rubella vaccination does not meet with ethical objections, despite the fact that it, too, could be seen as treating the mother for the sake of the baby. The issue of ART for HIV-infected people must be considered separately from the issue of ART for prevention of MTCT. It requires debate and policy decisions outside the scope of MTCT policy-making. When adopting ART and replacement feeding, however, it becomes a point of principle that HIV-positive pregnant women be assured the best possible care available in their countries. In some places, ARVs will be available for therapy and prenatal VCT may help women to access ARV combinations; in others, such treatment will simply not be feasible.

EMERGENT ISSUES

PMTCT Plus

As PMTCT is becoming the universal standard of practice in Africa, there is a need for simple and acceptable interventions to incorporate care for the mothers and the entire family. A number of arguments have been raised to suggest that the mothers are neglected in the current scheme of events. Berer argues that a short course of zidovudine is an intervention that uses women's bodies to deliver preventive treatment to infants (150). Although the anti-HIV benefits to the infant are clear, there is no benefit to the women. Also arguing for better health care for HIV-infected pregnant women, Rosenfield and Fidgor (151) raised the following questions: Should we not be giving serious consideration to finding ways to offer women treatment simply because they are infected with HIV and not just because they are pregnant? Should we not value saving women's lives as an equal priority to decreasing transmission to infants?

The positions expressed above set the stage for a more inclusive approach to the management of care of HIV-infected women, their infants, couples, and the entire family.

Correspondingly, programs are now geared toward PMTCT Plus. The MTCT-Plus Initiative is designed to promote wellness and to improve the health care for HIV-infected mothers and their families by providing a continuum of services (152) from patient education to nutritional support, prophylaxis for opportunistic infections, and ART. MTCT Plus builds on successful PMTCT programs to create high-quality HIV care.

As Nigeria plans to expand its PMTCT programs, it is important to incorporate the concept of PMTCT Plus in order to promote the health of the entire family. The initiative also has the inherent advantage of prolonging the mothers' life and thus reducing the burden of orphanhood.

Integration and Linkages to Other Health Care Interventions

PMTCT should neither be construed as nor constructed to be a program implemented separate from other health-related issues. Experience from southern Africa shows that the benefits of services for PMTCT go far beyond providing antiretrovirals (153). This was realized by incorporating PMTCT into existing maternal/child health services, including antenatal care, delivery services, infant welfare clinics, and immunization programs. There is further synergy when the laboratories, family planning, and special clinics — such as chest clinics and STI clinics — are involved in the program.

By extension, community-based HIV/AIDS care and support initiatives should be part of the overall planning for PMTCT programs. Such a broad-based program approach has contributed to a more effective response to HIV/AIDS by motivating health care providers, improving HIV/AIDS knowledge in the community, getting male partners more involved in HIV prevention and the health of their families, and facilitating clients' access to HIV/AIDS care and support. The authors note that integration of family planning promotes barrier methods of contraception to clients seeking contraception and helps in the prevention of unwanted pregnancy in HIV-positive women (153). Similarly, it was observed that identifying HIV-infected women offers an opportunity to introduce rational simple HIV/AIDS care, including screening and prophylaxis for tuberculosis. Furthermore, antenatal HIV counseling and testing can help to involve women and their male partners in HIV/AIDS prevention activities, HIV/AIDS care, and child health promotion.

These linkages are still blurred in the current national program; however, with minimal effort, this anomaly can be corrected, as most of these units have the tradition of working together already.

CONCLUSION AND RECOMMENDATIONS

The data derived thus far from the national PMTCT program and other studies within the country are neither strong enough nor appropriately disaggregated for input into a definitive policy framework. Many questions remain unanswered, and both biomedical studies and operational analyses are needed. For issues of infant feeding, for example, Nigeria will need its own data from sociological, behavioral, and nutritional studies to incorporate into countrywide infant feeding patterns. Input from other areas of Africa particularly hard hit by HIV could be adapted for local use in determining certain policy recommendations.

Specifically, the PMTCT program in Nigeria needs the following urgently:
- Access should be increased and the approach should be both vertical and horizontal. A rapid scaling-up of implementation is crucial to drastically reduce the overall number of pediatric HIV/AIDS infections. Nigeria should continue to build the boat as it sails. This is necessary for ART access to be increased from less than 1% in 2005 to 50% in 2010. Effort to expand PMTCT should include provision of an enabling environment. Coordinating ministries—including NACA and Federal Ministry of Health—should produce and circulate guidelines on VCT, PMTCT, and ART. A visible national coordination program for implementation and monitoring and evaluation should be established and empowered. Coordinating bodies, donors, and implementing partners should ensure fairness and equity in establishing these new projects.
- Early incorporation of more holistic approaches—such as the concept of PMTCT Plus—will promote the health of the entire family unit. As more children are saved from HIV infection, the entire family will be healthy and economically productive enough to see the children through the early and difficult stages of life and thus reduce the burden of orphanhood.
- ART monotherapy is outdated because of the high likelihood of viral resistance; hence, a more pragmatic approach that uses triple therapy for HIV-infected women—preferably covering a short lactation period to reduce transmission through breastfeeding—is necessary.

- Capacity building should be intensified, and program planners at the ministries of health should try to forecast human-resource needs accurately enough to make the scale up effective.
- PMTCT should be fully integrated into the entire hospital system, especially the maternal and child health unit, the laboratory, the family planning clinic, and other ancillary medical and surgical specialties, such as adult and pediatric ART clinics, tuberculosis clinics, and STI clinics. This approach should build a comprehensive continuum of care, including access to ART for all members of affected families. Although the antenatal clinics remain a good source of contact with HIV-infected women, attempts should also be made to encourage partner participation, including testing and access to care for men.
- Even when PMTCT services are available, programs should be linked to innovative local community-based programs to create demand for the services. Such initiatives include partnering with faith-based organizations and other nongovernmental organizations and promoting universal counseling and confidential testing. Rapid testing should be considered to avoid missed opportunities and the failure of many individuals to return for their test results.
- Monitoring and evaluation efforts ensure greater understanding of the program for the implementers and other stakeholders; therefore, efforts should be directed toward building strong results-based monitoring and evaluation systems.
- Resource mobilization should be vigorously pursued and barriers to resource utilization should be addressed and removed.
- Proactive coordination and sound logistics management system should be established before massive scale-up takes place to avoid an inconsistent supply of commodities and missed opportunities.

ACKNOWLEDGMENT

We wish to thank the APIN leadership for the opportunity to be part of this noble and educative effort.

REFERENCES

1. UNAIDS. *AIDS Epidemic Update.* Geneva: UNAIDS, December 2004.

2. Dabis F, Leroy V, Castetbon K, et al. Preventing mother-to-child transmission of HIV-1 in Africa in the year 2000. *AIDS*, 2000;14:1017–1026.

3. World Health Organization/UNAIDS. *HIV in Pregnancy: A Review.* (WHO/CHS/RHR/99.15) Geneva: World Health Organization/UNAIDS, 1999.

4. Dabis F, Ekpini ER. HIV-1/AIDS and maternal and child health in Africa. *Lancet*, 2002;359:2097–2104.

5. Chikwem JO, Mohammed I, Bwala HG, Ola TO. Human immunodeficiency virus (HIV) infection in patients attending a sexually transmitted diseases clinic in Borno State of Nigeria. *Trop Geogr Med*, 1990;42:17–21.

6. Nnatu SN, Anyiwo CE, Obi CL, Karpas A. Prevalence of human immunodeficiency virus (HIV) antibody among apparently healthy pregnant women in Nigeria. *Int J Gynecol Obstet*, 1993;40:105–107.

7. Sagay AS, Imade GE, Nwokedi EE. Human immunodeficiency virus infection in pregnant women in Nigeria. *Int J Gynecol Obstet*, 1999;66:183–184.

8. Federal Ministry of Health. *A Technical Report on the 2001 National HIV/Syphilis Sentinel Survey Among Pregnant Women Attending Antenatal Clinics in Nigeria.* Abuja: Federal Ministry of Health, 2001.

9. Federal Ministry of Health. *2003 National HIV Seroprevalence Sentinel Survey.* Abuja: Federal Ministry of Health, 2004.

10. UNAIDS. *Counseling and Voluntary HIV Testing for Pregnant Women in High HIV Prevalence Countries: Elements and Issues.* Geneva: UNAIDS, 1999;24.

11. Gray RH, Wawer MJ, Serwadda D, et al. Population-based study of fertility in women with HIV-1 infection in Uganda. *Lancet,* 1998;351:98–103.

12. Brettle RP, Raab GM, Ross A, Fielding KL, Gore SM, Bird AG. HIV infection in women: immunological markers and the influence of pregnancy. *AIDS,* 1995;9:1177–1184.

13. European Collaborative Study and the Swiss HIV Pregnancy Cohort. Immunological markers in HIV-infected pregnant women. *AIDS,* 1997;11:1859–1865.

14. Miotti P, Liomba G, Dallabetta GA, Hoover DR, Chiphangwi JD, Saah AJ. T lymphocyte subsets during and after pregnancy: analysis in human immunodeficiency virus type-1 infected and uninfected Malawian mothers. *J Infect Dis,* 1992;165: 1116–1119.

15. O'Sullivan MJ, Lai S, Yasin S, Helfgott A. The effect of pregnancy on lymphocyte counts in HIV infected women. *HIV Infection in Women Conference,* Washington, DC, February 22–24, 1995 (abstract S20).

16. Burns DN, Landesman S, Minkoff H, et al. The influence of pregnancy on human immunodeficiency virus type-1 infection: antepartum and postpartum changes in human immunodeficiency virus type-1 viral load. *Am J Obstet Gynecol,* 1998;178: 355–359.

17. French R, Brocklehurst P. The effect of pregnancy on survival in women infected with HIV: a systematic review of the literature and meta-analysis. *Br J Obstet Gynaecol,* 1998;105:827–835.

18. Alliegro MB, Dorrucci M, Phillips AN, et al. Incidence and consequences of pregnancy in women with known duration of HIV infection. Italian Seroconversion Study Group. *Arch Intern Med,* 1997;157:2585–2590.

19. Ryder RW, Temmerman M. The effects of HIV-1 infection during pregnancy and the perinatal period on maternal and child health in Africa. *AIDS,* 1991;5(Suppl 1):S75–S85.

20. Martin R, Boyer P, Hamill H, et al. Incidence of premature birth and neonatal respiratory disease in infants of HIV-positive mothers. The Pediatric Pulmonary and Cardiovascular Complications of Vertically Transmitted Human Immunodeficiency Virus Infection Study Group. *J Pediatr,* 1997;131(6): 851–856.

21. Leroy V, Ladner J, Nyiraziraje M, et al. Effect of HIV-1 infection on pregnancy outcome in women in Kigali, Rwanda, 1992–1994. Pregnancy and HIV Study Group. *AIDS,* 1998;12(6):643–650.

22. Brocklehurst P, French R. The association between maternal HIV infection and perinatal outcome: a systematic review of the literature and meta analysis. *Br J Obstet Gynaecol,* 1998;105(8):836–848.

23. Lambert JS, Watts DH, Mofensen L, et al. Risk factors for preterm birth, low birth weight, and intrauterine growth retardation in infants born to HIV-infected pregnant women receiving zidovudine. *AIDS,* 2000;14:1389–1399.

24. Lyman W, Kress Y, Kave K, et al. Detection of HIV in fetal central nervous system tissue. *AIDS,* 1990;4: 917–992.

25. Lapointe N, Michaud M, Pekovic D, et al. Transplacental transmission of HTLV-III virus. *N Engl J Med,* 1985;312:1325–1326.

26. Brossard Y, Aubin J, Mandelbrol L, et al. Frequency of early in-utero HIV-1 infection: a blind DNA polymerase chain reaction study on 100 fetal thymuses. *AIDS,* 1995;9:359–366.

27. Mayaux M, Burgard M, Teslas J, et al. Neonatal characteristics in rapidly progressive perinatally acquired HIV-1 disease. *JAMA,* 1996;275:606–610.

28. Bryson Y, Luzuriaga K, Wara D. Proposed definitions for in-utero versus intrapartum transmission of HIV-1. *N Engl J Med,* 1992;327: 1246–1247.

29. Biggar RJ, Cassol S, Kumwenda N, et al. The risk of human immunodeficiency virus-1 infection in twin pairs born to infected mothers in Africa. *J Infect Dis,* 2003;188(6):850–855.

30. Goedert JJ, Duliege AM, Amos CI, Felton S, Biggar RJ. High risk of HIV-1 infection for first-born twins. *Lancet,* 1991;338:1471–1475.

31. Rouzioux C, Costagliola D, Burgard M, et al. Estimated timing of mother to child human immunodeficiency virus type-1 (HIV-1) transmission by use of Markov model. The HIV Infection in Newborns French Collaborative Study Group. *Am J Epidemiol*, 1995;142(12):1330–1337.

32. Msellati P, Newell M-L, Dabis F. Rates of mother-to-child transmission of HIV-1 in Africa, America and Europe: Results from 13 perinatal studies. *J Acquir Immune Defic Syndr*, 1995;8:506–510.

33. De Cock KM, Fowler MG, Mercier E, et al. Prevention of mother to child HIV transmission in resource-poor countries: translating research into policy and practice. *JAMA*, 2000;283:1175–1182.

34. Lallemant M, Le Coeur S, Samba L, et al. Mother-to-child transmission of HIV-1 in Congo central Africa. *AIDS*, 1994;8:1451–1456.

35. Kind C, Rudin C, Siegrist CA, et al. Prevention of vertical HIV transmission: additive protective effect of elective caesarean section and zidovudine prophylaxis. *AIDS*, 1998;12:205–210.

36. Blanche S, Rouzioux C, Moscatao M-LG, et al. A prospective study of infants born to women seropositive for human immunodeficiency virus type 1. *N Engl J Med*, 1989;320:1643–1648.

37. Fiscus SA, Adimora AA, Funk ML, et al. Trends in interventions to reduce perinatal human immunodeficiency virus type 1 in North Carolina. *Pediatr Infect Dis J*, 2002;21:664–668.

38. Mandelbrot L, Landreau-Mascaro A, Rekacewicz C, et al. Lamivudine-Zidovudine combination for the prevention of maternal Infection transmission of HIV-1. *JAMA*, 2001;285(160):2083–2093.

39. Cooper ER, Charurat M, Mofenson L, et al. Combination antiretroviral strategies for the treatment of Pregnant HIV-1 infected women and prevention of perinatal HIV-1 transmission. *J Acquir Immune Defic Syndr Hum Retroviral*, 2002;29:484–494.

40. Anderson VA. The placental barrier to maternal HIV infection. *Obstet Gynecol Clin North Am*, 1997;24(2):797–820.

41. World Health Organization. *HIV in pregnancy: A review*. WHO/CHS/RHR/99.15. Geneva: World Health Organization, 1999;35.

42. Semba RD. Overview of the potential role of vitamin A in mother-to-child transmission of HIV-1. *Acta Paediatr Suppl*, 1997;421:107–112.

43. Fawzi WW, Msamanga GI, Hunter D, et al. Randomized trial of vitamin supplements in relation to transmission of HIV-1 through breastfeeding and early child mortality. *AIDS*, 2002;16:1935–1944.

44. Preble EA, Piwoz EG. *Prevention of Mother-to-Child Transmission of HIV in Africa: Practical Guidance for Programs*. Support for Analysis and Research in Africa (SARA) Project. Washington, DC: Academy for Educational Development, 2001;3.

45. Baba TW, Kock J, Mittler M, et al. Mucosal infection of neonatal rhesus monkeys with cell-free SIV. *AIDS Res Hum Retroviruses*, 1994;10:351–357.

46. Sellon RK, Jordan HL, Kennedy-Stokskopf SK, Tompkins MB, Tompkins WAF. Feline immunodeficiency virus can be experimentally transmitted via milk during acute maternal infection. *Virology*, 1994;8:3380–3385.

47. Featherstone C. M cells: portals to the mucosal immune system. *Lancet*, 1997;350:1230.

48. Amerongen HM, Weltzin R, Farnet CM, Michetti P, Haseltine WA, Neutra MR. Transepithelial transport of HIV-1 by intestinal M cells: a mechanism for transmission of AIDS. *J Acquir Immune Defic Synd*, 1991;4:760–765.

49. Dunn DT, Newell ML, Ades AE, Peckham CS. Risk of HIV 1 transmission through breastfeeding. *Lancet*, 1992;340:585–588.

50. Nduati R, John G, Mbori-Ngacha D, et al. Effect of breastfeeding and formula feeding on transmission of HIV: a randomized trial. *JAMA*, 2000;283:1167–1174.

51. Coutsoudis A, Pillay K, Spooner E, Kuhn L, Coovadia HM. Influence of infant-feeding patterns on early mother-to-child transmission of HIV-1 in Durban, South Africa: a prospective cohort study. South African Vitamin A Study Group. *Lancet*, 1999;354:471–476.

52. Coutsoudis A, Pillay K, Kuhn L, et al. Method of feeding and transmission of HIV-1 from mothers to children by 15 months of age: prospective cohort study from Durban, South Africa. *AIDS*, 2001;15:379–387.

53. Smith M, Kuhn L. Exclusive breastfeeding: does it have the potential to reduce breastfeeding transmission of HIV-1? *Nutr Rev*, 2000;58(11):333–340.

54. Mofenson LM, McIntyre JA. Advances and research directions in the prevention of mother-to-child HIV-1 transmission. *Lancet*, 2000;355:2237–2244.

55. Dabis F, Leroy V, Castetbon K, et al. 2000. Preventing mother-to-child transmission of HIV-1 in Africa in the year 2000. *AIDS*, 14:1017–1026.

56. Garcia PM, Kalish LA, Pitt J, et al. Maternal levels of plasma human immunodeficiency virus type 1 RNA and the risk of perinatal transmission. *N Engl J Med*, 1999;341(6):394–402.

57. Welles SH, Leroy V, Ekpini ER, et al. HIV-1 genotypic zidovudine drug resistance and the risk of maternal-infant transmission in the Women and Infants Transmission Study. The Women and Infants Transmission Study Group. *AIDS*, 2000;14:263–271.

58. Jackson JB, Berger-Pergola G, Guay L, et al. Identification of the K103N resistance mutation in Ugandan women receiving nevirapine to prevent HIV-1 vertical transmission. *AIDS*, 2000;14:F111–F115.

59. Renjifo B, Fawzi W, Mwakagile D, et al. Differences in perinatal transmission between HIV-1 genotypes. *J Hum Virol*, 2001;4:16–25.

60. Dickover R, Garraty E, Plaeger S, Bryson Y. Perinatal transmission of major, minor and multiple HIV-1 strains in-utero and intrapartum. *7th Conference on Retroviruses and Opportunistic Infections*, San Francisco, California, January 30–February 2, 2000 (abstract 181).

61. Meldrum J. *Preventing Mother to Child Transmission of HIV.* London: NAM Publications, 2003. Accessed at www.aidsmap.com.

62. Ayouba A, Nerrienet E, Menu E. Mother-to-child transmission of HIV-1 in relation to season in Yaounde, Cameroon. *Am J Trop Med Hyg*, 2003;69(4):447–449.

63. Cohen J. Mother's malaria appears to enhance spread of AIDS virus. *Science*, 2003;302:1311.

64. Plummer FA. Heterosexual transmission of human immunodeficiency virus type-1 (HIV): interactions of conventional sexually transmitted diseases, hormonal contraception and HIV-1. *AIDS Res Hum Retroviruses*, 1998;14(Suppl 1):S5–S10.

65. Taha T, Kumwenda N, Liomba G, et al. Heterosexual and perinatal transmission of HIV-1: association with bacterial vaginosis (BV). XII International Conference on AIDS, Geneva, Switzerland, June 28–July 3, 1998 (abstract 527/23347).

66. Lee MJ, Hallmark RJ, Frenkel LM, DelPriore G. Maternal syphilis and vertical transmission of HIV type-1 infection. *Int J Gynecol Obstet*, 1998;63:247–252.

67. Sperling RS, Shapiro DE, Coombs RW, et al. Maternal viral load, zidovudine treatment, and the risk of transmission of human immunodeficiency virus type 1 from mother to infant. *N Engl J Med*, 1996;335:1621–1629.

68. Blattner W, Cooper E, Charurat M, et al. Effectiveness of potent antiretroviral therapies on reducing perinatal transmission of HIV-1. *XIII International AIDS Conference*, Durban, South Africa, July 9–14, 2000 (abstract LbOr4).

69. Chuachoowong R, Shaffer N, Siriwasin W, et al. Short-course antenatal zidovudine reduces both cervicovaginal human immunodeficiency virus type 1 levels and risk of perinatal transmission. *J Infect Dis*, 2000;181:99–106.

70. Bulterys M, Landesman S, Burns DN, Rubinstein A, Goedert J. Sexual behavior and injection drug use during pregnancy and vertical transmission of HIV-1. *J Acquir Immune Defic Syndr Hum Retrovirol*, 1997;15:76–82.

71. Turner BJ, Hauck WW, Fanning R, Markson LE. Cigarette smoking and maternal-child HIV transmission. *J Acquir Immune Defic Syndr Hum Retrovirol*, 1997;14:327–337.

72. Read J for the International Perinatal HIV Group. Duration of ruptured membranes and vertical transmission of HIV-1: a meta-analysis from fifteen prospective cohort studies. *7th Conference on Retroviruses and Opportunistic Infections*, San Francisco, California, January 30–February 2, 2000 (abstract 659).

73. Goldenberg RL, Vermund SH, Goepfert AR, Andrews WW. Choriodecidual inflammation: a potentially preventable cause of perinatal HIV-1 transmission? *Lancet*, 1998;352:1927–1930.

74. Kuhn L, Steketee RW, Weedon J, et al. Distinct risk factors for intrauterine and intrapartum human immunodeficiency virus transmission and consequences for disease progression in infected children. Perinatal AIDS Collaborative Transmission Study. *J Infect Dis*, 1999;179:52–58.

75. Kuhn L, Coutsoudis A, Moodley D, et al. HIV-1 specific T-helper cell responses detected at birth: protection against intrapartum and breast-feeding-associated transmission of HIV-1. *7th Conference on Retroviruses and Opportunistic Infections*, San Francisco, California, January 30–February 2, 2000 (abstract 702).

76. MacDonald K, Embree J, Njenga S, et al. Mother-Child Class 1 HLA concordance increases perinatal human immunodeficiency virus type 1 transmission. *J Infec Dis*, 1998;177:551–556.

77. Philpott S, Burger H, Charbonneau T, et al. CCR-5 genotype and resistance to vertical transmission of HIV-1. *J Acquire Immune Defic Syndr*, 1999;21:189–293.

78. Mangano A, Gonzalez E, Catano G, et al. CCR5 haplotypes associated with enhanced or reduced transmission of HIV-1 from mother to child. *7th Conference on Retroviruses and Opportunistic Infections*, January 30–February 2, 2000 (abstract 448).

79. Kreiss J. Breast-feeding and vertical transmission of HIV-1. *Acta Paediatr*, 1997;421(Suppl):S113–S117.

80. Leroy V, Newell M, Dabis F, et al. International multicenter pooled analysis of late postnatal mother to child transmission of HIV -1 infection. *Lancet*, 1998;352:597–600.

81. Walker N, Schwartlander B, Bryce J. Meeting international goals in child survival and HIV/AIDS. *Lancet*, 2002;360:284–289.

82. UNAIDS/Government of Zimbabwe. *Situation Analysis in Zimbabwe — The Zimbabwe Mother-to-Child HIV Transmission: Prevention Project*. Geneva: UNAIDS, 1998;41.

83. Dray-Spira R, Lepage P, Dabis F. Prevention of infectious complications of Paediatric HIV infection in Africa. *AIDS*, 2000;14:1091–1099.

84. Dabis F, Leroy V, Castetbon K, et al. Preventing mother-to-child transmission of HIV-1 in Africa in the year 2000. *AIDS*, 2000;14:1017–1026.

85. Bureau of the Census. *HIV/AIDS in the Developing World*. Report WP/98-2. Washington, DC: U.S. Government Printing Office, 1999.

86. Pam SD, Sagay AS, Egah D, et al. Mortality of HIV-exposed infants in Jos, Nigeria. *3rd IAS Conference on HIV Pathogenesis and Treatment*, Rio de Janeiro, Brazil, July 24–27, 2005 (abstract TuPe5.2P19).

87. Downs AM, De Vincenzi I, for the European Study Group in Heterosexual Transmission of HIV. Probability of heterosexual transmission of HIV: relationship to number of unprotected sexual contacts. *J Acquir Immune Defic Syndr*, 1996;11:388–395.

88. Royce RA, Sena A, Cates W Jr., Cohen MS. Sexual transmission of HIV. *N Engl J Med*, 1997;15:1072–1078.

89. Padian N, Shiboski S, Vittinghoff E, Glass S. Heterosexual transmission of HIV: results from a ten year study. *Am J Epidemiol*, 1997;146:350–357.

90. UNAIDS. *Prevention of HIV Transmission from Mother-to-Child: Planning for Programme Implementation*. Geneva, UNAIDS, 1998;16.

91. United Nations General Assembly. *Final Declaration of Commitment on HIV/AIDS (A/s-26/L2)*. New York: United Nations General Assembly, 2001. Accessed at http://unaids.org/UNGASS/index.html.

92. Adeokun L, Mantell JE, Weiss E, Delano G, et al. Promoting dual protection in family planning clinics in Ibadan, Nigeria. *Int Fam Plann Persp*, 2002; 28(2):87–95.

93. Plan International. *MTCT in Resource Poor Countries: Integrating Mother to Child Transmission Risk Reduction into RH/FP*. Surrey, United Kingdom: Plan International, 2001.

94. Odutolu O, Adedimeji A, Odutolu OT, Baruwa O, Olatidoye F. Economic empowerment and reproductive behavior of young women in Osun State, Nigeria. *Afr J Reprod Health*, 2004;8:1.

95. Wilson TE, Massad LS, Riester KA, et al. Sexual, contraceptive, and drug use behaviors of women with HIV and those at high risk for infection: results from the Women's Interagency HIV Study. *AIDS*, 1999;13:591–598.

96. Smits AK, Goergen CA, Delaney JA, Williamson C, Mundy LM, Fraser VJ. Contraceptive use and pregnancy decision-making among women with HIV. *AIDS Patient Care STDs*, 1999;12:739–746.

97. Lindsay MK, Grant J, Peterson HB, Willis S, Nelson P, Klein L. The impact of knowledge of human immunodeficiency virus sero-status on contraceptive choice and repeat pregnancy. *Obstet Gynecol*, 1995;85: 675-9.

98. Strategic approaches to the prevention of HIV infection in infants: report of a WHO meeting, Morges, Switzerland. March 20–22, 2002.

99. U.S. Centers for Disease Control and Prevention. Guidelines for the use of antiretroviral agents in HIV-infected adults and adolescents. *MMWR*, 1998;47(RR-5):42–82.

100. Kapiga SH, Shao JF, Lwihula GK, Hunter DJ. Risk factors for HIV infection among women in Dar-es-Salaam, Tanzania. *J Acquir Immune Defic Syndr*, 1994;7: 301–309.

101. Stafford MK, Ward H, Flanagan A, et al. Safety study of nononynol 9 as a vaginal microbicide: evidence of adverse effects. *J Acquir Immune Defic Syndr Hum Retrovirol*, 1998;17:327–331.

102. Altman LK. Hopes for anti-HIV treatment dashed. *The New York Times* on the Web, July 13, 2000. (http://nytimes.gpass.com).

103. Sweat M, Gregorich S, Sangiwa G, et al. Cost-effectiveness of voluntary HIV-1 counseling and testing in reducing sexual transmission of HIV-1 in Kenya and Tanzania. *Lancet*, 2000;356:113–121.

104. UNAIDS. *Counseling and Voluntary HIV Testing for Pregnant Women in High HIV Prevalence Countries: Guidance for Service Providers*. Geneva: UNAIDS, May 1999.

105. Federal Ministry of Health. *National Guidelines on Prevention of Mother-to-Child Transmission (PMTCT) of HIV Infection*. Abuja: Federal Ministry of Health, 2005.

106. Shaffer N, Chuachoowong R, Mock PA, et al. Short-course zidovudine for perinatal HIV-1 transmission in Bangkok, Thailand: a randomized controlled trial. *Lancet*, 1999;353:773–780.

107. Moodley D, Moodley J, Coovadia H, Gray G, et al. A multi-center randomized controlled trial of nevirapine versus a combination of zidovudine and lamivudine to reduce intrapartum and early postpartum mother to child transmission of human immunodeficiency virus type-1. *J Infec Dis*, 2003;187: 725–735.

108. Lallemant M, Jourdain G, Le Coeur S, et al. Multi-center randomized controlled trial assessing the safety and efficacy of nevirapine in addition to zidovudine for the prevention of perinatal HIV in Thailand, PHPT-2 Update. *Antivir Ther*, 2003; 8(Suppl 1):S199.

109. Dabis F, Ekouevi DK, Rouet F, et al. Effectiveness of a short course of zidovudine + lamivudine and peripartum nevirapine to prevent HIV-1 mother-to-child transmission. The ANRS DITRAM Plus Trial. Abidjan, Cote d'Ivoire. *Antivir Ther*, 2000; 8(Suppl 1):S5236–S5237.

110. Cooper ER, Charurat M, Mofenson L, et al. Combination antiretroviral strategies for the treatment of pregnant HIV-1 infected women and prevention of perinatal HIV-1 transmission. *J Acquir Immune Defic Syndr Hum Retrovirol*, 2002;29:484–494.

111. Tonwe B, Tonwe-Gold B, Ekouev DK, et al. Highly active antiretroviral therapy for the prevention of perinatal HIV transmission in Africa: Mother-to-Child Transmission Plus Program, Côte d'Ivoire. *12th Conference on Retroviruses and Opportunistic Infections*, Boston, Massachusetts, February 22–25, 2005.

112. The International Perinatal HIV Group. The mode of delivery and the risk of vertical transmission of human immunodeficiency virus type-1. A Meta Analysis of 15 prospective cohort studies. *N Engl J Med*, 1999;340(13):977–987.

113. The European Mode of Delivery Collaboration. Elective Caesarean section versus vaginal delivery in prevention of vertical HIV-1 transmission: a randomized clinical trial. *Lancet*, 1999;353(9158): 1035–1039.

114. ACOG committee opinion scheduled Caesarean delivery and the prevention of vertical transmission of HIV infection. *Int J Gynecol Obstet*, 2001;73(3): 279–281.

115. Bell C, Devarajan S, Gersbach H. *The Long Run Economic Cost of AIDS: Theory and an Application to South Africa*. Working Paper No. 3152. Washington, DC: World Bank, 2003.

116. Sagay AS, Kapiga SH, Imade GE, Sankale J-L, Idoko JA, Kanki P. HIV infection among pregnant women in Nigeria. *Inter J Obstet Gynecol*, 2005;90:61–67.

117. Emuveyan EE. Findings of the formative research on PMTCT in Nigeria. *4th National AIDS Conference*, Abuja, Nigeria, May 3–5, 2004.

118. Federal Ministry of Health. *National Policy on HIV/AIDS, 2003*. Abuja: Federal Ministry of Health, 2003.

119. United Nations Development Programme/Swaziland. *Gender Focused Responses to HIV/AIDS: The Needs of Women Affected by HIV/AIDS*. Mbabane: United Nations Development Programme/Swaziland, August 2000.

120. Cartoux M, Meda N, Van de Perre, at al. Acceptability of voluntary HIV testing by pregnant women in developing countries: an international survey. *AIDS*, 1998;12:2489-2493.

121. Family Health International. *HIV/AIDS Prevention, Care and Treatment Resources for Use in Developing Countries.* Arlington, Virginia: Family Health International, 2004.

122. Connor EM, Sperling RS, Gelber R, et al. Reduction of maternal-infant transmission of human immunodeficiency virus type 1 with zidovudine treatment. *N Engl J Med,* 1994;331: 1173–1180.

123. Wiktor S, Ekpini E, Karon J, et al. Short course oral zidovudine for prevention of mother to child transmission of HIV-1 in Abidjan, Cote d'Ivoire. A randomized trial. *Lancet,* 1999;353:781–785.

124. Dabis F, Msellati P, Meda N, et al. 6-month efficacy, tolerance, and acceptability of a short regimen of oral zidovudine to reduce vertical transmission of HIV in breastfed children in Cote d'Ivoire and Burkina Faso: a double-blind placebo-controlled multi-centre trial. *Lancet,* 1999;353:786–792.

125. Saba J for the PETRA Trial Study Team. Interim analysis of early efficacy of three short ZDV/3TC combination regimens to prevent mother to child transmission of HIV-1. *6th Conference on Retroviruses and Opportunistic Infections,* Chicago, Illinois, 1999.

126. Van Dyke RB, Korber BT, Popek E, et al. The Ariel Project: a prospective cohort study of maternal-child transmission of human immunodeficiency virus type 1 in the era of maternal antiretroviral therapy. *J Infect Dis,* 1999;179:319–328.

127. Cooper ER, Nugent RP, Diaz C, et al. After AIDS Clinical Trial 076: the changing pattern of zidovudine use during pregnancy, and the subsequent reduction in the vertical transmission of human immunodeficiency virus in a cohort of infected women and their infants. *J Infect Dis,* 1996;174: 1207–1211.

128. Fiscus S, Adimora AA, Schoenbach VJ, Wilfert C, Johnson VA. Can zidovudine monotherapy continue to reduce perinatal HIV transmission? The North Carolina experience 1993-1997. *12th World AIDS Conference.* Geneva, June 28–July 3, 1998 (abstract 33162).

129. Lindergren ML, Byers RH, Thomas P, et al. The perinatal HIV/AIDS epidemic in the United States: success in reducing perinatal transmission. *JAMA,* 1999;282:531–538.

130. Guay L, Musoke P, Fleming T, et al. Intrapartum and neonatal single dose nevirapine compared with Zidovudine for the prevention of mother to child transmission of HIV-1 in Kampala, Uganda. HIVNET 012 randomized trial. *Lancet,* 1999;354: 795–802.

131. Jackson BJ, Musoke P, Fleming T, et al. Intrapartum and neonatal single-nevirapine compared with zidovudine for prevention of mother-to-child transmission of HIV-1 in Kampala, Uganda: 18-month follow up of the HIVNET 012 randomized trial. *Lancet,* 2003;362:859–868.

132. Knudtson E, Para M, Boswell H, Fan-Havard P. Drug rash with eosinophilia and systemic symptoms syndrome and renal toxicity with a nevirapine-containing regimen in a pregnant patient with human immunodeficiency virus. *Obstet Gynecol,* 2003;101:1094–1097.

133. Stern JO, Robinson PA, Love J, et al. Comprehensive hepatic safety analysis of nevirapine in different populations of HIV infected patients. *J Acquir Immune Defic Syndr,* 2003;34(Suppl 1):S21–S33.

134. Boehringer-Ingelheim Pharmaceutical Inc. Important new safety information for clarification of risk factors for severe life threatening and fetal hepatotoxicity with VIRAMUNE (nevirapine). 2004.

135. Eshleman SH, Mracna M, Guay L, et al. Selection and fading of resistance mutations in women and infants receiving nevirapine to prevent HIV-1 vertical transmission (HIVNET 012). *AIDS,* 2001;15: 1951–1957.

136. Kantor R, Lee E, Johnson E, et al. Rapid flux I non-nucleoside reverse transcriptase inhibitor resistance mutations among subtype C HIV infected women after single dose nevirapine. *2nd IAS Conference on HIV Pathogenesis and Treatment,* Paris, France, July 13–16, 2003 (abstract 78).

137. Beckerman KP. Long term findings of HIVNET 012: the next steps. Commentary. *Lancet,* 2003;362: 842–843.

138. Mandelbrot L, Landreau-Mascaro A, Rekacewicz C, et al. lamivudine-zidovudine combination for the prevention of maternal infection transmission of HIV-1. *JAMA,* 2001;285(160):2083–2093.

139. Tuomala RE, Shapiro D, Mofenson LM, et al. Antiretroviral therapy during pregnancy and the risk of an adverse outcome. *N Engl J Med,* 2002;346(24): 1863–1870.

140. Lange J, Stellato R, Brinkman K, et al. Review of neurological adverse events in relation to mitochondrial dysfunction in the prevention of mother to child transmission of HIV: PETRA study. *2nd Conference on Global Strategies for the Prevention of HIV Transmission from Mothers to Infants.* September 1–6, 1999, Montreal, Canada (abstract 250).

141. Public Health Service Task Force. *Recommendations for Use of Antiretroviral Drugs in Pregnant HIV-1 Infected Women for Maternal Health and Interventions to Reduce Perinatal HIV 1 Transmission in the United States.* Public Health Service Task Force, 2003. Accessed at http://AIDSinfo.nih.gov.

142. World Health Organization. *New Data on the Prevention of Mother to Child Transmission of HIV and Their Policy Implications: WHO Technical Consultation on Behalf of the UNFPA/UNICEF/WHO/UNAIDS Inter-Agency Task Team on Mother-to-Child Transmission of HIV.* Geneva: World Health Organization, October 11–13, 2000.

143. Adewole I, Jegede A, Adesina A, et al. The role of significant others in the management of discordant couples. Medimond International Proceedings. *XV International AIDS Conference,* Bangkok, Thailand, July 11–16, 2004;103–106.

144. National Action Committee on AIDS. The HIV/AIDS Emergency Action Plan (HEAP). Abuja: National Action Committee on AIDS, 2001.

145. Musoke P, Guay LA, Bagenda D, et al. A phase I/II study of the safety and pharmacokinetics of nevirapine in HIV-1 infected women in Uganda and their neonates (HIVNET 006). *AIDS,* 1999;13:478–486.

146. Federal Ministry of Health. *National Guidelines on Implementation of Prevention of Mother to Child Transmission of HIV Program in Nigeria.* Abuja: Federal Ministry of Health, 2001.

147. Mirochnick M, Fenton T, Gagnler P, et al. Pharmacokinetics of nevirapine in HIV-1 infected pregnant women and their neonates. *J Infect Dis,* 1998;178:368–374.

148. UNAIDS. Prevention of HIV Transmission from Mother-to-Child: Planning for Program Implementation — Conclusions of the Meeting. Geneva: UNAIDS, 1998;16.

149. UNAIDS. *Prevention of HIV from Mother to Child: Strategic Options.* Geneva: UNAIDS, 1999.

150. Berer M. Reducing perinatal HIV transmission in developing countries through antenatal and delivery care and breast feeding supporting child survival. *Bull World,* 1999;77:871–877.

151. Rosenfield A, Fidgor E. Where is the M in MTCT? The broader issues in mother to child transmission of HIV. *Am J Public Health,* 2001;91(5).

152. Rabkin M, El-Sadr W, Abrams E. *The MTCT-Plus Clinical Manual.* New York: Mailman School of Public Health, Columbia University, 2003.

153. Rutenberg N, Baek C, Kalibala S, Rosen J. UNICEF and Horizon. *Evaluation of United Nations–Supported Pilot Projects for the Prevention of Mother-to-Child Transmission of HIV: Overview of Findings.* HIV/AIDS Working Paper. New York: UNICEF, 2003.

17

TREATMENT AND CARE OF HIV DISEASE

John A. Idoko,* Babafemi Taiwo,[†]
and Robert L. Murphy[†]

The treatment and care of HIV-infected people requires comprehensive integration of patient-centered medical and social services. Essential elements of this approach include the provision of clinical care, nursing care, nutritional care and support, psychological support, health information and counseling, legal protection, and economic sufficiency. Notable components of successful clinical care include early diagnosis, access to care, antiretroviral therapy, symptom control, prophylaxis against opportunistic infections, treatment of opportunistic infections and malignancies, and end-of-life care. The achievement of these objectives requires multisectoral and multidisciplinary teams that are cross-linked to provide a continuum of care that involves patients, their families, healthcare providers, governmental and nongovernmental organizations, and society at large.

Prevention of new infections should be integrated into HIV/AIDS treatment and care programs as HIV infection remains incurable despite advances in antiretroviral treatment. Toward this end, "social immunization" — such as through community mobilization, widespread education, counseling and testing, sexual abstinence until marriage, monogamy, condom use, and female empowerment — must be strengthened, as we await the perfection of vaginal microbicides, HIV vaccines, and other currently investigational prevention strategies. Even if HIV transmission were to cease

*Jos University Teaching Hospital and AIDS Prevention Initiative in Nigeria, Jos, Nigeria
[†]Division of Infectious Diseases, Northwestern University Feinberg School of Medicine, Chicago, Illinois, USA

completely in Nigeria and other resource-limited countries, the existing burden of HIV/AIDS would continue to task all stakeholders into the foreseeable future.

THE CASE FOR ANTIRETROVIRAL THERAPY IN RESOURCE-LIMITED SETTINGS

Antiretroviral therapy (ART) has significantly reduced morbidity and mortality, prolonged life expectancy, and improved quality of life among people with HIV infection (1). ART has also been effective in the prevention of mother-to-child transmission of HIV (PMTCT) (2). The increasing availability of ART has created a major incentive to participate in voluntary counseling and testing (3), and has broadened and enhanced prevention efforts by reducing stigma and increasing uptake of behavior change communication messages. Effective ART may reduce overall transmission at the population level. Comprehensive care—including antiretrovirals (ARVs), treatment of opportunistic infections, and the use of prophylactic agents—benefits the individual, the community, and the country.

The provision of affordable, accessible, and good quality treatment and care on a global scale for people living with HIV is essential for tackling the epidemic, improving lives, and protecting the significant development gains of the past 20 years. Addressing the care and treatment needs of HIV-infected people is also a critical component of achieving the millennium development goals of the next decade. Until 2005, only 5% of the six million people who required ARVs in resource-limited countries could access these drugs. Between 2003 and the end of 2005, however, these numbers rose three-fold (4), mainly from the massive scaling up of programs supported by the 3 by 5 Initiative of the World Health Organization (WHO); the Global Fund to Fight AIDS, Tuberculosis, and Malaria; the World Bank; and the U.S. President's Emergency Plan for AIDS Relief (PEPFAR). Nigeria, with a national seroprevalence of 5% (5) and an estimated four to six million people living with HIV, has at least 800,000 people in urgent need of ART. Only about 5% of those in need are currently receiving ART, but this number is expected to rise sharply with the 2005 presidential directive to treat 250,000 individuals by the end of 2006.

It should be noted that ART has many risks and limitations. First, early and delayed adverse effects—such as metabolic disorders, mitochondrial toxicities, and numerous organ-specific adverse reactions—are continual concerns. The scope of these adverse effects is rather broad, and our understanding of their pathogenesis and clinical presentations continues to evolve. Second, many HIV clinicians and researchers now view the late 1990s as a period of irrational optimism about the possibility of a cure for HIV. During that era, mathematical models suggested HIV infection in an individual could be eradicated by many years of continuously suppressive ART (6). It has since become clear, however, that such a feat is unachievable because of the complexity of the regimens, the difficulties of maintaining long-term adherence, viral mutation, and toxicity. Even in the absence of systemic replication, latently infected resting CD4+ T cell populations persist in lymph nodes and other organs. Prolonged ART appears to impair the development of HIV-1–specific immune responses because it reduces systemic HIV that would otherwise serve as the antigenic stimulant of such responses. Therefore, plasma viremia inevitably rebounds whenever treatment is stopped.

ARVs do not cure HIV infection and therefore must be taken for life. They can result in major toxicities and drug interactions, and drug resistance can develop if adherence is poor. The cost of ARVs and laboratory monitoring pose major financial challenges, particularly in resource-poor countries. The lack of an adequate health infrastructure and insufficient human resources create serious obstacles to providing ART in an effective, durable, and sustainable manner. Furthermore, increased commitment to treatment and care may lead to the neglect of prevention efforts and programs aimed at reducing the social and economic impact of HIV.

NATURAL HISTORY AND CLASSIFICATION OF DISEASE

The natural history of untreated HIV infection can be divided into six stages: initial infection; acute retroviral syndrome, or primary HIV illness; recovery and seroconversion; asymptomatic chronic HIV infection; symptomatic HIV infection; and AIDS.

Acute retroviral syndrome develops two to six weeks after the initial infection and is characterized by an acute flu-like illness. The clinical features include fever, headache, malaise, joint pains, pain and tenderness in the muscles (myalgia), diarrhea, maculopapular rash, and generalized swollen lymph glands (lymphadenopathy). These symptoms may be accompanied by various self-limiting neurologic manifestations, such as atypical aseptic meningitis and acute encephalitis. Acute retroviral syndrome

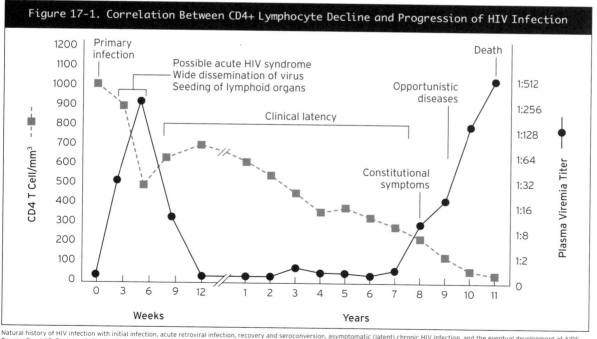

Figure 17-1. Correlation Between CD4+ Lymphocyte Decline and Progression of HIV Infection

Natural history of HIV infection with initial infection, acute retroviral infection, recovery and seroconversion, asymptomatic (latent) chronic HIV infection, and the eventual development of AIDS
Source: Fauci AS, Pantaleo G, Stanley S, Weissman D. Immunopathogenic mechanisms of HIV infection. *Ann Intern Med*, 1996;124:654-663.

Table 17-1. CDC Classification of HIV-Infected Individuals

CD4+ Cell categories	Clinical Classification		
	Asymptomatic	Symptomatic	AIDS related disease
> 500/mm³	A1	B1	C1
200 - 499/mm³	A2	B2	C2
< 200/mm³	A3	B3	C3

Table 17-2. WHO AIDS-Defining Diagnosis

Candidiasis–esophageal
Cervical cancer–invasive
Cryptococcosis–extrapulmonary
Cryptosporidiosis with diarrhea > 1 month
Cytomegalovirus: any organ except spleen, liver, or lymph nodes
Herpes simplex with mucocutaneous ulcer > 1 month or with bronchitis, pneumonia, or esophagitis
Histoplasmosis–extrapulmonary
HIV-associated dementia
HIV-associated wasting with involuntary loss of > 10% body weight + chronic (> 30 days) diarrhea, fatigue, or fever
Isosporosis with diarrhea > 1 month
Kaposi's sarcoma
Lymphoma of brain
Lymphoma–non-Hodgkin's
Mycobacterium avium or *Mycobacterium kansasii* disseminated
Mycobacterium tuberculosis–disseminated or pulmonary
Nocardia
Pneumocystis carinii pneumonia
Pneumonia, recurrent
Progressive multifocal encephalopathy
Salmonella septicaemia
Strongyloides extraintestinal
Toxoplasmosis of internal organ

goes unrecognized in many individuals perhaps because of a lack of suspicion or perhaps because it is difficult to distinguish these features from a host of other common tropical illnesses, such as malaria, typhoid fever, the common cold, and glandular fever. Acute retroviral syndrome is characterized by high plasma viremia and depressed CD4+ cell numbers and function (Figure 17-1). Acute retroviral syndrome has also been described in chronically HIV-infected patients who are reinfected with another strain of HIV, and a similar clinical syndrome occurs in some patients as a result of virologic rebound following withdrawal of suppressive ART (7).

During acute retroviral syndrome, tests that directly detect HIV — HIV RNA by polymerase chain reaction (RNA PCR), DNA PCR, and p24 antigen — are usually positive, but HIV antibody tests are negative. The sensitivity of RNA PCR for diagnosing acute retroviral syndrome approaches 100%, but the specificity is slightly lower (about 98%). HIV RNA level during this syndrome is usually greater than 100,000 copies/ml. The sensitivity of p24 antigen is lower compared to HIV RNA, but p24 is the most specific test (8). Other possible laboratory abnormalities during acute retroviral syndrome include: thrombocytopenia, lymphopenia, anemia, monocytosis, low-level atypical lymphocytosis, thrombocytosis, bandemia, and abnormal liver function tests.

The infected individual is most infectious during acute retroviral syndrome because of the high viral replication level. Reports from Malawi have shown that in areas of high HIV prevalence, up to 3% of individuals in high-risk populations, such as those with sexually transmitted infections (STIs), may have acute HIV infection and are potential sources of HIV transmission even though they have negative serology for HIV (9). This type of situation poses a major public health challenge in resource-limited countries where high-risk individuals may form a significant proportion of blood donors. This problem is compounded in such environments by the lack of screening tools that directly detect HIV.

Following seroconversion, infected individuals become HIV antibody positive and remain asymptomatic for five to ten years before developing clinical illness. During this asymptomatic period, some balance is established between the virus and the immune system, allowing the rate of HIV replication to remain relatively stable in the absence of treatment. The plasma viral load at which this relative equilibrium occurs has been termed "viral set-point." It is influenced by the pathogenicity of the infecting strain and the host immunologic repertoire; hence, it varies from one person to the next. However, continuous destruction of the immune system usually occurs, ultimately leading to an immunologic collapse with two major clinical consequences: the occurrence of opportunistic infections caused by microorganisms that the body's immune system normally holds in check, and the development of certain cancers. Symptomatic disease usually begins with minor opportunistic infections, progressing later to life-threatening disease—AIDS. This late stage disease is characterized by CD4+ counts of less than 200 cells/mm^3, AIDS-defining opportunistic infections and cancers, wasting syndrome, and neurologic complications (10). Less than 5% of HIV-infected people are long-term non-progressors, who escape this eventual immunologic and clinical collapse.

The staging of HIV and AIDS disease has important implications for clinical decision making and priority setting for treatment because patients with AIDS, symptomatic disease, and low CD4+ counts usually have more severe disease and therefore require more

Table 17-3. WHO Clinical Staging System for HIV Infection in Adults and Adolescents

Clinical Stage I: Asymptomatic
1. Asymptomatic
2. Persistent generalized lymphadenopathy
   And/or performance scale 1: asymptomatic, normal activity

Clinical Stage II: Early (Mild) Disease
1. Weight loss < 10% of body weight
2. Minor mucocutaneous manifestations (seborrheic dermatitis, prurigo, fungal nail infections, recurrent oral ulcerations, angular cheilitis)
3. Herpes zoster within the last five years
4. Recurrent upper respiratory tract infections (e.g., bacterial sinusitis)
   And/or performance scale 2: symptomatic, normal activity

Clinical Stage III: Intermediate (Moderate) Disease
1. Weight loss, > 10% of body weight
2. Unexplained chronic diarrhea > 1 month
3. Unexplained prolonged fever (intermittent or constant) > 1 month
4. Oral candidiasis (thrush)
5. Oral hairy leukoplakia
6. Pulmonary tuberculosis within the past year
7. Severe bacterial infections (e.g., pneumonia, pyomyositis)
   And/or performance scale 3: bedridden < 50% of the day during the past month

Clinical Stage IV:
1. HIV wasting syndrome
2. *Pneumocystis carinii* pneumonia
3. Toxoplasmosis of the brain
4. Cryptosporidiosis with diarrhea > 1 month
5. Cryptococcosis, extrapulmonary
6. Cytomegalovirus disease of an organ other than liver, spleen or lymph node (e.g., retinitis)
7. Herpes simplex virus infection, mucocutaneous (> 1 month) or visceral
8. Progressive multifocal leukoencephalopathy
9. Any disseminated endemic mycosis
10. Candidiasis of the esophagus, trachea, bronchi, or lungs
11. Atypical mycobacteriosis, disseminated
12. Non-typhoid salmonella septicemia
13. Extrapulmonary tuberculosis
14. Lymphoma
15. Kaposi's sarcoma
16. HIV encephalopathy
    And/or performance scale 4: bedridden > 50% of the day during the past month

Table 17-4. WHO Staging System for HIV in Children

Clinical Stage I:
1. Asymptomatic
2. Generalized lymphadenopathy

Clinical Stage II:
1. Chronic diarrhea > 30 days duration in absence of known etiology
2. Severe persistent or recurrent candidiasis outside the neonatal period
3. Weight loss or failure to thrive in the absence of known etiology
4. Persistent fever > 30 days duration in the absence of known etiology
5. Recurrent severe bacterial infections other than septicemia or meningitis (e.g., osteomyelitis, bacterial (non-TB) pneumonia, abscesses)

Clinical Stage III:
1. AIDS-defining opportunistic infections
2. Severe failure to thrive in the absence of known etiology
3. Progressive encephalopathy
4. Malignancy
5. Recurrent septicemia or meningitis

Table 17-5. CDC AIDS Case Surveillance Definition for Infants and Children

Immune Category	< 12 months		1-5 years		6-12 years	
	CD4+/mm	%	CD4+/mm	%	CD4+/mm	%
Category 1: No suppression	≥1,500	≥25	≥1,000	≥25	≥500	≥25
Category 2: Moderate suppression	750-1,499	15-24	500-999	15-24	200-499	15-24
Category 3: Severe suppression	<750	<15	<500	<15	<200	<15

urgent attention. The U.S. Centers for Disease Control and Prevention (CDC) classification (Table 17-1) employs a set of AIDS- and non-AIDS-related diseases, as well as CD4+ count, to determine disease severity. All patients in categories A3, B3, and C1–C3 are defined as having AIDS based on the presence of an AIDS-defining illness and/or a CD4+ count of less than 200/mm^3.

The WHO has developed a clinical definition of AIDS for surveillance, whereby adults with a positive HIV antibody test and one or more of the conditions listed in Table 17-2 are considered to have AIDS. The WHO has also developed an improved clinical staging system with four categories of clinical conditions believed to have prognostic significance (Table 17-3). A performance scale has also been incorporated into the system. Table 17-4 shows the WHO staging system for HIV infection and disease in children, while Table 17-5 shows the CDC AIDS case surveillance definition for infants and children.

GOALS OF HIGHLY ACTIVE ANTIRETROVIRAL THERAPY

The goals of HIV therapy are to provide optimal and individualized treatment for HIV-infected people at all stages of disease. ART for HIV became available in 1987 with the approval of AZT, a reverse transcriptase inhibitor and nucleoside analogue now known as zidovudine (11). While zidovudine monotherapy prolonged life, its beneficial effects were short-lived and within months the disease would again progress. Combination therapy with two nucleoside analogues offered some improvement. However, the benefits were again time-limited regardless of the specific combination (12). It was not until new classes of ARVs — the non-nucleoside reverse transcriptase and protease inhibitors — became available and were used in combination with two nucleosides that sustained results were achieved. The use of three ARVs from two drug classes has been termed triple-combination therapy or "highly active antiretroviral therapy" (HAART). HAART use is associated with sustained suppression of plasma HIV RNA (viral load) as measured by PCR, and significant improvement in immune status as measured by absolute and percentage CD4+ counts (13). These results have led to increased survival, reduced morbidity (14), and decreased vertical (15) and sexual transmission (16). HAART may also be used to prevent infection following inadvertent exposure to HIV (17).

Although HAART has produced dramatic benefits by increasing healthy survival, eradication of the virus in any individual has been elusive. The apparent invincibility of HIV, even in the face of HAART, has been aided by complex viral and cellular kinetics that allow it to persist in long-lived cells such as latently infected CD4+ T lymphocytes and tissue-bound macrophages. In addition, there are potential "sanctuary" sites such as the brain, testes (18), and retina (19), where the presence of blood-tissue barriers limits entry of otherwise potent ARVs.

Therapy must often be tailored to fit the needs of individual patients; however, the goals of ART remain the same:

- **Clinical:** Prevent progression of disease, prolong life, and improve the quality of life.
- **Virologic:** Maximally suppress plasma HIV RNA (viral load).
- **Immunologic:** Reconstitute the immune system with an increase in the quantity and quality of CD4+ cells.
- **Therapeutic:** Provide the most convenient HAART regimen with a low pill burden, few food requirements or limitations, and an infrequent dosing schedule, and enhance adherence.
- **Toxicity:** Select a regimen with the fewest acute and chronic adverse effects.
- **Pharmocokinetic:** Choose regimens with favorable pharmacokinetic properties and a high threshold for development of resistance.
- **Public health:** Reduce infectiousness in the population.

HAART has become the standard of care for treatment of HIV infection. The key to successful HAART in a resource-limited country such as Nigeria is the concept of durability. A durable regimen is one in which the potency of the drug—defined by its ability to suppress virus below levels of detection (< 50 or < 400 HIV RNA copies per ml, depending on the assays used—is maintained over a long period of time. A durable regimen can prevent the emergence of resistance, promote health, reduce the complexities of care, and ensure health cost savings. Current knowledge of the mechanisms of action, toxicity, drug resistance, and pharmacokinetic profile of available ARVs should inform the development of a durable regimen. Other key issues that will influence the development of durable regimens in resource-limited countries include knowledge of the effectiveness of available regimens, patterns of resistance, and the presence of comorbidities, such as tuberculosis and hepatitis B or C. Monitoring and evaluating ART programs to ensure they produce the desirable outcomes is also important for enhancing durability.

Table 17-6. Antiretroviral Drugs Available in 2005					
NRTIs	**NtRTIs**	**Nucleotide/NRTI**	**PIs**	**NNRTIs**	**Fusion Inhibitors**
Zidovudine	Tenofovir	Truvada®	Saquinavir	Nevirapine	
Didanosine			Ritonavir	Delavirdine	Enfuvirtide
Didanosine EC			Indinavir	Efavirenz	
Stavudine			Nelfinavir		
Stavudine XR			Amprenavir		
Abacavir			Lopinavir/ritonavir		
Lamivudine			Atazanavir		
Combivir®			Fosamprenavir		
Trizivir®			Tipranavir		
Epzicom®					
Emtricitabine					

Abbreviations: NRTIs: nucleoside reverse transcriptase inhibitors; NtRTI: nucleotide reverse transcriptase inhibitors; NNRTIs: non-nucleoside reverse transcriptase inhibitors; PIs: protease inhibitors
Notes: Combivir®=zidovudine + lamivudine; Trizivir®=zidovudine + lamivudine + abacavir; Epzicom®=abacavir + lamivudine; Truvada®=tenofovir + emtricitabine; lopinavir/ritonavir=Keletra®

Actions required to achieve durable ART include:

- Maximize adherence to the ARV regimen;
- Select sequential ARVs in a rational manner, starting with the most potent, locally proved combinations;
- Preserve future treatment options;
- Select drug combinations with high mutational thresholds;
- Use resistance testing in selected clinical settings;
- Select drugs with similar pharmacokinetic profiles;
- Limit the use of drug combinations with high toxicity;
- Use combinations with low pill burden, food requirements, and refrigeration storage needs; and
- Avoid adding single agents to a failing drug regimen.

CLASSES OF ANTIRETROVIRALS AND MODES OF ACTION

The major classes of ARVs are: nucleoside reverse transcriptase inhibitors (NRTIs); nucleotide reverse transcriptase inhibitors (NtRTIs); non-nucleoside reverse transcriptase inhibitors (NNRTIs); protease inhibitors (PIs); and fusion inhibitors (Table 17-6). The drugs in each of these classes interfere with specific steps in the HIV replication cycle.

NRTIs are synthetic nucleoside analogues that are inactive until taken up by infected cells and converted to the triphosphate compound through the action of cellular enzymes. The active triphosphate forms inhibit HIV-1 replication by incorporating into the viral DNA chain and competing with deoxynucleotide triphosphate (dNTP), which is the natural substrate for HIV reverse transcriptase (RT). This terminates the growing DNA strand, leading to incomplete replication of the virus.

The only NtRTI that is used for HIV

Table 17-7. Factors Determining the Choice of Antiretroviral Therapy	
Patient-Related Factors	**Drug-Related Factors**
• HIV RNA levels (viral load) • Baseline CD4+ cell count • Comorbidities (viral hepatitis, TB) • Lifestyle • Preference • Childbearing potential	• Potency • Convenience • Tolerability • Adverse events (toxicity) • Resistance profile • Cost • Refrigeration

treatment is tenofovir disoproxil fumarate (tenofovir DF). Tenofovir DF requires initial diester hydrolysis for conversion to tenofovir. Tenofovir is then taken up by cells and is phosphorylated to tenofovir diphosphate, which competes with the natural substrate (deoxyadenosine 5-triphosphate) for incorporation into viral DNA. This causes premature DNA chain termination and incomplete replication of the virus.

NNRTIs do not require intracellular phosphorylation to be active. Instead, these agents bind to a hydrophobic pocket of RT that is distinct, but close to the dNTP binding site. Thus, they do not compete with template or nucleoside triphosphates, but rather exert non-competitive inhibition of RT. These agents are active against HIV-1, but not HIV-2.

Normal HIV replication involves the action of two groups of proteases. First, there are cellular proteases that cleave envelope precursor polyprotein, leading to the formation of the glycoprotein spikes that are on the surface of the virus. Viral proteases are responsible for cleaving Gag and Gag-pol precursor polyproteins with formation of the remaining viral proteins, including RT, protease, and integrase. PIs act by inhibiting HIV protease, making the enzyme incapable of processing the Gag and Gag-pol polyproteins and resulting in the production of immature non-infectious HIV particles.

The only fusion inhibitor in use at this time is enfuvirtide (T-20). This agent inhibits the fusion between HIV and cellular membranes by binding to the gp41 portion of the HIV glycoprotein envelope, preventing the conformational changes that are necessary for the fusion of HIV to cellular membranes.

Currently investigational ARV drug classes include coreceptor antagonists and maturation inhibitors. CCR5 and CXCR4 are coreceptors for the binding of HIV to target cells; thus, agents that antagonize them have the potential to interfere with this critical step in the lifecycle of the virus. However, one potential limitation of CCR5 antagonists is that they are only likely to be effective against CCR5-tropic HIV, while CXCR4 antagonists are expected to be effective only against CXCR4-tropic virus. It is uncertain whether the use of CCR5 antagonists will cause selection of CXCR4-tropic virus, or conversely, whether selection of CCR5-tropic virus will occur with the use of CXCR4 antagonists.

CHOICE OF ANTIRETROVIRAL REGIMENS

While there are many effective HAART regimens that are used to treat HIV infection, the initial strategy must be based on specific drug and patient factors such as proven potency, ease of administration, potential drug toxicities, pharmacokinetics, resistance threshold, expense, and availability (Table 17-7). The current Nigerian ART guidelines recommend starting with an initial HAART regimen that includes two NRTIs plus one NNRTI or a PI (20). The preferred first-line regimen is zidovudine or stavudine, plus lamivudine; or emtricitabine, plus nevirapine or efavirenz. Three alternative first-line regimens are also recommended: tenofovir, plus lamivudine or emtricitabine, plus nevirapine or efavirenz; abacavir, plus lamivudine or emtricitabine, plus nevirapine or efavirenz; or zidovudine or stavudine, plus lamivudine or emtricitabine, plus tenofovir or abacavir.

Previous reports have shown that the potency of NNRTI-containing regimens was equivalent to that of PI-containing regimens (21). As an initial strategy, if a PI-containing regimen is chosen, most PIs can be combined with ritonavir for pharmacokinetic enhancement. Although enhancement of a PI-based regimen with ritonavir is likely to be more effective than using another PI alone, it may cause more side effects (22). A review of several clinical trials indicates that the most potent HAART regimens include efavirenz or lopinavir/ritonavir in combination with two NRTIs (23).

Based on a review of data from a number of studies, the preferred initial HAART combinations for adults are: efavirenz in combination with lamivudine and either zidovudine, stavudine, or tenofovir; or lopinavir/ritonavir in combination with lamivudine and either zidovudine or stavudine (24). A number of alternative regimens are less preferred because of the increased pill burden, potential adverse events, or limited efficacy data. Clinicians try to avoid stavudine as a first-line therapy because of its long-term, cumulative toxic effects.

NRTI Backbones

Multiple options are now available for the initial choice of dual NRTIs, the "NRTI backbone" (Table 17-8). The Nigerian guidelines recommend four of them: stavudine plus lamivudine, zidovudine plus lamivudine, tenofovir plus lamuvidine/emtricitabine, or abacavir plus lamuvidine (20). All of the backbone combinations are effective when combined with an NNRTI or PI, but their side effect profiles are different. Didanosine, although a very effective drug, should be avoided as an initial therapy because of the potential for developing neuropathy and pancreatitis, which can be fatal.

The NtRTI, tenofovir, plus either lamivudine or emtricitabine, has been shown to be well tolerated and as effective as stavudine plus lamivudine (24). To date, it appears that effects of long-term toxicity such as lipoatrophy and hypertriglyceridemia occur less frequently with tenofovir than with stavudine-based treatment (25). The coformulation of a tenofovir/emtricitabine (Truvada®) tablet means that this combination can be taken once daily with efavirenz with only two pills. Compared to Combivir®, the coformulation Truvada, when given in combination with efavirenz, had a superior virologic effect, less toxicity, and no tenofovir resistance. The Truvada/efavirenz combination is now widely used in Western countries because of its high virologic success and low toxicity rates (26).

Stavudine plus lamivudine is well tolerated in the short term; however, over time, some patients develop peripheral neuropathy and/or peripheral and facial lipoatrophy. Zidovudine plus lamivudine is associated with gastrointestinal side effects, anemia, and neutropenia; however, it is not associated with

Table 17-8. Nucleoside Combinations Used in HAART

NRTI Combination	Advantages	Disadvantages
Stavudine + lamivudine (a recommended combination)	Acutely well tolerated; inexpensive; readily available	Peripheral neuropathy; pancreatitis; lactic acidosis (rare); lipoatrophy; hypertriglyceridemia
Zidovudine + lamivudine (a recommended combination)	Inexpensive; readily available	Gastrointestinal effects; anemia; neutropenia; lipoatrophy (less so than stavudine-based); lactic acidosis (rare)
Tenofovir + lamivudine or emtricitabine (an alternative recommendation)	Acutely well tolerated; fewer long-term complications	Fewer long-term complications; expensive; limited availability; drug interactions more likely with tenofovir (i.e., atazanavir); tenofovir must be taken with food
Stavudine + didanosine (an alternative, not recommended initially)	Effective; inexpensive	Peripheral neuropathy; pancreatitis; lactic acidosis (rare); lipoatrophy; hypertriglyceridemia; didanosine must be taken without food
Zidovudine + didanosine (an alternative, not recommended initially)	Effective; inexpensive	Side effect profile not optimal: gastrointestinal effects; anemia; neutropenia; peripheral neuropathy; pancreatitis; lactic acidosis (rare); lipoatrophy
Abacavir + lamivudine	Effective and well tolerated	Abacavir hypersensitivity reaction
Zidovudine + stavudine (contraindicated)	None; should never be used	Antagonistic interaction; should never be used together

Abbreviations: HAART: highly active antiretroviral therapy; NRTI: nucleoside reverse transcriptase inhibitor

peripheral neuropathy and is associated with less peripheral and facial lipoatrophy than stavudine-containing regimens. Because of the high prevalence of anemia in Nigeria, the hemoglobin of all patients commencing treatment with zidovudine must be checked; zidovudine is contraindicated if the hemoglobin is less than 8 gm/dl.

The combination of abacavir and lamivudine is well tolerated, is usually not associated with mitochondrial toxicity, and can be dosed once or twice daily. A coformulation of the two drugs (Epzicom®) has been used successfully in a number of clinical trials (27). One major limitation of the widespread use of abacavir, however, is the occurrence of hypersensitivity reaction (HSR) in 5% to 10% of patients, which may occur in the first few weeks of therapy. Thus, physicians need to be trained to distinguish abacavir hypersensitivity rash from nevirapine-associated rash. Moreover, subsequent rechallenge after initial hypersensitivity can lead to death. HLA haplotype B-5701 has been associated with abacavir HSR, but the magnitude of the association is uncertain since many patients with the HSR lack HLA B-5701 (28). It has also been suggested that heat shock proteins (Hsp 70) represent an early component of the abacavir-specific immune response, which is sensitive to inhibition of type 1 alcohol dehydrogenase and influences interferon-gamma expression (29). It appears that African ethnicity, male gender, and CDC class C disease are associated with reduced risk (30). A preliminary report suggested that the incidence of severe HSR may be higher with once daily dosing compared to twice daily dosing (31).

Coformulated NRTI Combinations

There are currently three coformulated dual NRTI combinations: zidovudine/lamivudine (Combivir), abacavir/lamivudine (Epzicom), and tenofovir/emtricitabine (Truvada). When combined with an

Table 17-9. Antiretroviral Drugs Added to Dual Nucleoside Combinations in HAART

Third HAART Drug	Advantages	Disadvantages
Nevirapine (a recommended choice)	Can be used in pregnant women; inexpensive; available	Rash (can be severe but rarely fatal); hepatotoxicity (rarely fatal); unfavorable interaction with rifampicin
Efavirenz (a recommended choice)	Inexpensive; available; dosed once daily; can be used with rifampicin at higher dose (800 mg daily)	Central nervous system effects common (usually self-limited); rash (usually mild to moderate); potential fetal abnormalities—cannot be used in pregnancy
Lopinavir/ritonavir (Kaletra®) (an alternative choice)	Potent; relatively well tolerated	Gastrointestinal; hyperlipidemia; abdominal and truncal fat accumulation; expensive; requires refrigeration
Indinavir with or without ritonavir (an alternative choice)	Inexpensive relative to protease inhibitors	Without ritonavir, must be taken without food three times daily; nephrolithiasis; skin disorders; abdominal and truncal fat accumulation; glucose intolerance
Atazanavir with or without ritonavir (an alternative choice)	Once daily administration; a low-pill burden; no effect on serum lipids; unique resistance profile	Indirect hyperbilirubinemia; must be dosed with ritonavir (100 mg daily) if tenofovir co-administered
Nelfinavir (an alternative choice, not recommended for first-line therapy)	Relatively expensive favorable safety data available in pregnant women; low potency	Gastrointestinal effects common; less effective than other protease inhibitors that are given with ritonavir; should not be given with ritonavir; hyperlipidemia; abdominal and truncal fat accumulation
Saquinavir (an alternative choice, not recommended for first-line therapy)	Less effect on lipids than other protease inhibitors	Gastrointestinal; must be used with ritonavir rather than alone; abdominal and truncal fat accumulation

Abbreviation: HAART: highly active antiretroviral therapy

NNRTI or a PI, these formulations offer reduced pill burden, improved adherence, and preserved potency. A notable disadvantage is the lack of flexibility in dosing: if changes are needed, the patient must revert to the individual drugs. Unlike the traditional thymidine NRTI backbones, failures with the abacavir/lamivudine and tenofovir/emtricitabine backbones are associated with M184V mutations with or without the L74 or K65, which leaves some plausible sequencing options (32). Interestingly, individuals developing the K65R mutation who experience virologic failure are still able to maintain a mean viral load decrease of 0.9 log from baseline as observed in the Gilead 903 study (24). In this study, using both virtual phenotype and true phenotype, patients with K65R mutation were hypersensitive to zidovudine and stavudine and had full or partial susceptibility to abacavir, and in many cases, based on the results of testing resistance alone, remained sensitive to tenofovir and didanosine. This occurred in the absence or presence of the M184V mutation, which is known in vitro to hypersensitize the virus to tenofovir. Therefore, patients experiencing failure with a K65R mutation may have virologic success with a second regimen, including one containing tenofovir.

Other NRTI Combinations

Alternative double nucleoside choices exist; however, their use is limited by availability constraints or potential toxicity. The combination of stavudine plus didanosine has been shown to be quite effective. However, toxicity from the combination is unacceptable with excessive rates of pancreatitis, lipoatrophy, peripheral neuropathy, and lactic acidosis. Tenofovir plus didanosine is generally inappropriate for initial regimens, and should be avoided in salvage regimens, if alternatives are available. When used together, didanosine dose should be reduced. Tenofovir plus abacavir should be avoided; this combination has been associated with an increased risk of virologic failure, especially in patients with a viral load of more than 100,000 copies/ml and a CD4+ count of fewer than 200 cells/mm^3 (33). Even among some people who achieve viral suppression, a paradoxical decline in CD4+ count occurs, which is poorly understood. It is worth noting that inappropriate dosing of didanosine was a common finding in patients with adverse outcomes (34). Lamivudine plus didanosine has been demonstrated to be an effective NRTI backbone in many studies. However, potential problems with this regimen include pancreatitis and peripheral neuropathy due to didanosine and probably increased risk of some manifestations of mitochondrial toxicity. Thus, it is not used in initial regimens. Emtricitabine has also shown to be effective when combined with didanosine and efavirenz once daily in treatment-naive patients (35), but this combination is not used in initial regimens because of toxicity. Zidovudine plus didanosine is usually used in second-line regimens after failure of initial therapy. Table 17-8 outlines the advantages and disadvantages of different NRTI combinations.

Selecting the Third Drug

In addition to the NRTI backbone, the third drug of a HAART regimen is a critical choice and should be chosen based on potency, pharmacokinetics, adverse event profile, and availability (Table 17-9). The most common third drug added to a HAART regimen is a non-nucleoside, either nevirapine or efavirenz. Both drugs have favorable pharmacokinetic profiles, are dosed infrequently (typically once daily), and have been shown to be effective (36). Both drugs are inducers of the cytochrome P450 (CYP450) system and may lower the effective concentrations of hepatically metabolized drugs in the blood, although to different degrees (37). The largest study to date comparing efavirenz-containing and nevirapine-containing regimens (the 2NN trial) found that both had similar virologic and immunologic efficacy. The major difference between these drugs is their toxicity profiles. Efavirenz was better tolerated with lower incidence of severe hepatic and cutaneous toxicity (38). Delavirdine, a third approved non-nucleoside, is infrequently used because of a higher pill burden and a lack of central nervous system penetration. Delavirdine is an inhibitor of CYP450. Non-nucleoside drugs should not be used together and should only be used in combination with two other ARVs.

Nevirapine

Nevirapine, the first non-nucleoside to be approved, is associated with rash in approximately 17% of patients. One-half of the rashes are mild, characterized by intact skin and absence of blistering, skin desquamation, involvement of mucous membranes, angioedema, or systemic signs (body aches, arthalgias, myalgias, fevers, lymphadenopathy, or significantly elevated hepatic transaminases). It is usually self-limited and does not require discontinuation of the drug. Antihistamines may offer some symptomatic relief. In approximately 0.5% of patients, the rash can be serious and includes potentially fatal Stevens-

Johnson syndrome or toxic epidermal necrolysis. Following the recommended lead-in dosing reduces the likelihood of developing nevirapine-associated rash.

Mild asymptomatic liver enzyme elevations (LEE) are relatively common, often self-limited, and do not require treatment discontinuation. Liver enzymes should be checked regularly until they have returned to normal. Symptomatic elevations of ALT and hepatic failure also occur with nevirapine (39), particularly during the first six weeks of treatment. Reported symptoms, including nausea, vomiting, and abdominal pain, are similar to those that occur in patients with pancreatitis and lactic acidosis; therefore, these conditions should be excluded. About half of the patients with nevirapine-associated hepatotoxicity have rash with or without other manifestations of autoimmune disease, strengthening the theory that it is essentially a hypersensitivity phenomenon. Risk factors for this rash-associated hepatitis include female with CD4+ counts greater than 250 cells/mm³ and male with CD4+ counts greater than 400 cells/mm³ (40). Therapy should be discontinued in patients with symptomatic LEE (with or without manifestations of hypersensitivity), liver failure, or lactic acidosis. Therapy with ARVs that are less hepatotoxic may be cautiously restarted after resolution of the LEE. Required supportive therapy should be given. Fatal hepatic failure has been reported but is rare (41).

Although nevirapine is not absolutely contraindicated in patients coinfected with HIV and hepatitis C virus (HCV), it should be used with caution because of preliminary reports that suggest an accelerated rate of hepatic fibrosis in such patients (42). Choosing another agent may be prudent to reduce the risk of necroinflammation and fibrosis in some patients. Also, the use of nevirapine in post-exposure prophylaxis (PEP) regimens is discouraged because of its propensity to cause hepatotoxicity in patients with intact immune systems (39). For HIV-infected patients who are coinfected with hepatitis B virus (HBV) or HVC, it is usually difficult to distinguish liver enzyme abnormalities caused by ARV hepatotoxicity or hypersensitivity from those caused by a flare of HBV or HCV due to immune reconstitution. It is important to make this distinction correctly, however, since it directly impacts the decision to continue or interrupt HAART. A helpful strategy involves close monitoring of the patient's laboratory and clinical course: patients who remain asymptomatic and have improving liver enzymes while receiving the same ART regimen probably have immune reconstitution hepatitis flare, in which case therapy can be cautiously continued. Therapy should be interrupted in those who are symptomatic and those who experience progressive worsening laboratory results on ART, because they probably have hepatotoxicity or hypersensitivity. A distinct advantage of nevirapine is its lack of adverse effects on the fetus and newborn, hence its use for prevention of vertical transmission. A potential disadvantage is an interaction with rifampicin, which precludes the use of the two drugs together.

Efavirenz

Efavirenz also is associated with rash, but this is usually less severe than with nevirapine and only infrequently leads to drug discontinuation. The primary problems associated with efavirenz use are central nervous system side effects and potential fetal abnormalities, specifically neural tube defects. The neurologic effects associated with efavirenz include mood alterations, sleep disorders, unusual dreams, hypomania, and anxiety. Usually these effects are self-limited and resolve after several days or weeks. Because of the potential adverse effects on the fetus, efavirenz should not be administered during pregnancy or in women contemplating pregnancy. The interaction with rifampicin is less than that of nevirapine. When the drugs are used together, the efavirenz dose is usually increased from 600 to 800 mg daily, although this may not be necessary in all patients. In one randomized, controlled study among Thai patients with tuberculosis and an average body weight below 60 kilograms, there was no significant difference in virologic and immunologic outcomes between patients who received 600 mg of rifampicin and those who received 800 mg in combination with an efavirenz-containing HAART regimen (43). In another study conducted in Durban, South Africa, serial trough efavirenz levels were followed in HIV-infected patients (mean weight 59.7 kilograms) with smear-positive tuberculosis. The patients received HAART regimens of efavirenz, didanosine, and lamivudine, while tuberculosis was treated with a rifampicin-containing regimen. Although there was wide variability in its plasma concentrations, efavirenz at a dose of 600 mg/day was found to be efficacious, with virologic success, immunologic success, and weight gain (44). The rifampicin dose did not require adjustment.

Protease Inhibitors

An effective alternative to the non-nucleoside approach is the addition of a PI as the third drug in a HAART regimen. The most effective and practical PIs to be considered for first-line therapy include lopinavir/ritonavir (Kaletra®), indinavir with or without ritonavir, and atazanavir with or without ritonavir. Nelfinavir is also an option, but it has been demonstrated to be less effective than lopinavir/ritonavir-based therapy (45). Pharmacokinetic enhancement of nelfinavir with ritonavir is less effective than with the other PIs and is associated with unacceptable gastrointestinal intolerance. Saquinavir hard gel (Invirase®) is an alternative only when co-administered with ritonavir. Amprenavir and its newer prodrug form, fosamprenavir, are not yet available in Nigeria.

Unfortunately, at their regular doses many PIs have trough levels close to the lowest concentration at which they exert antiviral activity, thus providing opportunities for viral replication and resistance. Ritonavir is a unique PI in that at very small doses, it alters the metabolism of other PIs by inhibiting gastrointestinal and hepatic CYP450 enzyme system. This improves pharmacokinetic parameters of co-administered PIs such as peak plasma concentration (Cmax), half-life, and trough concentration (Cmin). The area under the plasma concentration versus time curve (AUC), which determines the overall viral exposure to the PI, is also increased, often allowing a reduction in the dose needed for effective treatment. Also, the inhibitory quotient — the ratio of Cmin to the concentration needed to inhibit viral replication by 50% (IC50), which influences the likelihood of developing resistance mutations — is improved with ritonavir-boosted PIs. For these reasons, ritonavir-boosted PIs generally have improved potency and greater pharmacokinetic barriers to resistance.

In contrast to some unboosted PI regimens, failure of ritonavir-boosted, PI-based regimens in previously PI–naive patients is unlikely to be due to development of resistance to the boosted PI. This was well illustrated when lopinavir/ritonavir plus two NRTIs was compared to nelfinavir plus similar NRTIs (45). The "anti-resistance" characteristic, which has been demonstrated with other boosted PIs, including atazanavir/ritonavir and fosamprenavir/ritonavir (46), underlies some of the strongest arguments in favor of boosted PI regimens. Also, ritonavir-boosting can be used to overcome low-level resistance to PIs.

Triple Nucleoside Regimens

Triple nucleoside combinations also have been studied as first-line HAART. These combinations allow sparing of NNRTIs and PIs. Although these combinations are convenient and cause fewer drug interactions, the potency of the fixed combination of zidovudine/lamivudine/abacavir has been inferior to non-nucleoside– and PI–based regimens (47). Therefore, triple nucleoside combinations should only be used in circumstances in which NNRTIs and PIs are either not available or not tolerated. Conversely, the combinations of tenofovir/lamivudine/abacavir or tenofovir/lamivudine/didanosine should be avoided because they failed in two studies (48,49). Resistance testing in both studies showed the emergence of both M184 and K65R mutations in patients with evidence of virologic failure.

Preliminary reports from the DART study of the evaluation of tenofovir/lamivudine/zidovudine have shown promising results (50). The good response with this particular regimen appears directly related to the presence of zidovudine and tenofovir, a combination that has bidirectional protection against resistance. One concern with the use of the DART regimen in some resource-limited settings, however, is the apparently increased risk of anemia (51). Nonetheless, the DART regimen is particularly promising in settings with high rates of tuberculosis coinfection, because it does not contain NNRTIs or PIs that are responsible for the drug interactions that complicate the management of both infections. Some quadruple NRTI regimens that contain zidovudine and tenofovir also have shown some promise in preliminary trials, but there are lingering concerns about broad NRTI resistance and a clear role for the regimen remains undefined. It should be noted that the DART study has no comparative treatment arm, and results must be interpreted with caution at this time.

STEPS TO INITIATE ANTIRETROVIRAL THERAPY

Assessment of the Patient

Several patient-related factors may influence the choice and outcome of ART in resource-limited countries. In Nigeria, many patients may delay visiting a clinic until they present with advanced HIV disease (WHO stage III or IV) because of the prevailing stigma and the absence of widespread counseling and testing. Patients may present with coexisting morbidities such as anemia, malaria, tuberculosis, or hepatitis, which may affect the choice of the drug regimen due to potential drug interactions and toxicities. A 2001 sentinel survey conducted by the Federal Ministry of Health found 23% of tuberculosis patients to be HIV positive (52). Most patients are poor, and financial constraints can cause treatment interruptions.

A detailed clinical evaluation of the patient should be made at baseline and every three to six months subsequently. Each visit should include a review of current symptoms and concomitant illnesses. Clinical features and diseases should be categorized as HIV-related or AIDS-defining. The patient should also be screened for the presence of coinfections, including malaria, tuberculosis, HBV, and STIs.

A detailed medical history, including a history of any high-risk sexual behavior and the number of sex partners, should be elicited from the patient. The history should also include the sexual and other relevant history of the patient's sexual partner or partners, as this information can be useful in determining the patient's relative risks for other infections, such as with the hepatitis B, hepatitis C, and human papilloma viruses. Other important information includes a history of any previous blood transfusions and, in women, the history of previous pregnancies, antenatal care, and deliveries. Many patients in Africa may be taking traditional medications for HIV-related disease. Identifying the remedies a patient may be taking is important, as these drugs may cause drug interactions or affect liver or kidney function, the ultimate pathways for the metabolism and excretion of most ARVs.

The initial physical examination of the patient should be detailed and should include: measuring weight, temperature, and vital signs; checking the skin for rashes, ulcers, and lesions; checking the oral cavity for thrush and sore throat; assessing mental and emotional status; and making appropriate assessments of the following organs or systems: lymph nodes, chest and cardiovascular, abdominal and gastrointestinal, genitourinary and rectal, gynecologic (women), neurologic, and ophthalmic.

Baseline laboratory investigations should include a chest X-ray for tuberculosis and pneumonia; microbiologic tests for tuberculosis, including a sputum smear and cultures; a full blood count; a fasting blood sugar; kidney and liver function tests; a lipid profile, including triglycerides and cholesterol; a pap smear for women; appropriate swabs for STIs; hepatitis B and C antibody tests; a syphilis test; a pregnancy test if indicated; a CD4+ count; and a HIV viral load if available.

After the initial work-up of the patient, the physician should have the information needed to determine the patient's stage of HIV disease and to assess other factors that will influence treatment decisions, such as the presence of HIV-related diseases and other concomitant illnesses, like hypertension or diabetes; the patient's weight profile; and concomitant medications, including any traditional medications. The decision of when to start ART and what regimen to choose in Nigeria is complicated by prevailing factors such as pregnancy, the presence of comorbidities (tuberculosis, HBV, or HCV), anemia, consideration of uninfected partners, and the availability and cost of the drugs. A successful HAART regimen should be tailored to the patient. For instance, in patients with a significant psychiatric history, efavirenz may not be the optimal choice because of its associated central nervous system effects. In women who are likely to get pregnant during treatment, efavirenz should be avoided because of the potential for fetal abnormality. Patients who are malnourished and anemic prior to treatment are not good candidates for therapy with zidovudine. Knowledge about the drugs and the full background of the patient is essential in designing the most acceptable and adhered to HAART regimen. The physician should see the patient at subsequent visits to discuss treatment options, including the risks and benefits of ART, and to choose the optimal ART regimen.

A treatment plan must be developed that the patient understands and to which he or she will be committed. Patient education and preparation are key to subsequent commitment and adherence to the administered regimen. There should be no rush to start patients on ART as this can lead to non-commitment, dropouts, and the generation of drug resistance. Clinicians should assess the patient's readiness for medication before initiation of therapy, potentially during multiple consultations. Patient education should include discussion of the goals of ART as well as the expected outcomes based on clinical, CD4+ cell, and viral load responses. It is critical for patients to understand that the first regimen has the best chance of long-term success. In addition, education and counseling should incorporate a detailed discussion of the need for adherence and possibly a detailed adherence plan, including the use of treatment partners. Adherence should be monitored and assessed at each clinic follow-up visit because there is evidence that adherence wanes over time (53).

Patients should be encouraged to join support groups as both peer education and support from members strengthen adherence among patients on ARVs. Furthermore, adherence goals should be built into all patients' treatment plans and interventions. Toxicities are the most common reasons for poor adherence to medications (54). When the treatment regimen is chosen, patients must be counseled on how to take the specific medications, what side effects could potentially occur, what to do in the event of an adverse effect, and where to go with any treatment or disease-related questions.

The criteria for commencement of ART according to the Nigerian guidelines (20) in both adults and adolescents are:

- WHO Stage IV disease (AIDS) irrespective of CD4+ count;
- WHO Stage III disease (symptomatic HIV) with CD4+ counts of less than $350/mm^3$; or
- WHO Stage I or II disease with CD4+ counts of less than or equal to $200/mm^3$.

Table 17-10. Suggested Monitoring Schedule for Patients Starting HAART							
	Pre-Treatment	Week 2	Week 4	Week 8	Every 12 Weeks	Every 4-8 Weeks	Every 24 Weeks
Physical exam	X	X			X		
Adherence counseling	X	X	X	X	X	X	
HIV RNA (if available)	X				X**		X
CD4+ cell count	X				X**		X
Complete blood count	X						X
Chemistry*	X						X

* includes serum lipids
** at first 12-week visit only
  Abbreviation: HAART: highly active antiretroviral therapy

MONITORING ANTIRETROVIRAL THERAPY AND PATIENT FOLLOW-UP

Before initiating therapy, the clinician and patient must agree on a schedule for monitoring the progress and effects of therapy (Table 17-10). At a minimum, the physician should evaluate stable patients every three months and order laboratory assessments twice annually. At treatment initiation, at the time of any treatment change, or with concurrent illnesses, monitoring should take place more frequently.

The first return visit to the clinic should be scheduled two weeks after the patient starts HAART. At this time, it is wise to assess the patient's tolerance of and adherence to the medications, especially any side effects related to nevirapine or efavirenz use, which occur in the first few weeks of therapy. A brief physical exam should be performed and, if indicated, a complete blood count and chemistry should be done to assess any potential adverse effects on blood count and hepatic function in particular. If the patient on a nevirapine-containing regimen does not have a rash or any medication-related side effects, the dose of nevirapine should be increased from 200 mg/day to 200 mg twice daily. If a rash is present in any form, the 200 mg dose should be continued until resolution, at which time the dose can then be increased.

The patient should again return to the clinic every four weeks to pick up drugs. This schedule ensures supervision of drug therapy and provides opportunities for adherence counseling and contact tracing for patients who miss their appointments. A brief and targeted physical examination should be performed. In resource-poor settings like Nigeria, it is not practical to carry out plasma HIV RNA (viral load) at four weeks to assess early efficacy because of costs and the unavailability of the tests in most ART centers. However, CD4+ counts and plasma HIV RNA levels should be monitored 12 weeks after commencing therapy and subsequently every 24 weeks if patients are stable. Unstable patients may require more frequent monitoring. The standard of care in Nigeria for monitoring ART is CD4+ cell enumeration and plasma viral load quantification. Plasma viral load correlates with disease progression (55) and is a critical parameter for assessing virologic failure. In tertiary and referral centers that have the necessary infrastructure and trained personnel to perform this assay, viral load quantification will provide the physician and patient with critical information on virologic status during ART and will indicate when virologic failure has occurred. In points of care where this assay is not available, CD4+ cell enumeration and clinical monitoring can be substituted.

Targeted physical examinations should be done every 12 weeks and a detailed examination every 24 weeks. Comprehensive laboratory monitoring should be done every 24 weeks for stable patients (Table 17-10). This should include a complete blood count and blood chemistry including liver enzymes, renal function, serum lipids, a CD4+ count, and plasma HIV RNA (where available). Every attempt should be made to discuss the laboratory results at follow-up visits, as this is an important part of promoting adherence and commitment to therapy. As much as possible, these results should be used in making decisions about drug management, as patients are often encouraged by a decline in HIV RNA and lack of toxicity.

Patients should be instructed to return to the clinic at any time between scheduled appointments if they have treatment-related questions or problems. In the event they believe they are experiencing a

Table 17-11. Adherence Factors for Antiretroviral Therapy	
Factors Associated with Improved Adherence	**Factors Associated with Poor Adherence**
• Patient knowledge of disease and drugs • Patient belief systems about HIV and modes of treatment • Clinician knowledge of disease and drugs • Low pill burden • Infrequent dosing schedule • No food effect on drugs • Continuous availability of drugs • Tracking treatment defaulters • Treatment support (directly observed therapy, family member, community and support group) • Develop linkage with local community-based organizations on adherence education and strategies	• Drug toxicity • Heavy pill burden and frequent dosing schedule • Active illicit drug and/or alcohol use • Untreated/uncontrolled psychiatric illness • Expense of drugs, monitoring, and travel • Inconvenient appointments with clinic • Lack of adequate transportation • Lack of food, clothing, and shelter • Poor nutritional support • Young age

drug-related serious adverse event and yet cannot visit the clinic, they should be instructed to stop all ARVs until they seek the advice of a professional in the clinic.

Adherence and Treatment Support

Success with any medication depends not only on the intrinsic properties of the drugs, but also on the ability of the patient to take the medications. HIV infection is one of the most difficult chronic diseases to treat optimally. Multiple drugs must be administered, the pill burden may be high, the regimen may be complicated, toxicities are common, drug interactions may occur, food restrictions may be required, medications are expensive, the regimen carries an enormous social and psychological burden for many, and therapy is lifelong. HAART is lifesaving, yet it is anything but easy and it is very unforgiving. Less than 95% adherence to a regimen can lead to viral resistance and ultimately treatment failure (56). It has been estimated that every 10% decrease in adherence leads to a corresponding 16% increase in mortality (57).

A number of factors affect adherence (Table 17-11). These include the patient's belief systems regarding the etiology (58), as well as their knowledge of the management and treatment of HIV infection (59). Other factors include the social, emotional, and financial status of the patient as well as the tolerability, dosing schedule, and pill burden of the drug regimen. Active use of injected drugs or alcohol, psychiatric disease, and depression are also important factors promoting non-adherence. Young people and those with a disruptive social life are also likely to be non-adherent to ART. Studies among HIV-infected patients have indicated a strong preference for once-daily dosing and compact regimens (60). Furthermore, several reports have observed a significant correlation between low pill burden and improved virologic response (61,62).

Despite the difficulties of taking lifelong treatment, improving patient adherence is possible. It is imperative to provide the patient with basic knowledge about ARVs and HIV disease and to stress the overall importance of adherence prior to initiating ART. Over the course of several visits before initiating therapy, clinicians can take a number of steps to improve the chances of good adherence, such as discussing cultural beliefs and myths about HIV and ART; discussing the risks and benefits of ART, including dosing schedules and side effects associated with different regimens; establishing readiness and full commitment to therapy; fostering trust in the health care team; recruiting family and friends for disclosure and treatment support; and developing support groups for people living with HIV/AIDS. Activities that engage family and community members in adherence education and treatment support can both promote adherence and minimize stigma.

Upon initiating ART, clinicians can take further steps to improve the likelihood of good adherence, such as tailoring the regimen to the patient's lifestyle; familiarizing the patient with the pills and dosing schedule; scheduling follow-up visits soon after initiation to discuss side effects and any other obstacles to taking the drugs; promptly responding to any problems by adjusting, changing, or stopping medications when needed; and treating associated conditions, such as depression, anxiety, psychotic disorders, and drug addiction. Facilitating family-based care — in which all infected members of the family are seen together at follow-up clinics for ART — is another useful strategy for enhancing adherence and successful ART.

The potential for improved adherence is also maximized when clinicians develop long-term plans for treatment and are careful to select regimens that will avoid drug interactions and side effects to the extent possible. Prescribing regimens with low pill burdens, infrequent dosing, minimal toxicities, and no food interactions are all associated with optimal adherence. Fixed dose combinations (63), pill boxes, and blister packs have all been found to be successful in increasing adherence to drugs in various resource-limited settings. Pagers and alarm clocks can also help to remind patients to take their medication. Tracking defaulters with pharmacy logs and home visits by clinic staff can be particularly useful in preventing prolonged periods of poor adherence and addressing potential problems with adherence as they arise. Other factors that may enhance adherence to ART include providing medications free of charge for those who cannot afford them. It has been suggested that a cost-sharing program could facilitate adherence to ART, although a recent report from Senegal does not support such an approach (64).

Directly observed therapy (DOT) is another way to ensure adherence, but the logistical requirements of this are often daunting, especially because HIV, unlike active tuberculosis, requires lifelong treatment. DOT is relatively easy to administer in controlled environments such as prisons, but it can also be implemented at the community level. For example, a large community-based ART program in Haiti used community health workers who visited patients daily. All patients gained weight, and fewer than 5% required medication changes due to side effects or toxicity. Among patients for whom viral load was tested, 86% had suppressed viral loads (65). Various cohort studies with DOT have observed that high therapeutic success can be achieved with PI- or NNRTI-based triple therapy regimens (66,67). The potential application of DOT-HAART in the Nigerian setting has shown promising preliminary results (68).

Adherence should be measured periodically; ideally, at every clinic visit. The most commonly used method is direct patient interview, which tends to overestimate adherence. Patient-reported poor adherence is usually accurate, however. A clinician's estimate of the likelihood of adherence is often unreliable.

DRUG RESISTANCE

With a virion half-life of 30 minutes and a daily production of up to 10^9 virions, HIV reverse transcriptase enzyme incorporates approximately one mutation per genome per replication cycle (69). The higher the viral replication, the more frequent the mutations, with almost every single point mutation occurring daily. These mutations produce a population of diverse, yet related viral variants referred to as "quasispecies," which are generated by the error-prone viral RNA-dependent polymerase. Whenever a mutation occurs, the fitness—or replicative capacity—of the altered virus may be enhanced, unchanged, or reduced, depending on the specific mutation and its interactions with the host immune system and the presence or absence of ARVs.

Approximately half of the virus population in plasma is cleared and replaced each day. The high turnover allows a rapid emergence of drug-resistant variants under selective pressure. To maximize its chances of survival, HIV, like other pathogenic organisms, evolves toward strains with the greatest ability to replicate in a given environment. Therefore, evolution toward wild-type virus, which typically has high replicative capacity, is favored in the absence of ARV pressure. On the other hand, when a patient is taking ARVs, viral evolution favors strains that are best able to replicate in that environment—that is, strains that are resistant to the particular drug or drugs. If the selected drug-resistant strain is of appropriate fitness, it may eventually become the dominant strain, although resistant variants are usually replaced by residual wild-type virus if the drug selective pressure is removed. Resting latently infected cells can, however, continue to harbor drug-resistant provirus.

The most effective way to interrupt the cycle of viral replication and mutation is to attain complete, durable viral suppression. Incomplete viral suppression encourages viral mutation and resistance. The factors contributing to incomplete suppression of virus replication include poor adherence, pharmacologic factors, host factors, inadequate ARV potency, and transmitted drug resistance. Mechanisms that result in HIV drug resistance include decreased drug binding, increased enzyme efficiency, nucleotide excision, increased target concentration, altered (co)receptor affinity, and altered drug transport. The factors linked to detection of resistance mutations are:

- A high baseline viral load or low baseline CD4+ count;
- Substantial but imperfect adherence (highest-risk patients);
- Injection drug use; and
- Use of drugs with low resistance development thresholds.

Drug resistance is a major problem for HIV-infected patients on ART. Among treatment-naive subjects initiating HAART, 25% developed drug-resistance mutations during a 30-month follow-up (70), while multi-class resistance was noted in about 10% (71). Resistance testing has been observed to improve treatment outcome in patients receiving ART (72). Mutations on the reverse transcriptase and protease genes can be mapped to specific codon changes that are often correlated with viral resistance to a specific drug, subclass of drugs, or class of drugs. While measuring resistance has become more common in the developed world, resistance testing is expensive and not available in many resource-poor countries like Nigeria. However, a fundamental understanding of viral resistance is required to treat patients, particularly those who have not responded to or failed a prior treatment regimen. Therefore, resistance testing should be embraced in tertiary health institutions as part of the process of monitoring individuals on ART in Nigeria.

Adherence is the most important factor in determining whether resistance emerges during treatment (73). The relationship between adherence and the accumulation of drug resistance is complex and variable. Drug resistance occurs at a range of adherence between 60% and 80% (74). Drug-resistance mutations that are associated with reduced viral fitness and virulence may lead to a fairly durable treatment benefit but also delay the need to modify therapy, thus allowing high-level resistance to emerge. Other mutations are associated with reducing (cross-resistance) or enhancing (hypersensitivity) the activity of some ARVs in the same or other classes.

Transmitted Drug Resistance

As ARV use becomes widespread in a given area, one might expect an increase in the proportion of patients who become infected with drug-resistant HIV strains. However, the emerging trend in places with a long history of ART is that transmitted resistance is low if HAART is comprehensive and widely available. Epidemiologic data from the CATCH study found the overall prevalence of HIV strains resistant to at least one ARV was 9.6% (75). The prevalence of drug-resistant HIV among patients infected for a year or less was 10.9%, compared to 7.5% among patients infected for more than one year. Data from the United States have demonstrated similar results (76). Among patients with primary HIV infection, 11.5% had resistance to at least one ARV compared to 7.5% among patients with chronic HIV infection. In both studies, the most common resistance was to NRTIs. Historical models have been used to predict that over the next decade, the rate of transmission of drug-resistant virus in Africa would remain below 5% and that most resistant strains would result from acquired, not transmitted, resistance (77).

Antiretroviral Therapy and Acquired Drug Resistance in Nigeria

The choice of HAART regimen may help to avoid resistance. Regimens that promote adherence by using pills with low toxicity, doses of one or two times a day, and fixed dose combinations will delay the onset of resistance. Other factors promoting a durable regimen include drugs that are potent, have favorable pharmacokinetic properties, and have a high barrier to resistance. The choice of the first regimen may determine future treatment options by determining the resistance pathways. There is, therefore, a need for studies to determine optimal regimens for the Nigerian ARV program. Nevirapine-containing regimens for PMTCT in the country also need to be evaluated in view of the reports of high-level resistance from the use of single-dose nevirapine (78) and the poor response—due to resistance—of these patients to subsequent nevirapine-containing HAART combinations (79).

Testing for Resistance

Drug resistance can be determined by two main techniques: genotypic and phenotypic testing. Genotypic testing detects specific mutations in the reverse transcriptase and/or protease genes. Phenotypic testing determines the relative amount of drug needed to suppress viral replication compared to a reference wild-type virus. These tests are most reliable when the viral load is greater than 1,000 copies/ml.

Genotypic tests are more readily available, have a quicker turnaround time, are less technically demanding to perform, and are relatively less costly. Another important advantage of genotyping is the ability to detect mutations that are in the process of back mutation (from resistant virus to wild-type, or "revertant" mutants), and whose amino acid sequences are between those of resistant virus and wild type virus. These partially revertant mutants may not influence phenotype, but their identification on genotypic testing offers valuable information. Genotyping has limited usefulness if the clinical significance of detected mutation has not been previously characterized, and if the mutations are multiple and complex, genotyping requires expert interpretation.

Phenotypic tests measure drug susceptibility directly. However, the assay is technically more demanding, limited in availability, and relatively expensive, and determining clinically relevant cut-offs or breakpoints is often difficult and variable. Advantages of phenotypic resistance assays include ease of interpretation and provision of meaningful information when multiple mutations are present in the same sample. Thus, phenotypic testing may be preferred to genotyping in heavily treatment-experienced patients, who harbor multiple, complex resistance mutations.

The usefulness of resistance testing is in the identification of drugs that are likely to work and, independently, not to work. These determinations may be imperfect, however, because clinically relevant mutations may not be detected by standard resistance tests if they constitute a very small proportion of the total viral pool. The more "active" drugs contained in a regimen, the greater the likelihood that the therapy will succeed.

The following situations warrant resistance testing consideration:

- Before initiating therapy in a patient exposed to possibly resistant virus, such as when a patient has been exposed to single-dose nevirapine or has had a sexual partner who was exposed;
- In patients who fail to adequately respond to first-line or second-line therapy; and
- In patients who experience viral "rebound" or a return of HIV RNA toward baseline.

Several caveats need to be considered about resistance testing: tests are most useful when the patient is on an ARV regimen; the absence of resistance to a drug that a patient has previously taken does not eliminate the possibility that the virus is resistant to that drug; if resistance to a drug is ever documented, it is assumed that the patient is likely to archive resistance virus indefinitely, regardless of subsequent test results; and expert advice is often required to interpret resistance test results.

TOXICITY

The use of ART for treating HIV-infected people in developing countries has increased significantly in the past few years and has already witnessed the gains of reduced mortality and morbidity seen in the developed world in the mid-1990s (80). Even though the adverse events of these drugs have been well documented (Table 17-12), experience in developing countries, particularly Nigeria, has been limited because of inadequate data gathering and the short duration of experience in the country.

Key Drug-Drug Interactions

The use of ARVs is complex. Drug-drug interactions can occur, posing a major challenge for treating HIV positive individuals. Interaction among drugs used in combination therapy, with other drugs, and even with food may affect the absorption, distribution, metabolism, and excretion of the various drugs used in the regimen. In general, clinically significant drug interactions occur when a change of not less than 25% of the drug concentration occurs.

Table 17-12. Adverse Events to Antiretroviral Therapy	
Drug	**Toxicity**
Nucleoside/Nucleotide Reverse Transcriptase Inhibitors	
Class Related	Lactic acidosis Hepatic steatosis Lipodystrophy (peripheral fat wasting)
Drug Specific	
Stavudine	Peripheral neuropathy, hepatitis
Zidovudine	Bone marrow suppression, myopathy, nausea, and vomiting
Didanosine	Pancreatitis, dry mouth, peripheral neuropathy
Lamivudine	Mild or no side effects
Abacavir	Hypersensitivity reaction, nausea
Tenofovir	Bone demineralization, renal failure
Non-Nucleoside Reverse Transcriptase Inhibitors	
Nevirapine	Rash, hepatitis, Stevens Johnson syndrome
Efavirenz	Rash, dysphoria, mood changes, vivid dreams, hypercholesterolemia, fetal abnormalities
Protease Inhibitors	
Class Related	Lipodystrophy (fat wasting/accumulation), hyperlipidemia, diabetes mellitus
Drug Specific	
Nelfinavir	Diarrhea, rash
Saquinavir	Few side effects
Indinavir	Hyperbilirubinemia, nephrolithiasis, nail changes, paronychia, dry skin, abdominal cramps
Ritonavir	Perioral dysathesia, flushing, hepatitis, diarrhea, nausea, vomiting, abdominal cramps
Amprenavir	Rash, nausea, diarrhea
Lopinavir	Diarrhea
Atazanavir	Hyperbilirubinaemia

The most studied interactions have been between drugs using the CYP450 enzyme system for drug metabolism in the liver. Because NNRTIs and PIs are metabolized through this system, many clinically relevant drug interactions occur with the use of these drugs. The interaction may take place via one of three pathways: as a substrate; as an inhibitor; or as an inducer. Rifampicin, rifapentine, and rifabutin all have significant interactions with NNRTIs and PIs by virtue of their ability to act as inducers of the CYP450 enzyme in the liver. Blood levels of NNRTIs and PIs are significantly reduced when combined with rifamycins.

However, the effect is least with rifabutin, hence the recommendation that rifabutin be used with NNRTIs and PIs in patients coinfected with HIV and tuberculosis. Rifabutin is metabolized by

CYP3A; therefore, its serum concentration is increased by PIs and delavirdine, which are inhibitors of the enzyme. As a result, rifabutin's dose has to be reduced if it is used with PIs or delavirdine. On the other hand, since efavirenz induces CYP3A and reduces serum concentrations of rifabutin, the dose of rifabutin has to be increased when they are used together. Rifampicin and rifapentine are not substrates for CYP3A, and their levels are not significantly affected by inhibitors or inducers of the enzyme. No significant interactions occur between rifamycins and NRTIs. Rifapentine is not recommended in HIV-infected patients with tuberculosis, because it is associated with rifamycin-monoresistant relapse.

Double-boosted PIs are now increasingly used to treat heavily experienced patients in whom it is critical to suppress viral load. Lopinavir/ritonavir should not be combined with amprenavir or fosamprenavir, because reports have indicated that this combination leads to profound reduction in plasma concentrations of the drugs (81). Similarly, the concentrations of lopinavir and indinavir are reduced when boosted lopinavir is used in the combination (82). It is not necessary to increase the dose of ritonavir when saquinavir is co-administered with lopinavir/ritonavir (83). Co-administration of a newer PI, tipranavir, lowers the concentrations of boosted saquinavir, lopinavir, and amprenavir (84).

A number of tenofovir-related interactions have also been observed. Tenofovir increases the concentration of didanosine (85). Therefore, the enteric-coated form of didanosine at a reduced dosage of 250 mg/day should be used in combination with tenofovir. Atazanavir and lopinavir/ritonavir each increase the levels of tenofovir (86,87); hence patients receiving HAART combinations of these drugs must be monitored because of possible adverse effects. On the other hand, tenofovir causes significant reduction in the plasma concentration of atazanavir, and ritonavir boosting is recommended whenever they are used together.

The absorption of atazanavir requires low gastric pH. Thus, it should not be used with proton pump inhibitors. However, preliminary results suggest that some H2-blockers such as famotidine can be safely administered with ritonavir-boosted atazanavir, although dosing may need to be altered (88).

The combination of tenofovir DF, lamivudine, and abacivir or tenofovir DF, lamivudine, and didanosine resulted in dramatic failures in virologic suppression (44,45), throwing into doubt the possible use of these drugs for once-daily regimens. Studies suggest that the drug interactions arising from the use of these combinations may arise from genetic barriers, rather than plasma (pharmacodynamic) interactions between the individual drugs (89).

SWITCHING DRUGS

Numerous reports have alluded to intolerability as the most common reason for failure of the first drug combination. A significant percentage (21%) of patients in the Italian ICONA study stopped their drugs because of toxicity (90). These observations — coupled with evidence linking PIs to lipid abnormalities and the effect of adherence on treatment outcomes — motivated physicians to switch patients already well suppressed from one class of ARVs to another.

The most frequent reasons for physicians to consider ARV switching are:

- to improve adherence by reducing the pill burden, removing food requirements, and reducing the dosing frequency of various drug combinations, which can be achieved by using a compact, once-daily regimen;
- to manage actual or possible toxicity; this includes not only morphologic and metabolic disturbance, but also other important adverse events, such as anemia, hypersensitivity reactions, and peripheral neuropathy;
- to reduce the risk of clinically important drug interactions, such as between nevirapine and rifampicin; and
- to take advantage of the more convenient new fixed dose formulations.

The main outcomes determining likely success of switching include: maintenance of virologic control; maintenance of CD4+ count response (and immune function); improvement, resolution, or prevention of toxicity; and improvement in patient adherence and quality of life.

People with HIV infection appear to have a strong preference for once-daily dosing and compact therapy (91). Clinical studies indicate that potential once-daily ARV regimens are as effective as past standard-of-care regimens (92). Once-daily therapy is not always superior to twice-daily regimens, however. One concern with once-daily dosing is the potential consequence of a missed dose, a phenomenon that has been described as "pharmacokinetic forgiveness." Pharmacokinetic forgiveness of a drug is the likelihood of maintaining therapeutic concentrations of the drug despite occasional missed doses. This concept is critical when comparing once-daily regimens with twice-daily regimens. Although once-daily regimens are associated with a higher overall adherence percentage than twice-daily dosing, an important difference is that those on once-daily regimens appear more likely to miss two consecutive doses (93). Since missing consecutive doses of ARVs may be a more significant factor for resistance development than missing single doses, it cannot be assumed that the higher adherence percentage of once-daily regimens makes them better than twice-daily regimens in all situations. The relevance of these preliminary observations to the clinical outcomes of patients is being investigated.

Thymidine analogues have an increased relative risk of adverse events within the NRTI class; hence, switching to a better-tolerated agent — abacavir or tenofovir DF — may help avoid or ameliorate thymidine-analogue–associated toxicities. In this regard, stavudine carries a higher relative risk than other NRTIs for mitochondrial toxicities, including morphologic changes from lipodystrophy and lactic acidosis. In contrast, lamivudine, emtricitabine, abacavir, and tenofovir DF do not appear to be associated with limb fat loss and are less likely to induce lactic acidosis.

Switching from stavudine to tenofovir DF, but not to abacavir, is associated with lipid improvements. A newly approved once daily PI, atazanavir, which has little or no effect on lipids (94), has added another switch option. These two strategies represent new treatment approaches to lipid management.

NRTIs are associated with few clinically important drug interactions, and most can be managed by dose modification rather than drug substitution. The exception is the switch from didanosine to an alternative

Table 17-13. Defining Success and Failure of Antiretroviral Therapy	
Defining Successful HAART Response	**Defining Treatment Failure**
HIV RNA decreases by > 1.0 log^{10} copies/ml after one month	HIV RNA does not decrease < 1.0 log^{10} copies/ml by one month
HIV RNA decreases to < 400 copies/ml by week 24	HIV RNA is > 400 copies/ml at week 24
If HIV RNA unavailable, CD4+ increase by > 50 cells/mm^3 from pretreatment levels by 24 weeks	HIV RNA increases to within 0.5 log^{10} copies/ml of pretreatment levels at any time
	CD4+ decreases to below pretreatment levels

Abbreviation: highly active antiretroviral therapy

NRTI in patients planning to start hepatitis C therapy with ribavirin. The fixed-dose coformulations of abacavir/lamivudine and tenofovir DF/emtricitabine are attractive not only for treatment initiation and switching for virologically suppressed patients but also for patients coinfected with HIV and HBV. Lamivudine, tenofovir, and emtricitabine all have dual activity on HIV and HBV, and these effects may be synergistic (95). Since all NRTIs except abacavir are mainly renally excreted, the dose of these drugs should be reduced in patients with renal insufficiency. Therefore, fixed-dose coformulations are usually inappropriate in such patients.

Treatment Failure and Indications for Change of Therapy

Defining Antiretroviral Success and Failure

Successful ART implies that a patient has taken his or her drugs and responded to treatment. A successful response is associated with a rapid decline in plasma HIV RNA and a corresponding increase in CD4+ count (Table 17-13). After one month of starting a successful HAART regimen, the plasma HIV RNA should have declined at least 10-fold, or one log^{10} copies/ml, while the CD4+ count should have risen above the starting point. Within 12 weeks of starting therapy, approximately 80% of patients will have HIV RNA less than 400 copies/ml and the CD4+ count should have increased by approximately 50 cells/mm^3 (96). The maximal effect of treatment should be observed in most patients by 24 weeks. More than 95% should have plasma HIV RNA below 400 or 50 copies/ml, depending on the assay used, and the CD4+ count increased by 50–100 cells/mm^3 (97). There is greater variability in the change in CD4+ count, especially early in treatment. Of note, approximately 10% of patients have a disconnection of response in HIV RNA and CD4+ counts in that HIV RNA declines, but the CD4+ count increase is blunted. Factors associated with such reduced CD4+ cell response include: older age, a lower baseline CD4+ count, and a very low nadir CD4+ count (98). Also, tuberculosis and, less strongly, malaria have been associated with decreased CD4+ cell counts. These patients may require continued prophylaxis with cotrimoxazle for opportunistic infections if the CD4+ cell count is below 200. If the plasma HIV RNA does not decrease steadily over the first three months or it rebounds to within 0.5 log^{10} copies/ml of pre-therapy values, then the HAART regimen is failing. By 24 weeks if the HIV RNA has not decreased to levels below detection (fewer than 400 copies/ml), the patient should be considered as having failed the therapy.

In addition to the laboratory changes in HIV markers, within the first few months of therapy, patients should feel better clinically if they were symptomatic prior to therapy. Typically patients describe an improved sense of well-being, weight gain, and less fatigue. They may note a decrease in oral or vaginal candidiasis, fewer herpes simplex outbreaks, improvement in skin and/or hair texture, regression of condylomata, and regression of Kaposi's sarcoma. Serum cholesterol levels may increase and triglycerides levels may decrease, corresponding to a return to pre-HIV infection status.

Patients who do not respond, or patients who have responded and are now experiencing a rebound in their plasma HIV RNA, are considered virologic or clinical treatment failures. Treatment failure has multiple causes. The most common cause is an ineffective treatment regimen either because the regimen prescribed in the first place was suboptimal or because the patient did not take the pills as instructed. Continued use of ARVs administered suboptimally will quickly lead to viral resistance and failure. Typical scenarios include: stopping just one medication because of drug intolerance or cost concerns; losing one or more medications; forgetting to take doses; sharing medications with family or friends; and selling parts of the regimen. The reason is not as important as the result: treatment failure and viral resistance.

Suboptimal adherence is not the only reason for treatment failure. Patients who fail to respond to the original regimen may actually have been infected with a resistant virus. This is particularly true in patients more recently infected in a community where ARVs are being used. For example, viral resistance to nevirapine may occur in areas where this drug is used to decrease mother-to-child transmission rates. Up to 23% of women who have taken single-dose nevirapine to decrease transmission rates may develop resistant virus, which can be transferred to their sexual partners and/or infants (99). In this setting, ideally, resistance testing should be done; if unavailable, treatment should be changed to a PI-based therapy as soon as possible.

Other reasons for treatment failure include suboptimal potency, such as triple nucleoside regimens like zidovudine/lamivudine/abacavir, stavudine/didanosine/lamivudine, tenofovir/lamivudine/abacavir, and tenofovir/lamivudine/didanosine. Studies have also observed that the combination of didanosine plus tenofovir plus an NNRTI results in high virologic failure rates in ARV-naive, HIV-positive patients (100). Failure rates were similar to those reported for triple-NRTI therapy with several resistance mutations identified; a didanosine plus tenofovir plus NNRTI combination therapy is therefore not recommended. Other less potent regimens include nelfinavir or saquinavir (unboosted)-based treatment. The most common situation involving suboptimal potency is prior use of regimens that do not qualify as HAART, such as single or dual nucleoside regimens, single PI regimens, or PIs given with just one nucleoside analogue. Non-HAART regimens should never be used except when administered in certain PMTCT strategies.

Poor pharmacokinetics with suboptimal drug concentrations can also cause treatment failure. Poor absorption, drug-drug interactions at the gut level, inappropriate food administration, and metabolic induction by CYP450 induced by concomitant medications are all potential causes of treatment failure. Examples include: rifampicin, nevirapine, and efavirenz decrease most PI concentrations; tenofovir decreases atazanavir concentrations; didanosine and indinavir taken with food results in low concentrations; lopinavir/ritonavir, atazanavir, and tenofovir must be taken with food or concentrations are reduced; lopinavir/ritonavir and amprenavir decrease each other's concentrations when taken together. In addition, the use of numerous traditional medicines in addition to HAART regimes may cause many yet unidentified drug interactions, which could affect the potency of the regimens.

Viral Blips

It is important to separate patients who are experiencing viral blips from those who have virologic failure. "Viral blip" refers to a transient increase in viral load to more than 50 copies/ml in a person with chronic viral suppression. It is usually random, fewer than 500 copies/ml — or fewer than 1,000 depending on the assay used — and readily returns to fewer than 50 (or fewer than 400) copies/ml without any change in treatment. The frequency of these blips is approximately 30% to 50% in patients on different chronically suppressive regimens, whether PI-based or NNRTI-based (101).

Possible explanations for the blips include: a transient release of drug-sensitive virus from latent reservoirs; an increase in target cells during infection or post vaccination; a transient increase in viral replication in relation to changes in ARV levels; and peculiar host factors. Viral blips were initially thought to represent release of resistant virus, but this notion has been disputed by the current consensus that they usually do not predict development of resistance or virologic failure. However, it has been suggested that viral blips are more common in people with very low CD4+ T cell counts at baseline (102). Moreover, patients with frequent blips have been found to have somewhat impaired CD4+ T cell recovery compared to those without blips (103). Like many aspects of the pathogenesis of HIV, our understanding of this phenomenon is evolving.

The best way to respond to these blips is still unclear because most patients who experience this phenomenon return to undetectable viral loads. The role of blips in predicting treatment failure also is not clear. The current recommendation for any rebound in viral load is to confirm the rise with a second test performed, two weeks or a month later, and in the interval to attempt to identify potential causes of the blip. Clinicians also recommend delaying viral load testing for at least two weeks to one month after vaccination or an infection.

Second-Line and Salvage Therapy

Changing therapy in patients already receiving treatment is done for one of two main reasons: toxicity or virologic failure. If patients become intolerant to a specific drug or regimen, substitutions can usually be found within the same class or from a different class. The more complicated situation involves switching from a virologic-failing regimen to a new and effective regimen, or "salvage therapy." The choice of which salvage therapy to use is even more difficult if drug resistance data are not readily available.

When treatment fails, a comprehensive evaluation of why a patient failed — including a thorough treatment history — must be performed. For instance, if a patient was non-adherent because the regimen was too complex, it is unlikely that that person would respond to an even more complex "salvage" regimen. This type of patient may require significant in-depth counseling prior to starting a new therapeutic approach.

The first treatment failure is the one that is easiest to salvage. Typically, patients are starting a non-nucleoside-based treatment. In Nigeria, that regimen would include nevirapine or efavirenz in most

Table 17-14. First- and Second-Line Regimens in Adults and Adolescents in Nigeria

First-Line Regimen	Second-Line Regimen RTI Component	PI Component
Zidovudine *or* stavudine + lamivudine *or* emtricitabine + nevirapine *or* efavirenz	Didanosine + zidovudine *or* tenofovir DF + zidovudine + lamivudine	
Tenofovir DF + lamivudine *or* emtricitabine + nevirapine *or* efavirenz	Didanosine + zidovudine *or* *or* didanosine + zidovudine + lamivudine	atazanavir/ritonavir *or*
Abacavir + lamivudine *or* emtricitabine + nevirapine *or* efavirenz	Didanosine + zidovudine + lamivudine *or* tenofovir DF + zidovudine + lamivudine	lopinavir/ritonavir *or*
Zidovudine *or* stavudine + lamivudine *or* emtricitabine + tenofovir disoproxil fumarate *or* abacavir	Efavirenz *or* nevirapine + didanosine *or* efavirenz *or* nevirapine + lamivudine	saquinavir/ritonavir

Notes: Nevirapine and atazanavir do not require cold chain. Tenofovir DF cannot be used with unboosted atazanavir. Lamivudine can be maintained in second-line regimens to reduce the viral fitness.

patients. When nevirapine fails, typically efavirenz will not work either, and vice versa. The alternative then is to initiate a PI-based treatment. Preferred at this junction is a ritonavir-boosted regimen, either lopinavir/ritonavir, indinavir/ritonavir, atazanavir/ritonavir, or saquinavir/ritonavir (Table 17-14).

The nucleosides may also need to be replaced. Lamivudine was likely to be included in the first regimen, and therefore the likely mutation associated with resistance is M184V. Thymidine analogue mutations, or TAMs, may also be present, particularly if the patient remained on the failing regimen for a prolonged period. A likely substitution in this situation with M184V and TAMs is the combination of abacavir plus didanosine or tenofovir plus zidovudine with or without lamivudine as an NRTI backbone. Although lamivudine loses its direct virologic potency in the presence of M184V mutation, it may be retained in the regimen as a third NRTI, because it allows for the persistence of M184V mutants that replicate poorly because of reduced viral fitness.

The second treatment failure is even more difficult to manage, especially without resistance testing. Typically, more than three drugs have to be taken. If possible, a new class of drug should be given, such as a fusion inhibitor like enfuvirtide. This drug, which is prohibitively expensive and in limited supply, is unlikely to be used in Nigeria in the near future. A newer PI, tipranavir-ritonavir, is active against many viral strains that are resistant to earlier PIs, but it is also unavailable in Nigeria at this time. In the same way, the promise of investigational drugs that are in advanced stages of development—such as CCR5 receptor antagonists TMC 114 and TMC 125—is unlikely to extend to Nigeria in the immediate future. Other strategies depend on how desperate the situation has become. "Giga-HAART"—or the administration of six or more drugs, regardless of susceptibility—has been used with modest success (104). In heavily treatment-experienced patients with multiple resistance mutations who are unable to achieve complete suppression of viremia, treatment goals become restricted to maintenance of immunologic function and prevention of clinical deterioration. In this population, ongoing HAART with even modest virologic suppression has been shown to reduce the fitness or replicative capacity of the virus and improve clinical outcomes (105). Structured treatment interruption is generally not recommended in patients with advanced HIV/AIDS because it is associated with rapid CD4+ decline. Most studies have shown similar adverse outcomes (106), although one CD4+ guided study demonstrated a good response to HAART in HIV-infected patients with high CD4+ cell counts (107). Vigilant prophylaxis against opportunistic infections, prompt management of treatable infections and malignancies, and palliative care may be the only remaining options in these situations for many such people.

Discontinuation of NNRTI-Based Regimens

Nevirapine and efavirenz have prolonged, steady-state half-lives — 25 to 32 hours for nevirapine and 40 to 55 hours for efavirenz. Both drugs remain in circulation at therapeutic concentrations for several days, and at subtherapeutic concentrations for several weeks after discontinuation. This phenomenon is subject to considerable racial and individual variability, appearing to be more prominent in people of African descent than European descent (108). Similar concerns about continued exposure to nevirapine, long after the drug had been discontinued, emerged in pharmacokinetic studies conducted on women who received single-dose nevirapine for PMTCT (109).

Simultaneous discontinuation of all the drugs in an NNRTI-based regimen is likely to lead to an undesired period of NNRTI monotherapy and predispose an individual to the development of NNRTI resistance. This risk is greatest among patients who have detectable plasma viremia at the time the NNRTI is discontinued. Although it is clear that the optimal strategy should involve discontinuation of the NNRTI first, followed by discontinuation of the NRTI backbone, less certain is the length of time that the "NRTI tail" should be continued before it is stopped as well (110). Recommendations have ranged from four to five days to as long as four weeks, but additional studies are ongoing. Another option is to switch the NNRTI to a PI and then to continue the PI plus the NRTIs for two weeks before stopping all drugs simultaneously.

ANTIRETROVIRAL THERAPY IN CHILDREN

The decision to initiate ART in a child depends on his or her age and the availability of virologic testing. Serologic diagnosis is unreliable in children younger than 18 months because maternally derived antibody may persist in the child. The clinical features of HIV infection may resemble those of many other prevalent conditions, such as malaria and malnutrition.

For HIV-seropositive children younger than 18 months with proven HIV status (DNA PCR), ART is recommended when the child has: WHO Pediatric Stage III disease irrespective of the CD4+ percentage; WHO Pediatric Stage II disease, with consideration of using CD4+ less than 20% to assist in decision-making; or WHO Pediatric Stage I (asymptomatic) and CD4+ less than 20%. If HIV seropositive status is not virologically proven but CD4+ cell assays are available, ART can be initiated when the child has WHO Stage II or III disease and CD4+ less than 20%. In such cases, HIV antibody testing must be repeated at 18 months of age to confirm HIV infection; only children with confirmed infection should continue with ART.

Table 17-15. First- and Second-Line Regimens in Children in Nigeria

First-Line Regimen	Second-Line Regimen	
	RTI Component	PI Component
Zidovudine *or* stavudine + nevirapine *or* efavirenz	Didanosine + zidovudine	Lopinavir/ritonavir *or* saquinavir/ritonavir *or* nevirapine
Abacavir + lamivudine + nevirapine *or* efavirenz	Didanosine + zidovudine	Lopinavir *or* saquinavir/ritonavir *or* nevirapine
Zidovudine *or* stavudine + lamivudine + abacavir	Didanosine + zidovudine *or* nevirapine	Lopinavir *or* saquinavir/ritonavir *or* nevirapine

Notes: Tenofovir DF is not currently approved for clinical use in children. Efavirenz is approved only in children older than three. Saquinavir/ritonavir is approved only in children weighing more than 25 kilograms. Nevirapine does not require cold chain.

For HIV-seropositive children aged 18 months or older, ART can be initiated when the child has: WHO Pediatric Stage III disease (clinical AIDS) irrespective of the CD4+ percentage; WHO Pediatric Stage II disease with CD4+ less than 15%; or WHO Pediatric Stage I (asymptomatic) and CD4+ less than 15. For children older than eight years, adult criteria for initiation of therapy are applicable.

The ideal goal of treatment is full suppression of virus to plasma HIV RNA to fewer than 50 or fewer than 400 copies/ml. This almost always means the use of HAART: an NNRTI (or a PI) and two NRTIs as recommended in the Nigerian ARV guidelines (Table 17-15) (20). Full suppression is not always attainable, particularly in children. Partial suppression is usually much better than no treatment at all. As in adults, pediatric treatment is lifelong. The first treatment regimen has the greatest chance of success, while subsequent regimens are usually more toxic and less tolerable. According to the Nigerian guidelines, the judgment about when to start ART depends on age, clinical staging, and CD4+ cell count, while the decision when to switch ARVs depends on clinical and laboratory staging, observation of toxicity, CD4+ cell count, and viral load (20).

A limited number of treatment options are available for children (Table 17-15). If children can be taught to take tablets or capsules, their options increase. Successful treatment also requires education of the parents or guardians. Successful treatment of older children may require disclosure to the child about his or her HIV status, drug education, and adherence counseling.

ANTIRETROVIRAL THERAPY DURING PREGNANCY

The decision to use ART in pregnancy is based on the premise that ART is beneficial to such women unless the adverse effects outweigh the benefits. The considerations for the use of ART should be based on four considerations: the need to use appropriate ARVs; the effects of ARV on pregnancy; the effect on transmission of HIV from the mother to the child; and the effect of the drug on the fetus. The major goal of ART in pregnancy is to achieve maximal suppression of plasma viral load to undetectable levels, even though there is evidence that women with plasma HIV RNA of less than 1,000 have minimal levels of transmission to their babies (111). Some evidence now supports the possibility of teratogenic effect of efavirenz in humans (112), in addition to the ample evidence in animal models (113). Therefore, efavirenz

Table 17-16. Antiretroviral Therapy in Individuals with Dual Infection with Tuberculosis

Category	Recommendation
Pulmonary tuberculosis and a CD4+ cell count of < 200 mm³ or extrapulmonary tuberculosis	Start tuberculosis treatment. Start antiretroviral therapy as soon as patient tolerates tuberculosis therapy: Zidovudine/lamivudine/efavirenz Stavudine/lamivudine/efavirenz Tenofovir DF/lamivudine/efavirenz Tenofovir DF/lamivudine/zidovudine
Pulmonary tuberculosis and a CD4+ cell count of 200-350 mm³	Start tuberculosis treatment. Start one of these combinations after completing two months of the induction phase of tuberculosis therapy with rifampicin: Zidovudine/lamivudine/tenofovir DF Stavudine/lamivudine/efavirenz Stavudine/lamivudine/nevirapine Tenofovir DF/lamivudine/efavirenz Tenofovir DF/lamivudine/nevirapine
Pulmonary tuberculosis and a CD4+ cell count of > 350 mm³	Treat tuberculosis and defer antiretroviral therapy. Monitor CD4+ cell counts.

is best avoided in early pregnancy. When there are no alternatives, an efavirenz-containing regimen may be instituted after the second trimester in pregnant HIV-positive women coinfected with tuberculosis.

HIV-positive pregnant women who meet the criteria for ART should begin therapy after the first trimester. According to the Nigerian PMTCT guidelines, zidovudine should be included as a component of ART whenever possible (114). Treatment should commence early enough to ensure good virologic control in patients enjoying HAART. The choice of drugs in pregnancy should include a review of prior exposure, drug resistance, and the clinical and immunological status of the mother. HIV-infected pregnant women already on ART should continue on therapy with a switch of treatment in the first trimester to include nevirapine but exclude efavirenz. HIV-positive pregnant women who do not meet the criteria for ART should have zidovudine prophylaxis from 28 weeks of pregnancy with chemoprophylaxis for the baby. (Other PMTCT interventions are discussed in Chapter 16, *this volume.*) The blood count of patients taking zidovudine should be monitored regularly because of the development of anemia, a common complication of pregnancy in Nigeria.

Of significant note is a warning by nevirapine's manufacturer, Boehringer Ingelheim, of an increased risk of hepatotoxicity in women with CD4+ cell counts above 250 cells/mm³. Other important issues include switching drugs to limit or prevent lipodystrophy, convenience of the regimen, adherence, and adverse events.

ANTIRETROVIRAL THERAPY IN HIV-INFECTED PATIENTS WITH TUBERCULOSIS

The incidence of tuberculosis has dramatically increased since the mid-1980s both in industrialized and developing countries. In Nigeria, reports from AIDS treatment centers in Jos and Lagos have observed high levels of tuberculosis coinfection among patients with HIV (115,116). Tuberculosis is the leading cause of morbidity and mortality among HIV patients in Nigeria (117). Without treatment, more than half of HIV-infected patients coinfected with tuberculosis are likely to die. With the correct treatment, such patients are cured after taking appropriate tuberculosis drugs for at least six months (Table 17-16). Proper treatment and isoniazid prophylaxis also prevents the spread of tuberculosis, because it makes people non-infectious. Concomitant treatment of tuberculosis and HIV is compounded, however, by the drug interactions between NNRTIs and PIs with rifampicin. Rifampicin is a potent stimulator of the P450 cytochrome enzyme in the liver and leads to dramatic reduction of the blood levels of NNRTIs and PIs to sub-therapeutic levels (118). Pharmacokinetic levels of efavirenz can be maintained by increasing the dose to 800 mg. The use of rifabutin in place of rifampicin has been recommended for people taking ART. Rifabutin is expensive, though, and scarce in resource-limited settings such as Nigeria. Other important issues in the treatment of tuberculosis/HIV–coinfected patients include pill burden, toxicity, and adherence issues. ARV use in patients coinfected with tuberculosis is shown in Table 17-16.

Paradoxical worsening of tuberculosis is defined as a transient worsening of disease at a pre-existing site or the development of new tuberculosis lesions while a patient is on appropriate antituberculosis therapy. It is thought to be due to improved *M. tuberculosis*–specific immune responses. Risk factors for paradoxical reaction include: a low baseline CD4+ T cell count, a high viral load, and initiation of ART within two months of initiating antituberculosis therapy. These reactions, which may be seen in 7% to 30% of patients, tend to occur within days to weeks of initiating ART, but may be delayed for several months. Moreover, they may occur in one-third of HIV-infected patients started on ART and tuberculosis therapy at the same time (119).

Possible manifestations are worsening adenopathy, enlarging central nervous system lesions, or increased pulmonary infiltrate. Patients may have an increase in the size of the cutaneous response to a tuberculin test, while those who were previously anergic may develop a marked cutaneous response to tuberculin. Other previously described manifestations are tenosynovitis, pleural effusion, meningitis, superior vena cava syndrome, and peritonitis. These reactions are indicative neither of drug resistance nor treatment failure, and they usually subside spontaneously after about 10 to 40 days. Moreover, non-steroidal anti-inflammatory agents may provide some relief (120). Severe cases may require temporary interruption of HAART; however, no change in tuberculosis treatment is needed except in the most severe cases.

The approach to tuberculosis diagnosis and treatment differ markedly between developed and resource-limited countries. In many resource-limited settings, positive sputum smear alone is used for tuberculosis diagnosis, and additional information is derived from chest X-ray. Mycobacterial culture and resistance testing are often unavailable, or are available but prohibitively expensive. Empiric treatment for tuberculosis is common. Routine laboratory tests to monitor the adverse effects of tuberculosis treatment may be unavailable. Instead, patients are educated about symptoms of drug toxicity to facilitate early reporting and appropriate treatment. Detailed information about treatment of tuberculosis in resource-limited settings can be obtained from WHO treatment guidelines.

Another significant difference between resource-limited and developed countries is the use of primary prophylaxis or secondary prophylaxis after full treatment for active tuberculosis. Primary prophylaxis is recommended in patients with positive Mantous test if active tuberculosis can be definitively excluded.

Table 17-17. Effects of HIV on HBV and HBV on HIV

Effects of HIV Coinfection on HBV	Effects of HBV Coinfection on HIV
• Markers of replicative HBV (high HBV DNA titer and HBeAg) are more commonly present • Lower transaminases, despite higher HBV DNA* • Decreased conversion from HBsAg and HBeAg positivity to anti-HBs and anti-HBe positivity • Poorer response to interferon • Increased risk of developing lamivudine resistance • Increased risk of liver cirrhosis • Increased liver-related mortality	• HBV increases HIV replication rate (controversial) • Lower CD4+ cell count due to hypersplenism in patients with cirrhosis • No proof that HBV influences the eventual outcome of HIV infection

*Lower transaminases occur because hepatic inflammation in HBV infection is not caused by direct cytopathic effect of the virus; rather, it correlates with host immunologic response. Thus, neonates and immune-compromised people tend to have lower transaminase levels.

However, several studies in resource-limited areas of tuberculosis endemicity have suggested that secondary tuberculosis prophylaxis may also be efficacious. The first study, conducted in Zaire, found decreased relapse rates when rifampin and isoniazid were given for an additional six months after completing a standard course of treatment (121). In a study in Abidjan, Côte d'Ivoire, HIV-infected patients who completed treatment for active tuberculosis were randomized to isoniazid plus sulphadoxine-pyrimethamine or placebo. Compliance with isoniazid was poorer than with sulphadoxine-pyrimethamine, but patients who received the combined prophylactic regimen had a significant decrease in tuberculosis recurrence, anemia, and wasting. There was also a trend toward improved survival (122). While these and other studies (123) suggest a potential beneficial effect of secondary prophylaxis, they do not provide answers to several critical issues, such as the impact of HAART on the apparent benefits, the optimal regimen for secondary prophylaxis, and the impact of secondary prophylaxis on the emergence of drug-resistant M. tuberculosis. The WHO does not yet endorse secondary prophylaxis, and additional studies are needed before secondary prophylaxis can be included in routine care standards.

ANTIRETROVIRAL THERAPY IN DUAL INFECTIONS WITH HIV AND HEPATITIS

Nigeria's high HIV-1 seroprevalence rate of 5.0% (5) and its high HBV carriage rate of 10.3% in the general population (124) have created opportunities for coinfection with HIV and HBV. This is made possible because HIV and HBV (and HCV) share the same modes of transmission. The prevalence of HBV in HIV-infected individuals ranges from 20% to 42% in Nigeria (125–127). Important virologic, epidemiological, and clinical interactions between HIV and HBV have been described. For example, people with HIV/HBV coinfection have a greater rate of chronic liver disease, higher viral loads of HBV, and accelerated progression of liver disease. (128). Table 17-17 summarizes these interactions.

Effects of Hepatitis B Virus on HIV Infection

The primary goal of treating chronic HBV is to halt progression of liver disease by suppressing viral replication. Until recently, the only antiviral agents available for treatment for HBV were lamivudine and interferon-alpha 2a and -alpha 2b. The availability of tenofovir, adefovir, and entecavir has expanded HBV treatment options. Tenofovir, lamivudine, and emtricitabine are effective against both HBV and HIV. Yet HBV lamivudine resistance occurs at a rate of approximately 20% per year, while resistance to tenofovir is much less frequent. Tenofovir is effective against lamivudine-resistant and probably emtricitabine-resistant strains of the virus. Preliminary studies have suggested that regimens that contain both lamivudine and tenofovir produce better HBV suppression than those with lamivudine alone (129). Emtricitabine plus tenofovir probably has similar effects. Thus, HAART regimens that contain tenofovir; emtricitabine or lamivudine; and a third agent have the potential to render multiple benefits for coinfected patients.

Since the introduction of suppressive combination ART, survival in HIV-infected people has been extended. Data are scarce on the clinical course of prolonged HIV/HBV coinfection and the effects of HAART in this setting. Nonetheless, a study of people coinfected with HIV and HBV has revealed that responses to HAART were inferior relative to those of people infected only with HIV (130). Although both patient groups achieved similarly significant immunologic responses to treatment, coinfection was associated with excess risk of virologic failure and of death. Virologic response was impaired in coinfected subjects, however, frequently as a result of interruptions in treatment driven by hepatic complications (Table 17-17). Furthermore, coinfected patients are more likely to develop hepatitis after HAART initiation (131,132), and they face a higher risk of hepatic decompensation and hyperbilirubinemia (133). The confluence of these events significantly contributes to the greater risk of liver-related mortality that occurs in coinfected people (134,135).

Patients with HIV/Hepatitis C Coinfection

HCV is a flavivirus with single-stranded RNA that is capable of very rapid replication, leading to the daily production of approximately 10^{12} virions. This replication rate is faster in HIV/HCV–coinfected people than in HCV mono-infected patients (136), and HAART has been shown to drive HCV's genetic diversity (137). Six genotypes have been characterized with significant geographic variation (138). Previous reports have observed that HIV/HCV–coinfected people experience more rapid progression of liver fibrosis and greater morbidity and mortality from liver disease than those infected with HCV alone (139). The accelerated pace of hepatic decline in HCV/HIV–coinfected patients occurs in part because they have diminished cellular immune responses to HCV infection, characterized by weak HCV-specific CD8+ T cell and CD4+ T cell immune activity (140). Thus, they are less able to clear HCV viremia after initial infection (141). Because of this, liver cirrhosis occurs in 15% to 25% of coinfected patients within 10 to 15 years after HCV infection compared to only 2% to 6% of people with HCV infection alone (142). Liver-related mortality is also greater in coinfected patients (143). Factors that predict progression to advanced liver fibrosis (the most prognostic indicator of the development of cirrhosis) in people coinfected with HIV and HCV include: CD4+ T cell counts of fewer than 200 cells/mm³; alcohol consumption; and an HCV infection duration of more than 40 years (144).

HCV does not appear to alter the natural course of HIV infection in any significant way. However, it was initially suggested that the recovery of CD4+ T cells in response to potent HAART was blunted in those who were HCV/HIV coinfected (145); subsequent studies failed to show similar findings (146). On the other hand, the initiation of HAART is often accompanied by a paradoxical increase in HCV viremia in coinfected patients, which explains some of the immune reconstitution hepatitis flare. It appears that an initial increase occurs in all patients, but it is prolonged only in those with low CD4+ cell counts (147). The biological explanation for this increase is still uncertain. Nonetheless, there is increasing evidence that immune restoration through HAART may slow the course of liver disease progression in individuals with HIV/HCV coinfection (148). It has therefore been recommended that hepatitis C should be treated aggressively in coinfected patients. Best results occur among those with a pretreatment CD4+ cell count of greater than 350 cells/mm^3. However, treatment of coinfected patients is complicated by drug interactions and poor tolerance of therapy. Potential toxicities may outweigh the benefits when the pretreatment CD4+ cell count is less than 200 cells/mm^3.

Three large randomized controlled trials of interferon-based therapy in patients who were coinfected with HIV and HCV have now been completed: the AIDS Clinical Trials Group study (149); the APRICOT (AIDS Peginterferon Ribavirin International Co-infection Trial) study (150); and the RIBAVIC study (151). These studies compared recombinant interferon alpha-2b plus ribavirin to peginterferon alfa-2b plus ribavirin. Overall, the results of these studies showed that patients who were treated with peginterferon had a better-sustained virologic response than with standard interferon. The sustained virologic response was less in coinfected patients than previously seen in HCV mono-infected patients. Treatment in the RIBAVIC study was discontinued in 42% of patients, and 31% had severe adverse events, suggesting that therapy was tolerated relatively poorly in this group. Toxicity may be enhanced in individuals treated with HAART, and even more in those treated concurrently with HAART and the combination of interferon and ribavirin. Ribavirin should not be coadministered with didanosine because of a drug-drug interaction that has been associated with potentially fatal hepatic decompensation, pancreatitis, and lactic acidosis (152).

HIV-2 INFECTION

HIV-2, the second HIV that causes immunodeficiency and AIDS, is found predominantly in West Africa, including Nigeria. Since the mid-1990s, HIV-2 prevalence in Nigeria seems to be diminishing, while various recombinant forms of HIV-1 are expanding rapidly in Nigeria (153). HIV-2 is five times less transmissible than HIV-1 (154), is associated with lower viral loads, and has a slower rate of disease progression (155).

Little is known about the best approach for treatment of HIV-2. Immunodeficiency develops slowly; therefore, it is unclear whether ART significantly slows progression. Some NRTIs such as zidovudine appear to be less active in HIV-2 than in HIV-1 (156). Moreover HIV-2 is not susceptible to NNRTIs and may have multiple pre-existing PI mutations leading to resistance (157). Monitoring infection by HIV-2 viral load assay is difficult due to the lack of a HIV-2-specific assay. It appears that triple-NRTI regimens—such as lamivudine, zidovudine, tenofovir (the DART regimen), or lamivudine, zidovudine, and abacavir — may be useful, although this has not been rigorously tested. More research and clinical experience are needed to determine the most effective treatment for HIV-2 infection.

POST-EXPOSURE PROPHYLAXIS

The magnitude of risk associated with a particular exposure to HIV tends to be influenced by the nature of the exposure and the status of HIV disease in the source patient. The risk of transmission following percutaneous occupational exposure is about 0.3% (158), which is lower than the risk of transmitting HBV or HCV. This risk can be reduced if ARVs are immediately administered and continued for the recommended one month. Post-exposure prophylaxis (PEP) is unnecessary if the exposed worker is already known to be HIV seropositive. For all others, baseline HIV tests should be performed and PEP initiated as soon as possible. Rapid HIV tests can be used to determine the HIV serostatus of the source person. However, the tests may be falsely negative during the window period, which is the time between detectable HIV antigens and the development of HIV antibody.

For occupational exposures, the health care worker and index patient should be tested for HIV before administration of PEP. A three-drug regimen should be provided as soon as possible to the health care worker for four weeks. Complete blood count and chemistry should be done after two weeks with HIV testing conducted at 12 and 24 weeks. If negative at 24 weeks, the health care worker can be considered to be uninfected. Rigorous evaluations of PEP programs have not been done, although such programs are not 100% efficacious in preventing infection. In an analysis of 57 voluntarily reported cases of occupationally acquired HIV infection, 14% of the health care workers acquired HIV infection despite receiving PEP (159). Although poor adherence due to the adverse effects of ARV drugs was implicated in some prophylaxis failures, other patients failed because the infecting virus was resistant to the prophylactic ARV drugs. Therefore, choosing the initial regimen should involve careful consideration, ideally with expert consultation, of the source patient's treatment experience and the local epidemiology of ARV resistance.

The choice of a PEP regimen should be based on the type of exposure and the status of the source patient (17). Also, drug resistance that is known or suspected to be present in the source patient should be considered. A three-drug regimen should be recommended when the source person is known to be infected with HIV and has markers of high infectiousness such as symptomatic disease, a high viral load, or a low CD4+ cell count. Three-drug regimens are also preferred if exposure involves a large-bore needle, deep injury, or visible blood on the needle, or if the needle was just removed from the source person's blood vessel. The three-drug regimens are generally similar to standard HAART regimens, but drugs with a high incidence of adverse reactions should be avoided. For example, nevirapine has been associated with severe cases of hypersensitivity reaction when used for prophylaxis (160). Since some of these reactions have been fatal, the use of nevirapine in PEP regimens should be avoided. The adverse events associated with nevirapine — including life-threatening rash and hepatic failure — are more common in HIV-uninfected, immunocompetent individuals (161). If possible, an alternative drug should be substituted, such as efavirenz, remembering that efavirenz cannot be used in patients who are pregnant or contemplating pregnancy. Alternative drugs include any PI-based three-drug regimens and even triple nucleoside regimens, such as zidovudine/lamivudine/abacavir (Trizivir®) or zidovudine/lamivudine/tenofovir.

A two-drug regimen may be considered if exposure is limited to a few drops or splash on mucous membrane or disrupted skin, provided the source patient does not have any marker of high infectiousness. The two-drug regimens typically consist of two NRTIs (such as zidovudine plus lamivudine). Even in relatively low-risk situations, some clinicians prefer three-drug regimens, although there are no proven advantages and toxicity may be increased. In situations in which the HIV serostatus of the source person is unknown, prophylaxis may be prudent after careful assessment of the specific situation.

A complete blood count and chemistry should be done after two weeks of PEP, and testing for HIV should be repeated at 12 and 24 weeks. If negative at 24 weeks, the health care worker can be considered to be uninfected. Low risk exposures such as body fluid contact with intact skin do not require prophylaxis. Although pregnancy is not a contraindication to PEP, it is necessary to closely monitor for adverse effects.

PEP following unprotected intercourse has not been studied in depth, although some health departments and treatment centers do provide such services. If clinically appropriate, the same regimen as the above should be employed. A similar approach has been taken in many areas of the world when a man suspected of being HIV positive has raped a woman.

The inability of PEP to prevent HIV transmission 100% of the time emphasizes the importance of using strategies that prevent exposure in the first place. Since accidental HIV exposure is a source of emotional turmoil, all patients should be offered psychological support and education on how to avoid future exposure. STI treatment, hepatitis prophylaxis, and emergency contraception may be important, depending on the nature of the exposure.

IMMUNE RECONSTITUTION INFLAMMATORY SYNDROME

Immune reconstitution or restoration, the improvement of previously compromised immune function, usually follows successful HAART (162). Although generally advantageous, it is sometimes associated with an inflammatory syndrome — called immune reconstitution syndrome, immune restoration disease (IRD), immune response reaction, or immune reconstitution inflammatory syndrome (IRIS) — especially in people who were severely immune compromised at baseline. Its onset is usually temporally related to the restoration of immunologic response to specific antigens in patients on HAART. Most cases occur within the first three to six months of treatment, but cases have been described as late as two years after initiation of HAART (163). IRIS occurs more commonly in patients who have CD4+ T cell counts of fewer than 50–100 cells/mm^3 at the time ARV therapy is initiated, especially if treatment leads to a greater than two- to fourfold increase in the CD4+ cell count (164). Additionally, the risk of IRIS is increased in patients who are ART naive, patients who start ART within 30 days of being diagnosed with an opportunistic infection, and those who have at least a 2 log^{10} drop in viral load within 90 days of initiating ART (165).

The clinical presentation depends on the antigen(s) against which the inflammatory response is directed. IRIS to cytomegalovirus, *M. tuberculosis*, *Cryptococcus neoformans*, *Pneumocystis carinii* pneumonia (PCP), and herpes zoster have well described (166). Other conditions that have been associated with IRIS include herpes zoster, HCV, progressive multifocal leukoencephalopathy, HBV, PCP, sarcoidosis, Guillain-Barre syndrome, toxoplasmosis, hemorrhagic cystitis due to BK virus, focal encephalitis probably due to parvovirus B 19, and leprosy.

Making a diagnosis of IRIS is often clinically challenging because it has to be differentiated from adverse drug reactions, natural progression of HIV/AIDS, and the worsening of underlying conditions not related to immune reconstitution. This is further complicated by the fact that its clinical presentation and course often differ from the typical findings in HIV-infected patients who have the same infection, but who are not on HAART. In tuberculosis, this may manifest as paradoxical clinical worsening while on tuberculosis treatment. The viral load is likely to be low and the CD4+ T cell count increased during IRIS, whereas the opposite is true in those with AIDS progression. However, increased CD4+ cell counts alone do not automatically indicate that a clinical syndrome is due to immune reconstitution. Conversely, the absence of a rise cannot be always used to exclude IRIS, because the syndrome can occur before the CD4+ cell count has risen significantly as long as there has been functional immune reconstitution. A decrease in the patient's viral load relative to the pre-HAART level, on the other hand, is a more consistent finding in IRIS (144). General steps in the management of IRIS are: treatment of the offending pathogen to reduce antigen load; continuation of HAART, except in extreme cases; and careful use of anti-inflammatory agents (steroids). Although patients with IRIS have higher hospitalization rates and undergo more invasive procedures during the acute illness, their long-term outlook is good (167). Compared to patients without IRIS, they have better virologic suppression and even show a tendency toward better survival (165).

CHALLENGES AND FUTURE DIRECTIONS IN TREATMENT AND CARE IN NIGERIA

In February 2001 the federal government of Nigeria launched a program aimed at providing HAART to adults and children nationwide. Private institutions such as oil companies, nongovernmental organizations, and state governments have offered additional access. By the end of 2005, about 50,000 individuals infected with HIV in Nigeria had received HAART from the Nigeria ART program with support from the U.S. President's Emergency Plan For AIDS Relief (PEPFAR) and the Global Fund for AIDS, Tuberculosis and Malaria. However, this number will still be less than 10% of the estimated 800,000 to 1,000,000 Nigerians who require access to ART. The recent presidential directive seeking to enroll 250,000 people on ART by 2006 will further increase the number of HIV-infected people on treatment.

A 2004 assessment of HIV/AIDS care in Nigeria by USAID (168) observed several key findings critical to scaling up the Nigerian ARV program. Their findings included: the current ART capacity fell far short of the number of patients requiring treatment; public facilities providing ART experienced severe budgetary constraints, limiting their ability to provide HIV services; the patient bore 35% of the financial burden of the ART, an enormous amount affordable only to a few Nigerians; and private sector ART services were limited because only a few patients could afford them. In addition, most public facilities were aware of national policies, guidelines, and protocols on HIV/AIDS service delivery and followed some of these guidelines and protocols; however, such documents were rarely obtainable at the sites where they were most needed. The authors suggested that all these components need to be addressed before any meaningful scaling up of ART services can take place.

Other obstacles to the scaling up and sustainability of ART in Nigeria include a lack of political commitment at the state and community levels, poor laboratory monitoring, a weak health infrastructure, a lack of well-trained personnel to deliver ART, a poor information management system, and the lack of adequate coordination in the implementation of ART.

The arrival of Global Fund, PEPFAR, and World Bank funding for the scale up of ART in Nigeria has dramatically increased the number of people accessing drugs. The cost of drugs, which had been a rate limiting factor in ART scale up, can further be reduced by purchasing drugs in bulk, using generic regimens, and taking advantage of parallel importation. In addition, local manufacture of ARVs is inevitable if delivery of ART is to cope with the huge numbers waiting to access these drugs. Tiered laboratory monitoring of patients is highly recommended. This allows for the use of simple monitoring tools, including manual CD4+ cell counts, at the level of community and secondary health institutions while reserving monitoring with plasma viral load and automated CD4+ cell counts for centers of excellence, medical research institutions, and tertiary health institutions. This will further reduce budgetary costs while preserving the quality of care. It is critical to address the weak laboratory and clinical infrastructure that exists in Nigeria, as ART is a comprehensive program. Hence, it is important that the capacity of the whole health system be improved to deliver not only ARVs, but also all related services, such as voluntary counseling and testing, treatments of STIs and opportunistic infections, and psychosocial support.

The lack of resources also demands that the implementation of new and innovative approaches to the monitoring of HAART—such as the use of DOT-HAART, peer education from support groups, and community involvement with education—support adherence and HIV prevention. The huge gaps in trained personnel requires a massive capacity building of all cadres of people involved in the delivery of ART, including physicians, pharmacists, laboratory staff, and counselors. Initiating programs with simple and limited drug options is also helpful, as it saves more complex regimens for failed therapy. An essential component of strengthening the health system is motivating and retaining trained and skilled personnel.

For an ART program in Nigeria to succeed, therefore, the following must be assured:

- A sustainable supply of adequate high-quality drugs (ART and opportunistic infection prophylaxis) and testing kits free of charge;
- Adequate resources to ensure the provision of drugs on a long-term basis;
- Adequate funds for training health care providers;

- Establishment of reference laboratories for monitoring drug toxicities, viral loads, and resistance. Monitoring of patients' blood chemistries, CD4+ cell counts, and viral load should be made free and done at least twice per year;
- Establishment of commodity management systems to prevent stock outs;
- A management information system to track programs, patients, and supplies, and to provide necessary data for evaluation; and
- The program must emphasize and carry out operational research, including the conduct of clinical trials to optimize current and future treatment options in Nigeria.

CONCLUSION

The decision to commence ART should be based on the degree of immunosuppression using symptoms and CD4+ cell counts as indicated in the Nigerian ART guidelines. Patients should not start therapy until they have received enough education to understand what HIV is, as well as how the treatment works and what the various treatment options are. They must also appreciate the importance of adherence and, as much as possible, the use of treatment-support partners should be encouraged to facilitate their adherence to ART. Patients should be motivated and ready to start ART before they begin the medication. ART must be provided as a comprehensive treatment embracing not only ARVs, but also regular counseling, psychological support, prophylaxis and treatment of opportunistic infections, and nutritional support.

Virtually all regimens with at least three drugs are effective. However, most triple NRTIs are less effective. The main differences are complications, pill burden, tolerability, toxicity, monitoring requirements, potency, drug interactions, refrigeration, pregnancy, and comorbid conditions. The choice of regimens should be based on considerations of potency, tolerability, convenience, long-term toxicity, and drug resistance. It is wiser to start from a simple but potent regimen and move on to complicated regimens later when resistance develops. It must be remembered that the first regimen remains the best opportunity for providing durable virologic response; therefore, the decision about the initial regimen for each individual patient must be carefully made.

The goal of treatment, particularly in ARV-naive patients, remains the maintenance of an undetectable viral load, a progressive rise in the CD4+ cell count, and a decline in the frequency and severity of opportunistic infections. Therefore, any progress short of these yardsticks may be associated with decreased durability and portend the development of drug resistance.

Community involvement through education, preparedness, support activities, and mobilization can greatly enhance drug adherence and must form a key strategy for achieving durable viral suppression. To succeed, an ART program must incorporate plans for sustainability, including: advocacy for political commitment (federal, state, and local, as well as private); involvement of the state and private sector; development of ART policies; updating of guidelines on ART and opportunistic infections; capacity building (infrastructure and personnel); and operational research with robust monitoring and evaluation.

Finally, the strategy that may prove useful with the massive scaling up of ART programs in Nigeria is one that encourages a community-based approach, with ART services provided at no cost to the patients in a tiered-delivery model that does not jeopardize the quality of care. This strategy provides the delivery of ART from zonal centers of excellence through tertiary centers to state and district facilities that meet minimum requirements for ART and to community-based facilities that do not meet minimum requirements for ART but can provide care and support services, such as voluntary counseling and testing and referrals.

REFERENCES

1. Palella FJ, Delaney KM, Moorman AC, et al. Declining morbidity and mortality among patients with advanced human immunodeficiency virus infection. HIV outpatient study investigators. *N Engl J Med*, 1999;338:853–860.

2. Ioannidis JP, Abrams EJ, Ammann A, et al. Perinatal transmission of human immunodeficiency virus type 1 by pregnant women with RNA virus levels <1000 copies/ml. *J Infect Dis*, 2001;83:539–545.

3. Weidle PJ, Timothy DM, Alison DG, et al. HIV/AIDS treatment and HIV vaccines for Africa. *Lancet*, 2002;359:2261–2267.

4. UNAIDS. *Progress on Global Access to HIV Antiretroviral Therapy: An Update on "3 by 5."* Geneva: UNAIDS, 2005.

5. Federal Ministry of Health. *National HIV Sentinel Survey*. Abuja: Federal Ministry of Health, 2003.

6. Finzi D, Blanckson J, Siciliano JD, et al. Latent infection of CD4+ T cells provides a mechanism for lifelong persistence of HIV-1, even in patients on effective combination therapy. *Nat Med*, 1999;5(5): 512–517.

7. Daar ES, Little S, Pitt J, Santangelo J, et al. Diagnosis of primary HIV-1 infection. Los Angeles County Primary HIV Infection Recruitment Network. *Ann Intern Med*, 2001;134(1):25–29.

8. Fiscus S, Pilcher C, Miller W, et al. Real time detection of patients with acute HIV Infection in Africa. *12th Conference on Retroviruses and Opportunistic Infections*, Boston, Massachusetts, February 22–25, 2005 (abstract 20).

9. Kilby JM, Goepfert PA, Miller AP, et al. Recurrence of the acute HIV syndrome after interruption of antiretroviral therapy in a patient with chronic HIV infection: a case report. *Ann Intern Med*, 2000; 133(6):435–438.

10. U.S. Centers for Disease Control and Prevention. 1993 Revised Classification System for HIV infection and Expanded Surveillance Case Definition for AIDS among Adolescents and Adults. *MMWR*, December 18, 1992;RR-17:1–9.

11. Yarchoan R, Klecker RW, Weinhold KJ, et al. Administration of 3'-azido-3'-deoxythymidine, an inhibitor of HTLV-III/LAV replication to patients with AIDS or AIDS-related complex. *Lancet*, 1986;1: 575–580.

12. Fischl MA, Stanley K, Collier AC, et al. Combination therapy and monotherapy with zidovudine and zalcitabine in patients with advanced HIV disease. *Ann Intern Med*, 1995;122:24–32.

13. Hammer SM, Squires KE, Hughes MD, et al. A controlled trial of two nucleoside analogues plus indinavir in persons with human immunodeficiency virus infection and CD4+ cell counts of 200mm³ or less. ACTG 320 Study Team. *N Engl J Med*, 1997;33:725–733.

14. Morcroft A, Vella S, Benfield TL, et al. Changing patterns of mortality across Europe in patients with HIV-1. *Lancet*, 1998;352:1725–1730.

15. Dorenbaum A. Report of the results of PACTG 316: an international phase III trial of standard antiretroviral prophylaxis plus nevirapine for the prevention of perinatal HIV transmission. *8th Conference on Retroviruses and Opportunistic infections*, Chicago, Illinois, February 4–8, 2001 (abstract LB7).

16. Roland M, Myers L, Chuunga R, et al. A prospective study of postexposure prophylaxis following sexual assault in South Africa. *12th Conference on Retroviruses and Opportunistic Infections*, Boston, Massachusetts, February 22–25, 2005 (abstract 539).

17. U.S. Centers for Disease Control and Prevention. Updated US Public Health Service guidelines for the management of occupational exposures to HBV, HCV and HIV and recommendations for post exposure prophylaxis. *MMWR*, 2001;50(RR-11):1–52.

18. Zhang H, Dornadula G, Beumont M, et al. Human immunodeficiency virus type 1 in the semen of men receiving highly active antiretroviral therapy. *N Engl J Med*, 1998;339(25):1803–1809.

19. Pomerantz RJ, Kuritzkes DR, de la Monte SM, et al. Infection of the retina by human immunodeficiency virus type I. *N Engl J Med*, 1987;317(26):1643–1647.

20. Federal Ministry of Health. *Guidelines for the Use of Antiretroviral Drugs in Nigeria.* Abuja: Federal Ministry of Health, 2005.

21. van Leeuwen R, Katlama C, Murphy RL, et al. A randomized trial to study first-line combination therapy with or without a protease inhibitor in HIV-1-infected patients. *AIDS*, 2003;17:987–999.

22. Cameroon DW, Japour AJ, Xu Y, et al. Ritonavir and saquinavir combination therapy for the treatment of HIV infection. *AIDS*, 1999;13:213–224.

23. Department of Health and Human Services. Guidelines for the use of antiretroviral agents in HIV-1 infected adults and adolescents. March 23, 2005. Accessed at http://aidsinfo.nih.gov/guidelines on August 2, 2005.

24. Staszewski S, Gallant JE, Pozniak AL, et al. Efficacy and safety of tenofovir DF (TDF) versus stavudine (d4T) when used in combination with lamivudine and efavirenz in antiretroviral naïve patients: 96 week preliminary interim results. *12th Conference on Retroviruses and Opportunistic Infections*, Boston, Massachusetts, February 22–25, 2005 (abstract 564b).

25. Gallant JE, Staszewski S, Pozniak AL, et al. Efficacy and safety of tenofovir DF vs stavudine in combination therapy in antiretroviral-naive patients: a 3-year randomized trial. *JAMA*, 2004;292(2):191–201.

26. Gallant JE, DeJesus E, Arribas Jr, et al. Tenofovir DF, emtricitabine, and efavirenz vs. zidovudine, lamivudine, and efavirenz for HIV. *New Engl J Med*, 2006;354(3):251–260.

27. Gallant JE, Rodriguez AE, Weinberg W, et al. Early non response to tenofovir DF (TDF) + abacavir (ABC) and lamivudine (3TC) in a randomized trial compared to efavirenz (EFV) + ABC and 3TC (ESS30009) unplanned interim analysis. *43rd Interscience Conference on Antimicrobial Agents and Chemotherapy*, Chicago, Illinois, September 14–17, 2003 (abstract 1722a).

28. Mallal S, Nolan D, Witt C, et al. Association between presence of HLA-B*5701, HLA-DR7, and HLA-DQ3 and hypersensitivity to HIV-1 reverse-transcriptase inhibitor abacavir. *Lancet*, 2002;359(9308):727–732.

29. Martin A, Almeda C, Nolan D, et al. Abacavir stimulates Hsp 70 redistribution in antigen-presenting cells of patients with hypersensitivity: association with type 1 alcohol dehydrogenase activity. *12th Conference on Retroviruses and Opportunistic Infections*, Boston, Massachusetts, February 22–25, 2005 (abstract 834).

30. Brothers C, Cutrell A, Zhao H, et al. Once-daily administration of abacavir is not a clinical risk factor for suspected hypersensitivity reactions in clinical trials, and rash alone is not sufficient to diagnose the reaction. *12th Conference on Retroviruses and Opportunistic Infections*, Boston, Massachusetts, February 22–25, 2005 (abstract 836).

31. James A, Johann-Liang R. Increased rate and severity of abacavir-associated hypersensitivity reaction in randomized controlled clinical trials. *12th Conference on Retroviruses and Opportunistic Infections*, Boston, Massachusetts, February 22–25, 2005 (abstract 835).

32. McColl DJ, Parkin NT, Miller MD, et al. Genotype and phenotypic patterns and replication capacity (RC) of HIV-1 containing the K65R or L74V mutations in reverse transcriptase (RT). *7th International Congress on Drug Therapy in HIV Infection*, Glasgow, United Kingdom, November 14–18, 2004 (abstract P112).

33. Khanlou H, Yeh V, Guyer B, et al. Early virologic failure in a pilot study evaluating the efficacy of therapy containing once-daily abacavir, lamivudine, and tenofovir DF in treatment-naive HIV-infected patients. *AIDS Patient Care STDS*, 2005;19(3):135–140.

34. Lacombe K, Pacanowski J, Meynard J-L, Trylesinski A, Girard P-M. Risk factors for CD4 lymphopenia in patients treated with a tenofovir/didanosine high dose-containing highly active antiretroviral therapy regimen. *AIDS*, 2005;19(10):1107–1108.

35. Saag MS, Cahn P, Raffi F, et al. Efficacy and safety of emtricitabine vs. stavudine in combination therapy in antiretroviral-naive patients: a randomized trial. *JAMA*, 2004;292(2):180–189.

36. Staszewski S, Morales-Ramirez J, Tashima KT, et al. Efavirenz plus zidovudine and lamivudine, efavirenz plus indinavir, zidovudine and lamivudine in the treatment of HIV-1 infections in adults. *N Engl J Med*, 1999;341:1865–1873.

37. Carr A, Vella S, de Jong MD, et al. A controlled trial of nevirapine plus zidovudine versus zidovudine alone in p24 antigenaemic HIV infected patients. *AIDS*, 1996;10(6):635–641.

38. Van Leth F, Phanuphak P, Ruxrungthan K, et al. Comparison of first-line antiretroviral therapy with regimens including nevirapine, efavirenz, or both drugs, plus stavudine and lamivudine: a randomized open-label trial, the 2NN study. *Lancet*, 2004;363:1253–1263.

39. Puro V, Soldani F, De Carli G, et al. Drug-induced aminotransferase alterations during antiretroviral HIV post-exposure prophylaxis. *AIDS*, 2003;17(13): 1988–1990.

40. Sanne I, Mommeja-Marin H, Hinkle J, et al. Severe hepatotoxicity associated with nevirapine use in HIV infected subjects. *J Infect Dis*, 2005;19:825–829.

41. Frenkel L, Stek AM, et al. Maternal toxicity with continuous nevirapine in pregnancy: results from PACTG 1022. *J Acquir Immune Defic Syndr*, 2004;36: 772–776.

42. Macias J, Castellano V, Merchante N, et al. Effect of antiretroviral drugs on liver fibrosis in HIV-infected patients with chronic hepatitis C: harmful impact of nevirapine. *AIDS*, 2004;18(5):767–774.

43. Manosuthi A, Sungkanuparph S, Vibhagool A, et al. A randomized controlled trial of efavirenz 600 mg/day versus 800 mg/day in HIV-infected patients with tuberculosis to study plasma efavirenz level, virological and immunological outcomes: a preliminary result. *XV International AIDS Conference*, Bangkok, Thailand, July 11–16, 2004 (abstract MoOrB1013).

44. Friedland G, Jack C, Khoo C, et al. Efavirenz levels and clinical outcomes in patients with TB and HIV treated concomitantly with ART and rifampin-containing TB regimen. In: *12th Conference on Retroviruses and Opportunistic Infections*, Boston, Massachusetts, February 22–25, 2005 (abstract 891).

45. Wamsley S, Berstein B, King M, et al. Lopinavir-ritonavir versus nelfinavir for the initial treatment of HIV infection. *N Engl J Med*, 2002;346:2039–2046.

46. MacManus S, Yates PJ, Elston RC, et al. GW433908/ritonavir once daily in antiretroviral therapy-naive HIV-infected patients: absence of protease resistance at 48 weeks. *AIDS*, 2004;18(4):651–655.

47. Gulick RM, Ribaudo HJ, Shikuma CM, et al. ACTG 5095: a comparative study evaluating the efficacy of abacavir, lamivudine and tenofovir in treatment-naïve HIV infected patients. *2nd International AIDS Society Conference on Pathogenesis and Treatment*, Paris, France, July 13–16, 2003 (abstract 43).

48. Farthing C, Khanlou H, Yeh V. Early virologic failure in a pilot study evaluating the efficacy of abacavir, lamivudine and tenofovir in treatment naïve HIV infected patients. *Antir Ther*, 2003;8(Suppl 1): S195.

49. Jemsek H, Hutcherson P, Harper E. Poor virologic responses and early emergence of resistance in treatment naïve, HIV-1 infected patients receiving a once daily triple nucleoside regimen of didanosine, lamividune and tenofovir DF. *11th Conference on Retroviruses and Opportunistic Infections*, San Francisco, California, February 7–11, 2004 (abstract 52).

50. Kaleebu P, DART Team. 48 week virologic response to a triple nucleoside/nucleotide analogue regimen in adults with HIV infection in Africa within the DART trial. *3rd IAS Conference on HIV Pathogenesis and Treatment*, Rio de Janeiro, Brazil, July 24–27, 2005 (abstract WeOaLB0203).

51. Cissy KM, Walker S, Kaleebu P, et al. Short term virologic response to triple nucleoside/nucleotide analogue regimen in adults with HIV infection in Africa within the DART trial. *12th Conference on Retroviruses and Opportunistic Infections*, Boston, Massachusetts, February 22–25, 2005 (abstract 22).

52. Federal Ministry of Health. *HIV/Syphilis Sentinel Survey*. Abuja: Federal Ministry of Health, 2001.

53. Mannheimer S, Fredland G, Matts J, et al. The consistency of adherence to antiretroviral therapy predicts biologic outcomes for human immunodeficiency virus infected persons in clinical trials. *Clin Infect Dis*, 2002;34:1115–1121.

54. d'Arminio MA, Cozzi LA, Rezza G, et al. Insights into reasons for the discontinuation of the first highly active antiretroviral therapy (HAART) regimen in a cohort of antiretroviral naïve patient. *AIDS*, 2000;14:499–507.

55. Mellors JW, Rinaldo CR Jr, Gupta P, et al. Prognosis in HIV-1 infection predicted by the quantity of virus in plasma. *Science*, 1996;272: 1167–1170.

56. Paterson DL, Swindells S, Mohr J, et al. Adherence to protease inhibitor therapy and outcomes in patients with HIV infection. *Ann Intern Med*, 2000; 133:21–30.

57. Friedland GH, Williams A. Attaining higher goals in HIV treatment: the central importance of adherence. *AIDS*, 1999;13:S61–S72.

58. Janz NK, Becker MH. The health belief model: a decade later. *Health Educ Q*, 1984;11:1–47.

59. Chesney MA, Ickovics JR, Chambers DB, et al. Self reported adherence to antiretroviral medications among participants in HIV clinical trials: the AACTG adherence instruments. *AIDS Care*, 2000; 12:255–266.

60. Claxton AJ, Cramer J, Pierce C. A systematic review of the associations between dose regimens and medication compliance. *Clin Ther*, 2001;8: 1296–1310.

61. Bartlett JA, DeMasi R, Quinn J, Moxham C, Rousseau F. Overview of the effectiveness of triple combination therapy in antiretroviral-naïve HIV-1 infected adults. *AIDS*, 2001;15:1369–1377.

62. Maggiolo F, Migliorino M, Maswrati R, et al. Virologic and immunologic responses to a once-a-day antiretroviral regimen with didanosine, lamivudine and efavirenz. *Antiviral Ther*, 2001;6: 249–253.

63. Gullick RM, Ribaudo HJ, Shikuma CM, et al. Triple nucleoside regimens versus efavirenz containing regimens for the initial treatment of HIV-1 infection. *N Engl J Med*, 2004;350:1850–1861.

64. Desclaux A, Laniece I, Ndoye I, et al. *The Senegalese Antiretroviral Drug Access Initiative*. Paris: ANRS, UNAIDS, WHO, 2004.

65. Farmer P, Leandre F, Mukherjee J, Gupta R, Tarter L, Kim JY. Community-based treatment of advanced HIV disease: introducing DOT-HAART. *Bull World Health Organ*, 2001;79(12):1145-1151.

66. Farmer P, Leandre F, Mukherjee J, et al. Community-based approaches to HIV treatment in resource poor settings. *Lancet*, 2001;358:404–409.

67. Altice FL, Mezger J, Hodges J, et al. Directly observed therapy (DOT) for HIV+ drug users (IDUs). *2nd IAS Conference on HIV Pathogenesis and Treatment*, Paris, France, July 13–16, 2003 (abstract 40).

68. Idoko JA, Agbaji O, Kanki P, et al. DOT HAART in a resource limited setting: the use of community treatment support can be effective. *12th Conference on Retroviruses and Opportunistic Infections*, Boston, Massachusetts, February 22–25, 2005 (abstract 629).

69. Mansky LM, Temin HM. Lower in vivo mutation rate of human immunodeficiency virus type 1 than that predicted from the fidelity of purified reverse transcriptase. *J Virol*, 1995;69:5087–5094.

70. Harrigan PR, Hogg RS, Dong WW, et al. Predictors of HIV drug-resistance mutations in a large anti-retroviral-naive cohort initiating triple antiretroviral therapy. *J Infect Dis*, 2005;191:339–347.

71. UK Collaborative Group on Monitoring the Transmission of HIV Drug Resistance. Analysis of prevalence of HIV-1 drug resistance in primary infections in the United Kingdom. *BMJ*, 2001;322: 1087–1088.

72. Panidou ET, et al. Resistance testing: impact on treatment outcomes. *AIDS*, 2004;18:2153–2161.

73. Bansberg DR, Hecht FM, Charlebois ED, et al. Adherence to protease inhibitors, HIV-1 viral load, and development of drug resistance in an indigenous population. *AIDS*, 2000;14:357–366.

74. Bansberg DR, Charlbois ED, Grant RM, et al. High levels of adherence do not prevent accumulation of HIV drug resistance mutations. *AIDS*, 2003;17: 1925–1932.

75. Wensing AMJ, van de Vijver DAMC, Asjo B, et al. Analysis from more than 1600 newly diagnosed patients with HIV from 17 European countries shows that 10% of the patients carry primary drug resistance: the CATCH Study. *2nd IAS Conference on HIV Pathogenesis and Treatment*, Paris, France, July 13–16, 2003 (abstract LB01).

76. Bennett D, Smith A, Heneine W, et al. Geographic variation in prevalence of mutations associated with resistance to antiretroviral drugs among drug-naive persons newly diagnosed with HIV in ten US cities, 1997–2001. *2nd IAS Conference on HIV Pathogenesis and Treatment*, Paris, France, July 13–16, 2003 (abstract 787).

77. Blower S, Bodine E, Kahn J, McFarland W. The antiretroviral rollout and drug-resistant HIV in Africa: insights from empirical data and theoretical models. *AIDS*, 2005;19(1):1–14.

78. Guay L, Musoke P, Fleming T, et al. Intrapartum and neonatal single dose nevirapine compared with zidovudine for the prevention of mother to child transmission of HIV-1. *New Engl J Med*, 2001;343: 982–991.

79. Jourdain G, Ngo-Giang-Huong N, Tungyai P, et al. Response to d4T/3TC/NVP in mothers based on previous history of single-dose NVP. *11th Conference on Retroviruses and Opportunistic Infections*, San Francisco, California, February 7–11, 2004 (abstract 41LB).

80. Coetzee D, Hildebrand K, Boulle A, et al. Outcomes after 2 years of providing antiretroviral treatment in Khayelitsha, South Africa. *AIDS*, 2004;18: 887–895.

81. Mauss S, Scholten S, Wolf E, et al. A prospective controlled study assessing the effect of lopinavir on amprenavir concentrations boosted by ritonavir. *HIV Med*, 2004;5:15–17.

82. Harris M, Alexander C, Ting L, et al. Rescue therapy with indinavir 600 mg twice daily and lopinavir/ritonavir: baseline resistance, virologic response and pharmacokinetics. *6th International Congress on Drug Therapy in HIV Infection*, Glasgow, United Kingdom, November 17–21, 2002 (abstract P170).

83. Stephan C, Henting N, Kourbeti I, et al. Saquinavir drug exposure is not impaired by the boosted double protease inhibitor combination of lopinavir/ritonavir. *AIDS*, 2004;18:503–508.

84. Leith J, Walmsley S, Katlama C, et al. Pharmacokinetics and safety of tripanavir/ritonavir (TPV/r): interim analysis of BI1182.51. *5th International Workshop on Clinical Pharmacology on HIV Therapy*, Rome, Italy, April 1–3, 2004 (abstract 5.1).

85. Kearney BP, Damle B, Plummer A, et al. Tenofovir DF (TDF) and didanosine EC (ddI EC) investigation of pharmacokinetic (PK) drug-drug and drug-food interactions. *XIV International AIDS Conference*, Barcelona, Spain, July 7–12, 2002 (abstract LBPE9026).

86. Kearney BP, Mittan A, Sayre J, et al. Pharmacokinetic drug interaction and long term safety profile of tenofovir DF and lopinavir/ritonavir. *43rd Interscience Conference on Antimocrobial Agents and Chemotherapy*, Chicago, Illinois, September 14–17, 2003 (abstract A-1617).

87. Kaul S, Bassi K, Kamle B, et al. Pharmocokinetic evaluation of the combination of atazanavir (ATV), enteric coated didanosine (ddI EC), and tenofovir disoproxil fumarate (TDF) for a once-daily antiretroviral regimen. *43rd Interscience Conference on Antirmicrobial Agents and Chemotherapy*, Chicago, Illinois, September 14–17, 2003 (abstract A1616).

88. Agarwala S, Eley T, Villegas C, et al. Pharmacokinetic effect of famotidine on atazanavir with and without ritonavir in healthy subjects. *6th International Workshop on Clinical Pharmacology of HIV Therapy*, Quebec City, Quebec, April 28–30, 2005 (abstract 11).

89. Landman R, Peytavin G, Descamps D, et al. Low genetic barrier to resistance is a possible cause of early virologic failure in once-daily regime of abacavir, lamivudine, and tenofovir: the TONUS Study. *11th Conference on Retroviruses and Opportunistic Infections*, San Francisco, California, February 7–11, 2004 (abstract 52).

90. d'Arminio Monforte A, Lepri AC, Rezza G, et al. Insights into the reasons for discontinuation of the first highly active antiretroviral therapy (HAART) regimen in a cohort of antiretroviral naive patients. *AIDS*, 2000;14:499–507.

91. Stone VE, Jordan J, Tolson, et al. Potential impact of once-daily regimens on adherence to HAART. *40th Annual Meeting of the Infectious Diseases Society of America*, Chicago, Illinois, October 24–27, 2002 (abstract 486).

92. Gathe J, Podzamczer D, Johnson M, et al. Once daily versus twice daily lopinavir/ritonavir in antiretroviral-naïve patients: 48 week results. *11th Conference on Retroviruses and Opportunistic Infections*, San Francisco, California, February 8–11, 2004 (abstract 57).

93. Vrijens B, Comte L, Tousset E, et al. Once-daily versus twice-daily regimens: which is best for HIV infected patients? *6th International Workshop on Clinical Pharmacology of HIV Therapy*, Quebec City, Quebec, April 28–30, 2005 (abstract 3).

94. Squires KE, Thiry A, Giordano M, et al. Atazanavir (ATV) QD versus efavirenz (EFV) QD with fixed dose ZDV + 3TC BID: comparison of antiviral efficacy and safety. *42nd Interscience Conference on Antimicrobial Agents and Chemotherapy*, San Diego, California, September 27–30, 2002 (abstract H-1076).

95. Dore GJ, Cooper DA, Pozniak AL, et al. Efficacy of tenofovir disaproxil fumarate in antiretroviral therapy-naïve and experienced patients coinfected with HIV-1 and hepatitis B virus. *J Infect Dis*, 2004; 189:1185–1192.

96. Garcia F, De Lazzari E, Plana M, et al. Long-term CD4+ T cell response to highly active antiretroviral therapy according to baseline CD4+ T cell count. *J Acquir Immune Defic Syndr*, 2004;36:702–713.

97. Phillips AN, Staszewski S, Weber R, et al. HIV viral load response to antiretroviral therapy according to the baseline CD4 cell count and viral load. *JAMA*, 2001;286:2560–2567.

98. Florence E, Lundgren J, Dreezen C, et al. Factors associated with a reduced CD4 lymphocyte count response to HAART despite full viral suppression in the EuroSIDA study. *HIV Med*, 2003;4(3):255–262.

99. Eshleman SH, Mracna M, Guay G, et al. Selection of nevirapine resistance (NVPR) mutations in Uganda women and infants receiving NVP prophylaxis to prevent HIV-1 vertical transmission (HIVNET-012). *8th Conference on Retrovirus and Opportunistic Infections*, Chicago, Illinois, February 4–8, 2001 (abstract 516).

100. León A, Martinez E, Mallolas J, et al. Early virological failure in treatment-naive HIV-infected adults receiving didanosine and tenofovir plus efavirenz or nevirapine. *AIDS*, 2005;19:213–215.

101. Easterbrook P, Ives N, Peters B, et al. The natural history and clinical significance of intermittent virological "blips" in patients who attain an initially undetectable viral load (VL) on HAART. *13th International AIDS Conference*, Durban, South Africa, July 9–14, 2000 (abstract WeOrB610).

102. Di Mascio M, Markowitz M, Louie M, et al. Viral blip dynamics during highly active antiretroviral therapy. *J Virol*, 2003;77(22):12165–12172.

103. Martinez V, Marcelin AG, Morini JP. HIV-1 intermittent viraemia in patients treated by nonnucleoside reverse transcriptase inhibitor-based regimen. *AIDS*, 2005;19(10):1065–1069.

104. Montaner JS, Harrigan PR, Jahnke N, et al. Multiple drug rescue therapy for HIV-infected individuals with prior virologic failure to multiple regimens. *AIDS*, 2001;15(1):61–69.

105. Deeks SG, Wrin T, Liegler T, et al. Virologic and immunologic consequences of discontinuing combination antiretroviral-drug therapy in HIV-infected patients with detectable viremia. *N Engl J Med*, 2001;344(7):472–480.

106. Dybul M. Structured treatment interruptions: approaches and risks. *Curr Infect Dis Rep*, 2002;4: 175–180.

107. Boschi A, Tinelli C, Ortolani P, Moscatelli G, Morigi G, Arlotti M. CD4+ cell-count-guided treatment interruptions in chronic HIV-infected patients with good response to highly active antiretroviral therapy. *AIDS*, 2004;18:2381–2389.

108. Taylor S, Allen S, Fidler S, et al. Stop study: after discontinuation of efavirenz, plasma concentrations may persist for 2 weeks or longer. *11th Conference on Retroviruses and Opportunistic Infections*, San Francisco, California, February 7–11, 2004 (abstract 131).

109. Johnson J, Li JF, Morris I, et al. Resistance emerges in majority of women provided intrapartum single dose nevirapine. *12th Conference on Retroviruses and Opportunistic Infections*, Boston, Massachusetts, February 22–25, 2005 (abstract 100).

110. Mackie NE, Fidler S, Tamm N, et al. Clinical implications of stopping nevirapine-based antiretroviral therapy: relative pharmacokinetics and avoidance of drug resistance. *HIV Med*, 2004;5(3):180–184.

111. Garcia PM, Kalish LA, Pitt J, et al. Maternal levels of plasma human immunodeficiency virus type 1 RNA and the risk of perinatal transmission. Women and Infants Transmission Study Group. *N Engl J Med*, 1999;34:394–402.

112. Fundaro C, Genovese O, Rendeli C, et al. Myelomeningocele in a child with intrauterine exposure to efavirenz. *AIDS*, 2002;16:299–300.

113. Bristol-Myers Squibb. Package insert: Sustiva™ (Efavirenz) capsules and tablets. Princeton, New Jersey: Bristol-Myers Squibb, January 2002.

114. Federal Ministry of Heath. *National Guidelines on Prevention of Mother to Child Transmission of HIV in Nigeria*. Abuja: Federal Ministry of Heath, 2005.

115. Idoko JA, Anteyi EA, Idoko LO, Agbaji OO, Ibrahim T. Human immunodeficiency virus (HIV) associated tuberculosis in Jos. *Niger Med Pract*, 1994;28:48–52.

116. Idigbe O, Sofola T, Odiah F, et al. Pulmonary TB and HIV infection among prison inmates in Lagos, Nigeria. *12th International AIDS Conference*, Geneva, Switzerland, June 28–July 3, 1998 (abstract 13256).

117. Ekong EE, Akinlade O, Uwah A. Trends and spectrum of mortality among HIV patients in the era of HAART — the Nigerian experience. *XIV International AIDS Conference*, Barcelona, Spain, July 7–12, 2002 (abstract MoPe3328).

118. Burman WJ, Jones BE. Treatment of HIV-related tuberculosis in the era of effective antiretroviral therapy. *Am J Respir Crit Care Med*, 2001;164:7–12.

119. Narita M, Ashkin D, Hollender ES, et al. Paradoxical worsening of tuberculosis following antiretroviral therapy in patients with AIDS. *Am J Respir Crit Care Med*, 1998;158(1):157–161.

120. Blumberg HM, Burman WJ, Chaisson RE, et al. American Thoracic Society/Centers for Disease Control and Prevention/Infectious Diseases Society of America: treatment of tuberculosis. *Am J Respir Crit Care Med*, 2003;167(4):603–662.

121. Perriens JH, St Louis ME, Mukadi YB, et al. Pulmonary tuberculosis in HIV-infected patients in Zaire—a controlled trial of treatment for either 6 or 12 months. *N Engl J Med*, 1995; 332(12):779–784.

122. Haller L, Sossouhounto R, Coulibaly IM, et al. Isoniazid plus sulphadoxine-pyrimethamine can reduce morbidity of HIV-positive patients treated for tuberculosis in Africa: a controlled clinical trial. *Chemotherapy*, 1999;45(6):452–465.

123. Churchyard GJ, Fielding K, Charalambous S, et al. Efficacy of secondary isoniazid preventive therapy among HIV-infected Southern Africans: time to change policy? *AIDS*, 2003;17(14):2063–2070.

124. Idoko JA, Njoku MO, Sirisena ND, et al. Carriage rate of HBV surface antigen in an urban community in Jos, Plateau State, Nigeria. *Nig Postgr Med J*, 2001;9:7–10.

125. Idoko J, Njoku O, Idoko H, et al. Seroprevalence of HBV and HCV in people living with HIV/AIDS. *13th International Conference on AIDS and STDs*, Nairobi, Kenya, September 21–26, 2003 (abstract 590603).

126. Baba MM, Gashau W, Hassan AW. Detection of HBV surface antigen in patients with and without the manifestations of AIDS in Maiduguri, Nigeria. *Nig Postgr Med J*, 1998;5:125–127.

127. Halim NKD, Offor E, Ajayi O. Epidemiologic study of the seroprevalence of hepatitis B surface antigen (HBsAg) and HIV-1 in blood donors in Nigeria. *J Clin Pract*, 1999;2:42–45.

128. Thio CL, Seaberg EC, Skolasky R Jr, et al. HIV-1 hepatitis B virus, and risk of liver-related mortality in the Multicentre Cohort Study (MACS). *Lancet*, 2002;360:1921–1926.

129. Dore G, Cooper D, Pozniak AL, et al. Anti-hepatitis B virus (HBV) activity in HBV/HIV coinfected patients treated with tenofovir DF (TDF) and lamivudine (Lam) versus lamuvidine alone; 144 week follow up. *XV International AIDS Conference*, Bangkok, Thailand, July 11–16, 2004 (abstract 3308).

130. Sheng WH, Chen MY, Hsieh SM, et al. Impact of chronic hepatitis B virus (HBV) infection on outcomes of patients infected with HIV in an area where HBV infection is hyperendemic. *Clin Infect Dis*, 2004;38:1471–1477.

131. Sukowski MS, Thomas DL, Chisson RE, et al. Hepatoxicity associated with antiretroviral therapy in adults infected with human immunodeficiency virus and the role of hepatitis C or B virus infection. *J Am Med Assoc*, 2000;283:74–80.

132. Aceti A, Pasquazzi C, Zechini B, De Bac C. The LIVERHAART Group. Hepatotoxicity development during antiretroviral therapy containing protease inhibitors in patients with HIV: the role of hepatitis B and C virus infection. *J AIDS*, 2002;29:41–48.

133. Benhamou Y, Dominguez S, Quioc J, et al. Effect of HIV infection in chronic Hepatitis B related liver decompensation. *12th Conference on Retroviruses and Opportunistic Infections*, Boston, Massachusetts, February 22–25, 2005 (abstract 933).

134. Chung R, Kinm A. HIV/hepatitis B and coinfection: pathogenic interactions, natural history and therapy. *Antivir Chem Cheomother*, 2001;12:73–91.

135. Konopnicki D, Mocroft A, de Wit S, et al. Hepatitis B and HIV: prevalence, AIDS progression, response to highly active antiretroviral therapy and increased mortality in the EuroSIDA cohort. *AIDS*, 2005;19(6):593–601.

136. Sherman KE, O'Brien J, Gutierrez AG, et al. Quantitative evaluation of hepatitis C virus RNA in patients with concurrent human immunodeficiency virus infections. *J Clin Microbiol*, 1993;31: 2679–2682.

137. Polyak SJ, Sullivan DG, Austin MA, et al. Comparison of amplification enzymes for hepatitis C virus quasispecies analysis. *J Virol*, 2005;2(1):41

138. Schreier E, Roggendorf M, Driesel G, et al. Genotypes of hepatitis C virus isolates from different parts of the world. *Arch Virol Suppl*, 1996;11: 185–193.

139. Rosenberg PM, Farrell JJ, Abraczinskas DR, et al. Rapidly progressive fibrosing cholestatic hepatitis—hepatitis C virus in HIV coinfection. *Am J Gastroenterol*, 2002;97:478–483.

140. Lauer GM, Nguyen TN, Day CL, et al. Human immunodeficiency virus type 1-hepatitis C virus coinfection: intraindividual comparison of cellular immune responses against two persistent viruses. *J Virol*, 2002;76(6):2817–2826.

141. Martinez-Sierra C, Arizcorreta A, Díaz F, et al. Progression of chronic hepatitis C to liver fibrosis and cirrhosis in patients coinfected with hepatitis C virus and human immunodeficiency virus. *Clin Infect Dis*, 2003;36:491–498.

142. Soto B, Sanchez-Quijano A, Rodrigo L, et al. Human immunodeficiency virus infection modifies the natural history of chronic parenterally-acquired hepatitis C with an unusually rapid progression to cirrhosis. *J Hepatol*, 1997;26(1):1–5.

143. Darby SC, Ewart DW, Giangrande PL, et al. Mortality from liver cancer and liver disease in haemophilic men and boys in UK given blood products contaminated with hepatitis C. UK Haemophilia Centre Directors' Organisation. *Lancet*, 1997;350(9089):1425–1431.

144. Benhamou Y, Bochet M, Di Martino V, et al. Liver fibrosis progression in human immunodeficiency virus and hepatitis C virus coinfected patients. The Multivirc Group. *Hepatology*, 1999;30(4):1054–1058.

145. Greub G, Ledergerber B, Battegay M, et al. Clinical progression, survival, and immune recovery during antiretroviral therapy in patients with HIV-1 and hepatitis C virus coinfection: the Swiss Cohort Study. *Lancet*, 2000;356:1800–1805.

146. Chung R, Evans S, Yang Y, et al. Immune recovery is associated with persistent rise in hepatitis C virus RNA, infrequent liver test flares, and is not impaired by hepatitis C virus in co-infected subjects. *AIDS*, 2002;16(14):1915–1923.

147. Anderson KB, Guest JL, Rimland D. Hepatitis C virus coinfection increases mortality in HIV-infected patients in the highly active antiretroviral therapy era: data from the HIV Atlanta VA Cohort Study. *Clinic Infect Dis*, 2004;39:1507–1513.

148. Qurishi N, Kreuzberg C, Luchters G, et al. Effect of antiretroviral therapy on liver related mortality in patients with HIV and hepatitis C virus coinfection. *Lancet*, 2003;362:1708–1713.

149. Chung R, Andersen J, Volberding P, et al. A randomized, controlled trial of PEG-interferon-alfa-2a plus ribavirin vs interferon-alfa-2a plus ribavirin for chronic hepatitis C virus infection in HIV coinfected persons: follow up results of ACTG A5071. *11th Conference on Retroviruses and Opportunistic Infections*, San Francisco, California, February 7–11, 2004 (abstract 110).

150. Torriani FJ, Rockstroh J, Rodriguez-Torres M, et al. Final results of APRICOT: a randomized, partially blinded, international trial evaluating peginterferon-alfa-2a + ribavirin vs interferon-alfa-2a + ribavirin in the treatment of HCV in HIV/HCV coinfection. *11th Conference on Retroviruses and Opportunistic Infections*, San Francisco, California, February 7–11, 2004 (abstract 112).

151. Perronne C, Carrat F, Bani-Sadr F, et al. Final results of ANRS HC02-RIBAVIC: a randomized controlled trial of pegylated-interferon-alfa-2b plus ribavirin vs. interferon-alfa-2b plus ribavirin for the initial treatment of chronic hepatitis C in HIV coinfected patients. *11th Conference on Retroviruses and Opportunistic Infections*, San Francisco, California, February 7–11, 2004 (abstract 117LB).

152. Lafeuillade A, Hittenger G, Chadapaud S, et al. Increased mitochondrial toxicity with ribavirin in HIV/HCV coinfection. *Lancet*, 2001;357:280–281.

153. Abimuku AG, Zwandor A, Gomwalk N, et al. HIV 1, not HIV 2 is prevalent in Nigeria: need for consideration in vaccine plans. *Vaccine Research*, 1994;2: 101–104.

154. Kanki P, Travers K, Hernandez-Avila M, et al. Slower heterosexual spread of HIV-2 compared with HIV-1. *Lancet*, 1994;343:943–946.

155. Marlink R, Kanki P, Thior I, et al. Reduced rate of disease development with HIV-2 compared to HIV-1. *Science*, 1994;265:1587–1590.

156. Reid P, MacInnes H, Cong ME, et al. Natural resistance of human immunodeficiency virus type 2 to zidovudine. *Virology*, 2005;336(2):251–264.

157. Rodes B, Holguin A, Soriano V, et al. Emergence of drug resistance mutations in human immunodeficiency virus type-2 infected subjects undergoing antiretroviral therapy. *J Clin Microbiol*, 2000;38:1370–1374.

158. Public Health Laboratory Service. AIDS and STD at the Communicable Diseases Surveillance Centre. Occupational transmission of HIV. Summary of published reports in June. Hamilton, Ontario: Public Health Laboratory Service, 1999:9–11.

159. Do AN, Ciesielski CA, Metler RP, et al. Occupationally acquired human immunodeficiency virus (HIV) infection: national case surveillance data during 20 years of the HIV epidemic in the United States. *Infect Control Hosp Epidemiol*, 2003;24(2):86–96.

160. Johnson S, Baraboutis JG. Adverse effects associated with use of nevirapine in HIV postexposure prophylaxis for 2 health care workers. *JAMA*, 2000;284(21):2722–2723.

161. U.S. Centers for Disease Control and Prevention. Serious adverse events attributed to nevirapine regimens for postexposure prophylaxis after HIV exposures worldwide; 1997–2000. *MMWR*, 2001;49:1153.

162. Stoll M, Schmidt RE. Immune restoration inflammatory syndromes: the dark side of successful antiretroviral treatment. *Curr Infect Dis Rep*, 2003;5(3):266–276.

163. Shelburne SA 3rd, Hamill RJ, Rodriguez-Barradas MC, et al. Immune reconstitution inflammatory syndrome: emergence of a unique syndrome during highly active antiretroviral therapy. *Medicine (Baltimore)*, 2002;81(3):213–227.

164. Cooney EL. Clinical indicators of immune restoration following highly active antiretroviral therapy. *Clinic Infect Dis*, 2002;34:224–233.

165. Shelburne, S, Visnegarwala F, Darcourt Jorge, et al. Incidence and risk factors for immune reconstitution inflammatory syndrome during highly active antiretroviral therapy. *AIDS*, 2005;19(4):399–406.

166. Domingo P, Torres OH, Ris J, et al. Herpes zoster as an immune reconstitution disease after initiation of combination antiretroviral therapy in patients with human immunodeficiency virus type-1 infection. *Am J Med*, 2001;110(8):605–609.

167. Jenny-Avital ER, Abadi M. Immune reconstitution cryptococcosis after initiation of successful highly active antiretroviral therapy. *Clin Infect Dis*, 2002;35(12):e128–133.

168. Kombe G, Galaty D, Nwagbara C, Partners for Health Reformplus. *Scaling up Antiretroviral Treatment in the Public Sector in Nigeria: A Comprehensive Analysis of Resource Requirements*. Bethesda, Maryland: Abt Associates, Inc., 2004.

18

RESEARCH AND THE KNOWLEDGE BASE FOR HIV/AIDS CONTROL

Phyllis J. Kanki* and Oni E. Idigbe†

Science and technology have become critical factors in economic and social development globally (1,2), and the springboard of science and technology is research. Research involves the systematic collection of data, the logical organization and analysis of facts, and the design and conduct of experiments to test specific hypotheses in such a way as to generate verifiable observations and evidence-based principles (3,4).

Research is relevant to every sector of society, but especially the health sector, and medical research has provided the strongest support for preventive and curative medicine. Globally, it has become generally accepted that improvement in health care delivery is closely associated with advances in medical research (5,6). Indeed, strengthening medical research capacities at the national level has constituted the most powerful, cost-effective, and sustainable means of advancing health and development (7).

Developed countries have successfully harnessed science to promote the health of their populations. These countries carefully direct medical research toward the most prevalent and unsolved health problems within their populations (3). They identify health problems and find new solutions, providing the most up-to-date information to modify health policies and develop new strategies,

*AIDS Prevention Initiative in Nigeria, Harvard PEPFAR, and Harvard School of Public Health, Boston, Massachusetts, USA
†Nigerian Institute of Medical Research, Lagos, Nigeria

monitoring the response to interventions, and promoting more research to identify new problems. Their efforts have helped to eradicate or control some long-standing health problems, reduce mortality and morbidity of predominantly communicable diseases in their communities, and extend the life expectancies of their citizens.

In contrast, most developing countries have made minimal investments in medical research. Research organizations tend to be underdeveloped, and scientists face serious constraints that limit their productivity. These constraints can be broadly classified into the lack of a critical mass of personnel, an inadequate work environment, and an uncooperative macroenvironment. Medical researchers in most developing countries tend to be intellectually isolated. Their training is often insufficient, and they usually have limited career paths, restricted research choices, and poor salaries. Their work environments tend to be characterized by a lack of access to scientific information, inadequate support staff, institutional instability, and inadequate facilities. The macroenvironment often has a lack of demand for research, the absence of an appropriate and robust scientific culture, insufficient public support, bureaucratic rigidity, and political instability. At the same time, developing countries face an estimated 90% of the global disease burden (8). To remedy this situation, urgent global efforts should be directed toward enhancing human and infrastructural capacities for medical research in developing countries.

RESEARCH AND AIDS

Fundamental to our understanding of AIDS were the early efforts of biomedical research. At the early stage of the epidemic, the need to identify the etiologic agent to better understand the epidemiology of the disease was urgent. Among the suspected agents were cytomegalovirus because of its association with immunosuppression, Epstein-Barr virus because of its known ability to populate lymphoid tissues, and hepatitis B virus because it was transmitted by blood and sex (9). Scientists recognized, however, that these viruses would have needed to have mutated significantly to cause such a new disease as AIDS. Comparative research focused on seroprevalence studies ultimately demonstrated no convincing association between AIDS and any of these viruses or a score of other agents (10).

In 1983, Montagnier and his colleagues first reported the association of this clinical syndrome with a candidate retrovirus (11). In 1984, Montagnier and Gallo provided conclusive virologic and epidemiologic evidence that the virus now known as the human immunodeficiency virus (HIV) was the causative agent of AIDS (12). It should be noted, however, that decades of earlier research in animal retrovirology were critical to the ability of the biomedical community to identify the etiologic agent of AIDS so quickly (13). Essex and colleagues had first proposed that a human retrovirus could be the etiologic agent of AIDS (9). It was soon established that HIV belonged to the lentivirus subfamily of retroviruses, known for their protracted course of infection and latency. In 1986, a new type of HIV was isolated from people in West Africa (14). Subsequent studies found this type to be less virulent than the first, and the two viruses differed in 60% of their genomic sequences (15). The earlier identified virus was designated HIV-1, while the West African virus was designated HIV-2.

Upon identification of HIV, scientists—through intensive efforts in the broad areas of basic, applied, and operational research—made major strides in the basic understanding and therapeutic management of all stages and manifestations of HIV infection. Basic research led to a full description of the biological structure of the virus, the natural history and pathogenesis of infection, the genomic structure, and the existence of several subtypes of HIV-1 and HIV-2 distributed within different geographic areas (16,17). Through the efforts of applied and operational research, information generated from basic research allowed investigators to develop laboratory techniques—both antibody and antigen based—for diagnosing infection, devising techniques for monitoring disease progression and responses to interventions, developing antiretrovirals (ARVs) for the clinical management of the infection, defining the clinical characteristics of the opportunistic diseases and cancers associated with HIV infection, and creating various treatment options for these opportunistic infections and cancers (18–21). Social science research also generated important information on the social, economic, cultural, and behavioral factors that influence transmission of the virus within various populations and communities (22–24).

Thus, the efforts of biomedical and social science research have not only contributed significantly to the knowledge of HIV/AIDS but have also helped investigators develop effective strategies for preventing transmission of the virus and treating those already infected. Figure 18-1 shows a graphic representation of the role of biomedical research in the understanding of HIV/AIDS.

HIV/AIDS IN NIGERIA

After Nigeria's first AIDS case was reported in 1986 (25), the virus began its insidious spread through the country's various populations and communities. By the end of 1999, cases of HIV infection or AIDS had been diagnosed in all of the country's 774 local government areas (26). The virus systematically permeated the entire Nigerian social fabric, affecting men and women in urban and rural areas and cutting across all social strata. Data from national HIV sentinel surveys indicated a rapid transition from near zero prevalence in 1990 to an overall 5.0% seroprevalence rate among the adult population (15 to 49 years) in 2003 (26). A review of infection rates and available clinical data in the country between 1990 and 2003 indicated an escalating epidemic that had spread beyond the "high-risk groups." By 2003, with an estimated three-and-a-half to four million infected individuals, Nigeria ranked second in sub-Saharan Africa and fourth globally in the absolute number of adults living with the virus (27). A year later, the pool of people living with the virus was still growing enormously and hundreds of thousands of people were dying of AIDS. Health systems and social coping mechanisms in the country were stretched and overburdened. In addition, with more than two million, Nigeria has the highest number of AIDS orphans in the world. The country's annual AIDS mortality figure has been projected to increase from 209,000 cases in 2001 to 700,000 in 2005 and 850,000 in 2010.

Initially, the impact of the epidemic was more pronounced on the health sector, and HIV/AIDS was viewed solely as a health problem. As the epidemic evolved, though, its impact broadened and became more of a burden for young men and women, who constitute the mainstay of agriculture, education, commerce,

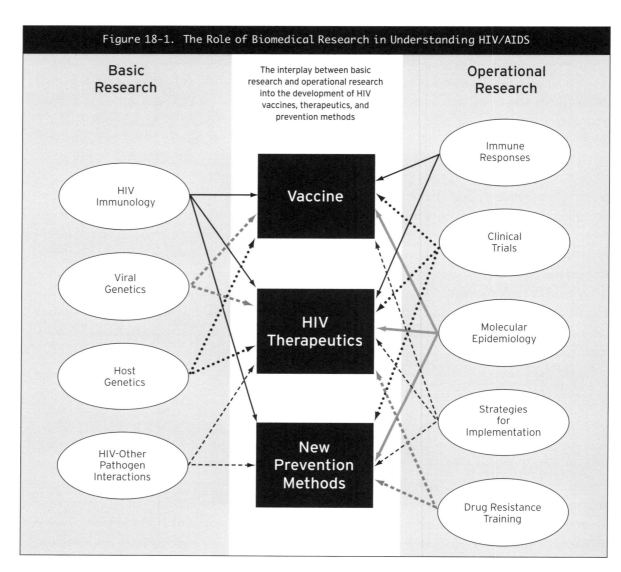

Figure 18-1. The Role of Biomedical Research in Understanding HIV/AIDS

Basic Research

The interplay between basic research and operational research into the development of HIV vaccines, therapeutics, and prevention methods

Operational Research

HIV Immunology

Viral Genetics

Host Genetics

HIV-Other Pathogen Interactions

Vaccine

HIV Therapeutics

New Prevention Methods

Immune Responses

Clinical Trials

Molecular Epidemiology

Strategies for Implementation

Drug Resistance Training

and industry. By 1999, it was clear that the impact of the epidemic had transcended the health sector to include the socioeconomic and development sectors. HIV/AIDS thus became Nigeria's most important health and development problem, requiring urgent attention and immediate response. The shift to the multisectoral impact of the epidemic underscored the fact that, despite all the preventive interventions, the need to mount an expanded program for care and support of the millions already living with HIV/AIDS had grown critical. The situation called for an expanded, multisectoral national response to the epidemic.

In 2000, President Olusegun Obasanjo exercised commendable political will to curb the epidemic by establishing a Presidential Committee on AIDS (PCA) with himself as the chairman. The PCA is thus the highest political body for HIV/AIDS in the country, with the role of the committee being absolutely advisory. The president further established an implementing organ, the National Action Committee on

AIDS (NACA), which has the corporate mandate to initiate and coordinate a multisectoral response to the epidemic on a national level. NACA was set up to work with essential federal ministries, international donor and development partners, nongovernmental organizations (NGOs), the organized private sector, and state and local government agencies. In line with the structure of the three tiers of government in the country, NACA is still expanding to establish the multisectoral response at the state level, through the state action committees on AIDS, and at the local level, though the local action committees on AIDS. With these structures in place, the country has been able to mount a multisectoral response to the epidemic and implement a number of HIV/AIDS prevention, care, and support programs.

In 2002, the federal government initiated a national ARV program designed to treat 10,000 adults and 5,000 children living with the virus. Since then, several other stakeholders in the country have also begun implementing ARV treatment programs. With the number of HIV-infected people rising, significant efforts in HIV control in Nigeria are being directed at care and support of infected individuals. ARVs are being provided only to a limited number of HIV-infected individuals who meet established clinical eligibility criteria. For HIV-infected people not yet eligible for ARVs, various palliative care strategies are being implemented. These include adequate nutrition, provision of mineral supplements and micronutrients, provision of immune boosters and antioxidants, and prompt diagnosis and treatment of opportunistic infections. Several international initiatives are also aimed at enhancing these care and support programs, most notably the Global Fund for HIV/AIDS, Tuberculosis and Malaria; the U.S. President's Emergency Plan for AIDS Relief (PEPFAR); the 3 by 5 Initiative of UNAIDS, whose goal has been to place three million HIV-infected people in resource-poor countries on ARV treatment by the end of 2005; and the AIDS Prevention Initiative in Nigeria (APIN), which is funded by the Bill & Melinda Gates Foundation. With these various initiatives, it is estimated that an estimated 250,000 Nigerians living with the virus will soon be on ARV therapy.

RESEARCH EFFORTS ON THE HIV EPIDEMIC IN NIGERIA

In the early 1980s, after the first AIDS cases were reported in the United States and later in other countries, there was a high level of uncertainty and anxiety about whether cases of HIV infection were present in Nigerian communities. The wider response was that of denial; HIV infection was non-existent in the country. Thus, the earliest efforts on the HIV epidemic were essentially focused simply on establishing whether there were HIV/AIDS cases in the country.

Subsequently, surveillance systems were put in place to track cases of the infection in the country. The first case of full-blown AIDS was identified in a 16-year-old girl by a team of scientists at the Nigerian Institute of Medical Research in Lagos. This case was reported at the International AIDS Conference in Paris in 1986 (25). Subsequently, a few cases of HIV seropositive but asymptomatic individuals were identified, as well as a few cases of AIDS-related complex (28). These early reports were clouded by sensationalism, panic, and politics, as the level of available information on HIV/AIDS during this period was low. In a study carried out among students in secondary and tertiary institution in Lagos, 98.5% of the respondents had heard about AIDS, although 85% did not know how the infection was transmitted and 74% viewed

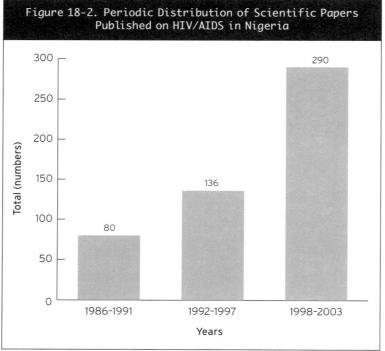

Figure 18-2. Periodic Distribution of Scientific Papers Published on HIV/AIDS in Nigeria

Source: Idigbe EO, Harry TO, Ekong EE, Audu RA, Musa AZ, Funsho-Adebayo EO, eds, *Nigerian Contributions to Regional and Global Meetings on HIV/AIDS/STIs, 1986-2003*. Lagos: Niyi Faniran Publishers, 2003.

AIDS as a disease of foreigners (29). Despite this, the few reported cases of AIDS-related complex foretold the urgent need for surveillance in the various populations and communities in the country.

The earliest efforts on systematic research on HIV/AIDS in Nigeria were based primarily on descriptive epidemiology. As the epidemic matured, however, the tempo and scope of the research activities progressively increased to embrace broad areas of basic, clinical, and social sciences as well as human rights, legal issues, and advocacy. Data from several studies on the evaluation of research inputs on HIV/AIDS in Nigeria indicated that the pattern of research efforts in the country was significantly influenced by the various stages of the evolution of the epidemic (30,31). This initial research focused on epidemiology and prevention, with little attention paid to the social and human right issues and only minimal effort on the basic, biomedical, and clinical sciences. As the number of HIV-infected people grew, however, the control efforts expanded from prevention to the provision of a continuum of care and support strategies. This shift equally stimulated efforts on HIV-related basic, clinical, and social science research.

In 2000, the government developed a bibliographic database for HIV in Nigeria (30). The study, which covered all 36 states and the Federal Capital Territory, focused on the retrieval and collation of all scientifically published and documented data on HIV/AIDS in the country between 1986 and 1999. A total of 506 publications were eventually retrieved from various libraries, educational institutions, research institutes, private sector establishments, and NGOs. Eighty, or 16%, of these publications were published between 1986 and 1991, 136 (27%) between 1992 and 1997, and 290 (57%) between 1998 and 2003 (Figure 18-2). A breakdown of these publications based on subject areas showed that 26 (5%) were in the area of basic sciences; 31 (6%) on human rights, politics, and advocacy; 94 (18%) on clinical sciences; 175 (35%) on social sciences; and 180 (36%) on epidemiology and prevention (31).

In 2003, another project developed a compendium of all abstracts of scientific papers presented by Nigerians in international conferences on HIV/AIDS (31). The compendium comprised of 365 abstracts presented by Nigerians in 17 regional and global conferences between 1986 and 2003. The abstracts were grouped into subject areas and period of publication. The data obtained from the project clearly indicated that the number of scientific papers presented by Nigerians in these conferences increased progressively between 1986 and 2003 (Figure 18-3).

Of the 365 abstracts, 8% were presented between 1986 and 1991, 12% between 1992 and 1997, and 80% between 1998 and 2003. The overall data indicated a considerable increase in research efforts on the HIV epidemic in the country between 1998 and 2003. The distribution of the abstracts based on

Figure 18-3. Distribution of Abstracts of Papers Presented by Nigerians in Regional and International HIV/AIDS Conferences

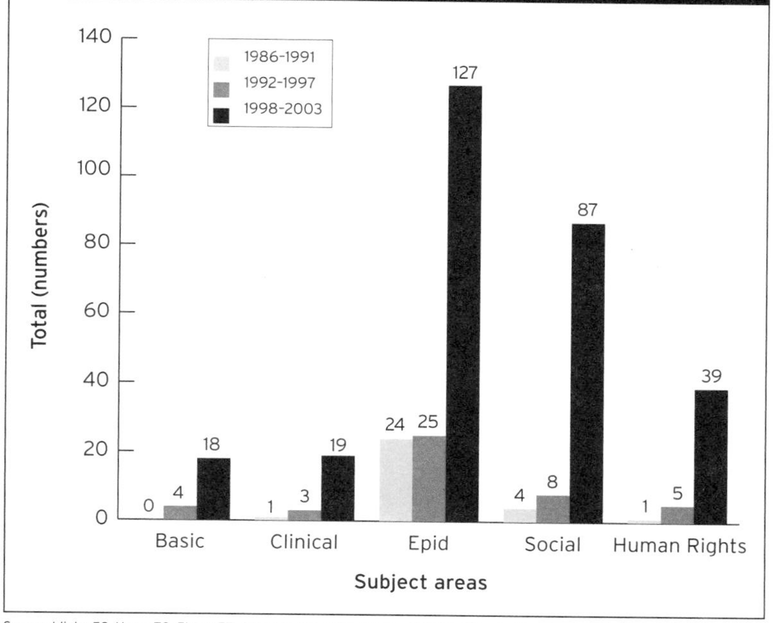

Source: Idigbe EO, Harry TO, Ekong EE, Audu RA, Musa AZ, Funsho-Adebayo EO, eds, *Nigerian Contributions to Regional and Global Meetings on HIV/AIDS/STIs, 1986-2003.* Lagos: Niyi Faniran Publishers, 2003.

the subject areas showed that 22 (6%) focused on basic sciences, 23 (6%) on clinical sciences, 45 (13%) on human rights and advocacy, 99 (27%) on social sciences, and 176 (48%) on epidemiology and prevention (Figure 18-3). Although these data did not differ much from the findings of the earlier study (30), information from the later study showed that between 1986 and 1991, no papers were presented on basic science, with only one each in clinical sciences and human rights and four papers from the social sciences. Between 1998 and 2003, however, the number of papers presented had risen to 18, 19, 87, and 39, respectively, in basic sciences, clinical sciences, social sciences, and human rights.

Specific data presented in these abstracts indicated that research efforts between 1986 and 1991 were geared toward establishing the magnitude, dynamics, and trends of the epidemic within various populations, as well as developing better strategies for the prevention of new infections. With the number of cases increasing and many patients beginning to manifest with opportunistic infections, research efforts were enhanced between 1992 and 1997, to generate more data for a better understanding of the pathogenesis of the infection, the profile of associated opportunistic infections, and the human, viral, cultural, and environmental factors driving the epidemic within the various populations and communities. Between 1998 and 2003, when hundreds of thousands began dying of AIDS, the workforce started shrinking, the number of AIDS orphans increased astronomically, and the socioeconomic impact retarded the national developmental process. As a result, substantial efforts were directed at operational research. Research efforts within this period focused essentially on how to implement the best practices and interventions that had worked on the national, regional, or global levels in the areas of care and support of people living with the virus, and the mitigation of HIV/AIDS on the national developmental process.

RESEARCH CAPACITIES ON THE HIV EPIDEMIC IN NIGERIA

Nigeria's level of capacity for basic, applied, and operational HIV/AIDS research evolved over three time periods: 1986–1991; 1992–1997; and 1998–2004.

1986–1991

At the early stage of this period, Nigeria's capacity for HIV research was minimal. Soon after the first AIDS case was diagnosed, the government responded by establishing the National Experts Advisory Committee on AIDS and the National AIDS and STDs Control Program (NASCP), both within the Federal Ministry of Health. These bodies pioneered the initial control strategies and research efforts on HIV/AIDS in Nigeria.

The major preoccupation at this stage was surveillance for the detection of infected cases. In developed countries, research efforts had contributed considerably to the generation of data on the clinical signs and symptoms associated with HIV infection, as well as the major modes of transmission of the infection. With some enhanced knowledge and awareness of the modes of transmission of the infection, the early national response focused primarily on prevention of transmission. The surveillance efforts at this period focused on detection of people already infected, particularly those considered high risk, such as sex workers, long-distance truck drivers, and migrant workers.

The World Health Organization (WHO) (32) and the U.S. Centers for Disease Control and Prevention (CDC) (33) had developed clinical surveillance and case detection systems based on broadly grouped major and minor signs of HIV infection. These were passive AIDS case definition systems, in which clinicians observed patients prospectively presenting at health facilities or retrospectively from hospital records. The presence of two major signs and one minor sign provided a presumptive diagnosis of AIDS. Clinicians were required to notify the federal and state health ministries of diagnosed and recorded cases. This system failed to capture the true picture of the epidemic, however, for several reasons: the long incubation of the virus meant that infected people were often asymptomatic; most health facilities had poor records because of underreporting, delayed reporting, or no reporting; HIV-infected people had inadequate access to health facilities; and, most important, health care providers tended to have little knowledge of the major and minor signs associated with AIDS. This surveillance system, used in Nigeria between 1986 and 1990, recorded only 52,962 AIDS cases, while the actual cumulative number of cases was estimated to be 850,000. Thus, the country's human and infrastructural capacities to implement this surveillance system were inadequate at that time.

When serologic tests for screening and confirming HIV-specific antibodies became available, however, HIV surveillance improved dramatically. These tests allowed investigators to obtain direct laboratory diagnoses of HIV infection. Between 1984 and 1985 the Nigerian Institute of Medical Research in Lagos developed the initial capacity to use these serologic tests, which were based on the enzyme-linked immunosorbent assay (ELISA) and were conducted with equipment Abbott Laboratories had donated from the United States. Confirmatory test kits were based on the Western blot; at that time, the tests were performed with equipment from the Kenyan Medical Research Institute. It was through these initial efforts that the country's first "true" AIDS case was diagnosed and reported (25).

In 1987, the WHO, working in collaboration with NACA and the NASCP, established nine additional HIV antibody-screening centers within health institutions. Six were located in the southern part of the country: University College Hospital in Ibadan; the University Teaching Hospital in Ife; the University of Nigeria Teaching Hospital in Enugu; the University Teaching Hospital in Calabar; the University Teaching Hospital in Benin City; and the Federal Vaccine Production Laboratory in Lagos. Three additional screening centers were in the north: the University of Maiduguri Teaching Hospital; the Ahmadu Bello University Teaching Hospital in Zaria; and the Jos University Teaching Hospital. From these centers, limited HIV seroprevalence surveys were carried out among specific groups, including sex workers, blood donors, patients with sexually transmitted infections (STIs), and pregnant women. Samples screened positive in these nine centers were sent to the University College Hospital in Ibadan and the University of Maiduguri Teaching Hospital for confirmation. At the time, these were the only two centers in the entire country with the capacity to perform the Western blot, the necessary confirmatory test to prove HIV infection.

In 1988, the WHO established an additional 12 screening centers across the country, bringing the total number to 22. Seven of these new centers were established in the north (Yola, Sokoto, Kano, Kaduna, Makurdi, Minna, and Katsina), while five were established in the south (Lagos, Port Harcourt, Owerri, Uyo, and Ilorin). The number of centers with the capacity to perform Western blot confirmatory tests also increased, from two to five. During this period, screening for HIV infection was anonymous and unlinked. Some level of human capacity for research was developed within this period as laboratory staff members were trained on the laboratory screening and confirmatory tests for HIV serostatus. Although the only major tool available for clinical and biomedical research at the time was HIV serology, several scientists used this limited capacity to carry out a few research studies. Most of these studies sought to estimate seroprevalence rates in various groups, especially populations engaged in high-risk behaviors for HIV acquisition or manifesting HIV-related disease conditions. Some of these early studies, although based essentially on serologic tests, generated important data on the epidemiology of HIV/AIDS in Nigeria. For instance, HIV seroprevalence rates of 0.7% to 1.8% were reported for blood donors; 2.9% to 4.5% among sex workers; 0.2% to 1.7% among pregnant women; 0.3% to 1.7% among STI clinic patients; and 2.0% to 4.0% among tuberculosis patients. Some of these studies also reported HIV-1 and HIV-2 coinfection cases within these groups (34–40).

During this period social science research increased as well, particularly in the development of strategies to prevent HIV transmission in the general population. Several research efforts were based on questionnaires designed to assess the knowledge, attitudes, practices, and beliefs among different population groups. Better strategies for advocacy and increasing awareness through health education—based mainly on various media of information, education, and communication—also kept evolving within this period. Research into preventive strategies hinged on three major modes of transmission and included promotion of protected sex, screening of blood before transfusion, and discouraging the use of contaminated sharp objects.

Although the capacity for social research on HIV infection was minimal, most of the studies yielded data that gave insight into possible social factors driving the epidemic, including local traditional and cultural practices, poverty, and low condom uptake (41–43). This information facilitated the development of better prevention strategies targeting the biological and social factors fueling the epidemic at the time.

Support for HIV programs during this early period was essentially government driven. The later period, however, witnessed the coming on board of some international donor and developmental agencies, NGOs, and several other private sector organizations, including the United Nation agencies, the WHO, the Department for International Development, the Canadian International Development Agency, the Japan International Cooperation Agency, the U.S. Agency for International Development (USAID), the Ford Foundation, the CDC, the U.S. National Institutes of Health, and the Institut Pasteur. The collaborative efforts of these various organizations contributed immensely to the development of the initial human and infrastructural capacities for research on HIV infection in the country.

1992–1997

From 1992 to 1997, biomedical and social research in the developed world added considerably to our understanding of various aspects of the global epidemiology, as well as the socioeconomic factors fueling the epidemic in different geographic locations. Some of the findings translated into the development and production of cheaper, efficient, easy-to-use, and rapid testing kits for HIV infection. Investigators also described the existence of multiple circulating subtypes of HIV-1 and HIV-2, the natural history of HIV infection, and the profile of opportunistic diseases associated with HIV infection in different parts of the world. Moreover, issues of stigmatization, discrimination, and ethical considerations for people living with the virus began to emerge.

These global data greatly influenced Nigeria's capacity for HIV research between 1992 and 1997. Serologic tests for HIV became more widely used, and the number of centers with HIV screening capacity increased extensively throughout the country. More people were diagnosed with HIV, and the reported number of infected people rose. Serologic data strongly suggested a progressive increase in transmission and the emergence of new cases. By the end of 1993 an estimated 800,000 adults were living with the virus. In 1997, the number of adults living with the virus was estimated at 1.9 million, an increase of more than 50% (26). As the situation worsened, more international agencies and NGOs came on board and enhanced support for the various HIV/AIDS control programs. This increased support remarkably enhanced the level of human and infrastructural capacities for basic and applied research on HIV/AIDS.

Issues of pre- and post-test counseling for HIV tests also emerged during this period. People started giving informed consent to be tested, which stimulated clinical research, as infected patients could be directly identified and followed up both clinically and biologically through laboratory tests.

Several research efforts centered on more in-depth laboratories studies on the epidemiology of the infection in various populations, identification of biological parameters for diagnosis, and the array of opportunistic infections associated with HIV infection. Levels of coinfection with HIV and tuberculosis were documented at 7% to 15%. The involvement of typical mycobacteria strains and fungal agents — including histoplasma, cryptococcus, and aspergillus — in HIV-associated respiratory diseases also was reported. Data from some of the studies showed that the prevalence of HIV and tuberculosis was much higher among prison inmates than among the general population (44–52).

Because the human and infrastructural capacities for HIV research were still developing, Nigerian scientists conducted most of their sophisticated and cutting-edge HIV research in conjunction with institutions in developed countries. Through these collaborations, researchers were able to establish the national prevalence of HIV-2 and identify the various subtypes of HIV-1 and HIV-2 circulating in Nigeria. Working with laboratories in the United States, Britain, Germany, and France, Nigerian researchers established the demographic characteristics of retroviral infections—including HIV-1, HIV-2, and human T-cell lymphotropic virus I (HTLV-I)—among female sex workers (53–55) and isolated and characterized a new variant of HIV-1 (56). A further study on the genomic structure and nucleotide sequence of a new HIV-1 strain classified it as a variant of HIV-1 subtype A (56–58), now known as CRF02_AG.

In estimating the national prevalence of the virus, of course, it was not feasible to screen the entire population. The WHO, though, introduced the sentinel surveillance system to monitor the dynamics of infection in various countries. The sentinel groups included those with tuberculosis and STIs; those whose behavior put them at higher risk of HIV infection, such as sex workers, migrant workers, and long-distance truck drivers; and antenatal clinic attendees, who were considered representative of the general population.

Nigeria adopted the sentinel surveillance survey in 1991 to serve as an active system to complement data generated from the passive AIDS case reporting system in use since 1986. Investigators used the sentinel surveillance system to estimate and monitor the magnitude and trend of the infection in various groups over time. The median seroprevalence rates from antenatal attendees were extrapolated to estimate national rates in the general adult population, those aged 15 to 49 years. Six anonymous, unlinked, and confidential seroprevalence surveys among antenatal clinic attendees were carried out at the national level between 1991 and 2003. Based on these studies, the estimated national HIV seroprevalence rates among the adult population showed a progressive increase from 1.8% in 1991 to 5.4% in 1999, 5.8% in 2001, and a slight drop to 5.0% in 2003 (26).

These surveillance data enabled estimates of the number of people infected with the virus at various stages of the epidemic and enhanced efforts at developing newer preventive strategies based on sexual, behavioral, and cultural practices. Within this period, researchers began to address gender, as well as the social and demographic status of people living with HIV/AIDS. Health education and awareness programs on HIV increased and were targeted toward various strata of the Nigerian society. Several seminar programs on HIV infection and its prevention strategies were organized for public and private sector organizations as well as the general population. Various print media published information on HIV prevention and broadcast media aired reports as well. Billboards on HIV were introduced in different strategic locations across the country. Research efforts also targeted the care of those living with the virus, while palliative care that focused on nutrition and strategies for prompt management of opportunistic infections started to emerge.

During this period, international agencies had severed support for government agencies for HIV research and control programs because of the country's military rule. Most of the capacity development for research and the research programs were supported by international agencies working through

NGOs. In general, meaningful capacities for research were developed within this period but were not sufficient to allow studies on the cutting edge of research.

At the same time, researchers in developed countries had analyzed the genome of the virus, identified biologic markers to track the natural progression of the infection, explored vaccine design issues, developed ARVs, and initiated small treatment trials for the clinical management of HIV infection as well as for various opportunistic infections. These researchers also made progress in developing more sensitive diagnostic techniques based on detection of HIV antigens in clinical samples. Knowledge of the HIV genome prompted several molecular biology studies, opening up new areas of global research and attracting attention to the molecular epidemiology of HIV/AIDS.

Despite the establishment of laboratories with the capacity to detect HIV infection, Nigeria's human and infrastructural resources were not advanced enough to allow molecular biology studies. The newer molecular biology and immunologic techniques required highly trained personnel and sophisticated equipment that was too expensive for resource-poor countries, including Nigeria. At the time, no laboratory in the country had the capacity to conduct the tests needed to monitor the progression of HIV infection, including those aimed at determining viral load and CD4+ cell counts. This situation significantly diminished Nigeria's overall research capacity.

1997–2004

From 1997 to 2004, the level of information on the global HIV/AIDS pandemic rose tremendously, enhancing the efforts of basic, applied, and operational research on the HIV epidemic worldwide. In Nigeria, this period witnessed a significant development of human resources and infrastructural facilities for HIV research. HIV screening and confirmatory tests became available in nearly every part of the country. Several organizations had dramatically enhanced their capacities for improved and sustainable prevention strategies, counseling, and testing, as well as for hospital-, home-, and community-based care for people living with the virus. Issues of the human rights of people living with HIV/AIDS also attracted attention. Several international agencies provided financial and technical support for establishing new laboratories and upgrading existing ones to enhance their capacities for research. Notable among these agencies were the WHO, UNAIDS, UNICEF, the United Nations Population Fund, the Canadian International Development Agency, the Department for International Development, USAID, the Ford Foundation, the Bill & Melinda Gates Foundation, the John D. and Catherine T. MacArthur Foundation, and the David and Lucile Packard Foundation. These organizations not only helped establish laboratories, but they also provided funds and technical support for research in such other areas as social sciences and impact mitigation studies.

The human capacity development for HIV research also grew considerably during this period. Several international organizations and NGOs developed modules for training health care providers. Moreover, a critical mass of clinical and biomedical scientists were trained at both the national and international levels. Several social scientists were also trained in socioeconomic research and human right issues.

The output of research within this period was significant, as investigators generated important in-country data. In 2001, the Ford Foundation established the first national reference laboratory with a full capacity for HIV research at the Nigerian Institute of Medical Research. This laboratory became the first in the country with facilities for estimating viral load and CD4+ cell counts based on automated techniques.

Since then, other organizations, most notably APIN and the USAID, have established HIV research laboratories in several other centers. APIN established laboratory facilities at teaching hospitals in Lagos, Ibadan, Jos, and Maiduguri, as well as at the Military Hospital in Lagos; it also enhanced facilities at the Nigerian Institute of Medical Research in Yaba, Lagos. More recently, the USAID established laboratory facilities at the National Hospital in Abuja and the teaching hospitals in Benin City, Nnewi, Port Harcourt, and Kano.

Most of these centers have trained personnel for determining CD4+ cell counts as well as other immunologic, hematologic, and clinical parameters. With these facilities now equipped, staffed, and functional, scientists have been able to conduct meaningful basic, applied, and operational research on various aspects of HIV/AIDS, generating significant information on the epidemic in Nigeria. Some studies have also been carried out on the molecular epidemiology of the virus and the emergence of circulating recombinant forms of the virus (46–52).

In 2000, the WHO advocated adoption of the second-generation surveillance system, which offers behavioral surveillance surveys alongside sentinel surveillance surveys. With the support of such organizations as Family Health International, the Society for Family Health, and APIN, Nigerian researchers were able to conduct several behavioral science studies at the national level (26). Until 2003, however, it was not possible to carry out the behavioral surveys alongside the sentinel surveys. It is hoped that this capacity will be developed in the near future to implement the second-generation surveillance system more effectively.

Globally, this period also witnessed a major breakthrough in the clinical management of HIV infection. Clinical trials confirmed that ARVs reduced mortality and morbidity among infected people, and several developed countries adopted ARVs in the clinical management of HIV. At first, the ARVs were not readily available in developing countries because of their high costs and the lack of other infrastructural requirements for the proper and effective implementation of ARV treatment programs. Over time, though, less expensive, generic brands of ARVs became available, and developing countries that could afford these cheaper drugs initiated ARV therapy programs.

In 2002, the Federal Government of Nigeria initiated a national ARV treatment program, under which 10,000 adults and 5,000 children living with HIV/AIDS were to be treated. The program is currently being implemented in 25 health centers across the country's six geopolitical zones. At its inception, the relevant clinical and biomedical health personnel were minimally trained on the use of ARVs and the laboratory monitoring tests for the treated patients. Since then, however, several state governments, NGOs, faith-based organizations, and private sector establishments started implementing ARV therapy programs in various health facilities.

Nigeria's immediate challenge during this period was to develop a critical mass of health personnel trained in implementing and sustaining these ARV programs. The biomedical personnel needed to learn the various laboratory techniques to monitor people undergoing treatment. Social scientists had to be trained to provide crucial psychosocial support to the patients during treatment. Despite the urgent need for this training, no adequate training tools, manuals, or modules were available. The immediate need was to develop appropriate training tools, then organize and implement those training programs across the country.

In 2003, APIN provided support for the development of training modules on ARVs for health personnel, including doctors, pharmacists, nurses, counselors, laboratory scientists, and data managers. With these training modules and additional support from the USAID and the Global Fund for AIDS, Tuberculosis and Malaria, several training programs took place in 2003 and 2004. By the end of 2004, 200 doctors, 98 pharmacists, 320 nurses, 270 counselors, and 268 laboratory scientists from more than 50 health facilities had been trained in the proper use of ARVs, the effective management of opportunistic infections, the relevant laboratory techniques for monitoring the outcomes of treatment, and counseling tools to ensure sustainable psychosocial support. These training programs significantly enhanced the participants' knowledge base and aided in developing the human resources for operational research.

As the use of ARVs grew, the need to enhance laboratory facilities to monitor patients on treatment became urgent. By the end of 2004, four government laboratories—the Nigerian Institute of Medical Research, the Jos University Teaching Hospital, the University College Hospital in Ibadan, and the University of Maiduguri Teaching Hospital—had acquired the capacity to test for viral load, as had an NGO-based laboratory, the Gede Foundation. In addition, 20 laboratories had acquired the capacity for automated CD4+ cell counts; 35 acquired the capacity for using manual techniques to estimate CD4+ cell levels. More than a hundred other laboratories enhanced their capacities for hematological, clinical chemistry, and microbiological tests.

Laboratory equipment and reagents were expensive, and the costs of various laboratory tests were high. While the government subsidized the patient costs for drugs under the Nigerian national ARV program, there was no provision for the costs of the laboratory tests. As a result, only the few patients who could afford them were monitored for their response to treatment; most other patients were monitored simply using clinical parameters. Thus, the data were inadequate to facilitate the monitoring and evaluation of the ARV treatment program on a national level. One of the few studies carried out at the institutional level, however, revealed the effectiveness of the national ARV program, as more than 80% of the patients achieved suppression of viral replication and improved immune status within 48 weeks of treatment (59).

The period of 1997 to 2004 also witnessed the launch of several initiatives geared toward boosting Nigeria's national response to the epidemic. Nearly all these initiatives provided for the development of adequate human and infrastructural capacities for HIV/AIDS research. Prominent among these initiatives are the Global Fund for HIV, Tuberculosis and Malaria; the U.S. President's Emergency Plan for AIDS Relief (PEPFAR); APIN; and the UNAIDS 3 by 5 Initiative.

In 2003, the Global Fund provided Nigeria's federal government with substantial grant support to provide ARVs to infected people and to accommodate other logistical support, such as laboratory facilities and services for the ARV programs. The Global Fund initiative has also provided support for establishing tools and other facilities for monitoring ARV resistance. Prior to this, there had been no articulated national study to establish the level of primary and acquired resistance to ARVs. With Global Fund support, however, a team of experts has been able to conduct a national survey on ARV resistance. This project is expected to stimulate the establishment of additional facilities for ARV resistance testing.

Also in 2003, the president of the United States launched PEPFAR, which provides US$15 billion to support HIV/AIDS for five years in 22 developing countries, including Nigeria. In the latter part of 2003, a few stakeholders in the United States were able to access the PEPFAR funds on behalf of Nigeria. These included the Harvard School of Public Health in Boston, the Catholic Relief Services, and the Consortium of USAID, Family Health International, the Institute of Human Virology in Baltimore, and the POLICY Project. With PEPFAR funding until 2009, these stakeholders will expand Nigeria's ARV treatment program to provide free drugs and free laboratory monitoring tests to more than 100,000 HIV patients. These programs are also expected to play a substantial role in strengthening the country's HIV research capacity over the next five years.

In 2004, the Harvard School of Public Health launched the PEPFAR program in six centers: the Nigerian Institute of Medical Research in Lagos; the University Teaching Hospital in Jos; the University College Hospital in Ibadan; the 68 Military Hospital in Lagos; the University Teaching Hospital in Lagos; and the University Teaching Hospital in Maiduguri. Before this program began, the Harvard School of Public Health had, through APIN, carried out various human capacity development programs for personnel working in these centers. In addition, APIN had significantly strengthened laboratory facilities in these centers, including the establishment of facilities for viral load estimation in four centers, automated techniques for CD4+ cell counts in six centers, and automated techniques for hematology and clinical chemistry in five centers.

The Catholic Relief Services, another PEPFAR grant recipient, has established an ARV treatment center in the Faith Alive Hospital in Jos. The third recipient of the PEPFAR grant—the Consortium of USAID, Family Health International, the Institute of Human Virology, and the POLICY Project—has also established ARV treatment centers with laboratory facilities in the following institutions: the University of Benin Teaching Hospital; the University of Calabar Teaching Hospital; the Nnamdi Azikiwe Teaching Hospital in Nnewi; the Aminu Kano University Teaching Hospital in Kano; the National Hospital Abuja; the Lagos State University Teaching Hospital; the General Hospital Broad Street in Lagos; the Mainland Hospital in Yaba, Lagos; and the University of Uyo Teaching Hospital.

These programs have enormously enhanced the research capacities of these centers, enabling them to conduct significant basic, applied, and operational research on HIV/AIDS in Nigeria. The entire system has also set an adequate platform for effective implementation of care and support programs for Nigerians living with HIV/AIDS. Although the UNAIDS 3 by 5 Initiative has yet to be implemented, it will form a significant component of the proposed scaling up plan for the national ARV treatment program in Nigeria.

CONCLUSION

Over the past 18 years, Nigeria's capacity for HIV research has increased remarkably. The level of this capacity still falls short, however, and several factors have been identified as responsible for its limitations. Most significant among these factors is inadequate research funding, which has hampered the ability of research to stay abreast of the evolving epidemic. Today, modern equipment and experienced personnel are needed to implement scientific programs, especially those at the cutting edge. Unfortunately, this equipment is often beyond the reach of the country's meager research funding. For this situation to improve dramatically, the various tiers of government and the organized private sector must contribute substantially to health research funding. This should, by statute, be a major component of the health budgets of the federal and state governments. During the past two decades, in fact, more than 85% of Nigeria's research funding came from developmental partners, foreign organizations, and international NGOs.

It is also imperative that the government and international partners actively implement the training and capacity building of health care workers with a vision toward sustaining such programs for the foreseeable future. Incorporation of such training into medical and nursing schools would exponentially increase the workforce needed for these critical HIV/AIDS prevention and treatment programs.

Research has also been conducted on other barriers for prevention of infection. Notable among these is the development and clinical trials of microbicides. Again, this is an area in which Nigerian scientists have made little contribution to global efforts. Although a small number of microbicide clinical trials are being conducted, much remains to be done to enhance the research capacity for developmental and clinical trials of newer agents for the prevention and care of HIV/AIDS.

As of 2005, several ARV treatment programs are being implemented in health facilities throughout Nigeria. Efforts to monitor the outcome of these programs are minimal, however, because of inadequate human and infrastructural capacities. With the proposed scaling up of these programs, efforts must be made to ensure adequate capacities for the various monitoring tests, especially viral load estimation, CD4+ cell counts, hematology, and clinical chemistry. When ARV therapy programs are improperly implemented, they run the risk of having both treatment failure and the development of resistant viral strains. Nigeria does not yet have a center with adequate capacity for drug resistance testing. As a matter of urgency, Nigeria should ensure that some centers develop the capacity to test for viral drug resistance. The few ARV resistance studies to date have been conducted in collaboration with laboratories in developed countries.

We now recognize that HIV has a great propensity for phenotypic and genotypic variation, resulting in the emergence of several subtypes of HIV-1 and HIV-2, as well as recombinant forms. These subtypes and recombinants are circulating in various locales globally. HIV subtypes may have important implications for disease pathogenesis, virulence, vaccine development, and treatment outcomes. These factors have made it mandatory for countries to monitor the subtypes and recombinant forms circulating in various communities. Unfortunately, Nigeria lacks the facilities and capabilities for HIV subtyping and molecular epidemiologic tracking. The federal government and other stakeholders should therefore ensure the timely development of such centers.

Scientists worldwide are seeking to develop therapeutic and preventive HIV vaccines. Thus far, Nigerian scientists have made only minimal contributions to this area, and although the government has developed an HIV vaccine plan, it has yet to be implemented. The need to develop human and infrastructural capacities in this area has grown urgent, to allow Nigeria to support vaccine development or vaccine trial initiatives. As a leader in West Africa, Nigeria could make a valuable contribution to vaccine development by researching the HIV subtypes predominant in the region: CRF_02/A/G, subtype G, and CRF_06. Further studies of various host and immune determinants of HIV infection would also inform rationale vaccine development, while building the capacity to evaluate immunologic responses to vaccine candidates.

During the past 20 years, Nigeria has progressed in its capacity and need for HIV/AIDS research. Research efforts have helped describe the epidemic and characterize the disease. As prevention and treatment programs have launched, clinical research efforts have determined the efficacy of such programs and will continue to inform their modification and improvement. Vaccine research will continue to play a critical role in the national and international response to HIV/AIDS. Nigeria's ability to capitalize on its benefits for intervention development and evaluation will no doubt contribute to its goal of achieving an evidence-based prevention and control program for HIV.

REFERENCES

1. Adebimpe OI, Tamuno OG. Science, technology, information and documentation. In: Maduemezia A, Okonkwo SNC, Okon EE, eds. *Science Today in Nigeria*. Abuja: Kayinade Nigeria Enterprises, 1995;25–60.

2. Tamuno OG. Availability and accessibility of biomedical information for teaching, research and service in Nigeria. In: *Access to Science and Technology Information in Nigeria*, 1992;17–31.

3. Lucas AO. Research for national health. In: Essien EM, Idigbe EO, Olukoya DK, eds. *International Conference on Health Research Priorities for Nigeria in the 1990s and Strategies for Their Achievement. February 19-21, 1991, Proceedings and Recommendations*. Lagos: Gabumo Press, 1991;19–21.

4. Che-Ho W. 2000 *National Science Council Review*. Taipei: Enyoy Enterprise Co. Ltd., 2001.

5. World Health Organization. *Strategic Health Research Plan, 1999–2003 for the WHO African Region, Zimbabwe*. (AFR/RC48/11). Geneva: World Health Organization, 1999.

6. World Health Organization. *Advisory Committee on Health Research: Report to the Director-General on the 39th Session*. (ACHR39/01.12). Geneva: World Health Organization, 2001.

7. Vallanjon M, ed. *Scaling Up the Response to Infectious Disease: A Way Out of Poverty*. Geneva: World Health Organization, 2002.

8. Alliance for Health Policy and Systems Research. *Strengthening Health Systems: The Role and Promise of Policy and Systems Research*. Geneva: Alliance for Health Policy and Systems Research, 2004.

9. Essex M. The etiology of AIDS. In: Essex M, Mboup S, Kanki PJ, Kalengayi MR, eds. *AIDS in Africa*. New York: Raven Press, 1994;1–20.

10. Rogers MF, Morens DM, Stewart JA, et al. National case-control study of Kaposi's sarcoma and *Pneumocystis carinii* pneumonia in homosexual men: part 2, laboratory results. *Ann Intern Med*, 1983;99:151–158.

11. Barre-Sinoussi F, Chermann JC, Rey F, et al. Isolation of a T-lymphotropic retrovirus from a patient at risk for acquired immune-deficiency syndrome (AIDS). *Science*, 1983;220:868–871.

12. Gallo RC, Salahuddin JC, Popovic M, et al. Frequent detection and isolation of cytopathic retroviruses (HTLV-III) from patients with AIDS and at risk of AIDS. *Science*, 1984;224:500–503.

13. Fauci AS. Basic immunology: the path to the delineation of the immunopathogenic mechanisms of HIV infection. *Trans Assoc Am Physicians*, 1988;101:160–173.

14. Barin F, Mboup S, Denis F. Serological evidence for virus related to simian T-lymphocyte retrovirus III in residents of West Africa. *Lancet*, 1985;ii:1387–1390.

15. Montano M, Williamson C. The molecular virology of HIV. In: Essex M, Mboup S, Kanki, PJ, Marlink RG, Tlou SD, eds. *AIDS in Africa*. 2nd ed. New York: Kluwer Academic Press, 2002.

16. Louwagie J, McCutchan FE, Peeters M, et al. Phylogenetic analysis of gap genes from 70 international HIV-1 isolates provides evidence for multiple genotypes. *AIDS*, 1993;7:769–780.

17. Chen Z, Luckay A, Sodora DL, et al. Human immunodeficiency virus type 2 (HIV-2) seroprevalence and characterization of a distinct HIV-2 genetic subtype from the natural range of simian immunodeficiency virus-infected sooty mangabeys. *J Virol*, 1997;71(5):3953–3960.

18. Steckelberg JM, Cockerill F, Cockerill FR. Update: serologic testing for antibody to human immunodeficiency virus. *MMWR*, 1988;36:833–840.

19. Pitchenik AE, Rubinston HA. The radiographic appearance of tuberculosis in patients with acquired immune deficiency syndrome (AIDS) and pre-AIDS. *Am Rev Respir Dis*, 1985;131:393–396.

20. Levine AM. Reactive and neoplastic lymphoproliferative disorders with HIV infection. In: Devita VT, Hellman S, Rosenberg SA, eds. *AIDS: Etiology, Diagnosis, Treatment and Prevention*. Philadelphia: Lippincott, 1988;263–275.

21. Fischl MA, Richman DD, Grieco MH, et al. The efficacy of AZT in the treatment of patients with AIDS and AIDS-related complex. *N Engl J Med*, 1987;317:185–191.

22. Becker MH. AIDS and behavior change. *Public Health Rev*, 1988;16(1-2):1–11.

23. National Commission on AIDS. *Behavioral and Social Sciences and the HIV/AIDS Epidemic*. Washington, DC: National Commission on AIDS, 1993.

24. O'Reilly KR, Piot P. International perspectives on individual and community approaches to the prevention of sexually transmitted diseases and human immunodeficiency virus infection. *J Infect Dis*, 1996; 174:S214–S222.

25. Nasidi A, Harry TO, Ajose-Coker OO, et al. Evidence of LAV/HTLV III infection and AIDS related complex in Lagos, Nigeria. *II International Conference on AIDS*, Paris, France, June 23–25, 1986 (abstract FR86-3).

26. Federal Ministry of Health. *2003 National HIV Seroprevalence Sentinel Survey in Nigeria*. Abuja: Federal Ministry of Health, 2003.

27. UNAIDS. *2004 Report on the Global AIDS Epidemic*. 4th Ed. (UNAIDS/04.16E). Geneva: UNAIDS, 2004.

28. Okpara RA, Akinsete I, Williams EE, et al. Antibodies to human immunodeficiency virus (HTLV-III/LAV) in people from Lagos and Cross River States of Nigeria. *Acta Haematol*, 1988;79:15–18.

29. Ezefili E, Williams E, Akinsete I. AIDS awareness and sexual experience among secondary and tertiary female students in Lagos, Nigeria. *V International Conference on AIDS in Africa*, October 10–12, 1990, Kinshasa, Zaire (abstract 90).

30. Idigbe EO, Ibrahim MM, Ubuane TA, et al., eds. *HIV/AIDS in Nigeria: Bibliography Report*. Lagos: Niyi Faniran Enterprises, 2000.

31. Idigbe EO, Harry TO, Ekong EE, Audu RA, Musa AZ, Funsho-Adebayo EO, eds. *Nigerian Contributions to Regional and Global Meetings on HIV/AIDS/STIs: 1986–2003*. Lagos: Niyi Faniran Enterprises, 2003.

32. World Health Organization. *Workshop on AIDS in Central Africa. Bangui, Central African Republic*. WHO/CDS/SIDA/85-1. Geneva: World Health Organization, October 22–24, 1985.

33. Centers for Disease Control. Mortality attributable to HIV infection/AIDS — United States, 1981–1990. *MMWR*, 1991;40:41–44.

34. Chikwem JO, Mohammed I, Oyebode-Ola T, et al. Prevalence of human immunodeficiency virus (HIV) infection in Borno State of Nigeria. *East Afr Med J*, 1988;65(5):342–346.

35. Harry TO, Nasidi A, Mohammed I. Unexplained immunoblot patterns seen in Nigeria: evidence of HIV-2 related virus infecting humans. *X International Conference on AIDS and Associated Cancers in Africa*, October 18–20 1989, Marseille, France (abstract 098).

36. Williams EE, Mohammed I, Chukwem JO, et al. HIV-1 and HIV-2 antibodies in Nigerian populations with high and low risk behaviour patterns. *AIDS*, 1990;4(10):1041–1042.

37. Chikwem JO, Mohammed I, Bwala HG, et al. Human immunodeficiency virus (HIV) infection in patients attending a sexually transmitted diseases clinic in Borno State of Nigeria. *Trop Geogr Med*, 1990;42: 17–22.

38. Ogunwande SA. The prevalence of oral ailments that are common in HIV infection in a Nigerian dental practice. *J Acquir Immune Defic Syndr*, 1990;3(11): 1117–1118.

39. Olusanya O, Lawoko A, Blomberg J. Seroepidemiology of human retroviruses in Ogun State of Nigeria. *Scand J Infect Dis*, 1990;22(2):155–160.

40. Dada AJ, Ajayi J, Ransome-Kuti O, et al. Prevalence survey of HIV-1 and HIV-2 infections in female prostitutes in Lagos State, Nigeria. *VII International Conference on AIDS*, June 16–21, 1991, Florence, Italy (abstract T91).

41. Nasidi A, Wali S, Onafalujo MO, et al. HIV infection in polygamous families in Nigeria. *IV International Conference in AIDS and Associated Cancers in Africa*, October 18–20 1989, Marseille, France (abstract 089).

42. Ademuwagen ZA. AIDS in Nigeria: socio-cultural and behavioural research components of AIDS prevention and control programme. *VI International Conference on AIDS in Africa*, December 16–19, 1991, Dakar, Senegal (abstract 913).

43. Chikwem JO, Ola TO, Gashau W, et al. Impact of health education on prostitutes' awareness and attitudes to AIDS. *J Public Health*, 1988;102:18–21.

44. Obi CL, Ogbonna BA, Igumbor EO, et al. HIV seropositivity among female prostitutes and non-prostitutes: obstetric and perinatal implications. *Viral Immunol*, 1993;6(3):171–174.

45. Nnatu SN, Anyiwo CE, Obi CL, et al. Prevalence of human immunodeficiency virus (HIV) antibody among apparently healthy pregnant women in Nigeria. *Int J Gynaecol Obstet*, 1993;40(2):105–107.

46. Adebajo AO, Smith DJ, Hazleman BL, et al. Sero-epidemiological associations between tuberculosis, malaria, hepatitis B and AIDS in West Africa. *J Med Virol*, 1994;42:366–368.

47. Harry TO, Kyari O, Mohammed I. Prevalence of human immunodeficiency virus infection among pregnant women attending ante-natal clinic in Maiduguri, north-eastern Nigeria. *Trop Geogr Med*, 1992;44:238–241.

48. Idigbe EO, Nasidi A, Anyiwo CE, et al. Prevalence of human immunodeficiency virus (HIV) antibodies in tuberculosis patients in Lagos, Nigeria. *J Trop Med Hyg*, 1994;97:91–97.

49. Idigbe EO, Nasidi A, John EKO, et al. Profile of respiratory opportunistic diseases associated with HIV infections in Lagos, Nigeria. *Biomedical Letters*, 1995;51:247–260.

50. Salako LA, Idigbe EO, Erinosho MA, et al. Malaria and human immunodeficiency virus (HIV) infections among adults in Ogun State, South-Western Nigeria. *Nigerian Q J Hosp Med*, 1996;6(4):279–283.

51. Idigbe EO, Nasidi A, Sofola T, et al. Pulmonary tuberculosis and HIV infections among prison inmates in Lagos, Nigeria. *Nigerian J Med Res*, 1997;1(2):17–21.

52. Akenami Fo, Koskiniemi M, Ekanem EE, et al. Seroprevalence and co-prevalence of HIV and HBsAg in Nigerian children with/without protein energy malnutrition. *Acta Trop*, 1997;64(4):167–174.

53. Dada AJ, Oyewole F, Onofowokan R, et al. Demographic characteristics of retroviral infections (HIV-1, HIV-2 and HTLV-1) among female professional sex workers in Lagos, Nigeria. *J Acquir Immune Defic Syndr*, 1993;1358–1363.

54. Kline Rl, Dada A, Blattner W, et al. Diagnosis and differentiation of HIV-1 and HIV-2 infections by two rapid assays in Nigeria. *J Acquir Immune Defic Syndr*, 1994;7:12–16.

55. Olaleye DD, Bernstein L, Sheng Z, et al. Type-specific immune response to human T-cell lymphotropic virus (HTLV) type 1 and type 11 infections in Nigeria. *Am J Trop Med Hyg*, 1994;50:7–11.

56. Olaleye DD, Sheng Z, Howard TM, et al. Isolation and characterization of a new subtype. A variant of human immunodeficiency virus type 1 from Nigeria. *J Trop Med Int Health*, 1996;1:10–15.

57. Howard TM, Rasheed S. Genomic structure and nucleotide sequence analysis of a new HIV type 1 subtype A strain from Nigeria. *AIDS Res*, 1996;12:18–21.

58. Akpede OO, Ambe JP, Rabasa AI, et al. Presentation and outcome of HIV-1 infection in hospitalized infants and other children in North-Eastern Nigeria. *East Afr Med J*, 1997;74(1):21–27.

59. Idigbe EO, Adewole TA, Eisen G, et al. Management of HIV-1 infection with a combination of nevirapine, stavudine and lamivudine: a preliminary report on the Nigeria ARV Program. *J Acquir Immune Defic Syndr*, 2005;40(1):65–69.

60. Howard TM, Olaleye DO, Rasheed S. Sequence analysis of the glycoprotein 120 coding region of a new HIV type 1 subtype A strain (HIV-11bNg) from Nigeria. *AIDS Res Hum Retroviruses*, 1994;10:1755–1757.

61. Abimiku AG, Stern TL, Zwandor A, et al. Subgroup G HIV-type 1 isolates in Nigeria. *AIDS Res Hum Retroviruses*, 1995;10:1581–1583.

62. McCutchan FE, Carr JK, Bajani M, et al. Subtype G and multiple forms of A/G intersubtype recombinant human immunodeficiency virus type 1 in Nigeria. *Virology*, 1999;254:226–234.

63. Peeters M, Esu-Williams E, Vergne L, et al. Pre-dominance of subtype A and G HIV type 1 in Nigeria with geographical differences in their distribution. *AIDS Res Hum Retroviruses*, 2000;16(4):315–325.

64. Agwale SM, Robbins KE, Odama L, et al. Development of an env gp41-based heteroduplex mobility assay for rapid human immunodeficiency virus type 1 subtyping. *J Clin Microbiol*, 2001;39:2110–2114.

65. Vicente AC, Agwale SM, Otsuki K, et al. Genetic variability of HIV-1 protease from Nigeria and correlation with protease inhibitors drug resistance. *Virus Genes*, 2001;22(2):181–186.

66. Agwale SM, Zeh C, Robbins KE, et al. Molecular surveillance of HIV-1 field strains in Nigeria in preparation for vaccine trials. *Vaccine*, 2002;20(16):2131–2139.

III

FUTURE POLICIES AND STRATEGIES

From the Trenches

AT FIRST DR. SUNDAY PAM REFUSED; HE couldn't possibly start a clinic for HIV-infected children. He lacked the staff, the funding, the time. But even as he was explaining to his department chairman the pressures on his overburdened neonatology practice, already he knew the practical would yield to the idealistic. Already he knew he would find a way to achieve the impossible. ■ For years the parents of Dr. Pam's newborn patients had entreated

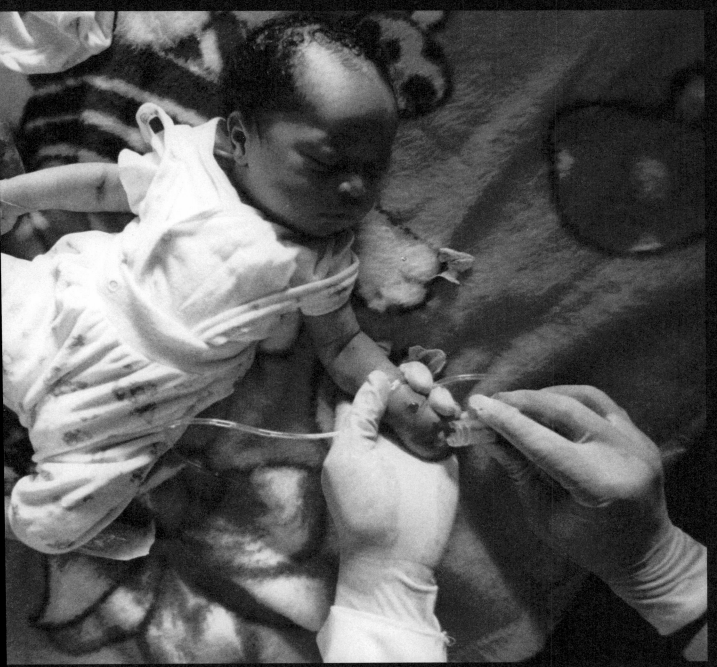

Many HIV-infected infants in Africa die within their first year of life.

him to care for their infected children. The adults were receiving care at an HIV/AIDS clinic that Professor John Idoko had been running at Jos University Teaching Hospital since 1997; the clinic has since evolved into an APIN Plus/Harvard PEPFAR clinic. But no organized care services existed for children living with HIV in Jos. Diagnoses were difficult to come by and support services were nonexistent.

"To start the clinic, first I enlarged my team by recruiting other pediatricians and nurses," Dr. Pam says. "I had to explain that this new component of our clinic would not be grant supported, and we would be undertaking those extra hours without pay. My colleagues all remained enthusiastic and, with tremendous support from the APIN leadership in Jos, we launched the Pediatric Infectious Diseases Clinic."

Dr. Pam deliberately avoiding using "HIV" or "AIDS" in the clinic's name. "We figured that if we labeled it 'AIDS,' " he says, "parents might keep their children away for fear of stigmatization."

The clinic opened in May 2002 with limited hours. A year later a dedicated full-day clinic was instituted, and more recently the clinical team supplemented those hours with an additional afternoon to accommodate the expanded patient load. The clinic now has two wings, one for HIV-exposed infant follow-up and another for antiretroviral treatment. Nearly 400 babies are registered in the first wing and more than 200 HIV-infected children are enrolled in the second.

"When we first began seeing HIV-infected children, our biggest challenge was in providing them with antiretrovirals," Dr. Pam says. "The federal program subsidized the drugs for adults, who would pay 1,000 naira—about eight U.S. dollars—a month. But subsidized antiretrovirals were not available for pediatric patients. Even when parents could obtain antiretrovirals for their children, the drugs cost as much as a hundred dollars a month."

Such a high expense can lead parents to compromise a child's adherence to the antiretroviral regimen, and such lapses allow viral resistance to develop, Dr. Pam adds.

"Some parents, in the hope of getting price breaks, went to pharmaceutical representatives directly and stopped bringing their children to our clinic. I suspect many of those children already have developed resistance, and I know many have died."

Dr. Pam remains haunted by the children whom he could not save when the program first began. He recalls in particular one eight-year-old girl with a beautiful smile, "Dije," who had contracted the virus several years earlier from a blood transfusion. She had developed not only the characteristic lesions of Kaposi's sarcoma, but symptoms of tuberculosis as well. With her CD4$^+$ count plummeting, Dije needed immediate antiretroviral therapy. But her mother could not afford the drugs.

"The child was deteriorating daily, and we desperately tried everything we could to get her the antiretrovirals," Dr. Pam recalls. "Finally, her mother was able to raise some money and buy the drugs. But this shy, intelligent girl received the medication for only two weeks before she died. We all felt devastated."

The situation has since improved dramatically, Dr. Pam says. "One major change is that the federal government has begun subsidizing antiretrovirals for children. And now, through the Pediatric Clinical Care Program, which started in the fall of 2005, the government is providing the drugs and the APIN Plus/Harvard PEPFAR program is providing the care and monitoring."

Dr. Pam can now take inspiration from the transformation of his patients. After just two months of antiretroviral therapy, eight-year-old "Tik" saw her viral load drop to an undetectable level. "I was so excited," Dr. Pam says, "because it confirmed that achieving undetectable viral loads in Nigerian kids was indeed possible. This is a good sign of adherence to therapy and it gives credibility to the work of our team."

19

INFLUENCING HIV/AIDS POLICIES AND PROGRAMS THROUGH A PARTICIPATORY PROCESS

Iyabo Obasanjo* and Modupe D. Oduwole†

In most African nations, the commitment of the leadership to all aspects of HIV/AIDS prevention and management has been crucial to the success of intervention programs (1). In countries in which the HIV epidemic has taken hold and surpassed the 5% prevalence rate, a lack of political will has been a major contributory factor. With an estimated 5% prevalence rate, Nigeria is on the cusp of either controlling its epidemic—and even reversing its HIV rate—as Uganda and Tanzania succeeded in doing, or having the rate exceed 20%, as has occurred in South Africa and Botswana. Political will and action are critical ingredients in any country's battle against the epidemic, and Nigeria is no exception.

This chapter discusses the processes in policy formulation, with analysis of the processes undertaken to produce HIV/AIDS policy instruments used in implementing the national response to the epidemic in Nigeria. A number of key considerations will be explored. Who, for example, were the actors? What were the power relationships and the extent of the exchange involved in the processes? Was policy formulation by fiat or consultative? Were documents prepared by experts for review or based on workshops? Did the policy go through a state review process? And how were people living with HIV/AIDS (PLWHAs) involved? Case studies on two Nigerian HIV/AIDS policy and

*Ministry of Health, Ogun State, Abeokuta, Nigeria
†Ogun State AIDS Control Program, Abeokuta, Nigeria

program documents will highlight principal lessons learned about the influence of stakeholder involvement in the formulation and implementation of policies and programs in Nigeria.

THE POLICY PROCESS: THEORETICAL CONSIDERATIONS

Policies are created through a process of problem identification, analysis, and solution that involves a wide spectrum of stakeholders (2). Participatory policy development is a process that enables those experiencing the particular problem for which the policies are being developed to be more directly involved in designing policy at each different stage (2,3). This wider involvement improves the odds that weaknesses will be identified and rectified before implementation and that the policies will therefore be more effective. In addition the process leads to greater accountability through direct engagement as well as through greater understanding (4).

Policy is not shaped simply on the basis of "good" research or information, nor does it emerge simply from bargaining among actors on clearly defined options. Rather, it is a more complex process through which particular considerations come to frame what matters and which voices count in policy deliberations in particular political and institutional contexts (5). Making sense of participation in policy processes requires an analysis of ways in which power and knowledge define policy spaces for engagement, privileging certain voices and excluding others (6).

The sheer complexity of the webs of actors engaged in policy processes, whose connections and interactions weave across and within the artificial divide between "citizens" and "state," make the process of understanding the nature of policy change in the context of stakeholders involvement so much more complicated. Different actors within the state as within civil society may take up a range of subject positions and represent a constellation of competing interests (7). It therefore follows that the process of policy making involves interactions between complex constellation of actors with conflicting interests and negotiating in policy arenas that are often conceptualized as policy spaces (8).

Policy spaces are moments in which interventions or events throw up opportunities, reconfiguring relationships between actors within these spaces or bringing in new actors and opening up possibilities for a shift in direction (9). Opportunities provided within these spaces allow for negotiations and consensus building to accommodate diverse views and interests.

THE NIGERIAN CONTEXT

The Structure

Nigeria follows a three-tier presidential system of governance, with a president elected every four years heading the federal government in Abuja, the capital. Elected along with the president are 109 members of the Senate and 363 members of the House of Representatives. The president appoints ministers, advisers, and others to assist in the administration of different sectors. The health minister is charged with primary oversight of HIV/AIDS.

Nigeria is a federation of 36 states, each with an elected governor and house of assembly, whose number varies by state. The governors appoint commissioners and advisers for different sectors. The health commissioner is charged with primary oversight of HIV/AIDS. Each of the 774 local government areas has an elected chairman who appoints supervisors. The health supervisor is charged with primary oversight of HIV/AIDS.

The Nigerian government, like most others, is responsible for establishing policies to govern the country's HIV/AIDS programs and services. Policy development is not simply a technical issue but is also one of governance, requiring the accommodation of varying interests with the ultimate purpose of the common good. This process can be either through fiat or by consultation.

The federal government policy on tackling the HIV/AIDS epidemic is to fight the disease multisectorally with the health sector as the arrowhead. Under the charge of the president, the National Action Committee on AIDS (NACA) creates and directs government policy on all aspects of HIV/AIDS, from prevention, to treatment, to ethical issues. Each state has a multisectoral state action committee on AIDS (SACA) whose membership derives from several line ministries other than health, and each local government is supposed to have a local action committee on AIDS (LACA).

In general, Nigeria has had a fluctuating experience in its HIV/AIDS response. Following the restoration of democratic rule in 1999, political commitment increased and the federal response to the epidemic changed dramatically (10–12). The critical shift in the national response followed the more coordinated manner in which all the relevant actors were involved, resulting in a truly multisectoral intervention. Line ministries, international agencies, civil society organizations, the UN Expanded Theme Groups, partnership forums, inter-faith forums, and youth forums were some of the various interest groups involved in the conceptualization, development, implementation, and assessment of these programs under NACA's coordination (11).

This was the setting under which the HIV/AIDS Emergency Action Plan, or HEAP, was produced. The implementation of HEAP witnessed an increase in coordinated HIV/AIDS activities in the country with networks formed for civil society organizations, PLWHAs, and other interested stakeholders, such as government agencies and researchers (11,12).

One immediate gain of the desire for a truly multisectoral response to the epidemic has been the involvement of a broad-based network of stakeholders in policy processes. Typically these processes have involved production of several drafts that were critically reviewed by different stakeholders through consultative processes often at national and subnational levels (12–14). There has been concern, however, about how truly representative the actors in the policy formulation processes have been and how much feedback they receive from their constituencies. The ineffective communication of policies from the federal to the lower levels of government and the agencies that are charged with implementing those policies has been cited as a shortcoming needing remedial action (15). Experts believe that extensive consultations with stakeholders have helped improve the quality of most of the documents now guiding Nigeria's response to the HIV/AIDS epidemic (10–12).

The degree of constructive engagements involving all stakeholders demonstrated in the development of the various HIV/AIDS policy documents in Nigeria will be expected over time to lead to more effective and results-driven programs. This is because all the interests will be expected to have been taken into account in the development of these tools and a sense of ownership will allow for critical appraisal at the different stages of implementation. We will await the evaluation of these policy instruments to be certain of the value of stakeholder participation in the effectiveness of these policies and programs.

Policy Milestones

During the late 1980s, HIV/AIDS was globally regarded as a purely health issue. The government agency responsible in Nigeria for coordinating HIV/AIDS and drafting policies was the Federal Ministry of Health (FMOH), which drafted the first national policy on HIV/AIDS. That period also witnessed a predictably low response to the epidemic partly because of the cynicism of most stakeholders and partly because of the basic denial about the problem and the enormous stigmatization and discrimination associated with the epidemic.

The period from 1993 to 1999 marked the emergence of strong and credible nongovernmental organizations (NGOs) in HIV prevention programs. Among other accomplishments, these NGOs widened the policy space by engaging in intense advocacy and agenda setting in the policy and program arenas. These organizations included Family Health International (FHI) and other NGOs supported by the British Department for International Development (DFID) (12).

Since 1999 HIV/AIDS has been recognized globally as a development issue needing a multisectoral response. In Nigeria, the roles of coordinating the national response and facilitating policy development processes shifted to NACA, which has since taken over these functions. Also during this era the faith-based community and PLWHA networks emerged as important actors. A stronger attention was also paid to networking and coalition building among NGOs, and many programs started with a particular focus on vulnerable populations such as members of the armed forces and men who have sex with men (16).

The foregoing discussion of national contexts and institutions reveals a steady increase in an enabling environment and adequate policy space for enhanced participatory policy processes. Anecdotal evidence will suggest that these have positively influenced HIV/AIDS policies and programs in Nigeria (11,12,16). As stated earlier, a controlled evaluation of these policies in the future will be more affirmative of these early impressions.

STRATEGIES FOR INFLUENCING POLICIES AND PROGRAMS

The forces driving the HIV/AIDS epidemic require all players, all stakeholders, and those even remotely affected by the epidemic to participate in the development of policies, planning, and implementation of HIV/AIDS prevention and care programs. Three main activities converge to produce changes in policies and programs: identifying the problem; finding solutions using a participatory approach; and providing advocacy to decision makers and those who influence them—the primary and secondary audiences. The systematic involvement of community members and structures is crucial to the success of the policy formulation process and the implementation of policies and programs.

Community involvement in HIV/AIDS programs is a process by which partnership is established between government or developmental partners and local communities in the planning, implementation, and use of HIV prevention and care activities in order to benefit from increased local self-reliance and social control of these services. This definition suggests that countries should not only provide resources when possible, but also contribute intellectually and participate in decision-making.

Community participation means involving people in as many decisions as they can handle, recognizing that some communities may be more ready and able to become involved than others. As a result of increased access to information and a greater degree of politicization, urban communities are in a better position to become involved than rural communities.

A number of time-tested and effective ways of involving community members in the process of policy formulation and program implementation have been identified. These methods are variously called participatory learning and action, participatory rural appraisal, participatory action research, and rapid rural appraisal. Program managers in many government agencies and NGOs are finding it more and more useful and effective to carry out investigations using local community members to collect information and conduct analyses to determine their own problems (17).

NIGERIA'S HIV/AIDS POLICY INSTRUMENTS

Policy instruments are essential for guiding a country's response to the HIV/AIDS epidemic. They not only express the government's commitment and priorities, but they also set the framework for an effective and coordinated response to the epidemic. In Nigeria, these instruments include national policies, strategic plans, and technical guidelines.

National Policies
In 1997, the government of Nigeria, through the Federal Ministry of Health, adopted the first national HIV/AIDS policy. In recognition of the dynamic nature of the epidemic and control strategies, NACA launched the second policy in 2003. The revised national policy both acknowledges the importance of a multisectoral approach to the control of HIV/AIDS and emphasizes the responsibility that all Nigerians must accept for the care and support of those infected with and affected by the virus (12).

Strategic Plans
Nigeria's first strategic plan, HEAP, covered a three-year timeframe, from 2001 to 2004, with a focus on three major areas: removal of sociocultural, informational, and systematic barriers to community-based responses; prevention; and care and support. When HEAP expired, NACA took the opportunity to review the national HIV/AIDS response and to develop a new strategic framework. In operation from 2005 to 2009, the National HIV/AIDS Strategic Framework is expected to benefit from the lessons learned in the implementation of HEAP for a better results-based operational plan.

Technical Guidelines

Several technical policies and guidelines also exist. The Federal Ministry of Health is responsible for providing technical leadership for the health-related response and developing policies and guidelines. This covers program components ranging from prevention, care, and support to treatment and includes policies and guidelines for voluntary counseling and testing, antiretroviral therapy, and prevention of mother-to-child transmission. NACA also coordinated the development of a strategy document for behavior change communication (BCC).

The development of these policy instruments was participatory, with different actors well represented. This broad representation has also become obvious in the implementation of the various guidelines, as different stakeholders, particularly PLWHAs, have participated as members of the various task teams for such interventions as prevention of mother-to-child transmission. As these programs progress, it is expected that evaluating them will reveal causal relationships between stakeholder involvement and positive outcomes.

POLICY FORMULATION PROCESS: THE NIGERIAN EXPERIENCE

Over the years, the process of developing HIV/AIDS policies in Nigeria has followed several stages, from the start-up phase to the consensus-building, preparation, drafting and review, ratification, and dissemination phases.

The Start-Up Phase

The development of policy and strategic plan on HIV/AIDS in Nigeria has usually been initiated by government in response to civil society, donors, development partners, and changes in the global response.

The Consensus-Building Phase

Nigeria's federal government leads the formulation process from the planning stages all the way through to the ratification stage. However, it recognizes that no single agency or civil society can respond to all aspects of the HIV epidemic by itself. It becomes important, therefore, for all players to come together to develop and agree on envisaged national policy instruments. In developing these policies, the government has partnered with a broad range of stakeholders, including government agencies at all levels, civil society organizations, PLWHA organizations, development partners, and donor agencies. This coordination has been achieved by seeking technical assistance from development partners with expertise in policy development. The USAID-funded POLICY Project has being the lead agency supporting the government of Nigeria in this regard, while UNAIDS provided lead support for the development of the National HIV/AIDS Strategic Framework (11,12).

To foster collaboration, a policy or planning committee and sub-committees are set up under the leadership of NACA. The broad range of stakeholders has included representatives from federal and state ministries of health, education, labor, defense, information, youth, women, and sports as well as the planning commission. Universities, research institutions, tertiary hospitals, and the private sector have been involved, as have donor communities, including the World Bank, USAID, and DFID. Development partners have included UNICEF, WHO, and the AIDS Prevention Initiative in Nigeria. The civil society sector has been represented by the Civil Society Consultative Group on HIV/AIDS in Nigeria, other NGOs, community-based organizations, women's groups, faith-based organizations, and youth groups. Representation of PLWHAs has been through support groups and the Network of People Living with HIV/AIDS in Nigeria (NEPWHAN).

Although challenging, this multisectoral approach has been fruitful and promoted ownership of the process. It has also enabled input from the different constituencies with negotiated trade-offs as necessary. With the new impetus by NACA to involve all actors even in implementation, programs are expected to become even more effective in addressing the needs of people infected with or affected by HIV.

The Preparation Phase

Preparing for policy development requires a broad-based participatory process, including a situation and response analysis. The strategies employed include rapid assessment, program review, and independent consultations with input from all stakeholders. Similar programs from other countries are also usually reviewed at this stage and then preliminary concept papers are circulated to all stakeholders in preparation for the drafting and review process (11,12,18,19).

The Drafting and Review Phase

This stage of the development process usually involves working as sub-committees for the respective components and issues. At this stage stakeholders are able to influence the content of the policies and negotiate and reach consensus on contentious issues. The draft is presented at several workshops and stakeholders are able to debate and agree on issues. The consultations at this level usually involve organizing zonal workshops at which views from different zones are received and deliberated upon. This is particularly crucial in a country like Nigeria, which has considerable religious and cultural diversity. Views and feedback are then collated and amendments are made as appropriate (12,15).

The Ratification Phase

At the national level, a final draft document is presented to the chairperson of NACA for any amendment. The chairperson then presents the final document to the president for endorsement. At the sectoral level, however, the sponsoring minister presents the final document to the Federal Executive Council for amendment and ratification for dissemination and use.

The Dissemination Phase

Different mechanisms are employed in disseminating new policy instruments. They are either presented nationally or at subnational levels depending on logistical convenience. The media play significant roles in ensuring that key messages are disseminated. Web-based disseminations are also becoming important channels for getting policy documents to the target audiences.

CASE STUDIES

Two documents—the National HIV/AIDS Behavior Change Communication Strategy (2004–2008) and the National HIV/AIDS Strategic Framework (2005–2009)—illustrate the processes through which the development of some HIV/AIDS policy instruments have passed in Nigeria. Lessons derived from these analyses will likely apply to most other policy tools, since NACA coordinated the formulation of these tools and applied the same methodologies.

The National HIV/AIDS Behavior Change Communication Strategy

Prior to 2003, BCC actors and activities had no defined coordination framework and little quality control regarding BCC messages (13). This need for coordination and quality control provided the impetus for the development of Nigeria's National HIV/AIDS Behavior Change Communication Strategy.

As NACA coordinated the development process, it involved various stakeholders, including government institutions, national and international NGOs, national and international BCC experts, NEPWHAN members, and international development agencies (15).

Activities undertaken to develop the strategic framework included:

- A review of best practices from across Africa in HIV/AIDS prevention, care, and support to identify successful, innovative, and evidence-based practices;
- A review of existing national data on epidemiology of HIV/AIDS in Nigeria;
- A review of past, current, and future HIV/AIDS activity plans and materials collated from diverse stakeholders; and
- Consensus building about the priority audiences and approaches as well as roles and responsibilities of all stakeholders.

The document eventually developed was the product of an extensive and detailed participatory process involving stakeholders from the BCC field. Many groups and individuals contributed to this process, particularly during the three workshops between February and November 2003, where the strategy was developed, reviewed, and finalized.

This document was also widely disseminated and it is thus hoped that it will meet the expectation of empowering all stakeholders to coordinate comprehensive, audience-responsive, and culturally appropriate BCC programs as important strategies for HIV/AIDS control in Nigeria.

The participatory process for this framework also extends to the implementation phase. Its operational framework corresponds with the existing structure for HIV/AIDS control activities in Nigeria, enabling many actors to work simultaneously in their areas of comparative advantage in a decentralized manner. The long-term success of BCC programs needs community involvement and ownership, a notion confirmed during the participatory approach adopted in the development of this framework. If all confounding variables could be held constant, the participatory process would likely result in effective programs.

Table 19-1. Activity Timeline for the Development of the National HIV/AIDS Strategic Framework (2005–2009)	
Timeframe	**Steps**
August to November 2004	Request for information for the national response review from stakeholders
November to December 2004	Desk review
December 2004	Technical working groups of eight thematic groups with 20 to 25 members per group covering all stakeholders
January to February 2005	Fact-finding visits to states
January to February 2005	First draft of the framework written
January to February 2005	Wide dissemination of first draft to stakeholders
February 2005	Constituent consultative entities review first draft and incorporate comments
March 2005	Second draft of the framework written
March to April 2005	Wide dissemination of second draft among stakeholders and collation of comments
April 2005	Incorporation of final comments
April 17, 2005	Final draft of the framework completed

The National HIV/AIDS Strategic Framework

A coordinating committee made up of NACA members, federal ministry representatives, and development partners served as the consultative group for developing the National HIV/AIDS Strategic Framework. These experts solicited the support of relevant stakeholders to help ensure the success of the policy development.

Working with consultants to collate views obtained through field visits to the states, two consultative processes — involving about 200 members of the technical thematic working groups and more than 150 members of constituent-coordinating entities — provided feedback, strengthening the final draft of the strategic framework (12). Table 19-1 details the activity timeline adopted for these processes.

Many actors were involved at different stages of developing the strategic framework, and adequate policy space was created, allowing constructive engagements and consensus building. The process of policy development was always consultative, and though experts were engaged in these processes, they usually acted only as facilitators at workshops and consensus-building meetings. NEPWHAN members, for example, were major actors and have continued to make significant contributions, not only to the design and production of policy documents, but to their implementation as well.

CONCLUSION

Studies have provided ample evidence that broad-based stakeholder participation in policy design and implementation leads to increased effectiveness of programs (20–22). As Nigeria responds to the HIV/AIDS epidemic with the help of its various policy instruments, it will need robust evaluations at the expiry of its frameworks to assess accomplishments and compare outcomes with particular attention to the contributions of the participatory process.

REFERENCES

1. UNAIDS. *Acting Early to Prevent AIDS: The Case of Senegal.* UNAIDS Best Practice Collection. Geneva: UNAIDS, 1999.

2. Brock K, Cornwall A, Gaventa J. *Power, Knowledge and Political Spaces in Framing of Poverty Policy.* IDS Working Paper 143. Brighton, United Kingdom: Institute of Development Studies, 2001.

3. McGee R, Brock K. *From Poverty Assessment to Policy Change: Processes, Actors and Data.* IDS Working Paper 133. Brighton, United Kingdom: Institute of Development Studies, 2001.

4. UK Poverty Programme. *Participatory Policy Development.* Oxford, United Kingdom: Oxfam GB, 2004.

5. Cornwall A. *Beneficiary, Consumer, Citizen: Perspectives on Participation for Poverty Reduction.* Stockholm: Swedish International Development Cooperation Agency, 2001.

6. Holland J, Blackburn J, eds. *Whose Voices? Participatory Research and Policy Change.* London: Intermediate Technology Publications, 1998.

7. Norton A, Bird B, Brock K, Kakande M, Turk C. *A Rough Guide to PPAs: Participatory Poverty Assessment: An Introduction to Theory and Practice.* London: Department for International Development, 2001.

8. Brock K, McGee R, Ssewakiryanga R. *Poverty, Knowledge and Policy Processes: A Case Study of Ugandan National Poverty Reduction Policy.* IDS Research Report 53. Brighton, United Kingdom: Institute of Development Studies, 2002.

9. Grindle M, Thomas J. *Public Choices and Policy Change.* Baltimore: John Hopkins University Press, 1991.

10. Federal Ministry of Health. *HIV/AIDS Emergency Action Plan.* Abuja: Federal Ministry of Health, 2001.

11. National Action Committee on AIDS. *Nigeria National HIV/AIDS Response Review: 2001–2004.* Abuja: National Action Committee on AIDS, 2005.

12. National Action Committee on AIDS. *National HIV/AIDS Strategic Framework.* Abuja: National Action Committee on AIDS, 2005.

13. National Action Committee on AIDS. *National HIV/AIDS Behavior Change Communication Strategy.* Abuja: National Action Committee on AIDS, 2004.

14. Federal Government of Nigeria. *National Policy on HIV/AIDS.* Abuja: Federal Government of Nigeria, 2003.

15. Federal Government of Nigeria. *Report of the National Evaluation Committee on HIV/AIDS on the National Response to the Medium Term Plan II (1993–1997).* Abuja: Federal Government of Nigeria, 2000.

16. Touray KS. *Mapping of Support Groups for People Living with HIV/AIDS in Nigeria: National Report.* Abuja: National Action Committee on AIDS, 2005.

17. Sharma RR. *An Introduction to Advocacy: Training Guide.* Washington, DC: Health and Human Resources Analysis for Africa, USAID, 1997.

18. Partners for Health, Reformplus Project/Abt Associates Inc., DELIVER/John Snow, Inc., POLICY Project/Futures Group. *Nigeria: Rapid Assessment of HIV/AIDS Care in the Public and Private Sectors.* Bethesda, Maryland: Partners for Health. Reformplus Project and Abt Associates Inc., 2004.

19. ActionAid, Nigeria. *Mapping Civil Society's Involvement in HIV/AIDS Programs in Nigeria.* Abuja: Action Aid, 2001.

20. Falobi O, Akanni O, eds. *Slow Progress: An Analysis of Implementation of Policies and Action on HIV/AIDS Care and Treatment in Nigeria.* Lagos: Journalists Against AIDS, 2004.

21. Federal Government of Nigeria/USAID. *Nigeria: Rapid Assessment of HIV/AIDS Care in Public and Private Sectors.* Abuja: Federal Government of Nigeria/USAID, 2004.

22. Department for International Development. *Benue Impact Studies.* London: Department for International Development, 2004.

20

PROSPECTS FOR AN HIV VACCINE

Abdoulaye Dieng Sarr,* Lateef Salako,†
and Souleymane Mboup‡

More than two decades have passed since researchers identified HIV as the cause of AIDS. HIV vaccine research has received more money than other vaccine effort in recent years, and at least 50 different vaccine preparations have entered clinical trials. Yet an effective HIV vaccine, which could prevent millions of new HIV infections each year, remains a distant dream.

Nonetheless, HIV vaccine researchers have strong reason to believe they will eventually succeed. Encouraging data from monkey experiments have shown that vaccines can protect animals from simian immunodeficiency virus (SIV), a relative of HIV (1,2). Several studies have also identified people who remain uninfected despite repeated exposure to the virus, suggesting that certain host genetic and virologic determinants can influence the probability of HIV infection (3–6). Additional studies have shown that a small percentage of HIV-infected people never develop AIDS, while others may control viral replication at low levels for at least a decade without damaging their immune systems; these people are called long-term non-progressors (7–10).

AZT, or zidovudine, the first antiretroviral (ARV) for the treatment of HIV infection, was licensed in 1987. Subsequent ARVs have been used in combination as highly active antiretroviral

---

*Department of Immunology and Infectious Diseases, Harvard School of Public Health, Boston, Massachusetts, USA
†Federal Vaccine Production Laboratory, Lagos, Nigeria
‡Laboratoire de Bacteriologie Virologie, Université Cheikh Anta Diop, Dakar, Senegal

therapy (HAART), which has dramatically improved the prognosis of people living with HIV/AIDS, particularly in developed countries, where most HIV-infected people can afford such treatments (11–13). It is well proven that such therapy prolongs suppression of viral replication, allows for significant immune reconstitution, and improves quality of life for people living with HIV/AIDS. Yet HAART has not been effective in eradicating latent reservoirs of virus, which contribute to viral resurgence when the therapy is discontinued (14,15).

It is now widely accepted that vaccination offers the best prospect for long-term control of HIV/AIDS in Africa, where current preventive and treatment strategies have proved insufficient and people maintain a strong belief in the ability of vaccines to eradicate endemic infectious diseases (14,16–19). When the leaders of African countries convened in Abuja in 2001 and adopted the Abuja Declaration on HIV/AIDS, Tuberculosis and Other Related Infectious Diseases, they affirmed the gravity of the HIV/AIDS epidemic in Africa and committed themselves to the pursuit of an HIV vaccine.

THE NEED FOR AN HIV VACCINE IN AFRICA

Treatment of HIV/AIDS can include ARVs that directly reduce viral load, treat co-morbidities, or treat opportunistic infections. In all these cases, treatment slows disease progression rather than leading to a cure. In some developed countries, where ARV therapy has been available for several years, HIV may now be considered a chronic infection with only a limited effect on life expectancy.

Although many African countries now have HIV/AIDS treatment programs, the treatment numbers are still small and there are many limitations. Therefore, AIDS treatment is not widespread enough to make a significant impact on the incidence of new HIV infections under the present circumstances. These limitations in treatment have led African nations to devote most efforts to prevention efforts, including behavior change communication initiatives, programs to prevent mother-to-child transmission of HIV, voluntary counseling and testing services, and prevention and treatment programs for other infections such as sexually transmitted infections and tuberculosis.

Despite these efforts, HIV continues to spread at alarming rates in Africa, underscoring the need to explore new approaches to current strategies and to adopt completely new measures. Vaccination is one such obvious measure.

In Africa, vaccines carry a strong reputation for endemic and epidemic disease control. Smallpox—which was so dreaded in many African countries that it was accorded the status of a deity with its own priests and devotees—was eradicated by vaccination, a feat that would have been unimaginable to traditional belief. Yellow fever is close to being eradicated; through vaccination it is no longer the dreaded killer that used to explode uncontrollably until a few years ago. Neonatal tetanus and postpartum tetanus in the mother are gradually yet steadily being consigned to history, once again because of vaccination. With the huge success of the global Expanded Programme on Immunization in preventing several childhood infectious diseases and the impending elimination of poliomyelitis, it can be understood why many Africans place hope on the future availability of a safe, effective, and affordable HIV vaccine.

THE ROLE OF VACCINES IN CONTROLLING INFECTIOUS DISEASES

A vaccine is a substance that contains immunogens; when given to a person, these immunogens are "seen" by the immune system. This exposure results in an immune response that mounts a defense against the pathogen (20). The goal of an HIV vaccine is to stimulate the immune system to create strong responses targeting two arms of the immune system; the humoral response consists of antibody production of the neutralizing type, and the cellular immune response results in the generation of cytotoxic T lymphocytes (CTLs) that specifically target and eliminate HIV-infected cells.

The main goal of a candidate vaccine is to either prevent or control an infection. An HIV vaccine may succeed in preventing infection by stimulating "sterilizing immunity." Successful vaccines, however, seldom, if ever, achieve sterilizing immunity. Virtually no vaccine has ever succeeded in giving complete protection from a virus. Reinfection occurs in an immunized person, but the infection is eliminated both by the individual's immune response and the self-limiting nature of most of the viruses for which we have vaccines. Additionally, these viruses kill the cells they infect; they do not set up a reservoir in the host (20–22).

Another scenario would be a preventive vaccine that may not prevent primary infection entirely, but rather would decrease the probability of HIV transmission from an infected individual to another person. The primary action of such a vaccine would be to prevent HIV infection in an exposed person. To achieve this, replication of the virus is eventually prevented in the vaccinated person with the result that the infection fails to take hold. The vaccines currently in Phase III clinical trials are not expected to block HIV infection completely. Nonetheless, given our limited options, they would be considered acceptable and worthy of deployment for HIV prevention, at least in Africa, if they either lowered viral load and subsequently reduced the infectiousness of the disease, or reduced transmission of HIV. This "non-sterilizing" scenario is an acceptable objective in the short term; however, the long-term goal aims for a completely sterilizing HIV vaccine. Both policy makers and vaccine recipients in Africa found the low efficacy of early vaccines disappointing, as their experience with previous vaccines had led them to believe an HIV vaccine would be a magic bullet.

A "therapeutic" vaccine, on the other hand, would not prevent primary infection at all. Rather, this type of vaccine would slow disease progression among people already infected with HIV. With such a vaccine strategy, the hope is that vaccinated individuals would remain asymptomatic and healthier for a longer period of time (1,22,23).

With regard to HIV, proven vaccine approaches used for other pathogens in the recent past have either failed—such as with whole-killed virus and subunit vaccines—or faced seemingly insurmountable regulatory hurdles—such as with live, attenuated vaccines. Recently therapeutic vaccines have received renewed interest as an alternative to current treatment options for HIV. The first immunotherapeutic vaccine trial was published in 1993. Since then, several therapeutic vaccine trials have been conducted. The results have consistently shown that, although in vitro–measured HIV-specific immune responses were evident as a result of vaccination, there was little evidence of clinical efficacy or clinical improvement (1,12,14,20,24,25).

PROPERTIES OF AN IDEAL HIV VACCINE

In a 2005 interview, the president and founder of the International AIDS Vaccine Initiative, Seth Berkley, listed the properties of an ideal HIV vaccine (26):

- **Efficacy.** The vaccine should be able to stimulate the production of a durable, functional, and protective immune response against most—if not all—subtypes to which an individual is likely to be exposed and from all potential routes of exposure. That is, it should be able to protect against genetically diverse HIV-1 strains and subtypes.
- **Safety.** The vaccine should have no early, intermediate, or late toxicity, and it should be well tolerated regardless of route of administration. It must be safe in infected and non-infected persons, thus removing the need for HIV screening before dosing. In addition, the vaccine should be safe in pregnancy, therefore removing the need for pregnancy screening. It should also be safe for use in people with tuberculosis, sexually transmitted infections, or cardiovascular, renal, or hepatic disease. The vaccine should have no adverse interactions with commonly used medications, including oral contraceptives, antimicrobials, antidiabetics, and antihypertensives. Finally, if the vaccine is also intended for children, it should be compatible with other childhood vaccines.
- **Delivery.** Commercial production should be restricted to only a few sites because of the complexity of vaccine manufacturing procedures, the need to comply with the good manufacturing practice requirements set forth in the quality system, and the high cost of setting up manufacturing facilities (up to US$150 million). Initially, only large manufacturing companies would be involved with production. Ideally, the goal would be to simplify production procedures sufficiently to allow only one or two West African countries to participate in vaccine production. As Nigeria and Senegal have experience with vaccine production, one or both of these countries should start planning for eventual participation in the commercial production of an HIV vaccine.
- **Stability.** The vaccine should be heat stable and have a long shelf life.
- **Route of administration.** The vaccine should be active orally; if injection is necessary, it should be possible to deliver the vaccine with an injection gun.
- **Duration of action.** The ideal vaccine would have a long-lasting effect with only a single dose. Alternatively, it should require two or three doses at most.
- **Efficacy indicator.** A cheap, simple, rapid, and sensitive test that can clearly distinguish between post-vaccination seroconversion test and post-infection seroconversion should be available.
- **Cost.** The vaccine should be affordable—or a special differential costing should be negotiated to make it affordable—to resource-poor countries. Distribution costs should also be reduced to affordable levels.

HIV VACCINE CANDIDATES UNDER INVESTIGATION

Vaccine design methods for a range of infectious diseases, as well as techniques for identifying and evaluating immune correlates of protection, have undergone substantial changes since the reorganization and better understanding of the science of vaccinology. Different generations have approached vaccine design and development with varying levels of success. First-generation vaccines were exclusively live, attenuated vaccines. Safety concerns, however, led scientists to develop second-generation vaccines, which contain chemically or physically inactivated pathogens. For instance, the live, attenuated Edmonston B strain measles vaccine, which was licensed in 1963, has changed several times. Distribution of the live Edmonston B vaccines ceased after 1975. A live, further attenuated preparation of the Enders-Edmonston virus strain, which is grown in chick embryo fibroblast cell culture and was licensed in 1968, is the only measles virus vaccine now available in the United States. This further attenuated vaccine causes fewer adverse reactions than the original Edmonston B vaccine (27,28). Purified or synthetic proteins represent a third-generation of vaccines, while recent advances in molecular biology and genetic engineering have led to the development of fourth-generation vaccines, including DNA, recombinant viral-vector–based vaccines, and pseudovirion vaccines, also known as virus-like particles.

As a vaccine against HIV remains the best hope for bringing the epidemic under control, an intensive global effort is under way to develop such a vaccine. The challenges, however, are considerable. To coordinate the research effort, the HIV Vaccine Trials Network (HVTN), an international collaboration of scientists and educators searching for an effective and safe HIV vaccine, was created in 1999 by the Division of AIDS of the National Institute of Allergy and Infectious Diseases, a component of the National Institutes of Health. The HVTN's mission is to facilitate the process of testing preventive HIV vaccines by conducting all phases of clinical trials, from evaluating experimental vaccines for safety and the ability to stimulate immune responses to testing vaccine efficacy.

Researchers have attempted many different strategies in their efforts to find an effective HIV vaccine. The experimental vaccines do not use whole or live HIV and cannot cause HIV or AIDS. The vaccines being tested have been designed to produce neutralizing antibodies and/or CTLs in order to fight infection. Historically, HIV vaccine development efforts have fluctuated between targeting the different arms of the immune system. Initially, emphasis was placed on the humoral response. Then, the focus shifted toward generating both humoral and cell-mediated immune responses, thus eliciting both neutralizing antibodies and CTLs. A more recent approach has placed more emphasis on eliciting CTLs rather than antibody responses (4,29–35).

Different types of candidate vaccines are being studied; based on the technology involved in their production, they can be classified into four major groups: recombinant subunit proteins; synthetic peptides; recombinant viral vectors; and DNA vaccines. Nearly 30 of these are undergoing clinical trials in human populations worldwide (Figure 20-1). These vaccines contain only some of the many genes that HIV requires for replication. The different types of HIV vaccines can be used either alone or in combination

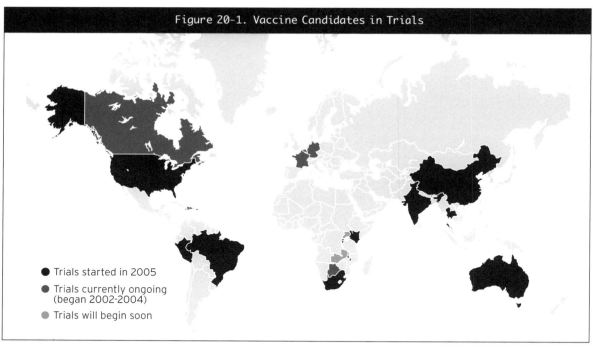

Figure 20-1. Vaccine Candidates in Trials

● Trials started in 2005
● Trials currently ongoing
  (began 2002-2004)
● Trials will begin soon

Source: Adapted from the International AIDS Vaccine Initiative, *The IAVI Report*, 2006; 4(1).

with another type of HIV vaccine. One approach to HIV vaccination is called the prime-boost strategy, which combines two of the same or two different types of HIV vaccines (30,36).

Subunit Vaccines

Subunit vaccines, also known as "component" vaccines, consist of individual HIV proteins or peptide epitopes rather than the whole virus. Peptide epitopes are defined as the specific site on an immunogen that stimulates specific immune responses, such as the production of antibodies or the activation of immune cells like CTLs. These proteins or peptides are typically made by genetic engineering techniques, rather than large-scale virus preparations. Most HIV subunit vaccines are based on HIV envelope proteins that coat the outside of the virus. These envelope proteins can prompt the body to produce an anti-HIV immune response, which will often include a strong neutralizing antibody and a weak to moderate CTL response.

Recombinant subunit protein vaccines are made of bigger pieces of proteins from the virus. Examples of recombinant subunit proteins include gp120, Gag, and Nef.

The pseudovirion type of subunit vaccine consists of virus-like particles that are non-infectious but structurally similar to HIV proteins.

An example of an HIV subunit vaccine is the Wyeth RC-529-SE, currently in Phase I clinical trials in the United States (HVTN 056). It is a multi-epitope (subtype B Env, Gag, and Nef) peptide HIV vaccine formulated with RC529-SE adjuvant, with or without granulocyte monocyte colony stimulating factor, or GM-CSF, which targets CTLs. GlaxoSmithKline has another candidate vaccine, which is composed of HIV subunit proteins (subtype B Nef and Tat fusion protein and subtype B gp120 Env subunit; HVTN 041).

Modified Bacterial Toxins

Modified bacterial toxins have been studied extensively as intracellular delivery agents because of their unique ability to translocate antigens across the cell membrane without affecting cell viability. Modified anthrax toxin lethal factor (LFn) protein can be used to deliver HIV antigens into the cell. The modified anthrax toxin lethal factor protein, once fused to HIV (LFn-HIV), is able to effectively induce anti-HIV CTLs in the absence of protective antigen. This fusion construct is being evaluated as a vaccine candidate (37–39). The LFn-p24 vaccine candidate produced by Avant Immunotherapeutics is now in Phase I clinical trials in collaboration with the Walter Reed Army Institute of Research and the National Institute of Allergy and Infectious Diseases in the United States.

Recombinant Viral Vectors

Recombinant viral vector vaccines are constructed by inserting HIV genes into live and infectious yet non-disease-causing viruses, such as poxviruses—including canarypox, vaccinia, and fowlpox—and adenovirus. These vectors provide a broad spectrum of uses in both basic and clinical sciences in allowing both the transient and long-term expression of almost any gene of interest in specific tissues. In addition, these vectors can accommodate substantial amounts of foreign DNA and can infect mammalian cells, resulting in expression of a large amount of foreign protein. These vaccines can be engineered to express one or more viral genes that cause infected cells to produce the protein in its native form.

Recombinant viral vectors enter cells and direct expression of the inserted HIV genes inside the cells; the proteins are then presented to the immune system in the same way that proteins from a virus-infected cell would be. As a result, they can induce both humoral and cellular immune responses. Subsequent boosting with recombinant subunit protein vaccines can substantially augment the antibody response to some live vector vaccines (30,40,41). Importantly, immune responses can be generated against the delivery vector, as well as to the incorporated antigens. Thus immune responses to the vector could limit the effectiveness of subsequent immunizations using the same vector.

Modified Vaccinia Ankara (MVA) Vector Vaccines

Modified vaccinia virus Ankara (MVA) is a highly attenuated strain of vaccinia virus produced after hundreds of passages of the virus in chicken cells (42,43). While MVA has lost about 10% of the vaccinia genome, it retains the ability to replicate efficiently in primate cells and provides similar levels of recombinant gene expression compared to replication-competent vaccinia viruses (44). MVA has been shown to be safe in a number of species, including monkeys, mice, pigs, sheep, and horses, with no local or systemic adverse effects. In addition, studies in mice and nonhuman primates have further demonstrated the safety of MVA under conditions of immune suppression (42,44). To date, thousands of human volunteers have been safely and successfully vaccinated against smallpox with MVA (45). Unfortunately, however, smallpox vaccination is sometimes associated with cardiovascular problems, though it has not yet been proved that smallpox vaccination was responsible for angina or heart attacks (46).

In animal models, MVA vaccines have been found to be immunogenic and protective against various infectious agents, including immunodeficiency viruses, influenza, parainfluenza, measles virus, flaviviruses, and smallpox (47). Macaque studies have yielded important data on MVA vector vaccines. Challenge studies in primates have shown that immunization regimens consisting of a prime DNA vaccine followed by boosting with recombinant MVA-based vaccine provided some protection in nonhuman primates upon challenge with an immunodeficiency virus. While vaccination did not prevent infection in these studies, it did result in a lower viral load setpoint, increased CD4+ counts, and less morbidity and mortality in vaccinated animals than in controls (47–49). The International AIDS Vaccine Initiative is conducting several Phase I studies on the use of MVA as a recombinant HIV vaccine (20,30).

Fowlpox Vector Vaccines

Fowlpox virus (FPV) is a member of the Poxviridae family. Productive infection by FPV is restricted to avian species. However, inoculation of mammalian cells with avipox-based recombinants results in expression of foreign genes (4). Some studies have shown that immunization of mammalian species by recombinant FPV can stimulate both humoral and cell-mediated immunity without local or systemic adverse effects (4,50). FPV vaccines are safe in many species, including chickens, mice, rabbits, ferrets, and monkeys. Because fowlpox cannot replicate in non-avian species, concern over potential systemic infection is much lower than for replication-competent vaccine vectors (51). Multiple Phase I and II clinical studies conducted in cancer patients using different fowlpox-based vaccines have supported the safety of this vector (52).

In animal models, FPV vaccines have been found to be immunogenic and protective against various infectious agents, including HIV (53). Challenge studies in primates have shown that immunization regimens, which incorporate priming with a DNA vaccine followed by boosting with a recombinant fowlpox-based vaccine, provide some protection in nonhuman primates following challenge with an immunodeficiency virus. One study showed protection of four vaccinated macaques, while all control animals became infected. In another study, various vaccination regimens were compared and none prevented infection; however, some vaccine regimens did result in lower viral load setpoints, increased CD4+ counts, and less morbidity and mortality in vaccinated animals than in controls. The most promising containment of challenge infections was achieved by intradermal vaccination with a DNA vaccine followed by recombinant FPV booster (4,36,40). Examples of this vaccination approach include HVTN 055 trials from Therion of Fowlpox Vector Vaccines (subtype B Env, Gag, Tat, Rev, Nef, and Pol).

Nonreplicating Adenoviral Vector Vaccines (AVV)

Nonreplicating viral vector vaccines using adenoviruses, also called adenovectors, were originally developed as delivery vehicles for use in gene therapy trials. To make an adenovector, scientists deleted one or more genes from the adenovirus genome and then replaced the deleted genes with segments of DNA that encode HIV proteins, or transgenes. This resulted in replication-incompetent adenoviral vectors that carry HIV transgenes into cells, where they are expressed as HIV proteins and then processed for presentation on the cell surface in association with MHC class I. Antigens presented in this way to CD8+ T cells can elicit an HIV-specific CTL response (1,12,54).

Adenovirus vector vaccines for HIV have elicited good immune responses, including both high-titer antibody production and high-frequency CTL responses in animal models, and have conferred protection in primate challenge studies (41). Rhesus macaques immunized with SIV Gag-based Ad5 vectors showed potent CTL responses that correlated with protection—reduced CD4+ loss, contained acute and chronic viremia, and reduced morbidity and mortality—following challenge with a pathogenic strain of SIV (55). In Phase I human studies, an adenoviral vector vaccine containing the HIV *gag* gene, administered as a series of injections or as a boost following priming with DNA vaccines, induced appreciable Gag-specific CD8+ responses in humans (56,57). An example of this vaccine approach includes the Merck-produced non-replicating adenoviral vectors (subtype B Gag, Pol, and Nef) being tested in HVTN 502.

Preexisting vector immunity appears to attenuate responses to adenovirus serotype 5 (Ad5) vaccines. Ad5 is endemic in many areas of the world. Different studies have detected neutralizing antibodies to Ad5 in 30% to 70% of U.S. participants, with up to one-third of vaccine trial participants having pre-vaccination neutralizing antibody titers of 1:200 or higher (54,58). In sub-Saharan Africa, the seroprevalence of neutralizing antibodies to Ad5 approaches 90% (41).

Some safety issues have been raised with regard to adenoviral vector vaccines, such as local and systemic reactions as well as moderate and sporadic malaise and body aches. However, these side effects frequently resolved spontaneously within 24 to 48 hours following injection (59).

The 1999 death of an 18-year-old in a gene therapy trial using an adenoviral vector at the University of Pennsylvania prompted extensive reviews of safety data from both human and animal studies of these agents. A National Institutes of Health report summarizing a review of clinical data from the case concluded that the young man's death was most likely due to a systemic adenovirus vector-induced shock syndrome (59). In that study, 19 patients suffering from ornithine transcarbamylase deficiency received E1/E4-deleted adenovirus vector particles infused directly into hepatic circulation. Almost all of the study subjects experienced one or more systemic symptoms, including fever, myalgia, nausea, and occasional emesis. Nearly all subjects showed a mild and transient thrombocytopenia without consistent abnormalities in coagulation, and higher-dose levels were associated with subsequent abnormal liver function studies. Animal studies have yielded similar results (59).

Some scientists have raised concerns about the potential for adenovirus vectors to become replication competent. Adenovirus vectors currently used in HIV vaccine studies are deleted in the E1 region and, in some cases, the E3 or E4 regions. It is theoretically possible that a vaccine containing an adenovirus vector could undergo recombination with a wild-type adenovirus that happens to be concurrently infecting a vaccinee. While there is little reason to expect such an event to result in any safety risk, participants in adenovirus vector vaccine trials who develop upper respiratory symptoms should undergo precautionary monitoring for shedding of recombinant adenovirus.

DNA Plasmid Vaccines

DNA vaccines contain circular plasmids that include a gene encoding the target antigen or antigens under the transcriptional control of a promoter region that is active in human cells. Unlike recombinant vector vaccines, DNA vaccines do not rely on a viral or bacterial vector. Instead, "naked" DNA, consisting of HIV genes, is injected directly into the body. DNA vaccines are generally less expensive to produce than peptide or protein vaccines and are chemically stable under a variety of conditions. DNA vaccines are generally administered intramuscularly, using either a needle and syringe or a needle-free injector. Cells take up the DNA and use it to produce HIV proteins. The proteins trigger the body to produce an anti-HIV immune response.

DNA vaccines were first tested in HIV-infected people and subsequently in uninfected people as preventive vaccines against HIV and malaria (13,25,60,61). While immune responses to DNA alone have been relatively weak in humans, combinations with adjuvants or with recombinant viral vectors in prime-boost approaches have resulted in appreciable HIV-specific CD8+ responses and have induced protective responses in primate models (62).

Several important safety issues have been raised with regard to DNA vaccines:

- Integration into cellular DNA could result in insertional mutagenesis through the activation of oncogenes or inactivation of tumor suppressor genes. In addition, an integrated plasmid DNA vaccine may in theory result in chromosomal instability through the induction of chromosomal breaks or rearrangement (63).
- DNA vaccines may influence the development of autoimmunity. Therefore participants in human trials of DNA vaccines are followed for possible signs and symptoms of autoimmunity. To date, there has been no convincing evidence of DNA vaccine-associated autoimmunity (64,65).
- Induction of antibiotic resistance has been a concern because part of the DNA plasmid production process involves selection of bacterial cells carrying an antibiotic resistance plasmid. Concern has been raised that resistance to the same antibiotic might be introduced in participants when the plasmid is used in clinical trials. It is important to know, however, that vaccinologists typically use antibiotics in these plasmids that are not commonly used to treat human infections.

The immune response to DNA vaccines results from uptake of plasmids into cells (including dendritic and muscle cells), expression of the target antigen and processing as intracytoplasmic antigens, and production of peptides that bind to class I MHC molecules to stimulate CD8+ T-lymphocyte responses. Antibody responses to plasmid-encoded proteins are also observed, suggesting that plasmid-encoded protein antigens stimulate B lymphocytes as well. Thus, DNA vaccines mimic viral infection by inducing both cellular and humoral immune responses.

The magnitude of these responses is generally modest when DNA is used alone. Data from primate studies and preliminary results of human trials suggest that more potent specific immune responses may be induced by combining DNA with adjuvants, by boosting with a recombinant viral vector or protein, or using both adjuvant and boost (25,56,62).

Challenge studies in primates using immunization regimens that include a DNA vaccine provide protection—prevention of infection, or control of viral replication with improved clinical outcomes—following challenge with an immunodeficiency virus. An example of this DNA plasmid vaccine is Epimmune (poly-epitopic: Gag, Pol, Vpr, Nef, Rev, and Env) being tested in HVTN 048.

Prime-Boost Strategies

A prime-boost strategy requires administration of one type of HIV vaccine, such as a DNA or recombinant vector vaccine, followed by a second type of vaccine, such as a subunit or recombinant vector vaccine. The goal of this approach is to stimulate different arms of the immune system and to enhance the body's overall immune response to HIV.

Combinations of different viral vector vaccines have been employed successfully in the past. For instance, studies in mice show that fowlpox-based and MVA-based vaccines used in combination induce immunity and protection against challenge with Plasmodium parasites (66). In macaques, DNA-based HIV vaccines can be effectively boosted with recombinant MVA-based vaccines expressing HIV antigens (67).

In macaques, Ad5 responses induced by primary vaccination appear to limit the usefulness of boosting with the same adenovirus vector. This attenuation may be overcome by increasing the vaccine dose, by using a heterologous prime-boost approach, or by taking both approaches (68). In macaques, boosting with adenovirus vectors based on alternative serotypes (such as Ad24) appears to improve cellular immune responses following Ad5-adenovector priming (54,68). In addition, preliminary reports from a macaque trial suggest that boosting with a canarypox vector (ALVAC vCP 205) following Ad5-adenovector priming results in superior cellular immune responses to HIV compared to boosting with the same adenovector (41).

DOES HIV STRAIN VARIATION REALLY MATTER?

Viral diversity poses a major barrier to the design of a successful HIV vaccine. The virus continually evolves because of genetic mutations and recombinations. Researchers must consider strain variation within individuals and among populations when developing HIV vaccines. Whenever a drug or immune response controls one variant, a distinct yet related resistant variant can emerge. In addition, certain variants may thrive in specific tissues or become dominant in an individual because they replicate more efficiently than others. Any of these changes may yield a virus that can escape identification and attack by the immune system (69,70).

The first HIV vaccines were derived from laboratory-adapted versions of a particular strain of virus known as the LAI strain (also known as IIIB or LAV), a subtype B virus. Other vaccines have been based on the SF-2 and MN isolates, which also belong to subtype B, the prominent HIV subtype in the United States and Europe. It has been shown that these as well as other laboratory-adapted viruses are more sensitive to neutralization than viruses in nature because of the laboratory adaptation process.

Newly developed vaccines are now based on wild-type HIV-1 strains, and many vaccines are being designed based on the subtypes most prevalent in Asia and Africa. This diversity is most evident in the HIV envelope glycoprotein, the usual target of neutralizing antibodies (nAb). An antibody generated to one envelope glycoprotein may not recognize an isolate with a slightly different envelope glycoprotein because of extensive variation within the nAb epitope. Thus, single-envelope glycoprotein vaccines have generally only protected against homologous, but not heterologous, challenge (71,72).

It is likely that a vaccine that overcomes HIV diversity will require the design of a cocktail of envelope glycoprotein antigens. Delivery of an array of envelope glycoproteins should elicit a broad immune response that can recognize the diverse population of HIV-1 that exists both within an individual and within a population. This strategy should take into account the main subtypes circulating in a particular geographic area. It would be difficult to design an effective candidate vaccine in Nigeria, for example, without considering the main circulating recombinant form, CRF02_AG, which is the dominant viral subtype in the country. Antigenic diversity has been addressed in the design of vaccines for other pathogens by the preparation of polyvalent vaccines. The poliovirus vaccine, for example, comprises three serotypes of poliovirus, while Pneumovax presents a cocktail of 23 pneumococcal variants, a feature that was essential in providing full protection against infection (21,27).

Another interesting strategy to reduce the impact of genetic diversity between HIV vaccines and circulating viruses would be to build a vaccine based on a consensus or ancestral viral sequence that bears a closer genetic similarity to all circulating viruses. A key question would be whether an artificially constructed gene sequence can encode a functionally and structurally intact and immunogenic protein.

The debate about how best to organize, or classify, different HIV strains is ongoing. For vaccine design, it may prove more useful to organize HIV diversity using categories other than subtypes. For instance, an alternative approach might be to organize the different variants of HIV by the immune responses they cause in people, or immunotype; this type of classification scheme might provide better clues about how to raise strong immune defenses against HIV.

CORRELATES OF HIV VACCINE PROTECTION

Most vaccine candidates undergo clinical trials despite their designers' limited knowledge about the vaccine's ability to induce immune responses or clear understanding of the exact immunologic components needed to protect an individual from infection.

The immune correlates of protection against a range of human viruses are usually provided through the generation of neutralizing antibodies, cell-mediated virus-specific immune responses, or both.

Vaccinologists tend to agree that vaccines capable of preventing establishment of chronic infection during natural infection are associated with the generation of virus-specific neutralizing antibodies, whereas cell-mediated responses, such as CTLs that destroy target cells expressing specific viral antigens, can potentially control the infection in instances where chronicity is not abrogated (47,71,76).

Vaccine-induced immune responses can vary substantially depending on the nature of the immunogen. The immune response generated by live, attenuated vaccines is generally very similar to that elicited by natural infection and thus includes both antibodies capable of preventing infection of target cells (neutralizing antibodies) and cell-mediated immunity. Subunit vaccines and purified synthetic proteins preferentially induce neutralizing antibodies and CD4+ T-cell responses, but not CD8+ CTLs. DNA vaccines and replication-defective virus-based vectors predominantly induce CTLs and CD4+ T-cell responses, but usually generate a poor antibody responses (47,60,66).

TECHNIQUES FOR DETECTING IMMUNE RESPONSES

Various techniques can be used to investigate the components of the immune system that confer protection as a result of vaccination. These detection techniques include the enzyme-linked immunospot assay (ELISPOT); tetramer staining; the chromium release assay; the limiting dilution assay; the proliferation assay; and FACS-based methods, which can provide additional information by allowing staining of cell surface markers and neutralizing antibody assays. Nevertheless, precise and quantitative assays are needed to identify and compare relevant immune responses induced in response to diverse vaccine candidates. In addition, as HIV infection is a global problem and different vaccine candidates are being tested worldwide among the different international vaccine trial sites (Figure 20-1), critical issues must be addressed about logistics, training issues, and the reliable performance of assays.

ELISPOT

The gamma interferon ELISPOT assay is a relatively simple technology that is fast (24 to 36 hours) and highly sensitive. The expression of gamma interferon is considered a proxy for the cell-mediated response. The ELISPOT does not require a high-tech platform, can be adapted for use in vaccine sites in developing countries, and can be used on fresh or frozen cells.

The assay does have disadvantages. High background can be a problem with some samples, making it difficult to distinguish low responders. The ELISPOT is also a qualitative test, and therefore does not produce quantifiable results. Also, whether ELISPOT can serve as a surrogate of functional T cells responses and enable meaningful decisions about vaccine efficacy is still a concern. Thus, assay variability validations are significant challenges to comparing multi-site trial results.

Chromium Release Assay

The chromium release assay is still the gold standard for CTL detection and evaluation, as it targets autologous or HLA-matched B cells lines. The main advantage of this assay is that it measures T cell function. Its disadvantages are that it is cumbersome to perform, insensitive, best with fresh cells, and not qualitative, and it often underestimates the true results. The assay also needs several weeks to be completed and involves the use of radioactive materials.

The Proliferation Assay

The T-cell proliferation assay is also a simple technology that is applicable for use in resource-poor settings. This assay works by evaluating the proliferation capacity of the CD4+ T cells. The limiting factors are that it usually takes days to a week to obtain results and it usually involves the use of radioactive materials.

Neutralization Assay

The neutralization assay is still the gold standard for broad screening of neutralizing antibodies. It is a functional assay and can be used on fresh or frozen serum samples. The assay is still cumbersome, not well optimized, and has considerable inter-laboratory variation. Neutralization assays require virus culture and highly trained personnel familiar with cell culture and biosafety level 3 facilities.

FACS-Based Methods

One of the FACS-based methods—intracellular cytokine cell staining—is very fast, requiring only about six hours, and can be used on whole blood and frozen peripheral blood mononuclear cells. Furthermore, several markers can be stained at the same time (cell phenotype and intracellular). The technique is very expensive, requires use of a FACS machine, needs highly trained personnel, and generates results that can be subjective. Another FACS-based method—tetramer staining—is relatively fast and does not require prior stimulation of cells. It is highly quantitative and sensitive and can use fresh or frozen cells. The technique requires prior knowledge of HLA type and epitope, however, and it does not distinguish between functional and non-functional responses. The technique is expensive, requires use of a FACS machine, needs highly trained personnel, and cannot be used for broad screening.

STAGES OF VACCINE TESTING IN HUMANS

After an experimental vaccine has been rigorously tested in laboratory and animal studies to determine its safety and immunogenicity, the vaccine must successfully complete three stages of testing in people before it can be licensed for widespread use. The HVTN Phase I trial, as well as Phase II and III trials, are randomized and double-blinded to participants and clinicians (Table 20-1).

A Phase I trial involves administering an experimental HIV vaccine to 20 to 100 HIV-negative volunteers. This Phase I trial collects information primarily on safety, looking for any vaccine-related side effects. In this phase of testing, the vaccine candidate is compared to a placebo, which is a known inactive substance. A Phase I trial can also provide initial data on the dose and administration schedule (the time between vaccinations) required to achieve the optimal immune response.

Once a Phase I trial has shown that the experimental HIV vaccine is safe, the vaccine candidate can advance into Phase II trials, which enroll as many as several hundred people. In these trials researchers

Table 20-1. Phases of Clinical Trials			
Phase	**Number of Participants**	**Primary Rationale**	**Duration**
I	20 to 100	Safety	12 to 18 months
II	Hundreds	Safety, dosing, and immunogenicity (required for Phase III)	2 to 3 years
III	Thousands	Safety and effectiveness (required before licensing)	3 to 5 years

Source: The International AIDS Vaccine Initiative, *The IAVI Report*, 2005;9 (1).

focus on safety while gathering more in-depth information about the human immune response to vaccination and further determining the optimal dosing and administration schedule.

The most promising experimental vaccines move into Phase III trials. These trials are designed to answer the question of whether a vaccine is effective in preventing HIV infection in thousands of HIV-negative volunteers. Data indicating a vaccine's safety and effectiveness in large numbers of people are required to support a license application. Such trials are extremely complex and costly. Only one Phase III trial of an HIV vaccine has been conducted thus far.

Phase IIb is an intermediate-sized trial, also known as "proof of concept" or probe of efficacy. Pharmaceutical companies often use this type of trial to gather better information on the efficacy of a vaccine candidate before undertaking highly demanding and costly Phase III trials. The VaxGen's two Phase III trials cost as much as US$300 million, and the current prime-boost trial in Thailand will cost more than US$100 million. Phase IIb trials are smaller than Phase III, but significantly larger than Phase II trials. Their intermediate size gives them statistical power to provide valuable preliminary information about vaccine efficacy, though they are generally not designed toward securing product licensure unless the data show strong evidence of efficacy. In most cases a product that showed moderate efficacy in a Phase IIb would be tested again in a confirmatory efficacy trial before seeking licensure; but if the efficacy was high, a Phase IIb trial could be used as the basis for a licensure application to regulatory authorities.

In measuring the risks and benefits of intermediate-sized trials, one example of a best-case scenario came from results announced in 2002 from Merck's human papillomavirus (HPV) vaccine candidate targeting HPV-16. (HPV has more than 100 strains, some of which can cause genital warts and cervical cancer.) The trial tracked roughly 1,500 volunteers for an average of a year and a half following the final immunization and monitored them for persistent HPV-16 infection, a surrogate measure of the vaccine's ability to protect against cervical cancer. The trial showed 100% protection against persistent HPV-16 infection in vaccine recipients. Based on these encouraging data, the company went on to launch a full-scale Phase III trial designed to secure licensure for the polyvalent vaccine that targets strains 6, 11, 16 and 18.

Intermediate-sized trials may also generate ambiguous results. One example of a worst-case scenario is the SPf66 malaria candidate vaccine, which was tested in a series of trials in Africa and South America. These trials yielded varying results. The most notable case occurred in the first African trial, which tested the vaccine in nearly 600 Tanzanian children. Although the trial was conducted in a region with high rates of malaria, the vaccine was found to be 31% effective in preventing a first episode of clinical malaria, but the 95% confidence interval for efficacy ranged from 0% to 52%. Although a 31% efficacious malaria vaccine might have been beneficial, particularly in areas with high endemicity, the debate over the SPf66 trial data effectively grounded the development of the malaria vaccine candidate, which still has not been tested in a definitive trial (73–75).

ETHICAL ISSUES IN VACCINE CLINICAL TRIALS

When the vaccine to be tested is specifically targeted at an HIV strain or subtype found in the host country, but not in the sponsor's country, then it becomes an ethical imperative for the initial clinical trials to be done in the targeted host country. In this case, the sponsor should strengthen the capacity of the country to undertake the study, usually in collaboration with other stakeholders. Even when a vaccine has been submitted to Phase I/II trials in the sponsor's country, it is ethically desirable for additional Phase I/II trials to be done in the host country, where the Phase III study is to be conducted. This step has the advantage of eliminating any possibility of safety and immunogenicity issues that might be influenced by environmental, racial, or genetic differences. It would also strengthen the capacity of the host country for any future Phase III trial. As a rule, Phase III trials should be done in endemic countries after suitable scientific, ethical, and infrastructure strengthening to empower them for conducting the trials successfully and competently. It is the trial sponsor's responsibility to ensure that all trials are conducted in accordance with the principles of good clinical practice.

Ethical considerations are critically important in all investigations involving human subjects and these considerations assume particular importance in the case of HIV vaccine trials (77). This added importance stems from the unusual preponderance of the virus in the world's poorest countries and the need to undertake the trials in such countries with their insufficient physical infrastructure, susceptibility to exploitation, and lack of understanding of their rights, privileges, and entitlements (16).

From 1997 to 1999, UNAIDS convened a series of expert consultations to discuss and agree as much as possible on the main ethical issues in HIV vaccine research and development (78,79). The following account is based on the outcome of these consultations as prepared in a summary document by UNAIDS (80,81). It should be borne in mind that what can be given in a text like this is a general outline of the ethical issues of importance when considering clinical efficacy evaluation of a vaccine. The details, which may change from location to location, must be discussed and agreed upon with local stakeholders, including government policymakers and community leaders; the host scientific community; the sponsoring agents; and the development and donor agencies operating in the host country. All the facts must be laid open to these stakeholders before any decisions relating to the clinical trial are made and a consensus must be reached before the trial begins.

The principal ethical issues to be considered in an HIV vaccine efficacy trial include the need for a program on HIV preventive vaccine development, vaccine accessibility to countries with the greatest need, capacity building, developing the clinical evaluation protocol, scientific and ethical review, vulnerability of trial populations, adverse reactions, benefits of participation, use of control groups, informed consent, access to risk reduction and prevention interventions, care and treatment during trial, inclusion of women and children in the trial, and monitoring and evaluation.

Need for an HIV Vaccine Development Program

Given our present state of knowledge on HIV and the treatment and prevention strategies currently available, vaccines offer the best hope for the effective containment of the HIV/AIDS epidemic in Africa (19). The development of an effective HIV vaccine therefore is an ethical imperative. Failure to pursue it would be tantamount to neglect of millions of Africans. The global community is morally responsible for doing everything possible to encourage and support research that would lead to the development of these vaccines. Scientists in developed countries and major international pharmaceutical companies need to commit some of their enormous human and material resources toward this end. The governments of developed countries should create incentives for them to undertake this work and should provide assurances—particularly for the pharmaceutical companies—that their investments will have profitable returns.

The endemic countries of Africa are not in a position to engage in the type of strategic research that can lead to vaccine production. They should, however, be able to give assurance of their willingness to encourage and support clinical trials of these vaccines in their populations when they become available. They should encourage their citizens to participate in trials and should not take any measures that would discourage participation. In some states of Nigeria, for example, pregnant women are asked without prior counseling to undergo HIV testing. Those whose tests are positive are denied registration for antenatal care and face the accompanying stigmatization. This kind of situation would need to be avoided when screening volunteers for participation in HIV clinical trials. Indeed, this practice must be stopped, not only because it is unethical, but also because its continuation would militate against enrolling volunteers in future HIV vaccine trials. In the meantime, Nigeria should start developing south-south linkages with other potential trial host countries and north-south linkages with potential sponsoring countries with a view to expanding knowledge and strengthening capacity for research in the clinical, scientific, and ethical fields.

Vaccine Accessibility to Countries with the Greatest Need

Recent experience with the introduction of vaccines for endemic disease control has shown that it takes many years for a newly introduced vaccine to gain extensive distribution in Africa (14). The cases of the hepatitis B and *Haemophilus influenzae* vaccines are well-known examples of this. If the story of HIV vaccine is allowed to proceed in the same manner, then the vaccine may not be available for use in Africa for an appreciable time after it would have been shown to be effective and has been widely available in other countries. Hence a novel approach to making the vaccine available to populations in greatest need has to be developed. It would be unethical, for example, for a vaccine not to be immediately available for populations in which it was tested and found to be efficacious. Discussions on how a vaccine shown to be efficacious would be made available to the trial population should be finalized before the trial begins. The stumbling blocks would include procurement and distribution costs and logistics. Such discussions should involve all stakeholders and the source and modality of funding should be firmly agreed upon.

In trying to achieve this end, sponsors should not be discouraged from testing vaccines in large countries where HIV is endemic because of a disinclination to make the vaccine available at low cost to such populations. In the same vein, any temptation to exploit poor endemic countries willing to accept inappropriate or unsuitable vaccines for trial should be resisted.

Capacity Building

Leaders at the national and community levels of the host countries must understand the clinical, ethical, and scientific implications of all aspects of the clinical evaluation to allow them to participate in a full and meaningful manner in all decision-making processes about the trial. The level of understanding tends to be lower in host countries than in sponsoring countries, and it is the responsibility of the sponsors, development agencies, and donor organizations supporting the study to take steps to strengthen the knowledge base of the host stakeholders. Capacity building in the host country's scientific infrastructure should also be regarded as an ethical requirement.

Developing the Clinical Evaluation Protocol

The protocol used for a Phase III trial should meet international standards in terms of being scientifically sound and clinically relevant to the host population from which the participants are to be drawn. The expected benefits to the participants should be clearly set out on the basis of current knowledge of the disease and on data from previous laboratory studies on the candidate vaccine. The numbers to be included in the trial, HIV status, and risk potential should be agreed in pre-study discussions between the sponsors and hosts and the final document should be vetted nationally for scientific, clinical, and ethical validity. In the course of discussing the protocol details, disagreements are bound to arise between various stakeholders. Many of these arise from limitations in the host's understanding of scientific issues and in the sponsor's understanding of the host's cultural norms. All parties should make efforts to understand each other's points of view through education, information, and communication. The development and donor agencies, which likely already have an established relationship with both the hosts and sponsors, can play a leading role in achieving the required mutual understanding and equanimity.

Community Participation

The community in a host country covers several key groups, including social and religious leaders, the chiefs, various trade groups, people living with HIV/AIDS, health care providers, the local scientific community, and groups among whom the trial participants would be drawn. This last group should include female sex workers, men who have sex with men, injection drug users, and young adults who engage in unprotected heterosexual sex with multiple partners. Membership of committees responsible for planning and implementing the clinical trial should include people drawn from groups that are relevant to the particular committee's task, and their individual contributions and concerns should be duly recorded and addressed at the meetings.

Scientific and Ethical Review

The protocol for a vaccine trial, in whatever phase, should be submitted for the ethical and scientific review and approval of both the sponsoring and host countries. Therefore, it is imperative that potential host country and communities be identified early and their capacity for independent and competent scientific and ethical review of studies be assessed. Any deficiencies found should be systematically corrected so the host country and community can undertake all the needed reviews without undue influence or pressure from any other interested groups.

Vulnerability of Trial Populations

In some cases, the prevailing social and economic situations may expose potential trial participants to increased susceptibility to exploitation and harm, either physical or mental. Such factors include social marginalization of people living with HIV/AIDS and those engaged in high-risk activities, poverty, ignorance, lack of access to effective and affordable health care, poor infrastructural facilities for effective trial performance, and inability to give consent. The protocol should safeguard against all these unfavorable factors and, if overcoming them is impossible, the trial should not be undertaken in such populations.

Adverse Reactions

HIV vaccine trial participants may experience adverse reactions, including biological, psychological, or socioeconomic ones. Such reactions should be minimized and carefully explained to the participants prior to enrollment. Procedures to treat or overcome adverse reactions, when they occur, should have been agreed upon and these should be implemented without additional stress to the participants.

Psychological reactions may be as damaging as biological ones. Thus, the stigmatization and discrimination that could accompany recognition that someone is participating in a trial should be avoided as much as possible by guarding the confidentiality of participants. This task is not easy in small communities and justifies the need to have a minimum population size on which to base a trial. A procedure for compensation should be established in the event, for example, that a participant loses his or her job as a result of participating in the trial. Those who need treatment for adverse reactions should have access to treatment of the highest quality available in the area at no cost.

The HIV vaccines now in trial do not use live virus and thus cannot cause infection. It should be borne in mind, however, that live, attenuated vaccines have been used for other diseases, and this approach may one day be explored for HIV. If that should occur, the potential health risk would be a major consideration.

The possibility that, rather than prevent transmission, a vaccine might worsen the course of an infection in vaccinated people exposed to the virus should be considered and discussed with participants. In addition, vaccine programs requiring a series of injections or repeated follow-up tests may cause harmful effects, such as injection abscess.

Benefits of Participation

The rewards that participants would derive from taking part in the trial should be agreed upon beforehand and be clearly articulated in the protocol. Inducement to accept unreasonably high-risk conditions should be avoided. Some of the expected benefits would include easy accessibility to health care facilities and personnel, increased education on HIV risks, prevention and treatment, supply of preventive and treatment tools at no cost, financial compensation to cover transportation and loss of income from time spent in participating, and development of immunity, if the vaccine turns out to be efficacious.

Use of Control Groups

At present, it is ethically justifiable to have a placebo control group in a Phase III trial, as no effective HIV vaccine exists. When an effective vaccine exists, however, the existing vaccine should be used as control for trials of any new vaccines, as long as the conditions of the new trial do not significantly differ from the conditions under which the existing vaccine was tested and found to be efficacious. To ensure that the participants in the placebo group derive some reasonable benefit from the study, the placebo could be another effective vaccine for a sexually transmitted infection common in the area, such as hepatitis B, provided there is no contraindication to its use.

Informed Consent

Freely given, clearly understood informed consent should be obtained from each trial participant. At some stages, consent should be combined with voluntary counseling. It is important to obtain informed consent from participants at several stages: prior to the initial screening for eligibility to participate in the trial, before testing for HIV status, before enrollment, during the trial before further HIV tests to evaluate response to the vaccine, and during the trial to ensure the subject has not had second thoughts about continued participation in the trial.

The participants must be clearly informed that they can withdraw the consent at any time without suffering repercussions. The procedure for obtaining consent should follow broadly the rules established by various international conventions. In particular, it must be conveyed, in writing and orally, in language clearly understood by the subjects. Where minors are involved, third-party consent should be obtained from parents or guardians, but as much information as the minors can understand should be given directly to them. In some cultures, women are not allowed to make decisions like this on their own, and their parents or husbands may have to give approval for them. Nevertheless, the woman should be given all the information directly and her approval obtained even if the final consent rests with another person.

Phase II and III trials enroll people with high-risk behavior. Care should be taken that some indigent people do not make false claims of high-risk behavior in order to be selected for participation and thereby reap the financial and other benefits offered to participants. Skilled counselors who can detect false claims should take part in the screening.

Informed consent must be obtained by independent operators who must accurately explain the risks and benefits to the participants. No one with a possible conflict of interest should take part.

Access to Risk Reduction and Prevention Interventions

All vaccine trial participants should continue to be provided with all available risk reduction and prevention interventions, which should be upgraded as better ones become available. The fact of participation in a trial that may or may not be efficacious should not be a license for high-risk behavior. If unprotected exposure occurs, the best available post-exposure chemoprophylaxis should be provided to the affected participant.

Care and Treatment During Trial

Trial sponsors should accept responsibility for the care and treatment of participants who become HIV infected in the course of the trial. Before the trial begins representatives of all stakeholders should agree on the level of care and type of treatment to be provided. These levels may vary from country to country and between different parts of the same country, depending on the level of the health care system. In Nigeria, the minimum level of care should be the best available in the country, including immunological monitoring, accessibility to the physician in charge, preventive behavior counseling, prevention and treatment of opportunistic infections, palliative care, post-exposure chemoprophylaxis, and ARV therapy. These benefits should be provided at no cost to the participant and should be lifelong. Since any long-term benefits such as ARV therapy would outlast the trial period, the country's health policymakers should be party to this agreement so they can work out modalities for taking over the responsibility from the sponsors at the end of the trial.

Inclusion of Women and Children in the Trial

Women should be encouraged to participate in HIV vaccine trials for many reasons, including the possibility that they may respond to a vaccine differently than men. In addition, any vaccine that proved effective would be given to women, including potentially pregnant women and breastfeeding women.

In the same way, a future effective vaccine would need to be given to children and adolescents below the legal age of consent. Hence, it is ethically proper that they participate in a trial for safety, immunogenicity, and efficacy. Adolescents engaging in unprotected sex are at high risk for acquiring HIV. If they are found to be suitable candidates for the trial, consent must be obtained from one or both parents, as long as the minor has no objection. If the minor does object, then his or her wish should prevail.

Monitoring and Evaluation

The quality of the scientific content of a trial should constantly be monitored to ensure that the process complies with the approved protocol at all times. Failure to maintain scientific quality might mean an invalid trial in which the participants would have been needlessly exposed to risk. Similarly, the quality, adequacy, and appropriateness of the consent and counseling processes should constantly be monitored to ensure the trial is being conducted in accordance with the agreed-upon ethical standards. This monitoring should be independent and require the services of well-trained monitors who cannot be unduly influenced by the trial sponsors, trial scientists, or the host community. The trial committee should discuss any untoward findings and take steps to correct the faults and mitigate any harm.

AFRICA-SPECIFIC STRATEGIES FOR AN HIV VACCINE

Regional considerations are important in the development of HIV vaccines in Africa. Adaptive immune responses—in the form of neutralizing antibodies and virus-specific CD4+ and CD8+ T cells—are the principal correlates of immune protection for most infections and vaccines. In HIV, there is evidence for the association of strong and early CTL responses during primary infection with control of viral replication and establishment of low viral setpoint (35). It has also been shown that HIV subtypes differ in disease and transmission potential, and their antigenic variation could require subtype-specific vaccine design (70,82,83). Differences in population genetic makeup, such as HLA class I, across regions suggest that a vaccine based on subtypes circulating in the United States may not guarantee efficacy for all African regions. African populations from different regions have varying frequencies of HLA class I antigens needed to present CTL epitopes, although consensus sequence selection of CTL epitopes may be used to minimize the potential impact of variation within subtypes. More research is needed to define immunodominant epitopes within HIV and CTL responses that reflect regional viruses and human HLA allele frequencies in African populations.

An HIV vaccine development initiative in Africa would have to deal with several major obstacles:

- The heterogeneity of HIV and multiple modes of transmission provide several portals of entry between geographic locations;
- Molecular epidemiologic surveillance will be required, as multiple levels of HIV diversity—including types, subtypes, and recombinants—vary from region to region and are dynamic; and
- The correlates of protective immunity remain unclear.

As a result of these obstacles, researchers should match vaccines to the circulating viruses, take into consideration issues of cross-protection and interaction, determine HLA profiles in target populations, identify CTL targets, determine the role of immune activation in responses, and develop the capabilities to evaluate these responses at vaccine trial sites. Continued surveillance and molecular epidemiology will provide critical information on the dynamics and characteristics of the epidemic and assist in the development of appropriate vaccines and other interventions. Also, immunologic and pathogenesis studies will help identify potential correlates of protection and build capacity for vaccine trials.

CONCLUSION

Vaccines, which have a justifiably strong reputation for infectious disease control in Africa, have several key advantages in controlling viral spread. They are amenable to mass deployment, thus making coverage relatively easy to achieve. They are more cost-effective than treatment and other preventive interventions. Their delivery requires personnel who are less highly skilled, and both politicians and general populations accept them well. In addition, most developing countries already have considerable experience and trained personnel in vaccine delivery that can be drawn upon when the time comes to deliver an HIV vaccine to the general population. For all these reasons, an effective HIV vaccine would offer African nations the best hope for controlling and ultimately eradicating the virus, and global efforts need to be intensified to develop, produce, evaluate, and deploy a suitable vaccine in Africa as soon as possible.

REFERENCES

1. Desrosiers R. Prospects for an AIDS vaccine. *Nature Med*, 2004;10:221–223.

2. Nacsa J, Radaelli A, Edghill-Smith Y, et al. Avipox-based simian immunodeficiency virus (SIV) vaccines elicit a high frequency of SIV-specific CD4+ and CD8+ T-cell responses in vaccinia-experienced SIVmac251-infected macaques. *Vaccine*, 2004;22:597–606.

3. Kaul R, Rutherford J, Rowland-Jones SL, et al. HIV-1 Env-specific cytotoxic T-lymphocyte responses in exposed, uninfected Kenyan sex workers: a prospective analysis. *AIDS*, 2004;18:2087–2089.

4. Kent SJ, Stallard V, Corey L, et al. Analysis of cytotoxic T lymphocyte responses to SIV proteins in SIV-infected macaques using antigen-specific stimulation with recombinant vaccinia and fowl poxviruses. *AIDS Res Hum Retrovir*, 1994;10:551–560.

5. MacDonald KS, Fowke KR, Kimani J, et al. Influence of HLA supertypes on susceptibility and resistance to human immunodeficiency virus type 1 infection. *J Infect Dis*, 2000;181:1581–1589.

6. Rowland-Jones SL, Dong T, Dorrell L, et al. Broadly cross-reactive HIV-specific cytotoxic T-lymphocytes in highly-exposed persistently seronegative donors. *Immunol Lett*, 1999;66:9–14.

7. Mendila M, Heiken H, Becker S, et al. Immunologic and virologic studies in long-term nonprogressors with HIV-1 infection. *Eur J Med Res*, 2000;4:417–424.

8. Migueles SA, Sabbaghian MS, Shupert WL, et al. HLA B*5701 is highly associated with restriction of virus replication in a subgroup of HIV-infected long term nonprogressors. *Proc Natl Acad Sci USA*, 2000;97:2709–2714.

9. Propato A, Schiaffella E, Vicenzi E, et al. Spreading of HIV-specific CD8+ T-cell repertoire in long-term nonprogressors and its role in the control of viral load and disease activity. *Hum Immunol*, 2001;62:561–576.

10. Yamada T, Iwamoto A. Comparison of proviral accessory genes between long-term nonprogressors and progressors of human immunodeficiency virus type 1 infection. *Arch Virol*, 2000;145:1021–1027.

11. Krim M, Baltimore D, Ward DE. The emergence and early years of the HIV/AIDS epidemic. In: Ward DE. *The AmFAR AIDS Handbook: The Complete Guide to Understanding HIV and AIDS*. New York: WW Norton, 1999:167–191.

12. Coordinating Committee of the Global HIV/AIDS Vaccine Enterprise. The Global HIV/AIDS Vaccine Enterprise: scientific strategic plan. *PLoS Med*, 2005; 2(2):e25. (Available at www.plosmedicine.org).

13. Esparza J. The Global HIV Vaccine Enterprise. *Int Microbiol*, 2005;8:93–101.

14. Berkley S. The need for a vaccine. In: Essex M, Mboup S, Kanki PJ, Marlink RG, Tlou SD, eds. *AIDS in Africa*. 2nd ed. New York: Kluwer Academic/Plenum Publishers, 2002:584–594.

15. Rowland-Jones S. AIDS pathogenesis: what have two decades of research taught us? *Bull Mem Acad R Med Belg*, 2004;159:171–175.

16. Esparza J, Bhamarapravati N. Accelerating the development and future availability of HIV-1 vaccines: why, when, where and how? *Lancet*, 2000;355:2061–2066.

17. Morel C. Neglected diseases: under-funded research and inadequate health interventions. *EMBO*, 2003;4:535–538.

18. Stover J, Walker N, Garnett GP, et al. Can we reverse the HIV/AIDS pandemic with an expanded response? *Lancet*, 2002;360.

19. The Nairobi Declaration. *An African Appeal for an AIDS Vaccine*. Declaration from a joint WHO/UNAIDS/SADC/SAA/AfriCASO consultation, Nairobi, June 12–14, 2000.

20. Cohen J. AIDS vaccine still alive as booster after second failure in Thailand. *Science*, 2003;302:1309–1310.

21. Clements-Mann ML. Lessons for AIDS vaccine development from non-AIDS vaccines. *AIDS Res Hum Retrovir*, 1998;14:197–203.

22. Heillman CA, Baltimore D. HIV vaccines, where are we going? *Nature*, 1998;4:532–534.

23. Esparza J, Osmanov S. HIV vaccines: a global perspective. *Curr Mol Med*, 2003;3:183–192.

24. Burton DR, Moore JP. Why do we not have an HIV vaccine and how can we make one? *Nature*, 1998;4:495–498.

25. Cohen AD, Boyer JD, Weiner DB. Modulating the immune response to genetic immunization. *FASEB*, 1998;12:1611–1626.

26. Berkley S. Accelerating AIDS vaccine development (interviewed by Marilynn Larkin). *Lancet*, 2005;5:16–19.

27. Hilleman MR. Personal historical chronicle of six decades of basic applied research in virology, immunology and vacccinology. *Immunol Reviews*, 1999;15:369–383.

28. Liu MA. Vaccine developments. *Nature*, 1998;4:515–519.

29. Hess C, Altfeld M, Thomas SY, et al. HIV-1 specific CD8+ T cells with an effector phenotype and control of viral replication. *Lancet*, 2004;363:863–866.

30. Hodge JW, Poole DJ, Aarts WM, et al. Modified vaccinia virus ankara recombinants are as potent as vaccinia recombinants in diversified prime and boost vaccine regimens to elicit therapeutic antitumor responses. *Cancer Res*, 2003;63:7942–7949.

31. Letvin NL, Walker BD. Immunopathogenesis and immunotherapy in AIDS virus infections. *Nature Med*, 2003;9:861–866.

32. Norris PJ, Moffett HF, Brander C, et al. Fine specificity and cross-clade reactivity of HIV type 1 Gag-specific CD4+ T cells. *AIDS Res Hum Retrovir*, 2004;20:315–325.

33. Rowland-Jones SL, Pinheiro S, Kaul R, et al. How important is the "quality" of the cytotoxic T lymphocyte (CTL) response in protection against HIV infection? *Immunol Lett*, 2001;79:15–20.

34. Yang OO, Nguyen PT, Kalams SA, et al. Nef-mediated resistance of human immunodeficiency virus type 1 to antiviral cytotoxic T lymphocytes. *J Virol*, 2002;76:1626–1631.

35. Yu XG, Addo MM, Rosenberg ES, et al. Consistent patterns in the development and immunodominance of human immunodeficiency virus type (HIV-1)-specific CD8+ T-cell responses following acute HIV-1 infection. *J Virol*, 2002;76:8690–8701.

36. Robinson HL, Montefiori DC, Johnson RP, et al. Neutralizing antibody-independent containment of immunodeficiency virus challenges by DNA priming and recombinant poxvirus booster immunizations. *Nature Med*, 1999;5:526–534.

37. Lu Y, Friedman R, Kushner N, et al. Genetically modified anthrax lethal toxin safely delivers whole HIV protein antigens into the cytosol to induce T cell immunity. *Proc Natl Acad Sci USAm* 2000;97:8027–8032.

38. McEvers K, Elrefaei M, Norris P, et al. Modified anthrax fusion proteins deliver HIV antigens through MHC Class I and II pathways. *Vaccine*, 2005;23:4128–4135.

39. Sarr AD, Lu Y, Sankalé JL, et al. Robust HIV type 2 cellular immune response measured by a modified anthrax toxin-based enzyme-linked immunospot assay. *AIDS Res Hum Retrovir*, 2001;17:1257–1264.

40. Kent SJ, Zhao A, Dale CJ, et al. A recombinant avipoxvirus HIV-1 vaccine expressing interferon-gamma is safe and immunogenic in macaques. *Vaccine*, 2000;28:2250–2256.

41. Kostense S, Vogels R, Lemckert A, et al. Adenovirus serotype 35-based vaccination in the absence or presence of serotype 5 specific immunity. *Keystone Conference on HIV Vaccines*. Banff, Alberta, March 29–April 4, 2003 (abstract 321).

42. Mayr A, Hochstein-Mintzel V, HS. Passage history, properties, and applicability of the attenuated vaccinia virus strain MVA. *Infection*, 1975;3:6–14.

43. Meyer H, Sutter G, Mayr A. Mapping of deletions in the genome of the highly attenuated vaccinia virus MVA and their influence on virulence. *J Gen Virol*, 1991;72:1031–1038.

44. Sutter G, Moss B. Nonreplicating vaccinia vector efficiently expresses recombinant genes. *Proc Natl Acad Sci USA*, 1992;89:10847–10851.

45. Earl PL, Americo JL, Wyatt LS, et al. Immunogenicity of a highly attenuated MVA smallpox vaccine and protection against monkeypox. *Nature*, 2004;428:182–185.

46. Upfal M, Cinto S. Adverse cardiac events after smallpox vaccination. *Emerg Infect Dis*, 2004;10(5). Accessed at www.cdc.gov/ncidod/EID/vol10no5/03-0967_04-0235.htm.

47. Amara RR, Villinger F, Staprans SI, et al. Different patterns of immune responses but similar control of a simian-human immunodeficiency virus 89.6P mucosal challenge by modified vaccinia virus Ankara (MVA) and DNA/MVA vaccines. *J Virol*, 2002;76:7625–7631.

48. Hanke T, Neumann VC, Blanchard TJ, et al. Effective induction of HIV-specific CTL by multi-epitope using gene gun in a combined vaccination regime. *Vaccine*, 1999;17:589–596.

49. Stittelaar KJ, Kuiken T, De Swart RL, et al. Safety of modified vaccinia virus Ankara (MVA) in immune-suppressed macaques. *Vaccine*, 2001;19:3700–3709.

50. Kent SJ, Zhao A, Best SJ, et al. Enhanced T-cell immunogenicity and protective efficacy of a human immunodeficiency virus type 1 vaccine regimen consisting of consecutive priming with DNA and boosting with recombinant fowlpox virus. *J Virol*, 1998;72:10180–10188.

51. Taylor J, Weinberg R, Languet B, et al. Recombinant fowlpox virus inducing protective immunity in non-avian species. *Vaccine*, 1988;6:497–503.

52. Cavacini LA, Duval M, Eder JP, et al. Evidence of determinant spreading in the antibody responses to prostate cell surface antigens in patients immunized with prostate-specific antigen. *Clin Cancer Res*, 2002;8:368–373.

53. Yamanouchi K, Barrett T, Kai C. New approaches to the development of virus vaccines for veterinary use. *Rev Sci Tech*, 1998;17:641–653.

54. Emini EA. Potential HIV-1 vaccine using a replication-defective adenoviral vaccine vector (plenary). *9th Conference on Retroviruses and Opportunistic Infections*, Seattle, Washington, February 24–28, 2002 (abstract L5).

55. Baxby D, Paoletti E. Potential use of non-replicating vectors as recombinant. *Vaccine*, 1992;10:8–9.

56. Shiver JW, Fu TM, Chen L, et al. Replication-incompetent adenoviral vaccine vector elicits effective anti-immunodeficiency-virus immunity. *Nature*, 2002;415:331–335.

57. Tellez I. HIV-specific T-cell responses in seronegative volunteers immunized with an HIV-1gag-pol DNA vaccine. *7th Conference on Retroviruses and Opportunistic Infections*, San Francisco, California, January 30–February 2, 2000 (abstract Mo.C365).

58. Varnavski AN, Zhang Y, Schnell M, et al. Pre-existing immunity to adenovirus in rhesus monkeys fails to prevent vector-induced toxicity. *J Virol*, 2002;76:5711.

59. National Institutes of Health Recombinant DNA and Advisory Committee. Assessment of adenoviral vector safety and toxicity. *Hum Gene Ther*, 2002;13:3–13.

60. Bagarazzi ML, Higgins TJ, Baine Y, et al. Vaccination of seronegative volunteers with a human immunodeficiency virus type 1 env/rev DNA vaccine induces antigen-specific proliferation and lymphocyte production of beta-chemokines. *J Infect Dis*, 2000;181:476–483.

61. Horton H, Vogel TU, Carter DK, et al. Immunization of rhesus macaques with a DNA prime/modified vaccinia virus Ankara boost regimen induces broad simian immunodeficiency virus (SIV)-specific T-cell responses and reduces initial viral replication but does not prevent disease progression following challenge with pathogenic SIVmac239. *J Virol*, 2002;76:7187–7202.

62. MacGregor RR, Boyer JD, Ugen KE, et al. First human trial of a DNA-based vaccine for treatment of human immunodeficiency virus type 1 infection: safety and host response. *J Infect Dis*, 1998;178: 92–100.

63. Ledwith BJ, Manam S T, Roilo PJ, et al. Plasmid DNA vaccines: assay for integration into host genomic DNA. *Dev Biol (Basel)*. 2000;104:33–43.

64. U.S. Food and Drug Administration, Center for Biologics Evaluation and Research and Office of Vaccine Research and Review. Points to consider on plasmid DNA vaccines for preventive infectious disease indications. Accessed at www.fda.gov/cber/gdlns/plasmid.txt.

65. Smith HA, Klinman DM. The regulation of DNA vaccines. *Curr Opin Biotechnol*, 2001;12:299–303.

66. Anderson RJ, Hannan CM, Gilbert SC, et al. Enhanced CD8+ T cell immune responses and protection elicited against *Plasmodium berghei* malaria by prime boost immunization regimens using a novel attenuated fowlpox virus. *J Immunol*, 2004;172: 3094–3100.

67. Hirsch VM, Fuerst TR, Sutter G, et al. Patterns of viral replication correlate with outcome in simian immunodeficiency virus (SIV)–infected macaques: effect of prior immunization with a trivalent SIV vaccine in modified vaccinia virus Ankara. *J Virol*, 1996;70(6):3741–3752.

68. Emini E. Ongoing development and evaluation of a potential HIV-1 vaccine using a replication-defective adenoviral vector. *Keystone Conference on HIV Vaccines*, Banff, Alberta, March 29–April 4, 2003 (abstract 012).

69. Kaleebu P, Mahe C, Yirrell D, et al. Effect of human immunodeficiency virus (HIV) type 1 envelope subtypes A and D on disease progression in a large cohort of HIV-1-positive persons in Uganda. *J Infect Dis*, 2002;185:1244–1250.

70. Kanki PJ, Hamel D, Sankalé JL, et al. Human immunodeficiency virus type 1 subtypes differ in disease progression. *J Infect Dis*, 1999;179:68–73.

71. Belshe RB, Graham BS, Keefer MC, et al. Neutralizing antibodies to HIV-1 in seronegative volunteers immunized with recombinant gp120 from the MN strain of HIV-1. *JAMA*, 1994;272: 475–480.

72. Esparza J, Osmanov S. HIV vaccines: a global perspective. *Curr Mol Med*, 1983;3:183–192.

73. Bass E. IIb or not IIb? AIDS vaccine trial sponsors weigh the merits of intermediate-size efficacy trials. *IAVI Report*, February–April 2004.

74. Trape JF, Rogier C. Efficacy of SPf66 vaccine against *Plasmodium falciparum* malaria in children. *Lancet*, 1995;14;345(8942):134–135.

75. Alonso PL, Smith T, Schellenberg JR, et al. Randomised trial of efficacy of SPf66 vaccine against *Plasmodium falciparum* malaria in children in southern Tanzania. *Lancet*, 1994;344:1175–1181.

76. Beattie T, Rowland-Jones S, Kaul R. HIV-1 and AIDS: what are protective immune responses? *J HIV Ther*, 2002;7:35–39.

77. Bloom BR. The highest attainable standard: ethical issues in AIDS vaccines. *Science*, 1998;279:186–188.

78. Guenther D, Esparza J, Macklin R. Ethical considerations in international HIV vaccine trials: summary of a consultative process conducted by the joint United Nations Program on HIV/AIDS (UNAIDS). *J Med Ethics*, 2000;26:37–43.

79. UNAIDS, World Health Organization, Japanese National Institute of Infectious Diseases. *AIDS vaccine research in Asia: needs and opportunities. Report from a UNAIDS/WHO/NIID meeting, Tokyo, 28–30 October, 1998. AIDS*, 1999;13(11):1–13.

80. UNAIDS. Ethical considerations in HIV preventive vaccine research. (UNAIDS/00.07E). Geneva: UNAIDS, 2000.

80. World Medical Association (WMA) Declaration of Helsinki. *Ethical Principles for Medical Research Involving Human Subjects*. Adopted by the 18th WMA General Assembly, Helsinki, Finland, June 1964 and amended by the: 29th WMA General Assembly, Tokyo, Japan, October 1975; the 35th WMA General Assembly, Venice, Italy, October 1983; the 41st WMA General Assembly, Hong Kong, September 1989; the 48th WMA General Assembly, Somerset West, South Africa, October 1996; and the 52nd WMA General Assembly, Edinburgh, Scotland, October 2000.

82. Renjifo B, Mwakagile D, Hunter D, et al. Differences in perinatal transmission among human immunodeficiency virus type 1 genotypes. *J Hum Virol*, 2001;4:16–25.

83. Gao F, Robertson DL, Morrison SG, et al. The heterosexual human immunodeficiency virus type 1 epidemic in Thailand is caused by an intersubtype (A/E) recombinant of African origin. *J Virol*, 1996;70: 7013–7029.

21

DEVELOPMENT ASSISTANCE FOR BUILDING INSTITUTIONAL CAPACITY

Olusoji Adeyi* and Jane Miller†

In their quest to mount effective responses to the HIV epidemic, countries often face the challenge of ensuring that development assistance supports the capacity building of local institutions. "Development assistance" in this context refers to the transfer and use of resources to achieve and sustain effective programs that offer HIV prevention, treatment, or care, or that mitigate the impact of the epidemic on families, communities, and sectors of the economy. The scope of this definition includes institutional development, capacity utilization, improvement of the country's knowledge base for HIV/AIDS control, official development assistance, and development assistance for health (1).[1] "Institutional capacity" refers to the organized skills, systems, and components required to mount effective HIV/AIDS control initiatives in Nigeria.

For years a global debate has raged about the conditions under which development assistance can be effective. Considerable evidence has accrued that development assistance works best in the pres-

*World Bank, Washington, DC, USA

†Department for International Development (Government of the United Kingdom), Lusaka, Zambia

[1] According to the definition by the Development Assistance Committee of the Organisation for Economic Co-operation and Development, "official development assistance" includes grants and loans to developing countries and territories, with the promotion of economic development and welfare as the main objective, and on concessional financial terms. "Development assistance for health" is broader than "official development assistance"; it includes nonconcessional loans from development banks and funds from private foundations and nongovernmental organizations that contribute directly to the promotion of development and welfare in the health sector in developing countries. (WHO Commission on Macroeconomics and Health, 2002)

ence of strong policies and effective institutions (2), and yet development assistance can also help to nurture effective institutions. A more recent study suggests that development assistance engenders success in countries with weaker policy environments; the authors found that higher-than-average short-impact aid to sub-Saharan Africa raised per capita growth rates by half a percentage point over the growth that average aid flows would have achieved (3). The basic result depends on neither the recipient's level of income nor the quality of its institutions and policies; the authors found that short-impact aid causes growth, on average, regardless of those characteristics. The authors also found evidence that the impact on growth tends to be greater in countries with stronger institutions or longer life expectancies. This debate contains a circular element, in that development assistance may strengthen institutional capacity yet may not be forthcoming in the absence of a certain level of institutional capacity. The future of the market for development assistance continues to be a matter of intense discussion (4).

Data on health expenditures and aid dependency reveal that Nigeria spends less on health than is average for low-income countries. Nigeria also receives less foreign aid than is average for low-income countries, both in per capita terms and as a percentage of gross national income (5). (See Table 21-1.)

A full understanding of development assistance and sustainability in Nigeria would require analyses of domestic objectives, resource commitments, the structure and function of institutions, relationships among local and international institutions, past and current resource needs, allocations and expenditures, and projections of future resource requirements. Unfortunately, the lack of accurate and reliable data on yearly allocations to — and expenditures on — HIV/AIDS control in Nigeria and the difficulty in obtaining data in a timely fashion prohibit a quantitative analysis of HIV/AIDS financing in Nigeria in this chapter. We place emphasis, therefore, on the qualitative aspects of development assistance and sustainability. The absence of valid quantitative data limits the discussion to institutional and organizations aspects. Yet this limitation itself helps to identify the critical need for government to ensure that information on the main sources and quantities of public expenditures and development assistance for HIV/AIDS is available in the public domain.

THE NIGERIAN RESPONSE TO HIV/AIDS

The National HIV/AIDS Strategic Framework

In 2000, Nigerian President Olusegun Obasanjo formed both the Presidential Committee on AIDS — comprising ministers from all sectors and the president as chairperson — and the National Action Committee on AIDS (NACA). NACA, in turn, prepared the country's HIV/AIDS Emergency Action Plan (HEAP), which received approval in 2001 for a three-year period (6). HEAP was the first countrywide strategy providing a multisectoral framework for the control of HIV/AIDS in Nigeria. With approximately 700 performance indicators emerging from various interest groups, it was an ambitious document. Unfortunately, its weak strategic focus limited its potential as a framework for coordinating development assistance. Compounding this problem was the challenge of coordination among the various governmental levels — federal, state, and local — and their agencies.

Table 21-1. Selected Data on Health Expenditure and Aid: Nigeria and Low-Income Countries						
	Aid Dependency		Health Expenditure			
	Aid per capita, in US$ (2002)	Aid as % of gross national income	Total % of gross domestic product (2001)	Public % of gross domestic product (2001)	Public % total (2001)	Health expenditure per capita, in US$ (2001)
Nigeria	2	0.8	3.4	0.8	23.2	15
Low-income countries	12	2.7	4.4	1.1	26.3	23

Source: World Bank, World Development Indicators, 2004.

A review of HEAP began at the end of 2004, with the intention of developing a new National HIV/AIDS Strategic Framework for 2005–2009. The strategic framework was developed in partnership with many stakeholders. In line with the internationally endorsed approach of "The Three Ones" (one national strategic framework, one national coordination body, and one monitoring and evaluation system), development agencies reached consensus about the need to work on this single national strategic plan.

The strategic framework is set within the context of the National Economic Empowerment Development Strategy (NEEDS), which is Nigeria's framework for poverty reduction. NEEDS sets the stage for coordination of strategies toward the achievement of Nigeria's long-term vision for economic development. States have been developing their own strategies, known as SEEDS, and HIV/AIDS has been mainstreamed into both NEEDS and SEEDS.

National Action Committee on AIDS

NACA was envisioned as a multisectoral mechanism that could coordinate the country's HIV/AIDS response rather than as an implementing agency. The committee includes representatives from the public sector, the private sector, nongovernmental organizations (NGOs), faith-based organizations, and networks of people living with HIV/AIDS. NACA members meet regularly; the committee also has a secretariat that serves as its technical and management arm.

A credit from the World Bank provided funds to strengthen both the NACA secretariat and a National Project Team (7). While this was useful in view of the complexity of program coordination and management, it has become clear that two parallel structures were being developed. Confusion arose about roles and responsibilities, as well as the appropriateness of the structure and system in relation to needs. Under a consultancy financed by the Department for International Development (DFID), the coordinating structures of the national response were assessed, and a restructuring plan was formulated through a long participatory process. This involved bringing the National Project Team and NACA together, ensuring better clarity in job descriptions, terms of reference, and "measurable deliverables" for each staff member. The restructuring plan requires new staff and changes in the functions of some of the existing staff. Some new staff members have been recruited, and the transition into the new re-engineering plan was slated for completion in 2005.

If the National Assembly passes an enabling law, NACA will transition into an agency, in line with the National Policy on HIV/AIDS that the president launched in 2003 (8). This law, which had not been passed as of late 2005, would give NACA a legal mandate, a formal budget line, and greater protection from potential political interference if future leaders are less committed to the HIV response than current ones. The underlying assumption is that a suprasectoral body such as NACA would enable the country to mount a more effective response to HIV/AIDS than would a strengthened ministry of health. This assumption is plausible, but there is no cross-country evidence to support it.

State Action Committees on AIDS

State and local action committees on AIDS—the SACAs and the LACAs—are responsible for spearheading the multisectoral response to HIV/AIDS at the state and local levels. In principle, the roles of the SACAs and the LACAs resemble that of NACA at the federal level in that they provide coordination and oversight.

Between 2000 and 2002, all states but one inaugurated a SACA. In 2003, NACA commissioned a review of the SACAs, showing that some were active, with 40% of all SACAs meeting at least four times a year (9). Others, however, appear to exist in name only. Ten SACAs have at least one full-time staff member, yet only seven states have a SACA office. The equipment available to SACAs is extremely basic, with only nine SACAs even having access to a telephone. Two states in particular—Lagos and Plateau—appear to have vibrant and functional SACAS. Lagos State took early action to establish its HIV/AIDS coordinating body and received assistance from local and external sources. Plateau State also benefited from external assistance, including direct support from the AIDS Prevention Initiative in Nigeria (APIN). In the case of Plateau State, APIN funded the development of a statewide action plan for HIV/AIDS control.

The role of the SACAs appears poorly understood in many states. While 81% of SACAs have terms of reference, in most cases those terms were adopted from recommendations that NACA sent, without any adaptation or consideration of local context. In some cases, the terms of reference are not fully understood; 58% of the SACAs view their role as being directly responsible for implementing the state response rather than merely providing coordination and oversight.

A number of factors have contributed to the SACAs' confusion about their roles and responsibilities. First, the SACAs have often taken their membership from people within line ministries and civil society organizations (CSOs) who are themselves directly responsible for implementing activities. Therefore their role within the SACA is confused with their role outside the SACA. This staff mix of membership carries risks, as it is difficult, and a potential conflict of interest, to be both the implementer and the overseer. NACA recommends that the SACAs have senior representation by policymakers at the state level rather than representation from the desk officers or those directly responsible for daily implementation. Some SACAs argue that desk officers understand best what is happening and what needs to be done. Ultimately the decisions about SACA membership rest with the chairman of the SACA, the state governor.

Second, because the SACAs play key roles in providing oversight for development assistance within the states, they tend to maintain a tight control of resources by directly implementing the HIV/AIDS programs themselves. Given the complexity of large-scale implementation, the SACAs do not have the capacity to mount responses to the depth and breadth needed. Therefore, the SACAs need to be empowered to identify the priorities for action, allocate the responsibilities to various implementing agencies such as line ministries and CSOs, and then oversee and monitor the implementers.

And third, in reality many governors are too busy to attend all meetings, and the responsibility of chairing the SACA is often delegated to someone in the governor's office. In 2003, the health commissioner served as the SACA chairman in 40% of the states. While the health sector is a key component of the HIV/AIDS response, the risk to one line ministry holding the chairmanship is that it may compromise the multisectoral philosophy of SACAs. It is important to note, however, that expectations of a large-scale multisectoral approach are unrealistic in the short term; even more modest interventions in the health sector tend to be weak. Therefore, it is pragmatic to start with core health sector functions in HIV/AIDS control, particularly when the capacity for larger multisectoral approaches is poorly developed.

Another challenge the SACAs face is the fact that many development agencies bypass them. In addition, some line ministries represented within the SACA will implement activities without the knowledge of the SACA. No systematic study of the reasons for this has been undertaken. Among the possible causes are the real and perceived weaknesses of many SACAs, including the perception that they might serve more as bureaucratic obstacles than as facilitators.

While many SACAs report having a workplan, few are implementing those workplans to the degree originally intended. SACAs cite a lack of resources as a principal reason; many would argue, however, that a lack of capacity and political will is equally at fault. During 2004, the number of states benefiting from World Bank assistance increased significantly. Workplans within 16 states are therefore beginning to have additional resources made available, and 15 states have shown a noticeable increase in activity. APIN has provided technical assistance to enable SACAs to develop state-level programs of action in Oyo and Plateau States. Most SACAs would benefit from capacity building to enable them to gain a greater understanding of their important role of coordination and oversight rather than direct control and implementation. This capacity building needs to be linked to the development of budget lines for HIV at the state level, together with strategies for coordinating external development assistance.

Local Action Committees on AIDS

Nigeria has 776 local governments, and a SACA review in 2003 estimated that more than 500 of those had established LACAs, only 134 of which are considered active (9). This represents 17% of all local governments. Even those described as "active" often cite a lack of funding and an inadequate capacity.

The local government response desperately needs strengthening if Nigeria is to reach most of its citizens with HIV/AIDS messages. In 2004 NACA promoted the development of HIV/AIDS information centers to be managed by staff members from local governments. Each center is intended to provide a local information resource, materials, and such commodities as condoms. The information would be available both to the general public and to the line departments, NGOs, and other CSOs. These centers may eventually be used for voluntary counseling and testing (VCT) as well. The first stage, however, is to build the capacity of a core group of local government staff.

If Nigeria is to provide an effective grassroots response to the HIV/AIDS epidemic, it will be in part through the strengthening of the local government sector. Given the huge number of local governments, and the lack of capacity at that level, these fortifying efforts will require a substantial increase in resources and effort.

Other Coordinating Agencies

In recent years, Nigeria has developed a number of HIV/AIDS coordinating groups that represent the interests of various key constituencies. Nigeria has an active UN Expanded Theme Group, established in 1996, which meets bimonthly and represents development partners, government agencies, and CSOs. Among the many groups and networks that exist or are emerging are the Donor Coordination Group; the National Assembly Response to HIV/AIDS, which has participation from both the senators and representatives; the Civil Society Consultative Group on HIV/AIDS in Nigeria, or CISCGHAN, which provides a voice and capacity building for NGOs and community-based organizations throughout Nigeria; and the Network for People Living with HIV. The recently formed Nigerian Business Coalition for AIDS has members representing some of the largest businesses and multinational companies working in Nigeria. The country has many active Muslim and Christian groups, with the Interfaith Coalition on HIV/AIDS taking on an ever-expanding role. While the proliferation of actors indicates increasing activities, the strategic relevance and technical quality of their work have yet to be documented systematically.

THE RATIONALE FOR DEVELOPMENT ASSISTANCE TO SUPPORT INSTITUTIONAL CAPACITY

Despite the president's strong commitment and leadership in the national response to HIV/AIDS, one of the country's constraints has been its limited *organized* capacity to address the epidemic. This limitation has been recognized for both the suprasectoral coordination functions and the health sector. For example, in addition to funding shortfalls at the National AIDS and STDs Control Program (NASCP) of the Federal Ministry of Health (FMOH), the "managerial, organizational, logistic, and technical capacities within NASCP are inadequate to coordinate so many players and programs in a country of this size and complexity" (10). The situation analysis further noted a "clear and urgent need for institutional capacity strengthening as a pre-requisite to ensuring leadership of the health sector response" (10).

The rationale for external development assistance in HIV/AIDS control is multiple. The immediate purpose would be to support locally led efforts to control the epidemic. In the short term, since HIV spreads across national boundaries, it has the potential for negative externalities beyond the confines of a particular country. In the medium- to long-term, not only would an uncontrolled epidemic have a large and negative impact on the Nigerian economy, but it could also reduce the inter-generational transfer of human and intellectual capital. With Nigeria's share of the regional population and economic output so significant, an unraveling of the Nigerian economy and social structure could have a negative impact on much of West Africa, including its security. Finally, achieving one of the targets of the Millennium Development Goals on HIV/AIDS — to have halted and begun to reverse the spread of HIV by 2015 — would be impossible in West Africa without successful efforts in Nigeria. The HIV epidemic also has direct and indirect impact on many of the other Millennium Development Goals.

THE TYPES OF DEVELOPMENT ASSISTANCE REQUIRED

Financial

The level of development assistance per year to Nigeria is unknown. NACA, the body responsible for coordination, has not developed any publicly available documentation that provides the full picture of development assistance for HIV/AIDS control in Nigeria. This is due in part to difficulties the committee has encountered in collecting data from some development assistance sources. Public sector data on financing the HIV response are spotty.

Determining the amount of financial resources allocated to HIV/AIDS is complex because of its multisectoral nature. For example, resources allocated to NACA and the SACAs, or reported by these committees, is not a good proxy for the total allocation, as most resources are allocated directly to the implementing agencies. Therefore resources allocated and used by line ministries, NGOs, and private agencies often go through neither NACA nor the SACAs, and these organizations rarely receive full information about the allocations. At the same time, it seems unnecessary to spend a great deal of public sector resources on coordination of private sector efforts *if* those private sector efforts are effective and working.

In addition, the amount of development assistance from the international community is difficult to estimate due partly to the lack of coordination of information and partly to the large discrepancy between planned and allocated budgets. This is particularly true of two of the largest international HIV/AIDS funders — the World Bank and the Global Fund to Fight AIDS, Tuberculosis and Malaria — in which the actual allocation per year is less than 20% of that planned. In addition, the resources the private sector has made available to HIV/AIDS are unknown and largely uncoordinated. The same is true for the financing from private individuals, foundations, charities, and faith-based organizations.

Despite the lack of data, it seems likely that, until recent years, the government has underfunded the country's HIV/AIDS control effort. In a 2003 survey, 78% of the SACAs reported that their lack of financial resources had prevented them from implementing their workplans (9). Most had long since exhausted the 2 million naira that NACA had sent in 2002. While this allocation was well intended, it led to the impression in some states that the state-level HIV/AIDS response — included the SACAs — would be federally funded. It has taken some time for the states to realize that they must take the HIV epidemic seriously by allocating adequate resources to state-led activities.

At the federal level, NACA has received government resources. The FMOH also has received substantial federal funding to implement its antiretroviral program (850 million naira in 2003 and 2004) (11), resulting in one of Africa's largest publicly funded antiretroviral programs, with approximately 14,000 people on treatment. This program has been clouded, however, by the slow release of government funds and the oversubscription for treatment. Overall, inadequate planning and management resulted in interruptions of treatment for many patients at the end of 2003.

The picture is mixed at the state level. Some state governors have begun to take the epidemic seriously, allocating resources to control efforts. After a slow start, for example, 16 states have now committed counterpart funding of US$100,000 for the World Bank-assisted HIV/AIDS project. Most of these financial pledges followed the elections of new state governors in 2003, which may signal a new commitment to the epidemic. In addition, some states have dedicated additional resources to procure antiretrovirals.

At the local level, the lack of funds is cited as a critical reason activities have been hampered, not just for HIV/AIDS services, but for all services. Even so, the local government level is considered the main source of service delivery.

Another crucial funding issue has been the need for greater information collation and transparency of allocations and expenditures. Enhanced information will enable better planning and more directed and focused support.

One important development in 2005 was the creation of a single workplan construct for NACA and each state SACA. NACA and the SACAs are encouraging all partner agencies to declare their funding commitments and incorporate their activities into the workplans. For the first time, NACA and the states may be able to assemble a comprehensive picture of the activities being undertaken within their constituencies and therefore be able to coordinate efforts. The Nigerian government, the World Bank, and UN agencies have become the first to incorporate their activities into these plans, and bilateral organizations have begun to come on board.

Organizational and Individual Capacity-Building

Probably as important as direct financial assistance, the national, state, and local government HIV/AIDS response requires development assistance in terms of capacity building of individuals and institutions. Capacity development needs to be considered in broad terms, including ensuring the existence of functional organizational structures, physical infrastructures, functional systems, and a fit between the functions to be performed and the individuals assigned to perform those functions.

The skill areas required to tackle the full complexity of the HIV/AIDS epidemic also are extensive, from basic science to biomedical and clinical research, and from policy development to management and service delivery.

CURRENT DEVELOPMENT ASSISTANCE RESPONSE TO HIV/AIDS

External Development Assistance

The major multilateral sources of external development assistance include the World Bank (through a credit of US$90.3 million) and the Global Fund (through grants of US$41.7 million to scale up the government's antiretroviral treatment program, US$27.4 million for PMTCT, and US$1.7 million for the civil society response, all of which were signed in 2003). The major bilateral sources include the governments of the United Kingdom (through DFID-financed programs); the United States (through the President's Emergency Plan for AIDS Relief and projects funded through USAID); Canada; and Japan. United Nations agencies have provided assistance, both under the umbrella of UNAIDS and individually; examples include UNICEF, the United Nations Development Programme (UNDP), and the World Health Organization (WHO).

A major challenge for Nigeria is the effective coordination of international development assistance in a way that encourages the implementation of programs supported by external funders at the same time that it avoids gaps among those programs and a wasteful duplication of efforts.

Development Assistance for NACA

Several development agencies—including the World Bank, DFID, the UN system, and the U.S. government (through the POLICY Project)—have provided support for NACA since its inception. Neither the Revenue and Expenses Statement for NACA nor the full scope of development assistance for HIV/AIDS control is in the public domain. Since 2003, at the request of the Nigerian government, development partners have made significant efforts to strengthen NACA, by funding the appointment of senior staff, for example, and by furnishing the new NACA offices. While NACA does have a budget line, which has risen in recent years, NACA depends heavily on external development assistance, raising questions about the extent to which the country is fulfilling its basic responsibilities of financing its coordinating body. Enhancing NACA's ability to coordinate an effective countrywide response to HIV/AIDS will require significant development assistance.

Development Assistance for the SACAs and the LACAs

In recent years, a number of development partners—including the World Bank, UNDP, DFID, APIN, and the U.S. Centers for Disease Control and Prevention—have been working with the SACAs to develop workplans. While an encouraging 75% of all states have workplans, in reality only 26% are implementing those workplans. A lack of funding is a common reason cited for failure to implement a workplan.

The World Bank-assisted project has established offices in 16 states, yet many of these are new, and they must build their own capacity before they can provide significant support to their partners.

Development Assistance for CSOs

The burgeoning civil society response to HIV/AIDS in Nigeria has begun to develop strategies for capacity building and coordination. The social marketing program, supported by DFID and USAID, is an exception in having national coverage, a strong capacity, and a long track record in awareness raising and condom marketing.

The faith sector, which delivers an estimated 40% of all health care in some states, also has huge potential. The Christian Health Association Nigeria, or CHAN, a 30-year-old network with 358 health institutions and more than 4,000 health facilities, runs 120 VCT centers and provides antiretrovirals in ten facilities. These drugs are provided on a fee-for-service basis with little financial support from the government.

The private sector response to HIV is poorly coordinated, and little is known about its financial allocations. NACA established a Business Coalition on AIDS in 2003, however, and some businesses—notably UNILEVER, Coca-Cola, and Chevron—have well-documented workplace policies.

By the second quarter of 2005, the World Bank-assisted project had committed more than US$18 million to more than 550 CSOs, including networks and coalitions, NGOs, community groups, faith-based organizations, workers' unions, professional associations, and private sector groups. Anecdotal claims of the impact of the scale up of civil society financing have been considerable. There has been no publicly available review or assessment, however, of the strategic relevance or technical quality of activities being undertaken by CSOs and the business sector.

Development Assistance for Substantive HIV/AIDS Control Programs

Most agencies in the United Nations have engineered specific responses to HIV. UNAIDS, which coordinates the UN system's contribution to HIV/AIDS, has actively supported the expansion of Nigeria's HIV response in line with the principle of "The Three Ones." Since this principle was adopted only as recently as April 2004 (12), it is too soon to determine its impact on HIV/AIDS control in Nigeria.

UNAIDS also supports the WHO in its efforts to expand access to antiretrovirals and to pursue the 3 by 5 Initiative, whose goal is to place three million HIV-infected people in resource-poor countries on antiretroviral treatment by the end of 2005. The WHO has been a key stakeholder, supporting ministries of health at both the federal and state levels and working with the FMOH in a national situation analysis and development of a health strategic plan. The WHO, which has offices in all states, maintains a focus on building capacity, as well as surveillance and strategic planning.

UNDP conducts a US$7 million project (2003 to 2007) aimed at building the capacity of eight states. It has a strong multisectoral focus and has been at the forefront in helping states mainstream HIV into SEEDS. The United Nations Population Fund has a US$40 million budget (2003–2007) for population, development, advocacy, reproductive health, and HIV. It has assisted in establishing VCT centers in 15 states and commodity procurement and distribution. UNICEF is working to scale up the PMTCT program in six states. It also has a large HIV program with the National Youth Service Corps. The International Labour Organization has been active in supporting HIV/AIDS workplace policies. UNIFEM, or the United Nations Development Fund for Women, has played an important role in ensuring that women have a voice and in mainstreaming gender issues into the National Strategic Plan.

The World Bank has provided a US$90 million credit facility to build the capacity of both individuals and institutions to enable an effective architecture for a substantial and scaled-up HIV response. Credit resources are also being used to scale up the public sector response at the federal, state, and local government levels. An HIV/AIDS Fund has been established at the federal and state levels for civil society funding. Implementation of the World Bank–supported program has been slowed by such factors as delays in the initiation of activities at the state level, organizational arrangements at the federal level, and the complexity of the project structure.

The major bilaterals working on HIV in Nigeria are the U.S., British, and Canadian governments. As mentioned earlier, the U.S. government has given Nigeria HIV/AIDS support through the President's Emergency Plan for AIDS Relief. The plan is to work with many partners, including national and international groups, to strengthen government systems, with a substantial scale-up planned over the five years of the project; US$34.5 million was budgeted for 2004.

During its long relationship with Nigeria, DFID has provided substantial funds aimed at strengthening NACA. DFID also funds a £52-million social marketing project with the Society for Family Health that increases access to commodities, particularly condoms.

The Canadian International Development Agency (CIDA) has a Can$4.8 million project over five years to provide resources to CSOs, with a specific focus on gender and human rights and a geographic focus along some specifically defined transport routes and junction towns. CIDA also provides funds to UNICEF and the WHO. Other bilaterals, including the Japanese International Cooperation Agency, are discussing their involvement with Nigeria.

Two U.S. foundations—the Ford Foundation and the Bill & Melinda Gates Foundation—also have provided major assistance. The Ford Foundation has supported a number of CSOs and provided funds to the Nigerian Institute of Medical Research (NIMR) to establish a reference laboratory and clinical research center. The Gates Foundation–funded APIN works in Lagos, Oyo, Plateau, and Borno states, with an emphasis on knowledge-based aspects of virologic and epidemiologic surveillance, program design, capacity building for the SACAs, targeted support for CSOs, equipment and training of key personnel in laboratories, support for PMTCT programs, and selected operational research projects. APIN has also supported a range of federal-level activities, including national HIV serosurveillance and a capacity-building program focused on the social and economic aspects of the HIV/AIDS epidemic.

CHALLENGES TO DEVELOPMENT ASSISTANCE FOR BUILDING INSTITUTIONAL CAPACITY IN NIGERIA

A Late Start

Until democratic elections in 1999, Nigeria was largely isolated from the international community. Efforts to develop a comprehensive response to the HIV/AIDS epidemic began only in 2000, and many working in the field have encountered a steep learning curve since then. Initially, the response focused on sensitization, enlightenment, and awareness raising; only recently has there been a shift toward behavioral change communication, care and support, and impact mitigation.

As discussed earlier, NACA, the SACAs, the LACAs, and other coordinating structures are mostly new, and in many areas, they have yet to fully understand their roles and responsibilities. Building their institutional capacity will require significant support. At the same time, there has been a mismatch between the availability of private-sector planning, marketing, and management skills applicable to HIV/AIDS program management, and the persistently weak capacity of the health sector to manage effectively a countrywide HIV/AIDS control effort.

A Weak Health System

The health system is only one component of an effective HIV response, yet it is arguably the most important. Today, Nigeria's health care system is weak, particularly at the primary health care level. Indicators for some of the most basic of health services, such as immunization, are among the worst in the world (13), and in 2000, Nigeria's overall health care system performance ranked 187th among the 191 member states of the WHO (14).

The national response to the epidemic is therefore faced with the additional challenge of providing HIV services within the context of an already strained system. Effective use of additional resources will be possible if the underlying system is strengthened concurrently with increasing attention to HIV/AIDS. If this does not happen, the additional resources being earmarked for HIV/AIDS activities risk the development of a distorted health system. This could easily happen if human and other resources become directed toward HIV and away from other core health services, further straining an already weakened system. At the same time, care must be taken to avoid a simplistic view that a perfect system must be in place before the epidemic can be controlled. Some activities, such as behavior change communications and condom distribution, are less demanding of a strong health system than others, such as large-scale antiretroviral treatment programs.

A Lack of Systematic Documentation

One of the greatest challenges facing government and development partners working to curb the epidemic in Nigeria is the limited availability of information on what exactly is happening. Many individuals have tacit knowledge of the status of HIV/AIDS control, but little of this information has been documented systematically. This is particularly true at the state level, where few SACAs have full information on the activities within their state or updated documentation. The result of this lack of information is poor coordination. This is particularly serious given the inadequacy of local and external resources. In 2004, Nigeria launched its national monitoring and evaluation system, the Nigerian National Response Information Management System, or NNRIMS. This system is essential for collecting information on the services being provided. NACA also has plans to work with the states on developing a situation analysis of HIV initiatives throughout the country. This enormous undertaking is needed to enable prioritization of activities both geographically and thematically.

The Need for Sustained Support, Supervision, and Monitoring

The SACA review that NACA commissioned in 2003 found that while many states had developed action plans, few had implemented them (9). The support for implementation therefore remains a challenge. There has been an assumption that once an action plan was developed, implementation would follow.

Without significant additional resources, support for skills development, supervision, and monitoring, however, implementation is unlikely to occur. This is because the skills needed to develop workplans differ from those required to implement programs. In addition, resources do not necessarily flow, just because there is a workplan, and with so many priorities competing for resources, it is not surprising that some important issues fall off the agenda.

A Complex Epidemic Requiring a Multisectoral, Multipartner Response

Mounting an effective multisectoral HIV response requires the mobilization of all relevant sectors of government and civil society. This mobilization presents an enormous logistical challenge, not only in ensuring that all actors understand their roles, but also in building their skills, coordinating their efforts, and monitoring their impact. This challenge, though not unique to Nigeria, is particularly difficult given the country's size and diversity.

Nigeria's Image of Corruption

In 2004, Transparency International ranked Nigeria as the third most corrupt country in the world (15). Although this finding was not based on HIV/AIDS program management, the country's overall poor ranking probably decreases the amount of resources it can attract. The federal government is taking measures to address issues of corruption, to strengthen financial management systems, and to improve accountability and transparency.

CONCLUSION

This chapter, although exploratory in nature, helps to identify key issues that require action by the leading federal agencies working on HIV/AIDS. Specifically, NACA must address issues of policy formulation and coordination across sectors without engaging in program implementation. NACA and the SACAs should *support* efforts of multiple institutions rather than seeking to *control* them. These committees should be limited to convening sessions on the formulation of evidence-based policies; serving as clearinghouses of information on programs, including findings from routine and special studies, particularly those dealing with the impact of HIV/AIDS control; facilitating consultations among sectors; disseminating information, including that on resource mobilization and allocation; offering federal- and state-level advocacy; and, in the case of NACA, providing external representation in non-specialized fora that deal with continental or global issues on HIV/AIDS. These committees should also eschew coordination as an end unto itself and avoid the temptation to seek control of specific activities of program funders and managers.

Other specific recommendations include:

- **Distinguish between the means and the end.** The goals of HIV/AIDS control in Nigeria must be differentiated from the means of achieving them. A multisectoral approach is useful not as an end unto itself, but as a means to reaching the goals of preventing transmission, treating and caring for those already infected, and mitigating the impact of the epidemic. To this end, it is critical that measurable results be defined as the centerpiece of HIV/AIDS control. This approach would also help to clarify the roles of different actors.

- **Strengthen coordination systems.** The distinction between control and coordination must be clarified at the national and state levels. The lack of coordination is hindering the extent to which development assistance can be allocated and used effectively. Better coordination will ensure that the existing resources are channeled to priority activities and geographic areas with greatest need. All development partners have a responsibility to work with the existing structures — such as NACA and the SACAs — and empower them with the skills to coordinate activities effectively. The SACAs should not misinterpret this statement to mean that the resources should be channeled through them for implementation. This approach would not be appropriate, and when this situation arises, development agencies should invest resources in the capacity development of SACAs to ensure they understand their role as coordinators — rather than controllers or implementers — of activities.

- **Ensure transparency in reporting.** If Nigeria is to improve its image and attract additional resources, all coordinating structures and implementing partners must strengthen their reporting practices, particularly through transparency in financial reporting. All development partners must, in turn, insist on good and transparent reporting and provide technical assistance when a lack of expertise is the reason for inadequate reporting.

- **Develop outcome-driven budgets and plans.** The development of program budgets that are guided by desired outcomes and that take into account implementation constraints is essential. These budgets would include local and external financial sources on short-, medium- and long-term bases as inputs into discussions on the sustainability of HIV/AIDS control in Nigeria. A system of HIV/AIDS accounts at the federal and state levels would be particularly useful in this regard. It is important that these accounts be available in the public domain.

- **Enhance systems through technical assistance, skills building, and other support.** Nigeria needs additional financial resources for HIV/AIDS control. Yet financial resources alone will not solve the HIV/AIDS problem; skills building is also needed in evidence-based approaches to program design, implementation, monitoring, and evaluation.

- **Combine short-term goals with long-term sustainability.** Developing separate programs focused on HIV/AIDS, without full consideration of the broader health system, runs the risk of either creating an unimplementable dream or further undermining the weak health system. At the same time, it is important to take a pragmatic rather than ideological approach to the problem. A binary approach to policy analysis — such as "vertical programs" versus "integrated programs" — will not resolve the HIV/AIDS problem in Nigeria. In the short- to medium-term, the country most critically needs efforts that are highly effective in curbing HIV transmission and in caring for those already infected. At the same time it is essential to improve service delivery systems in all key sectors relevant to HIV/AIDS control.

Although the root causes and impacts of the HIV epidemic extend well beyond the health sector, much of the burden of diagnosis and treatment falls on that sector. Hence, the FMOH should both assume major leadership responsibility for addressing HIV/AIDS and receive the resources to meet that responsibility. Both the FMOH and NACA should work toward transparent planning, including the regular publication of the sources, amounts, and uses of development assistance for HIV/AIDS in the country. External partners should, in turn, support rather than supplant local leadership and plans.

REFERENCES

1. World Health Organization. *International Development Assistance and Health: Report of Working Group 6 of The Commission on Macroeconomics and Health.* Geneva: World Health Organization, 2002;10.

2. World Bank. *Assessing Aid: What Works, What Doesn't, and Why.* Washington, DC: World Bank, 1998;1–44.

3. Clemens M, Radelet S, Bhavnani R, et al. 2004. *Counting Chickens When They Hatch: The Short-Term Effect of Aid on Growth.* Working Paper Number 44. Washington, DC: Center for Global Development, 2004;33.

4. Klein M, Hartford T. *The Market for AID.* Washington, DC: International Finance Corporation, 2005.

5. World Bank. *World Development Indicators.* Washington, DC: World Bank, 2004.

6. National Action Committee on AIDS. *HIV/AIDS Emergency Action Plan: 2001–2004.* Abuja: National Action Committee on AIDS, 2001.

7. World Bank. Project Appraisal Document on a Proposed Credit of US$90.3 million equivalent to the Federal Republic of Nigeria for an HIV/AIDS Program Development Project. Report Number 21457-UNI. Washington, DC: World Bank, 2001. Accessed at www.worldbank.org on May 30, 2005.

8. Federal Government of Nigeria. *National Policy on HIV/AIDS.* Abuja: Federal Government of Nigeria, 2003.

9. National Action Committee on AIDS. *Capacity Review of SACAs and LACAs.* Abuja: National Action Committee on AIDS, 2003.

10. Federal Ministry of Health. *National Situation and Response Analysis of the Health Sector Response to HIV and AIDS in Nigeria.* Abuja: Federal Ministry of Health, 2005.

11. Federal Ministry of Health. Central Accounts. Abuja: Federal Ministry of Health.

12. "'Three Ones' agreed by Donors and Developing Countries." Accessed at www.who.int/3by5/newsitem9/en/ on May 30, 2005.

13. National Population Commission of Nigeria and ORC Macro. *Nigeria Demographic and Health Survey 2003.* Calverton, Maryland: National Population Commission of Nigeria and ORC Macro, 2004.

14. World Health Organization. *World Health Report.* Geneva: World Health Organization, 2000.

15. Transparency International. *The Corruption Perceptions Index 2001 Ranks 91 Countries.* Accessed at www.transparency.org/cpi/2001/cpi2001.html on May 30, 2005.

22

EXPENDITURES ON HIV/AIDS AND THEIR POLICY IMPLICATIONS

David Canning,* Ajay Mahal,*
Olakunle Odumosu,† Prosper Okonkwo,‡
and Adedoyin Soyibo§

With an estimated 5% of the adult population of Nigeria infected with HIV and financial resources limited, expenditures on HIV/AIDS and their implications for government, household, and donor budgets hold obvious policy relevance for Nigeria. For instance, if it emerges that health expenditures associated with HIV/AIDS are rising rapidly, that would point to a heightened burden on government and household budgets in the near future and the consequent need for both to increase the efficacy with which existing financial resources are being used and to find additional resources devoted to HIV.

In two earlier chapters, we highlighted the potential financial implications of HIV/AIDS for Nigerian firms and for households (see Chapters 8 and 9, *this volume*). Those chapters did not, however, examine the financial contributions of the federal, state, and local governments in Nigeria; international donors; or nongovernmental organizations (NGOs), including faith-based groups that operate health facilities. Neither did those chapters examine the inter-linkages between this spending and household and private sector spending on HIV/AIDS. Moreover, the earlier studies represented in those chapters focused primarily on expenditures associated with the treatment of people living with

*Department of Population and International Health, Harvard School of Public Health, Boston, Massachusetts, USA
†Nigerian Institute of Social and Economic Research, Ibadan, Nigeria
‡AIDS Prevention Initiative in Nigeria, Ibadan, Nigeria
§Health Policy Training and Research Programme, Department of Economics, University of Ibadan, Ibadan, Nigeria

HIV/AIDS (PLWHAs) and the financial implications of caregiving by household members to PLWHAs, with little attention devoted to prevention, capacity building, and other categories of expenditures. One goal of this chapter is to address these gaps.

The second goal of this chaper is to assess the level of aggregate expenditures on HIV/AIDS, their composition, and trends in expenditures over time, which can be useful information for managing and designing policy interventions. Allocations of spending into activities for prevention, treatment, or capacity building, when combined with information on the state of the HIV/AIDS epidemic and its projections, would have the obvious benefit of helping senior policy managers better target their expenditures to these activities. Indeed, information on costs and expenditures collected as part of the process of constructing HIV/AIDS accounts has been used for undertaking cost-benefit and cost-effectiveness analyses of HIV/AIDS treatment interventions (1).

Policy experts involved in health and development work can obtain valuable information from the way HIV/AIDS expenditures are financed. If household out-of-pocket spending accounts for a significant portion of HIV/AIDS-related expenditures, policy makers would need to identify ways to ameliorate the economic burden on households. This may include expanding support for income-generation schemes, or social safety nets. Because an excessive reliance on household out-of-pocket spending may also mean that resources are being used less efficiently—households could do better if they pooled resources and bought HIV-related health services in bulk—ways would have to be found to address this inefficiency. As another example, high levels of reliance on international funding, particularly on recurrent spending, may indicate problems with sustaining current levels of spending further down the road, particularly if the AIDS epidemic were to grow even more severe.

The third goal of this chapter is to demonstrate the application of the National Health Accounts (NHA) methodology in assessing expenditures on HIV/AIDS in resource-poor settings. Briefly, the NHA offers a systematic method for recording and analyzing financial flows related to health care: between different ultimate sources of funds, financing intermediaries, and the providers of health care (2).

Up until now most work in this area has been undertaken in Central and South America, and very little in sub-Saharan Africa, with Rwanda being an exception. In doing so, we hope to highlight the major gaps in data that currently exist in Nigeria and thereby establish an agenda for future research and analysis on the subject.

To explore these issues, this chapter estimates the expenditures on HIV/AIDS incurred in the Oyo and Plateau states of Nigeria and examines the ways these expenditures are currently being financed, based on the NHA methodology. A word on the choice of Oyo and Plateau states: although accounting for only about 6.3% of the total land area of Nigeria and a roughly similar share of its projected total population of more than 130 million, these states can provide insights for Nigeria as a whole on the following grounds.[1] First, Oyo and Plateau offer some geographic variation, with one located in southwestern

---

[1] The 1991 census data on population and geographic area for each state were obtained from the Nigerian Population Commission website and www.nigeriabusinessinfo.com/nigeria-population.htm. Projected population for 2003, owing to the lack of a census since 1991, was obtained from the United Nations website (http://esa.un.org/unpp/p2k0data.asp).

Nigeria and the other in central Nigeria. Second, they both have considerable variation in terms of the ethnic composition of their population. And third, the adult HIV prevalence rates in the two states are not too far from the national average of 5.0% — 3.9% for Oyo State, and 6.3% for Plateau State, or roughly 82,000 HIV-infected adults in Oyo State and 81,000 in Plateau State.[2]

HIV/AIDS FINANCING IN DEVELOPING COUNTRIES

Several previous studies have estimated the amount spent on HIV/AIDS-related activities. Some focused only on expenditures incurred by the public sector, whereas others provided more information on the sources and uses of funds for HIV/AIDS. Many earlier studies did not apply the full-fledged NHA methodology, although more recent studies have done so.

In the early 1990s, two studies sought to estimate expenditures on HIV/AIDS in Asia — one in Thailand for 1991–1992 (3), and the other in Sri Lanka for 1993 (4). The Thailand study highlighted HIV/AIDS expenditures by various sources of funds — the government, the donor community, and the private sector. However, the results were presented in a way that probably double-counted some categories of expenditures (5). This study also did not provide any estimates of out-of-pocket expenditures incurred by households, a key indicator of the economic burden of AIDS on families. It also failed to include, for example, expenditures linked to the management of HIV/AIDS–related activities and research. The Sri Lanka analysis, while it did include the latter category of expenditures, did not include estimates of household expenditures either, and was plagued by problems of double counting as well (5).

A later study for Thailand focused more specifically on public spending for HIV/AIDS (6). Public expenditures considered in the study included five categories of HIV/AIDS activities: health promotion and medical services, coordination, empowerment of individual and community, social and psychosocial services, and research. In view of its limited aims, the study did not include out-of-pocket health spending incurred by PLWHAs or by their families on their behalf.

The Harvard School of Public Health undertook a study on behalf of UNAIDS to track the level and flow of national and international resources to HIV/AIDS–related activities in developing countries during 1996 and 1997 (7). It relied mainly on mailed questionnaires to collect information on HIV/AIDS expenditures from 64 developing countries and transition countries (the latter in Eastern Europe), and provided information only on funds provided by governments and donor agencies. Data on expenditures by households, employers, and NGOs — and indeed the entire private sector — were not captured by the study and the authors themselves acknowledge that they underestimated national and international HIV/AIDS spending by nearly one-third. However, the study's omission of household and firm spending on HIV/AIDS meant that the undercount was likely much larger.

---

[2]HIV prevalence data was obtained from the National Action Committee on AIDS (NACA) website (www.naca.gov.ng). Estimates of adults with HIV in the two states are based on HIV prevalence rates reported by NACA, combined with age-distribution data from the National Population Commission, and projected populations in the two states from United Nations (see above).

Subsequent studies have been more comprehensive and technically sound than those previous analyses. For example, Shepard and others undertook a five-country study of the sources and uses of health expenditures linked to HIV/AIDS — in Brazil, Côte d'Ivoire, Mexico, Tanzania, and Thailand, respectively (8–13). These studies used a variety of sources—such as official documents and expert assessments—to bring together estimates of funds spent by the public, private, and international sectors on HIV/AIDS activities, and the broad purposes for which these funds were used. Expert assessments were used to estimate the health care utilization patterns of AIDS patients and per-case costs of treatment of AIDS, which were then multiplied by the estimated number of AIDS cases to obtain total treatment costs. When available, information about social insurance schemes was used to estimate the distribution of treatment costs between insurers, the public sector, employers, and out-of-pocket payments by households. The estimates of HIV/AIDS expenditures obtained in these studies typically did not include expenditures on "mitigation"—for example, caring for AIDS orphans. More generally, these studies did not distinguish between ultimate sources of funding and financing intermediaries, thereby leaving open the possibility of double counting some of the expenditures.

SIDALAC — the Regional AIDS Initiative for Latin America and the Caribbean — has served as a supporting body for a number of HIV/AIDS expenditure studies based on the NHA methodology. At least 10 such studies have been completed in the Latin America and Caribbean region and another 10 are under way (14). Available data suggest that in 18 of these countries a total of US$1.27 billion was spent on HIV/AIDS in the year 2000; 74% was public spending, 24% was private spending, and the remaining was funded by external agencies. Brazil, Argentina, and Mexico account for the bulk of these expenditures. The per capita spending on HIV/AIDS in these countries was about US$2.70 in the year 2000, with nearly two-thirds of all spending devoted to personal health care, including antiretroviral (ARV) therapy, hospitalizations, ambulatory care of PLWHAs, and diagnostic tests. ARV expenditures accounted for approximately 65% of the spending on personal health care. Preventive and public health expenditures amounted to roughly US$0.65 per person, with about 60% to condoms, followed by information, education, and communication programs, then by blood banks. Non-health activities — including training of personnel, research, economic support to PLWHAs, and empowerment — accounted for only 3% of the total. Out-of-pocket spending amounted to less than 20% of the total spending on HIV/AIDS, and external funds were significant only for some of the smaller countries of Latin America and the Caribbean (Bolivia, Nicaragua, Honduras, and Guyana). Eighty percent of the external support came from bilateral donors, with another 14% from multilateral agencies. Private external support was relatively small.

In Africa, the only comparable study thus far is the one Barnett et al. undertook for Rwanda (15). This study identified three sets of HIV/AIDS–related activities, namely those relating to prevention and promotion, such as raising awareness, effecting behavior change, and promoting safer sex campaigns; management, such as palliative care, surveillance, blood screening, and family support; and treatment, including hospital and ambulatory care expenditures, counseling, and alternative and traditional therapies.

DATA AND METHODOLOGY FOR NIGERIA

As noted earlier, applying a NHA methodology to HIV/AIDS essentially means describing expenditure flows on HIV/AIDS across three sets of agents: the ultimate sources of funds; the financial intermediaries; and the uses to which funds are put. These uses can be classified in a number of ways: by type of provider, such as government, private, or nonprofit, for example, or by functional classification of care and services, such as inpatient care, outpatient care, administration, training, and research. The data can be cut in other ways as well. In undertaking our analysis for Oyo and Plateau states, we limited ourselves to describing financial flows of only two types: from sources of funds to financial intermediaries and from financial intermediaries to providers of care. Given that a country has several sources of funds, multiple financial intermediaries, and a number of different providers and functions, these flows are best presented in the form of two matrices, each corresponding to a different cut on the financial flows related to health.

In the Nigerian context, four issues were of obvious concern:
- What are the appropriate boundaries of expenditures on HIV/AIDS?
- Who are the main ultimate sources of finance, financial intermediaries, and providers of services?
- Should all of Nigeria be covered in the analysis, or would it be better to focus on only a few geographic regions?
- What are the main sources of data for obtaining the information on expenditure flows associated with AIDS in Nigeria, and how accessible are those data?

Expenditure Boundaries

Table 22-1 summarizes the main activities associated with AIDS that were of concern for the purposes of this chapter. Specifically, and in line with much of the existing literature on the subject, such as by Barnett, et al. (15), we divided the activities of interest into three categories: prevention and health promotion activities; care, support, and management; and treatment.

Financial flows relating to some of the activities listed in Table 22-1 do not ordinarily enter into the calculus of a "standard" NHA analysis. We refer, in particular, to expenditures on family support programs — such as care and support for AIDS orphans and support for families of PLWHAs, including microcredit schemes. In the context of the HIV epidemic, however, it seems appropriate to include expenditures associated with these activities, which seek to address an important set of consequences of AIDS. At the same time, there are activities that one might consider relevant because of their impact on financial flows associated with AIDS, but that are actually excluded. In particular, informal/unpaid care and support provided by immediate and extended family members that do not show up in financial flows are excluded, just as in the rest of the NHA literature because of the definition of health expenditure as actual spending. Including a monetary value of such care would need a careful assessment of the opportunity costs involved and is a valuable research question in its own right, and we leave this as a topic of further work in Nigeria. Excluding this category, however, means that the estimates of the care and support expenditures reported here underestimate the true societal costs of HIV/AIDS in this category.

Table 22-1. Setting the Boundaries of Expenditure Flows Linked to HIV/AIDS

Prevention and Promotion Activities	Care, Support, & Management	Treatment
Awareness Raising and Behavior Change • Mass media campaigns • Peer education • School education programs • Small group and community-level education • Outreach to high-risk groups, such as sex workers **Safe Sex Campaigns** • Condom social marketing • Free distribution of condoms • Safe sex workshops **Prevention of Perinatal Transmission** • HIV testing and counseling of pregnant women • Provision of antiretrovirals during pregnancy and at the time of delivery • Breastfeeding interventions **HIV Counseling and Testing** • Anonymous HIV testing • Referrals for care • Counseling services **Management of Sexually Transmitted Infections** • Testing, counseling, referral, and treatment **Blood Screening Programs** • Screening of blood • HIV test kits • Notification and counseling of infected donors **Universal Precautions and Other Safety-Promoting Interventions in Medical Settings**	**Palliative Care** • Home-based care • Psychosocial support programs **HIV/AIDS Surveillance and Research** • Training data collectors • Epidemiologic data collection and analysis • Research **Family support programs** • Care for children orphaned by AIDS • Support for families of people living with HIV/AIDS	**Hospital and Ambulatory Care Expenditures** • Inpatient stays • Outpatient visits • Psychiatric services • Nutrition services • Diagnostic services (laboratory and radiology) • Antiretroviral therapy and other drug-based treatments **Counseling for HIV/AIDS Patients** **Alternative/Traditional Therapies**

Another important omission from our expenditure calculations were household expenditures on condom purchases and sexually transmitted infections (STIs) other than HIV that would otherwise get classified as preventive interventions.

Entities as Sources of Funds, Financial Intermediaries, and Providers of Services

Table 22-2 lists the major entities involved in financial flows associated with HIV/AIDS in Nigeria, whether as an ultimate source of funds, as a financial agent or intermediary, or as a provider of services.

There are five main ultimate sources of funds in Nigeria: governments at various levels, households, international organizations, private sector firms, and NGOs. Nigerian governments, particularly at the federal and state levels, are likely to serve as ultimate sources of funds. The federal government contributes to financing of HIV/AIDS flows in several ways: by its support to various ministries—including the Federal Ministry of Health—for their initiatives on AIDS and provision of health care services to

Table 22-2. Listing Sources of Funds, Financial Intermediaries, and Providers of HIV/AIDS–Related Services in Nigeria

Ultimate Sources of Funds	Financial Intermediaries	Providers of Services
Governments • Federal Government of Nigeria • State governments **Nonprofit Organizations** • Faith-based organizations • Trade unions • Other nongovernmental organizations **International Donor Agencies** • Multilateral (e.g., the World Bank and the World Health Organization) • Bilateral (e.g., the U.S. Agency for International Development and the Department for International Development) • Foundations (e.g., the Bill & Melinda Gates Foundation and the Ford Foundation) **Households** **Firms** • Private • Public	**Government Ministries and Agencies** • Ministries of Education (federal and state levels) • Ministry of Defense • Ministries of Health (federal and state levels) • Ministry of Internal Affairs • Ministries of Labor (federal and state levels) • Ministry of Women's Affairs (federal and state levels) • Ministry of Transportation • Departments of Health in local governing areas • National Youth Services Corp • Action committees on AIDS (federal, state, and local levels) **Insurance** • Private voluntary insurance • Social insurance **Firms** • Private • Public **Household Out-of-Pocket Payments** **Nonprofit Organizations** • Nongovernmental organizations • Community-based organizations • Trade unions	• Health facilities of the governments (federal, state, and local levels) • Health facilities of nongovernmental organizations and community-based organizations (including blood banks, diagnostic centers, and pharmacies) • Nongovernmental organizations providing education and counseling services • Health facilities of employers • Private-sector health care providers, including hospitals, individual practices, traditional healers, diagnostic centers, and blood banks • Print and electronic media providing health information services • Service providers of international nongovernmental organizations

PLWHAs; contributions to the National Action Committee on AIDS (NACA); subsidizing purchases of ARVs; and possibly support of state-level health initiatives.[3] State governments too, through their own facilities, contribute to providing services to PLWHAs, and they may support, from their own revenues, other state-level ministries, as well as local governing areas that provide services associated with HIV/ AIDS. According to a NHA analysis recently undertaken for Nigeria, local governing areas have independent and relatively substantial independent sources of funding, perhaps through the mechanism of fiscal transfers across different levels of government (16).

Households are a major source of funds for services related to HIV/AIDS. Their contributions may take the form of out-of-pocket payments for the treatment of opportunistic infections associated with HIV and, when not subsidized by the government, ARVs as well. Households may also be paying premiums to health maintenance organizations in Nigeria that provide health insurance, presumably some of it to cover care associated with HIV/AIDS. Even if HIV/AIDS is covered by exclusion clauses, there is the

---

[3]Note that any contributions to states through assignments of oil revenues — that are part of the standard federal-state resource transfer process without reference to health — count as state revenues, and *not* as federal government contributions.

technical possibility that individuals may be treated for opportunistic infections such as tuberculosis, without their HIV status being revealed to the insurer.

A third important source of funds is contributions by international organizations which, by a recent NHA estimate, amounted to about 6% of Nigeria's entire health spending (16). International funding agencies include multilateral institutions that support HIV/AIDS–related activities through financial support/loans to the government, whether for supporting NACA through its multi-year support of US$90.3 million, or by its support under the Health Systems Development Project, which may have contributed to improved health services for all users of the public system, including PLWHAs; the World Bank is an example of such an institution. International funding agencies also include bilateral agencies such as the Department for International Development (DFID) of the United Kingdom and USAID, whose funding is in the form of grants; the Global Fund on AIDS, Tuberculosis and Malaria; and private foundations such as the Bill & Melinda Gates Foundation, which has funded the AIDS Prevention Initiative in Nigeria (APIN), a US$25 million grant over a five-year period. Financial support is also available from various agencies of the United Nations and the World Health Organization, as well as the European Commission.

Private and public firms also contribute to HIV/AIDS–related expenditures in several different ways. These may include provision of funds for health care, HIV prevention, and health promotion programs. The precise way in which these funds are spent may vary across firms: whether health services are provided directly by firms through their own facilities, by contribution to premiums of insurance companies, by contracting with outside providers (private or nongovernmental), or by including a lump-sum amount in salaries. Firms may also pay for funeral expenses of employees (or their dependents), and that could also be included as an expenditure under the category of "management" of HIV/AIDS. The Nigerian Institute of Social and Economic Research (NISER) estimates a total of about 574 small, medium, and large firms, both public and private, in Oyo and Plateau states.

Finally, contributions are also likely from faith-based organizations and other NGOs, from their own sources of funds. These contributions may take the form of provision of free and/or subsidized prevention and treatment services; legal assistance to PLWHAs; or care and support for orphans and families affected by HIV/AIDS. It is well known that "mission" health facilities are a major provider of health services in Nigeria—indeed, the NHA study by Soyibo et al. suggests that 10% to 12% of all health spending in Nigeria is directed toward services provided by NGOs and mission facilities in Nigeria (16). We could not access data on the number of mission facilities, or their number of beds, or their personnel strength. However, the NACA website suggests that at least 20 NGOs are involved in HIV/AIDS prevention and care/support work in Plateau and Oyo states; their true number may actually be even higher.

Several of the entities that serve as sources of funds also enter the fray as financial intermediaries in the flow of funds associated with the HIV/AIDS epidemic. Specifically, within the government at the federal level, the ministries of defense, education, health, internal affairs, women's affairs, and labor function as intermediaries in the sense that the Ministry of Finance serves as the ultimate source of their funding. Many of these ministries are likely to be involved in HIV/AIDS-related activities by means of the health care that they provide through their own facilities, or education programs that they fund. The same should be true for state government ministries, especially health, education, labor, and women's affairs. In addition, action committees on AIDS at the national level (NACA), at the state level (SACAs), and the local level (LACAs) are involved in AIDS activities and channel funds for this purpose, whether from the federal government or international sources, although they themselves may not have any independent funding source.

When firms provide subsidized services through their own facilities, they are also acting as intermediaries. Similarly, NGO operations that involve the provision of subsidized services, or reimbursements, essentially describe NGOs in their role as financial intermediaries.

Finally, when households end up paying providers with out-of-pocket payments, they are acting in their capacity as financial intermediaries. In this connection, when payments by households are reimbursed by firms, the government, or insurance companies, it is these entities (and not the households) that are characterized as financial intermediaries. When using household survey data to calculate out-of-pocket payments, such reimbursements are deducted from household accounts and attributed as payments made to providers by the party that reimburses the household.

The end-target of financial flows is providers of various services associated with HIV/AIDS. As Table 22-2 indicates, the list of providers could be public, private for profit, or private not for profit, including faith-based organizations. International organizations could also be recipients of funding flows, if they undertake research (such as the POLICY Project, or the Harvard School of Public Health), or provide services such as technical help in administering ARVs.

Geographic Coverage

The present study of health spending on HIV/AIDS in Nigeria was limited to two out of the 36 Nigerian states — Plateau and Oyo. The primary reasons for limiting the analysis to two states were the extremely limited financial resources available to carry out the analysis and the fact that APIN has ongoing projects in these two states, which we believed would facilitate data collection. In addition, Plateau State has an estimated HIV infection rate among adults that is higher than the national average, whereas Oyo State has an estimated HIV infection rate that is somewhat lower than the national average, so together these two states might be taken as reasonably representative of the state of affairs in Nigeria.

Sources of Data and Data Limitations

In principle, a wide variety of sources of data were available to undertake this analysis. Table 22-3 indicates some of the major sources of data that the team expected to be able to use for the purpose of undertaking the study.

In practice, however, accessing financial flows linked to AIDS in the data described in Table 22-3 proved to be extremely difficult. In particular, HIV/AIDS–related data from government sources — be it NACA, the Federal Ministry of Health, or any of the other federal ministries — was either inaccessible or unavailable in a form immediately suited to the construction of expenditure flows using an NHA methodology. Some limited information on HIV/AIDS–related funding provided by international fund-

Table 22-3. Main Identified Sources of Data for National AIDS Accounts Work for Plateau and Oyo States, Nigeria		
Government	**Private Sector**	**International**
Federal Government of Nigeria • Approved budget of the Federal Republic of Nigeria • Report of the Accountant General of the Federation • Federal Office of Statistics • Reports and expenditure data from the National Action Committee on AIDS, Ministry of Defense, Ministry of Education, Ministry of Internal Affairs, Ministry of Women's Affairs, and Planning Commission **Governments of Plateau and Oyo States** • Approved budgets of state governments • Reports of the Accountant General of States • State statistical offices • Reports and expenditure data from state action committees on AIDS and various ministries • In-depth interviews with government representatives **Local Government** • Approved budgets of local governments • Report of the auditor generals of local governments • Reports and expenditure data from the local action committees on AIDS • In-depth interviews with government representatives	*Private Employers* • Records of the organized private sector associations (e.g., Nigerian Association of Chambers of Commerce) • Interviews and surveys of a sample of large and small firms *Insurers* • Surveys of insurance companies and health maintenance organizations *Households* • Surveys of AIDS patients and their families • Household health care utilization and expenditure surveys • Expert assessments of utilization and unit costs of care *Care Providers* • Provider (facilities) survey • Interviews with staff at selected facilities	• Interviews/surveys of donor agencies • Records of the National Action Committee on AIDS • Annual reports/ audited accounts of nongovernmental organizations/missions • Federal Ministry of Finance data

ing agencies was available from various published sources, although again not in a form that would have allowed for detailed breakdowns of expenditures by use. Repeated efforts by NISER to obtain detailed data from NACA and the international funding agencies did not prove very effective. We were able, though, to obtain health budget data for Oyo State; the state hospital management board that operates health facilities; and the Oyo Ministry of Health, which undertakes surveillance, research, training provision, and oversight activities. We were also able to obtain some information from the SACAs in Oyo and Plateau states.

The research team believed that LACAs and local governments were unlikely to be sources of significant financial information. Given the limited financial resources at hand to collect data, the following strategy was adopted: to estimate financial flows by undertaking sample surveys of different non-government entities and to infer at least some of the government and international agency contributions indirectly, from data derived from the surveys; data from other, independent studies that provided information on the cost of provision of HIV/AIDS–related services, whether government or other; and, when possible, Web searches.

Survey and Interview Data

Table 22-4 summarizes the total number of households surveyed and interviews with other entities that were undertaken for this report. Our surveys sampled six sets of respondents: general households (HIV status unknown); households with at least one member known to be infected with HIV; public and private firms; health care providers; NGOs; and insurance companies. We collected general household samples from four local government areas in each state, two predominantly urban and two predominantly rural.[4] We chose the local government areas to be as representative of the state as possible, but it was not random. At least one of the urban areas was the capital of the state.

The methods for sampling entities other than general households differed slightly from those mentioned earlier. All insurance companies operating in the states were sampled, and the sample of firms was obtained by randomly selecting from a sampling frame available with NISER. Major NGOs (excluding mission health facilities) working on HIV/AIDS in the two states were purposively sampled.

The data from firms, insurance com-

Table 22-4. Basic Information on Sample Surveys/Interviews

Population Surveyed	Sample Size	
	Oyo State	Plateau State
Enterprises	47	26
• State owned or parastatal	8	5
• Private (multinational)	38(3)	19(2)
• Other/not recorded	1	2
Insurance Companies	20	11
• State owned or parastatal	2	1
• Private	17	9
• Other/not recorded	1	1
Health Care Providers	42	20
• Private (non-traditional)	26	15
• Private (traditional)	2	0
• Public	6	2
• NGO	1	2
• Other (not specified)	7	1
Households (General)	591	409
• Individuals		
Households (with HIV)	161	322
• Individuals		
NGOs	3	6
• Faith based	1	6
• Women's groups	1	0
• Domestic	1	2

Abbreviation: NGO: nongovernmental organization

panies, and NGOs (including providers) yielded information on expenditures incurred on HIV/AIDS—related activities undertaken by these entities and the ways these expenditures were financed. Information from general household surveys yielded data on the health care utilization patterns in the general population, not necessarily associated with HIV/AIDS. Additional information was derived from surveys of PLWHAs, who were accessed through NGOs. Because of this procedure, we suspect that our survey of PLWHAs over-sampled HIV-positive individuals at an advanced enough stage of disease to need care—thereby biasing our results toward greater health care use and expenditures among PLWHAs than the average individual with HIV. Given our concern with expenditures on health care linked to HIV status, this is on its face a desirable outcome. On the other hand, it would have been incorrect to scale our sample-based per capita estimates of expenditures on HIV/AIDS—related care by the estimated numbers of HIV-positive people in each state to

---

[4]There are 32 local government areas in Oyo State and 17 local government areas in Plateau State (http://nigerianembassy-argentina.org/government/xstates.shtml).

obtain aggregates at the state level. To account for this possibility, we scaled up our estimates with the help of the UNAIDS estimate of roughly 520,000 adults with advanced HIV infection for all of Nigeria (17).

Details on Methodology

Households

We used household survey data on PLWHAs to obtain information on out-of-pocket spending on inpatient and outpatient care and by type of health facility or source (public, private, nongovernmental, traditional care providers, and pharmacies); expenditures incurred on drugs; the use of inpatient days in public, private, and mission facilities by PLWHAs; the proportion of out-of-pocket spending that employers and insurance companies reimbursed; and any support received from relatives and members of the community at large, including NGOs.

International Donors

We had access to aggregate resources allocated to HIV/AIDS in Nigeria by several — though by no means all — of the major international agencies: DFID; the Gates Foundation through APIN; the Global Fund for AIDS, Tuberculosis and Malaria; UNAIDS; UNICEF; the United Nations Development Program (UNDP); USAID; and The World Bank (18–21). Given our exclusion of other funding agencies, our analysis potentially underestimates donor contributions to HIV/AIDS in Nigeria, and by implication, Oyo and Plateau states. A bias may also have arisen in the other direction, however, since not all donors operate in all states. Unfortunately, except for World Bank, Global Fund, and Gates Foundation funding, our information on donor contributions specific to Oyo and Plateau states for HIV/AIDS was limited. Another issue that had to be resolved was the fact that aggregate funding data as officially reported cover several years and thus the expenditure for 2004 had to be isolated for Oyo and Plateau states.

For the World Bank, we disentangled year-by-year allocations and their use for: (a) capacity building in NACA, SACA, and governments; (b) support for prevention interventions in ministries; and (c) an HIV/AIDS intervention fund for NGOs to undertake HIV prevention work for Oyo and Plateau states based on the World Bank (21). It was assumed that all funds in categories (a)-(b) were provided to the government (federal, state, and local taken in the aggregate), which then allocated the funds to appropriate providers for capacity development and prevention activity. Unfortunately, further breakdown by type of provider was not possible in the absence of additional information and we did not attempt to do so. For (c) all funds were assumed to be allocated to NGOs, which were then allocated to activities based on information from the NGO survey. Given that APIN funding was US$25 million over a period of years, we assumed that US$5 million was spent in 2004, divided equally between the four states in which APIN was active in 2004 — so Oyo and Plateau received US$2.5 million. These funds were allocated to different providers and uses based on a formula that relied on surveys of NGOs.

Detailed information on Global Fund expenditures for 2004 was obtained from original grant documents on the Global Fund website (22). The grantee agency (NACA in two cases, and a NGO on the other) were taken as the original recipient of funds, and allocations to Oyo and Plateau states were taken as proportional to the share of Oyo and Plateau states in the number of advanced HIV cases among adults in Nigeria. The grant documents also offered some information on the type of uses to which chunks of grant money were likely to be put—capacity building for treatment and treatment support (we assumed this to be equal parts capacity building and treatment support); capacity building for PMTCT and PMTCT support (assumed to be equal parts capacity building and HIV prevention); and NGO coordination (assumed to be divided up as per NGO survey data).

USAID funds for 2004 were allocated to prevention and policy and strategy development heads based on details provided to USAID (20). Prevention funds were allocated to NGOs and the government (a share of half was assumed for both) and policy and strategy funds solely to the government. Again, because detailed breakdown of allocations by state was unavailable, allocations to Oyo and Plateau states were taken as proportional to the share of Oyo and Plateau states in the number of advanced HIV cases among adults in Nigeria. We would be overestimating allocations to Oyo and Plateau states if USAID does not work in these two states. Finally, allocations by recipient NGOs to providers and specific uses were based on the NGO survey and all of the government allocations were assumed to go for capacity building and strategy development.

Because DFID committed roughly US$130 million over eight years, we assumed an equal amount was spent each year—or US$16.25 million—with allocations to Oyo and Plateau states taken as proportional to the share of these two states in the number of advanced HIV cases among adults in Nigeria. Then, based on DFID (18) and UNAIDS (17), 60% of these funds were assumed to be allocated to NGOs and 40% to the government for strategy development and capacity-building work. Subsequent allocations to providers were made on the basis of the procedures described previously. Finally, all UN agency funds were allocated to the government, or prevention or capacity building work as outlined in UNAIDS (17).

Firms and Other Enterprises

Information on HIV/AIDS–related expenditures of enterprises came from two sources. The first was the household survey that provided data on whether households used employer-owned facilities, any out-of-pocket payments incurred on the use of these facilities, and reimbursements for any household out-of-pocket spending by enterprises. The second source was a survey of 70 small, medium, and large enterprises in Oyo and Plateau states in which we obtained information on the health expenditures incurred on employer-financed own facilities, employer-financed off-site facilities, payment for insurance premiums, reimbursements for out-of-pocket expenditures incurred by employees, and medical allowances included in salaries. The survey of enterprises also provided us with information on whether the firms excluded HIV-positive individuals from any of their health benefits, any preventive expenditures incurred by them, and any financial support from the government and external agencies for HIV-related expenditures.

The enterprise survey data provided us with evidence that not all firms support PLWHAs and that some private sector firms do not offer any health benefits. We assumed that the proportion of firms' employees with advanced HIV was the same as the adults in the general population. This could be biased upward since our survey suggests that many firms discriminate against PLWHAs and may not employ them. Per-employee spending was then allocated to employees with and without HIV, on the assumption that per-episode treatment costs for the latter were half those for employees with HIV. Finally, per-employee treatment costs by type of expenditure—such as employer facilities, offsite facilities, reimbursements, and premiums—were scaled up by using state-level data on the number of small, medium, and large firms in Oyo and Plateau, assuming that the average number of employees in the population of firms was the same as the sample average.

While many firms reported incurring self-financed expenditure on prevention programs, none responded to the corresponding question on the amount spent. Our estimates of HIV/AIDS expenditures do not include the amounts spent by firms, and thus are an underestimate of the true level of prevention expenditures. This is obviously an area in which further research could be useful.

Nongovernmental Organizations and Mission Health Facilities
Household surveys provided us with information on the use of mission health facilities by households and any out-of-pocket charges for the use of these facilities. In addition, a separate survey of nine NGOs provided us with information on expenditures on prevention activities (information, education, and communication programs, STI interventions, condom distribution, interventions targeted to high-risk groups, and media campaigns) and care/support and treatment (home-based care, legal support, income support, nutrition interventions, and treatment). Although we had information on the activities these NGOs were involved in, some did not report the actual amounts they spent. For NGOs undertaking an activity that did not report a corresponding amount, the missing amount was taken as being equal to the average for all organizations reporting undertaking it in the survey, after adjusting for employee strength. With these adjustments, the total spending of our sample NGOs on HIV/AIDS work amounted to about 70 million naira. Because this was only a small proportion of the total estimated funding to NGOs from donors and other sources, we scaled up total NGO spending to be equal to its incoming financial resources. However, these resources were assumed to be spent on activities in the proportions reported in the sample. We aggregated these expenditure categories into broadly three—prevention, care/support, and treatment—because we did not have such detailed information for any other agency or category. About 6% of all expenditures were allocated to treatment by NGOs, with the remainder to prevention and care/support activities in the ratio of 1:2.

We used information on the relative magnitude of the different sources of financing in the NGO survey, coupled with international donor allocations to NGOs, to derive the contributions of the government and user fee revenues. These were relatively small, as most of the NGO revenue sources appear to have been international donors—nearly 90%. User fee revenues were assumed to be from treatment services.

We also estimated any subsidies provided by mission facilities to individuals obtaining care. These subsidies were estimated as the difference of the cost of providing services *less* any facility charges reported as having been paid. The latter was obtained from household survey data. The former was estimated as being as the same as the cost of equivalent service provided in government facilities, calculated by the methods indicated later. We estimated these subsidies for PLWHAs to be roughly on the order of 50% of total treatment costs.

Drug Expenditures

We obtained estimates of drug spending from information provided in the household survey and contributions to ARV costs of the government. In our analysis, the estimated drug spending is closer to 30% of total spending, and possibly even higher if the cost of drugs used in public facilities—but not paid for by the general public—is considered. Our estimates are consistent with drug spending observed elsewhere in Africa, ranging from 30 to 70% of total health spending (23).

Government Spending

It proved difficult to reconstruct government spending associated with HIV/AIDS given the lack of complete information at the federal and local levels, and state government health spending data from only Oyo State. We did manage, however, to reconstruct some elements of this spending. First, we assessed the amounts allocated by the federal government to ARVs and associated delivery expenses in 2004 at about 1.5 billion naira (24). Based on additional information on the location of sites where the subsidized ARVs were provided to PLWHAs (2 out of the 25 sites were located in Oyo and Plateau states), and assuming equal allocations to all sites, we obtained estimates of federal ARV funding for Oyo and Plateau states. Since at least part of this spending was recouped by user fees, we estimated the federal government contribution to ARV provision to be the amounts spent *less* estimated user fees.

Information on another component of federal government spending on HIV/AIDS in Nigeria was obtained from World Bank documents that allocated some funds (16% of total approved funding on HIV/AIDS in World Bank to the federal government, including various federal ministries) (21). Moreover, the government was expected to contribute some matching funds (about 6.7% of the World Bank contribution) to HIV/AIDS activities as part of the some project. The corresponding federal "allocations" to Oyo and Plateau states were taken as proportional to the share of Oyo and Plateau states in the number of advanced HIV cases among adults in Nigeria. Moreover, the expenditures were assumed to be on the items identified under the World Bank project in the same proportion as identified in the project document. Given the nature of our calculations, it is possible that some spending incurred by the federal government is not captured by the above data. That would downwardly bias our calculations for Oyo and Plateau states, but only if some of this omitted spending could be considered as effectively being directed at these two states.

To estimate the allocations for the two state governments for HIV/AIDS we proceeded as follows. First we considered the amounts allocated by the Oyo State government to its state hospital management board, which operates government health facilities there. Correspondingly, we used the household survey to estimate the number of inpatient stays and outpatient visits by people with and without HIV at public facilities in Oyo State. Using the assumption that each outpatient visit is one-tenth the cost of an inpatient stay and that people with advanced HIV disease cost twice as much as people without HIV for a given visit or stay, we assessed that PLWHAs accounted for about 5.7% of all hospital spending in Oyo State. We validated this assumption first by comparing expenditures per visit or stay for people with and without HIV who sought care at private facilities. We also confirmed it by estimating a simple hospital cost function for a sample of health facilities that we surveyed as part of this exercise.

Table 22-5. Spending on HIV/AIDS in Oyo and Plateau States: Sources to Financing Agents (Naira/Millions)

	Government	Firms	Donors	Mission/NGO	HH (S)	HH (O)	Total
Government Ministries	236.91–470.29		537.92				774.83–1008.21
Firms		13.98					13.98
Insurance Companies		0.07					0.07
Mission/NGO	56.23		653.84	25.92			735.99
Households		15.24			790.28	207.14	1012.66
Total	293.13	29.29	1191.76	25.92	790.28	207.14	2537.52–2770.91

Source: Authors' calculations
Note: HH (S) means households with HIV-infected members who spend on their own care; HH (O) are households in the community, not necessarily with HIV-infected members, that support the health expenditures of HIV-positive individuals.

This exercise yielded the per stay/visit cost for people with and without advanced HIV disease, which we used to construct estimates of state government health spending for Plateau State using household survey data on public facility use and assumptions about the number of PLWHAs. To these we also added a share of Ministry of Health expenditures, which are not reflected in facility costs but should be considered as a sort of overhead expense in providing state-level health services. We used government expenditures *less* facility charges to define the net contribution of the government at the state level.

Even with this exercise, three issues were left unresolved. First, our household survey–based user charge estimates for Oyo are 70 times higher than reported in the state government budget, similar to the findings of Soyibo et al. (16). There is no easy way to resolve this anomaly unless there is some combination of unrecorded revenues, bribes paid at the level of the facility, or recall bias among household survey respondents. If the funding was in the form of bribes, then subtracting out-of-pocket payments from government expenditures to get at *net* government financial contributions is obviously incorrect, because it would downwardly bias our estimates of this contribution. Thus, we presented a *range* of estimates to reflect this uncertainty about the nature of out-of-pocket payments by households. Second, we do not consider expenditures of local governments, and to that extent, our HIV/AIDS expenditure estimates in Oyo and Plateau states are downwardly biased. Third, we are unable to account for government spending on orphans and care/support except to the extent that it is already accounted for through government-funded NGO providers of services. To fill these gaps with more careful government expenditure analysis is an obvious topic for future research in Nigeria.

FINDINGS AND DISCUSSION

Tables 22-5 and 22-6 contain our main findings. First, we estimate that Oyo and Plateau states spent between 2.54 billion and 2.77 billion naira on prevention, management, and treatment associated with HIV/AIDS during 2004. Based on our previous discussion, this range is a lower bound to the true levels of HIV/AIDS–related spending in these two states. Household out-of-pocket spending on HIV/AIDS in

	Government	Firms	Insurance	NGO	Households	Total
Treatment						
Public Facilities	27.67-261.05			3.43	233.38	497.86
Private Facilities		9.70	0.07	7.97	55.99	73.73
Traditional Care				1.44	16.18	17.62
Firms' Facilities		4.28			0.00	4.28
Pharmacies	105.6				481.76	587.36
NGO/Mission Facilities				36.36	36.48	72.84
Laboratories and Other					148.22	148.22
Prevention Service Providers	331.40			236.50		567.90
Care and Support Providers				450.29		450.29
Overheads	94.05					94.05
Strategy/Capacity	216.11				40.64	256.76
TOTAL	774.83-1008.21	13.98	0.07	735.98	1012.66	2537.52-2770.91

Source: Authors' calculations
Note: HH (S) means households with HIV-infected members who spend on their own care; HH (O) are households in the community, not necessarily with HIV-infected members, that support the health expenditures of HIV-positive individuals.

Oyo and Plateau states amounted to approximately 4% of overall out-of-pocket spending on all health services by the population in these two states.

Second, our analysis suggests that 36% to 39% of all spending on HIV/AIDS–related services was incurred by households, 43% to 47% by international donors, and 12% to 19% by the government (Figure 22-1). Firms and NGOs contributed roughly equal shares—about 1% of total spending—on HIV/AIDS. By way of comparison, the results of the NHA analysis that Soyibo et al. conducted on the overall health spending in Nigeria suggest a contribution of 22% for the government, 66% for households, 6% for international donors, and 6% for firms (Figure 22-2) (16). Our results for HIV/AIDS spending also differ from calculations that we separately carried out to estimate the major sources of overall health spending (both HIV- and non-HIV related) in Oyo and Plateau states. Those results, which are described in Figure 22-3, suggest that 69% of all health spending in these two states was incurred by households, 21% by the government, 6% by firms, and 4% by donors.[5] This points to how substantially different financing for HIV/AIDS is from other classes of health spending in Nigeria.

It is also interesting to note that our estimates of the share of out-of-pocket spending on HIV/AIDS expenditures in Oyo and Plateau states lie well between the range of estimates reported for Central

[5]Details on the methods used for estimating overall health spending in Oyo and Plateau states can be obtained from the authors upon request.

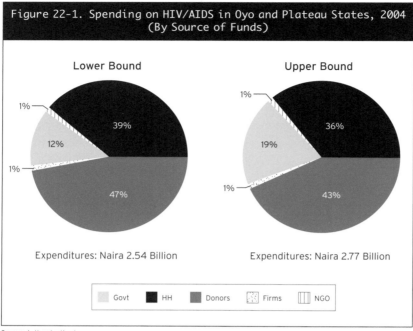

Figure 22-1. Spending on HIV/AIDS in Oyo and Plateau States, 2004 (By Source of Funds)

Lower Bound

39%
12%
1%
1%
1%
47%

Expenditures: Naira 2.54 Billion

Upper Bound

36%
19%
1%
1%
43%

Expenditures: Naira 2.77 Billion

Govt | HH | Donors | Firms | NGO

Source: Authors' estimates
Abbreviations: HH: households; NGO: nongovernmental organization

and South America (14). However, our estimates of the share of external contributions to HIV/AIDS spending are higher than average for SIDALAC countries. The only countries with a comparable share of external donor spending on HIV/AIDS in Latin America are Bolivia and Nicaragua, both of which are tiny compared to Nigeria.

A third major observation with regard to our analysis is the significance of HIV/AIDS–related drug expenditures that amount to 21% to 23% of overall HIV/AIDS spending and nearly 48% of out-of-pocket spending by households on HIV/AIDS services. One can imagine the share could become even higher if the HIV/AIDS epidemic worsens in the future and Nigeria's needs with respect to ARVs increase. Our estimates of drug shares are higher than those reported by Soyibo et al. (16), in which drug expenditures amounted to roughly about 13% of total spending. Because the Soyibo et al. study looked at all health spending and was not restricted to HIV/AIDS, our findings would suggest that drug expenditures account for a greater share of HIV/AIDS–related spending than for health services on average.

Fourth, estimates presented in Table 22-5 suggest that nearly 48% to 52% of all spending was directed to treatment, 20% to 22% to prevention, and 16% to 18% to care and support, perhaps pointing to a greater need to address HIV prevention in Nigeria. These estimates, however, need to be treated with caution because they exclude expenditures for prevention that households might already be incurring—such as for condom purchases or STI treatment. For instance, Nigerians currently use about 68 million condoms annually (25). Assuming a uniform distribution of condom use across the population, this translates into about 5.17 million condoms used annually in Oyo and Plateau states. Assuming an average payment for a condom of about 25 cents (or 35 naira), we get estimated out-of-pocket expenditures of 180 million naira for preventive action. Including this in our calculations of AIDS expenditures would raise the share of preventive spending to 25% to 28% and lower the share of expenditures and care/support to 45% to 49% and 15% to 17%, respectively. Unfortunately, our household survey estimates of STI cases were too low to allow for reliable estimates of STI treatment expenditures to be made at the state level. Estimates for Latin America, however, suggest that STI treatment expenditures tend to be small as a proportion of total spending on

HIV/AIDS, so excluding this category of expenditures should not affect our findings significantly (14).

Fifth, it is worth noting the relatively small role of formal insurance mechanisms such as insurance in financing HIV/AIDS–related health spending in Oyo and Plateau states, and the somewhat greater role of informal "mechanisms" such as relatives and the community at large, whose contributions to expenditures incurred by PLWHAs accounted for approximately 20% of household out-of-pocket spending and 8% of all health spending (Tables 22-5 and 22-6). While informal insurance is clearly better than no insurance at all, it may not be as efficient as formal pooling mechanisms that may be able to obtain better prices for health care in the marketplace.

It is worth noting that our estimates on the role of formal insurance in HIV/AIDS spending differ from the estimated expenditures supported by data in available NHAs for Nigeria (16). Given that Lagos State accounts for more than 75% of all health insurance enrollment in Nigeria, this should not be surprising. This finding is also consistent with data from our surveys that show that private insurance plays an insignificant role in protecting people in Oyo and Plateau states against the financial risk associated with ill health. It is possible that respondents missed insurance company payments for health services. In the case of households, this is understandable since such payments would not be reflected in out-of-pocket payments. In the case of firms too, such payments are unlikely to be reported, although ordinarily one would expect this to be reflected in premium payments for employees, unless most of it is paid by employees.

We sought to assess the implications of the possibility of data omissions with regard to insurance coverage. For this purpose, we used the results of a survey of all insurance companies (31 in total) with business in Oyo and Plateau states. Most of these companies offered general, life, and

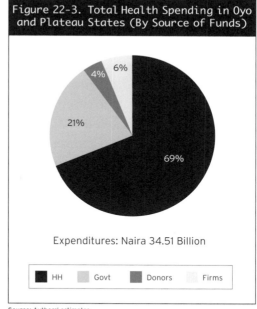

Figure 22-2. Total Health Expenditures in Nigeria, 2002 (By Source of Funds)

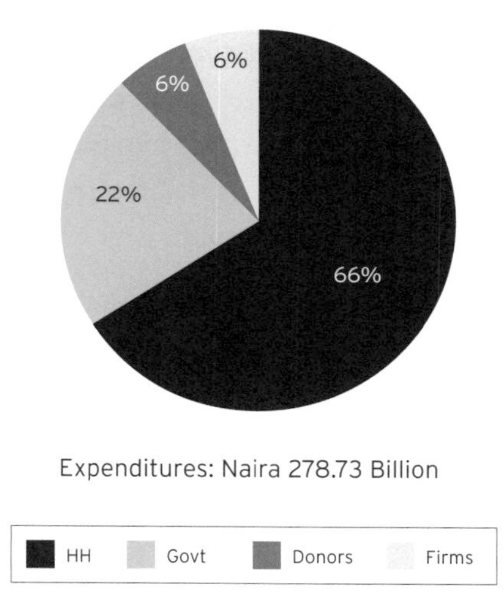

6%
6%
22%
66%

Expenditures: Naira 278.73 Billion

■ HH   Govt   ■ Donors   Firms

Source: Soyibo A, Odumosu O, Ladejobi F, Lawanson A, Oladejo B, Alayande S. National Health Accounts of Nigeria, 1998-2002. Draft report submitted to the World Health Organization. Ibadan, Nigeria: University of Ibadan, 2005.

Figure 22-3. Total Health Spending in Oyo and Plateau States (By Source of Funds)

4%
6%
21%
69%

Expenditures: Naira 34.51 Billion

■ HH   Govt   ■ Donors   Firms

Source: Authors' estimates

health insurance. The survey responses of insurance companies were plagued by substantial non-response and some doubt remains as to whether these companies provided us with data on premium income for all of Nigeria, or only for the two states of interest. Ignoring these concerns for the moment, we estimated that the entire group of companies had a total premium income from all of their business of about 15 billion naira annually. Only two of these companies responded to our queries about payments made directly to health care providers, and those estimates suggest that such payments accounted for about 10% of the premium income.

Using this proportion for all the insurance companies, we estimated the total direct payments made by insurance companies to health care providers in Oyo and Plateau states at 1.5 billion naira. That would amount to roughly 100 million naira in payments for PLWHAs based on assumptions underlying calculations made earlier in this chapter. Including these amounts in Tables 22-5 and 22-6 would, of course, raise our estimates of total spending on HIV/AIDS–related services by 4%, and the share of treatment to 50% to 54%. Including both the estimated condom expenditures by households and the direct payments by insurance companies would not change the shares of respective providers by much in Table 22-6. What would change, however, is the role of formal insurance in providing risk protection to households affected by HIV —with claim payments amounting to about 10% of out-of-pocket spending incurred by households.

CONCLUSION

The estimates reported in this chapter are possibly crude approximations of the extent of spending associated with HIV/AIDS in Nigeria. Our analysis is based on only two states for Nigeria and our data are relatively incomplete even to permit a full-fledged application of the NHA framework for the calculation of expenditures on HIV/AIDS care programs in even these two states. Furthermore, there are *prima facie* important areas where the differing results between our analysis and that of Soyibo et al. need to be sorted out (16). These are obviously fruitful areas for further work. They also imply that any guidance for policy in Nigeria emerging from this work must be treated with careful regard of the data gaps that currently exist on financing of HIV/AIDS in the country.

At the same time, several conclusions can be readily drawn if policymakers are concerned about developing sustainable policy action aimed at halting the spread of HIV and ameliorating its subsequent implications for poverty. First, HIV imposes a significant financial burden on Nigerian households. This is being ameliorated at least partially by contributions from the community at large, public sector subsidies on drugs, and, depending on the data, formal insurance. If the HIV epidemic were to expand significantly in Nigeria, however, it is unlikely that other households and the general community would be able to keep up with this level of support. Thus other resource-pooling mechanisms may have to be considered—including implementing with renewed vigor the much-delayed National Health Insurance Scheme. Promoting income generation among poor Nigerians would increase their ability to pay for services, but would not affect the inefficiency of resource use for health care that would require bulk purchasing of services.

Second, extending treatment to everyone who needs treatment will impose a significant financial burden on the government should it decide to do so. We illustrate this by the following calculation. Suppose that the government were to extend treatment to all of the roughly 36,000 people (about 7% of the estimated 520,000 people in Nigeria) who likely need such care in Oyo and Plateau estimates. That may amount to a nearly 30-fold increase in the ARV budget currently being allocated to these two states based on our estimate of 1,200 people currently receiving such treatment. A key message in our chapter is the need to make explicit and integrate into public expenditure frameworks the incremental resource requirements for AIDS therapy.

Third, the financial implications of extending treatment mean that attention to preventive measures will be crucial. A potentially effective way to do this would be by promoting condom use. According to one estimate, only 6% of the 989 million risky sexual interactions annually in Nigeria are intermediated by condom use. Assuming away, for the moment, the challenge of devising an effective strategy to promote condom use, extending condom coverage to even 50% of the risky sexual transactions would imply an increase in resources devoted to condom purchases by 700%! Taking the figure of 180 million naira derived in the previous section as an estimate of the current condom expenditures on Nigeria, this would mean an additional amount of resources—1.36 billion naira—devoted to this purpose. Of course, any advocacy or mass media campaigns required to achieve behavior change will require extra funds.

Finally, there is the issue of sustainability. Our data suggest a significant role for external funding, be it for treatment, care and support, or prevention. Given that such aid is not guaranteed forever, at some point the various levels of governments in Nigeria will face an even greater financial burden as aid agencies withdraw. Early action and possibly even greater efforts by the government to focus on prevention now may help address this concern, when later the government may have to deal with donor fatigue, a greatly expanded HIV epidemic, and much higher funding needs.

ACKNOWLEDGMENTS

We are grateful to a number of individuals and institutions for their encouragement, comments, and material help in undertaking this work. We are especially thankful to Professor Phyllis Kanki, Dr. Soji Adeyi, and Dr. Wole Odutolu of APIN and Professor Michael Reich of the Harvard School of Public Health. At NISER we greatly benefited from the guidance and advice of Dr. D. O. Ajakaiye, Dr. A. Sunmola, Ms. Nancy Nelson-Twakor, Mr. L. N. Chete, and Mr. A. O. Ajala. Dr. A. O. Okesola of the Oyo State AIDS Control Programme and Mr. Bala Mitok Rumtong of the Plateau State AIDS Control Programme provided us with access to data on HIV/AIDS expenditures. Seminar participants at Harvard and NISER provided several useful comments that benefited this study.

REFERENCES

1. Bloom D, Mahal A, Rosenberg L, Sevilla J, Weston W. *Asia's Economies and the Challenge of AIDS*. Manila: The Asian Development Bank, 2004.

2. Berman P. National Health Accounts in developing countries: appropriate methods and recent applications. *Health Econ*, 1997;6:1.

3. Viravaidya M, Obremsky S, Myers C. The economic impact of AIDS in Thailand. In: Bloom D, Lyons J, eds. *Economic Implications of AIDS in Asia*. New Delhi: Oxford University Press, 1993.

4. Bloom D, Mahal A, Christiansen L, et al. Socio-economic dimensions of the HIV/AIDS epidemic in Sri Lanka. In: Bloom D, Godwin P, eds. *The Economics of AIDS*. New Delhi: Oxford University Press, 1997.

5. Odumosu K, Adedoyin Soyibo A, Mahal A. *Plan of Action for a HIV/AIDS Accounts for Nigeria.* Ibadan: AIDS Prevention Initiative in Nigeria and Nigerian Institute of Social and Economic Research, 2002.

6. Pothisiri P, Tangcharoensathien V, Lertiendumrong J, Hanvoravongchai P. *Funding Priorities for the HIV/AIDS Crisis in Thailand.* Geneva: UNAIDS, 1998.

7. Ernberg G, Opuni M, Schwartlander B, Walker N. Level and flow of national and international resources for the response to HIV/AIDS, 1996–97. Draft Report. Boston, Massachusetts: Harvard School of Public Health, 1999.

8. Shepard D. Levels and determinants of expenditures on HIV/AIDS in five developing countries. In: Ainsworth M, Fransen L, Over M, eds. *Confronting AIDS: Evidence from the Developing World.* Washington, DC: World Bank, 1998.

9. Kone T, Silue A, Agness-Soumaharo J, Bail R, Shepard D. Expenditures on AIDS in Cote d'Ivoire. In: Ainsworth M, Fransen L, Over M, eds. *Confronting AIDS: Evidence from the Developing World.* Washington, DC: World Bank, 1998.

10. Izazola J-A, Saavedra J, Prottas J, Shepard D. Expenditures on the treatment and prevention of HIV/AIDS in Mexico. In: Ainsworth M, Fransen L, Over M, eds. *Confronting AIDS: Evidence from the Developing World.* Washington, DC: World Bank, 1998.

11. Iunes R, Campino A, Prottas J, Shepard D. Expenditures on HIV/AIDS in the state of Sao Paulo, Brazil. In: Ainsworth M, Fransen L, Over M, eds. *Confronting AIDS: Evidence from the Developing World.* Washington, DC: World Bank, 1998.

12. Tibandebage P, Wangwe S, Mujinja P, Bail R, Shepard D. Expenditures on HIV/AIDS in Tanzania. In: Ainsworth M, Fransen L, Over M, eds. *Confronting AIDS: Evidence from the Developing World.* Washington, DC: World Bank, 1998.

13. Kongsin S, Cameron C, Suebsaeng L, Shepard D. Levels and determinants of expenditure on HIV/AIDS in Thailand. In: Ainsworth M, Fransen L, Over M, eds. *Confronting AIDS: Evidence from the Developing World.* Washington, DC: World Bank, 1998.

14. SIDALAC (Regional AIDS Initiative for LAC). Flows of financing and expenditures on HIV/AIDS. *IAEN (International AIDS Economics Network) Annual Conference,* Washington, DC, April 24–25, 2003.

15. Barnett C, Bhawalkar M, Nandakumar AK, Schneider P. *The Application of the National Health Accounts Framework to HIV/AIDS in Rwanda.* Special Initiatives Report No. 31. Bethesda, Maryland: Abt Associates, 2001.

16. Soyibo A, Odumosu O, Ladejobi F, Lawanson A, Oladejo B, Alayande S. National Health Accounts of Nigeria, 1998–2002. Draft report submitted to the World Health Organization. Ibadan, Nigeria: University of Ibadan, 2005.

17. UNAIDS. *Country Situation Analysis: Nigeria.* Geneva: UNAIDS, 2004.

18. Department for International Development. 2004. Nigeria: Country Assistance Plan (CAP) 2004–08. Accessed at www.dfid.gov.uk/pubs/files/nigeria-cap.asp on October 15, 2005.

19. UNAIDS. *Country HIV and AIDS Estimates, End-2003.* Country Reports. Geneva: UNAIDS, 2004.

20. USAID. USAID's Strategy in Nigeria. Accessed at www.usaid.gov/locations/sub-saharan_africa/countries/nigeria on October 15, 2005.

21. World Bank. Project appraisal document on a proposed credit in the amount of SDR 71 million (US$90.3 million equivalent) to the Republic of Nigeria for a HIV/AIDS program development project. Report no. 21457-UNI. Human Development III, Country Department 12, Africa Regional Office. Washington, DC: World Bank, 2001.

22. The Global Fund for AIDS, Tuberculosis and Malaria. *Global Fund Disbursements by Region, Country and Grant Agreement.* Accessed at www.theglobalfund.org/en/files/disbursementdetails.pdf on October 15, 2005.

23. So A. Policies that promote fair pricing of pharmaceuticals. Draft Report. Boston, Massachusetts: Harvard School of Public Health, 1999.

24. Abt Associates, John Snow, Futures Group. *Nigeria: Rapid Assessment of HIV/AIDS Care in the Public and Private Sector.* Bethesda, Maryland: Abt Associates, 2004.

25. POLICY Project. *Coverage of Selected Services for HIV/AIDS Prevention, Care and Support in Low and Middle Income Countries in 2003.* Washington, DC: POLICY Project, 2003.

23

MONITORING AND EVALUATION OF HIV/AIDS IN NIGERIA

Oluwole Odutolu,* Jerome O. Mafeni,†
Prosper Okonkwo,* and Oluwole A. Fajemisin‡

"If you do not measure results, you cannot tell success from failure. If you cannot see success, you cannot reward it. If you cannot reward success, you are probably rewarding failure. If you cannot see success, you cannot learn from it. If you cannot recognize failure, you cannot correct it. If you can demonstrate results, you can win public support."

— DAVID OSBORNE AND TED GAEBLER IN *REINVENTING GOVERNMENT* (ADDISON WESLEY, 1992)

When the HIV epidemic first emerged in Nigeria, little was known about which interventions were likely to slow the spread of the virus. That lack of understanding, coupled with institutional and public denial of the existence of the epidemic, made measuring the success of the limited interventions then available extremely difficult. In Nigeria, as in most of Africa, monitoring and evaluation (M&E) efforts were limited to biological surveillance surveys conducted biennially. As program managers developed second-generation surveillance methodologies, they made halfhearted attempts to conduct behavior surveillance surveys and to evaluate high-risk population groups. Beset as they were with the challenge of mobilizing resources for their interventions, though, these managers failed to place emphasis on monitoring the success of their programs.

*AIDS Prevention Initiative in Nigeria, Abuja, Nigeria
†ENHANSE Project, The Futures Group, Abuja, Nigeria
‡World Health Organization, Minna, Niger State, Nigeria

Until the mid-1990s, most M&E in Nigeria took place in a relatively piecemeal fashion. An HIV surveillance system had been established, but it did not function effectively. Several isolated behavioral studies were conducted using different sampling methods and indicators, and research studies contributed additional information. Unfortunately, results were neither shared nor passed on to a central coordinating system for analysis and use in program planning and policy-making.

Since 2000 this situation has changed considerably. Much more is now known about how HIV spreads through populations and what changes are needed to slow its progression. Political commitment also has increased considerably, and Nigeria now receives substantial resources both from its own public coffers and from bilateral and multilateral donor organizations.

With many HIV/AIDS programs now scaled up, the need to track changes and be able to correlate them with interventions has become even more critical. The National Action Committee on AIDS (NACA) has established an M&E unit, which is appropriately staffed and supported by M&E working groups with membership from key stakeholders. The Federal Ministry of Health also has expanded its Epidemiological Unit for the Health Sector Response to the epidemic to strengthen other M&E elements. Other federal agencies have yet to develop similar M&E structures, however, and state and local governments have yet to establish equivalent structures to monitor and evaluate programs at those levels.

A country risks losing the utility of many of its HIV-related measurements when it lacks a comprehensive M&E system. Such a system confers several key advantages. It contributes to more efficient use of data and resources by ensuring, for example, that indicators and sampling methodologies stay comparable over time. It uncovers information that serves the needs of many constituents, including program managers, researchers, and donors. And it eliminates the need for those constituents to duplicate efforts by repeating baseline surveys and evaluation studies — an especially important asset when resources are scarce.

From the national perspective, a coherent M&E system helps ensure that donor-funded M&E efforts best contribute to national needs rather than simply serving the reporting needs of agencies or legislatures overseas. It also encourages communication among different groups involved in the national response to HIV. Shared planning, execution, analysis, and data dissemination can reduce programmatic overlaps and increase cooperation among the different groups, many of whom may work more efficiently together than in isolation.

The ultimate application of data for program planning and analysis is crucial in any M&E system. Analysts must avoid collecting data that cannot or will not be used. Countries have different M&E needs, dictated by the state of their HIV epidemics, their national response, and their available resources. Yet successful M&E systems share common elements, such as uncovering new information, limiting biases, providing clarity, enabling consensus, and fostering well-reasoned and meaningful actions that have broad-based ownership.

THE ROLE OF M&E IN HIV/AIDS PREVENTION AND CONTROL

In the past, M&E systems were designed to improve health and promote development. They tracked programmatic activity and results, and they allowed program managers to allocate resources wisely to achieve the best possible result.

The HIV epidemic differs from many other health and development issues because of its relative newness and uncertain course. New interventions are constantly proposed, and they must prove effective to justify their incorporation in a national or international response. Operations research can establish the effectiveness of a given intervention, such as sex education in selected high schools to reduce risk behaviors. For a strong national M&E system, though, much more is needed to track more generalized success. In the example of sex education, repeated behavioral surveys among a national sample of high-school students would be needed to reflect changes in risk behavior following the integration of sex education into the nationwide curriculum.

The epidemic itself continues to shift. For years, everyone focused on prevention. As HIV epidemics have turned into AIDS epidemics from one country to another, though, care of the sick and social support to people living with HIV/AIDS and their families have gained in importance. These programs are often both difficult to deliver and expensive. Based on work in South America and Rwanda, for example, the World Bank has estimated the cost of AIDS treatment per person at 1 to 2.7 times a country's per capita gross domestic product. This formula predicts that Nigeria will spend an annual $250 to $675 to care for each person living with HIV/AIDS (1). Monitoring and evaluating the impact of HIV/AIDS programs is critical in ensuring delivery of the best possible services.

HIV is politically charged in most countries. Important religious and political lobbies, along with the general population, may oppose interventions, and top-level decision-makers may therefore be reluctant to tackle the issue, preferring to focus on more politically neutral programs, such as maternal mortality and child nutrition. It is in this context that M&E is perhaps most useful. Only careful measurements of the success of existing initiatives can persuade reluctant policy-makers to expand program efforts.

To gain the public's and politicians' approval for public expenditure on development programs, the evaluation field has adopted performance or results-based M&E. In some countries, such as India, public service performance contracts are being used in government reforms to prove accountability and to learn from the process of project, program, or policy implementation. As a management tool that assesses how outcomes are being achieved over time (2), results-based M&E can:

- Provide crucial information about public sector performance;
- Track the progress of a project, program, or policy;
- Promote credibility and public confidence by reporting on program results;
- Help formulate and justify budget requests;
- Identify potentially promising programs and practices;
- Focus attention on achieving outcomes important to organizations and their stakeholders;
- Provide timely, frequent information to staff;
- Help establish key goals and objectives;
- Permit managers to identify and take action to correct weaknesses; and
- Support a development agenda that is shifting toward greater accountability.

The results-based M&E tool becomes extremely important in tracking an epidemic as dynamic as the HIV one. Both explicitly and implicitly, Nigeria has chosen to use results-based M&E for its national response, as illustrated by the measurable targets it set in its 2003 National Policy on HIV/AIDS and the Nigerian National Response Information Management System.

PROGRAM EXAMPLES FROM NIGERIA

The words "monitoring" and "evaluation" have often been used in HIV/AIDS programming in Nigeria, but there has been little evidence to suggest that M&E data have been used to ensure program accountability and sound decision-making. By 2002, under NACA leadership and with the support of its development partners, particularly UNAIDS, Nigeria undertook the design of a national M&E framework. The process was completed in 2003, with the establishment of the Nigerian National Response Information Management System (NNRIMS) (3). This framework was designed to track performance, provide feedback to program and project management, and ensure accountability based on the HIV/AIDS Emergency Action Plan (HEAP) and more appropriately the new National HIV/AIDS Strategic Framework (4). Thus Nigeria has adopted the principle of "The Three Ones" — one multisectoral coordinating and facilitating body, one national implementation framework, and one M&E framework — as stipulated by UNAIDS (5). Nigeria's M&E systems are thus in their formative stages; but it is imperative to note that the Nigerian multisectoral HIV control program aims to achieve at least a 25% reduction in HIV prevalence every five years (6).

The implication of that goal is that Nigeria should invest in high-impact prevention programs with targeted interventions to high-risk groups such as sex workers, long-distance truck drivers, and high-risk youths. Much can be gained by focusing on youths, for example; from the 2003 survey the highest age-specific prevalence was observed among women aged 20 to 24 years (5.6%) followed by those aged 25 to 29 years (5.4%) (7). Other dividend-yielding interventions include the policy of 100% condom use and peer education among high-risk groups, particularly young people. Such interventions are crucial, especially because each year a new cohort of young people becomes sexually active (8). They can and should be helped to remain HIV free through delay in sexual initiation, decrease in casual sex, and increased condom use (9). Purposive and aggressive programming is needed to diagnose and treat sexually transmitted infections (STIs), prevent mother-to-child transmission of HIV, provide voluntary counseling and testing, and ensure the safety of the blood supply.

Explicitly, Nigeria needs to set priorities and scale up prevention interventions. Critical to the goal of reducing the HIV prevalence rate by 25% are other determinants of incidence, especially those emanating from such structural and environmental factors as poverty, gender inequality, migration, internal displacement, and low levels of education (10). Achieving that goal will also require concerted structural shifts, such as poverty alleviation, gender equality, and a reduction in conflict situations.

It should also be noted that the increased access to antiretrovirals for people living with HIV/AIDS would likely enhance the length and quality of their lives. The implication is that the same group could be tested at several points, and repeated counts will be interpreted as a non-reduction in the prevalence rate. Essential to reducing prevalence, however, is the prevention of new infections and the reduction of incidence rates in both high-risk groups and the general population. To achieve these goals, Nigeria must identify resource needs and be able to mobilize both human and financial resources. Past efforts at resource mobilization produced good results, but more recently Nigeria has not been able to use such funds effectively or efficiently in a timely fashion, such as with the World Bank IDA credit and the Global Fund on AIDS, Tuberculosis and Malaria; donor reluctance may have been an issue here.

Nigeria needs a functional M&E system at national and subnational levels to track implementation and provide results for measuring success. This statement does not suggest that the country had a complete vacuum before; earlier M&E systems, which were largely driven by donors' desires to track their own activities, resulted in a proliferation of M&E indicators. Most of these indicators, however, were not harmonized and standardized for use by all stakeholders. As a result, the various M&E programs could not feed into a national M&E structure (3).

Similarly, nongovernmental organizations (NGOs) have carried out related project evaluation, which usually captures the inputs and outputs of the process rather than the outcome. Experience has shown that NGO projects are so small and fragmented that it is difficult for them to coalesce enough to enable a meaningful, measurable impact on the epidemic. The project evaluation reports are also difficult to account for at the national level. It is therefore important that NACA and other stakeholders consciously embrace the culture of accountability and learning, establish data and data management policies, and build systems of continuous documentation of the country's HIV-related activities.

Program Monitoring and Evaluation

Since 1991, Nigeria has carried out national HIV and syphilis sentinel surveys on a biennial basis. The surveys, based on two important biological markers, are conducted among women attending antenatal clinics in both rural and urban settings in all 36 states. Other evaluation activities based on biological markers include patients attending tuberculosis and STI clinics and high-risk populations such as sex workers, injection drug users, and military personnel. As identified in the NNRIMS, these outcome indicators are important to tracking the epidemic and its impact. Second-generation surveillance surveys—the Youth Behavioral Surveillance Survey, the National HIV/AIDS and Reproductive Health Survey, and the National Demographic and Health Survey (NDHS)—have been conducted to monitor behavior change in the general population and in high-risk groups. These surveys are critical for providing information for the outcome-level behavior indicators.

The NNRIMS identified 21 core outcome indicators, and these surveys have proved their worth by helping to verify 16 of the 21 indicators. The 2003 NDHS, for example, provided information on HIV-related knowledge, attitudes, and beliefs and high-risk sexual encounters that are listed as indicators in the NNRIMS (11). It is important to understand, of course, that there is programmatic information vital to understanding the dynamics of the epidemic that the outcome indicators cannot reveal. Such information can provide answers to observed changes in the trend of the epidemic. It has always been difficult in the Nigerian context, for example, to find evidence-based explanations for changes in prevalence levels from the sentinel surveys. Such ambiguity could result in black-box evaluations where program planners and other stakeholders "cannot adequately describe the nature of the program that produced, or failed to produce, the outcome of interest" (12). The other types of evaluation used in Nigeria include situation and response analysis, rapid assessment, evaluation of NGO projects, and behavioral studies.

Nigeria's demand for evaluation is increasing, yet the country's capacity to do the process justice remains weak. No institutions have been geared toward providing training in evaluation within the country. To date, donor agencies and other international organizations have supported M&E training outside Nigeria and have acted as catalysts for incorporating M&E into NGO programs.

The Need for a National Results-Based M&E System

The NNRIMS was designed to bridge the gaps in the country's evaluation practices. It was "developed to monitor the implementation of HIV/AIDS prevention and control activities and evaluate the impact of the various activities" (3). It focuses on the collection, collation, analysis, dissemination, and use of information from ongoing program efforts. It is also intended to harmonize, standardize, and operationalize national indicators and to popularize their use among stakeholders.

The twenty-one core outcome indicators that the NNRIMS recognizes include five for prevalence and impact of HIV/AIDS, eleven for behavioral outcomes, and five for policies and national commitment. The output-level indicators are subdivided into twelve for knowledge/beliefs and risk perception; four for availability and quality of products and services; and four for capacity building. NNRIMS is institutionalized in NACA and its operation is being developed to also capture information from subnational levels. NACA is currently pilot testing the framework in four states and two line ministries.

The ministries of health, defense, and internal affairs (through the prisons service), as well as the Armed Forces Programme on AIDS Control, have rudimentary M&E systems that feed into the national response. Although the other line ministries have ongoing activities, they lack an M&E system.

Building Results-Based M&E System
The 2003 National Policy on HIV/AIDS and NNRIMS have both established indicators and targets that are inherent parts of results-based M&E (Table 23-1). Once the expected results are fully defined and consensus is reached, a number of key steps will need to be taken to establish a viable M&E system. According to Rist (2) those steps are to:
- Select key performance indicators to monitor outcomes and agree on a performance evaluation methodology;
- Establish baseline data on indicators, including collection of data and documentation of sources;
- Quantify targets;
- Prioritize objectives by assigning weights that add up to 100% and, using a scale, define targets precisely (13);

Table 23-1. Core Indicators for HIV/AIDS Monitoring and Evaluation

Impact-Level Indicators	Targets	Source	Frequency
1. HIV prevalence among pregnant women Percentage of blood samples taken from pregnant women aged 15 to 24 who test positive for HIV during a routine sentinel surveillance at selected ANC clinics	**Baseline 2003:** 5.0% **Target 2005:** 15% reduction **Target 2007:** 25% reduction	Serosurveillance surveys	Biennially
2. Percentage of children who are AIDS orphans Percentage of children under 15 in a household survey whose mother and/or father had died of AIDS	**Baseline 2003:** Not yet released **Target 2005** **Target 2007**	NARHS DHS Special surveys	Biennially
3. Ratio of orphans to nonorphans who are in school The ratio of orphaned children aged 10 to 14 in a household survey who are currently attending school to non-orphaned children the same age who are attending school	**Baseline 2003:** Not yet released **Target 2005** **Target 2007**	MOE reports Special surveys	Annually
Outcome-Level Indicators			
1. Higher risk sex in the previous year Percentage of respondents who have had sex with a non-marital, non-cohabiting partner in the previous 12 months of all respondents reporting sexual activity in the previous 12 months	**Baseline 2003** All respondents: 14.8 Sexually active: 18.8 Had sex in the previous 12 months: 22.8 **Target 2005:** 5% reduction **Target 2007:** 10% reduction	NARHS/BSS	Biennially
2. Condom use at last higher risk sex Percentage of respondents who said they used a condom the last time they had sex with a non-marital, non-cohabiting partner in the previous 12 months of all respondents reporting sex with such a partner in the previous 12 months	**Baseline 2003:** 44.7% **Target 2005:** 60% **Target 2007:** 75%	NARHS/BSS	Biennially
3. Consistent condom use among commercial sex workers Percentage of sex workers reporting consistent condom use in the last one week of all sex workers reporting sex with clients in the previous week	**Baseline 2003:** 57.1% **Target 2005:** 75% **Target 2007:** 90%	Sex workers surveys	Biennially
4. Men and women seeking treatment for STIs Percentage of men and women with STI symptoms who have been treated in a health care facility/pharmacy in the last one year and whose providers have been trained in STI care in a population-based survey of all the people who reported symptoms	**Baseline 2003:** 39.7% **Target 2005:** 45% **Target 2007:** 50%	NARHS	Biennially
5. Population requesting an HIV test, receiving a test, and receiving the results Percentage of people aged 15 to 49 surveyed who ever voluntarily requested an HIV test, received the test, and received their result in the previous 12 months	**Baseline 2003:** 1.1% **Target 2005:** 5% **Target 2007:** 15%	Youth BSS/NARHS	Biennially
6. Pregnant women counseled and tested for HIV Percentage of pregnant women at public antenatal clinics offered VCT by trained staff or referred to VCT services of all pregnant women attending antenatal clinics	**Baseline 2003:** .... **Target 2005:** 25% **Target 2007:** 50%	Health care facility assessment FMOH reports	Biennially Quarterly
7. HIV-positive women provided with antiretroviral therapy in pregnancy Percentage of women testing positive at selected antenatal clinics in the previous 12 months who have received a complete course of antiretrovirals to prevent MTCT according to national guidelines of all women who tested positive at selected clinics	**Baseline 2003:** .... **Target 2005:** 30% **Target 2007:** 60%	FMOH reports	Quarterly
Output-Level Indicator (Political Commitment)			
1. Spending on HIV prevention This is defined as the amount of money allocated in national accounts for spending on HIV prevention and care programs per adult aged 15 to 49	**Baseline 2003:** .... **Target 2005:** .... **Target 2007:**	Special surveys (National AIDS Accounts)	Biennially

Source: Adapted from the Nigerian National Response Information System
Abbreviations: ANC: antenatal care; BSS: Behavioral Surveillance Survey; DHS: Demographic and Health Surveys; FMOH: Federal Ministry of Health; MOE: Ministry of Education; MTCT: mother-to-child transmission of HIV; NARHS: National HIV/AIDS and Reproductive Health Survey; NDHS: National Demographic and Health Survey; STI: sexually transmitted infection; VCT: voluntary counseling and testing

- Define the mode and frequency of data collection, analysis, and reporting for each input, output, and outcome indicator as well as the instruments for analysis and reporting;
- Determine the types, timing, and levels of evaluations;
- Define how the findings will be disseminated, used in decision-making, and incorporated into the improvement performance, such as through reports to the National Assembly; and
- Establish the roles and responsibilities for carrying out the various tasks for the M&E plan for its overall coordination.

Finally, building and running the system requires a champion—a committed person at the leadership level who can monitor the system and oversee its daily operation. That person must also be able to garner the highest political support.

Incentives for Better Use of Information from M&E System
Critical to the actualization of results-based M&E is the issue of incentives (13), especially in Nigeria, where the demand for evaluation is weak. A budget allocation should be established for M&E, and funds should be released when needed. Other incentives may include: tying fund disbursements for continuing projects and programs to successful achievement of results for every level of implementation; increasing budgetary allocations for good performances; universal usage of evaluation results and information for decision-making in program implementation, budgeting, and reporting to donors, the National Assembly, and the presidency; and rewarding evaluators and program personnel for good performance.

Monitoring and Evaluation of the National Response (1993–2004)
Under the Medium-Term Plan II (MTP II), from 1993 to 1998, the M&E problem became compounded by the lack of a coordinated plan and an inadequate M&E capacity within the National AIDS and STD Control Program (NASCP). A multidisciplinary committee later undertook an evaluation of the MTP II on an ad-hoc basis; the situation and response analysis included a desk review, interviews, collection and analysis of service records, facility inspection, and surveys.

The evaluation report provided a narrative of a constellation of findings from the six geopolitical zones (14). It also looked at the outcome of some prevention interventions conducted during the period, including promotion of safer sex behavior; diagnosis and treatment of STIs; blood safety measures; reduction of HIV transmission through injections and other skin-piercing instruments; and measures to increase health care accessibility for people with HIV. Others included the establishment of voluntary counseling and testing centers, local production of condoms, and advocacy to policy makers. The report contained an appraisal of the contributions of government, development partners, professional associations, and other civil society organizations toward the implementation of the plan.

Apart from the FMOH, other sectors were adjudged to have elicited negative responses (a lack of awareness), no responses (indifference), or weak responses. In fact the health sector response was considered weak because the government did not fund the plan and because donor participation was limited, as it occurred during an autocratic military rule, when Nigeria was under sanctions. Although NASCP was supposed to coordinate the plan, it was hindered not only by a lack of funds but also by logistical problems, poor political commitment, inadequate staffing, and a lack of full participation by the states. The report concluded among other things that the MTP II was poorly implemented; the report findings have since been used to help inform the design of HEAP.

HEAP, which covered 2001 to 2004, has not yet been evaluated. A 2004 situation and response analysis for the health sector under HEAP documented progress in program implementation (15). The health sector has initiated antiretroviral therapy, prevention of mother-to-child transmission (PMTCT), and voluntary counseling and testing at the national level. Antiretroviral therapy is now provided to more than 13,000 HIV-infected people from 25 public sector sites (16). PMTCT is provided from 11 sites and voluntary counseling and testing is provided from the PMTCT sites and numerous other sites in the private sector. Some states have started similar programs. M&E systems are being built around these programs and the data generated will feed into the national indicators for these services. The report documented the availability and quality of Nigeria's blood supply, which it considers uneven. Other running programs focus on tuberculosis and STIs. At the national level, clinical guidelines and protocols have been developed but not well disseminated. The report noted that limited training had been provided, but in the absence of widespread distribution of national guidelines, many states had developed their own.

In 2005 NACA conducted the Nigeria National HIV/AIDS Response Review (2001–2004), which identified two major challenges: a lack of gender sensitivity in the system and the failure of NNRIMS to address program evaluation (17). NNRIMS, though a good structure, is still in its early stages of implementation. NNRIMS was based on HEAP, which had a narrow focus on HIV/AIDS responses and thus needs to be reviewed in conjunction with the thematic areas in the National HIV/AIDS Strategic Framework. Among the issues identified were an inadequate baseline data, a current M&E plan not comprehensive enough to cover 2005–2009, and the gender insensitivity of NNRIMS. The major constraint to evaluation was identified as inadequate technical capacity for M&E at all levels.

With reference to meeting international commitment for evaluation, Nigeria was one of the 189 signatories to the United Nations General Assembly Special Session on HIV/AIDS (UNGASS) Declaration of Commitment. It met an important M&E commitment in 2003 by reporting on nine of the thirteen UNGASS indicators (Table 23-2) (18).

The Role of Donors and International NGOs and M&E in Nigeria

Donors and international NGOs have contributed to M&E activities in Nigeria in terms of capacity building and instituting project evaluation practices among local NGOs. Some large interventions have produced meaningful measures of success and impact on the epidemic, while others have operational dimensions that input into future program designs.

A participatory evaluation of the STD/HIV Management Project, Nigeria Phase II was conducted at the end of the project in March 2003 (19). The goal of the project, which was funded by the Department for International Development (DFID), was "to improve access of high risk and specific vulnerable groups to quality HIV/STD/TB health and support interventions in Benue and Ogun States." All key outputs were assessed as either largely or completely achieved, with the exception of strengthening multisectoral responses. The project was noted to have "increased the quality, access and utilization of HIV related services in project areas." High-risk and vulnerable groups were the target population for many of the preventive and outreach activities but care users were not classified by high-risk or vulnerability. The review team felt the data were insufficient to validate the extent to which the project has improved access for high-risk and vulnerable groups defined as specifically identifiable target groups within the community, such as sex workers, commercial motorcyclists, and long-distance truck drivers.

The Society for Family Health (SFH) is one of the few organizations that has invested heavily in evaluation in Nigeria. Apart from being involved in the National HIV/AIDS and Reproductive Health Survey, which provides information for measuring the HIV-related behavior indicators, SFH periodically evaluates the impact on behavior change of its various media campaigns. Its Future Dreams Radio Campaign, for example, resulted in a substantial increase in condom sales immediately after the campaign began (20). Monthly sales doubled from about 5.1 million condoms in June 2000 to more than 10.7 million by June 2001. Eighty percent of those who heard the message knew that condoms provided protection against HIV infection, compared to 62% of those who did not hear the message. The behavior data also showed that 51% of respondents who heard the program used condoms correctly and consistently with non-spousal partners in the preceding two months, compared with 33% of those who did not hear the program (20).

A survey of most-at-risk communities noted significant changes as reflected in an increased level of condom use in non-marital sex, increased parent-to-child communication on sexuality issues, less resistance to condom use by sex workers' clients, and increased feelings of self-worth among young people, sex workers, and married women (21). Similar evaluation reports have included the Boy/Girlfriend TV Adverts, the Radio Drama Evaluation Using Panel Listeners' Group, and the Femi and Fati HIV Billboard Campaign.

Similarly, USAID and DFID have conducted impact-related studies that have provided valuable information about the epidemic in the educational sector and rural Benue State. These studies form a benchmark for assessing the sectors in the future and have implications for programming. The Benue Impact Studies were conducted between July 2002 and June 2003 with the goal of analyzing the current and possible future impact of HIV/AIDS on rural livelihoods in Benue State (22). Among other findings the studies revealed that:

- Stigmatization was extensive in some communities and may have caused an underreporting of chronic illnesses and AIDS-associated symptoms.
- The HIV adult prevalence rate in Benue State was approximately 13.5% in 2001.
- A demographic analysis suggested a difference in population structures between AIDS-affected and non-AIDS–affected communities.
- The rural extended family still seems able to take care of the increased numbers of AIDS orphans, as 83% of them attend school while only 7% have been forced to work to support themselves.
- The trend over the past few years suggests an increase in poverty levels.

In 2004 USAID commissioned a study titled, "Assessing Educators' Views on the Impact of HIV/AIDS on Primary Education in Nigeria: Implications for Future Programs" (23). Conducted in Nassarawa, Kano, and Lagos states, the study noted variations across the states, with Nassarawa the most affected by the epidemic. Among the study's recommendations for future programming were the following:

- Operational guidelines should be developed to enable school administrators and educational planners to address HIV-related issues — such as stigmatization and absenteeism — among teachers and children affected by HIV/AIDS.
- The ongoing dissemination of the family-life-skills and HIV/AIDS curriculum developed by the Nigerian Educational Research and Development Council and the Universal Basic Education Commission should be scaled up to reach primary schools and be implemented with capacity-building workshops on HIV/AIDS issues for primary school teachers.
- More culturally appropriate and gender-sensitive resource materials on HIV/AIDS should be distributed to primary schools.
- The dialogue with teacher training institutions should be enhanced so that training on family life skills and HIV/AIDS can be incorporated into pre-service training curricula.

Although few HIV/AIDS programs have been evaluated in Nigeria, the national response is poised for more purposeful M&E, as evidenced by the progress being made in implementing the NNRIMS and enhancing the capacities of the agencies responsible for the sentinel and behavioral surveillance surveys. We are also beginning to see evaluative studies commissioned. But successfully monitoring and evaluating the epidemic will require expansive M&E capacity building, which can be done through identifying and developing training institutions within the country and by establishing evaluation associations to promote the culture and practice of evaluation. Collaboration with external evaluation associations and agencies—particularly the UN agencies—will go a long way toward improving the current capacity.

MEETING INTERNATIONAL OBLIGATIONS FOR M&E REPORTING

Nigeria has been a signatory to several key HIV/AIDS resolutions, including the Millennium Development Goals, adopted at the Millennium Summit in 2000, which calls for expanded efforts to halt and reverse the rate of HIV spread by 2015, and the Abuja Declaration on HIV/AIDS, Tuberculosis and Other Related Infectious Diseases in 2001, which declared regional and national commitments to confront the epidemic (24).

As noted earlier, in 2001 Nigeria became a signatory to the Declaration of Commitment on HIV/AIDS adopted by the United Nations General Assembly Special Session on HIV/AIDS, or UNGASS, which commits member states and the global community to taking strong and immediate action to address the HIV/AIDS crisis. The declaration calls for achieving a number of specific goals, such as reducing HIV prevalence among young men and women, expanding care and support, and protecting human rights.

The UNGASS declaration underscores the critical importance of compiling accurate information and disseminating it widely to all interested individuals and stakeholders. By identifying concrete, time-bound targets and requiring that efforts be undertaken to measure global success in reaching these targets, the member states envisioned that the declaration would promote greater urgency and solidarity in the campaign against the epidemic.

The member states formulated a number of indicators to measure the efforts of the various nations to reach their goals. To monitor progress toward the actualization of the targets, countries were requested to make biennial reports on their national response and the epidemic using those indicators. Countries therefore had to develop methods to ensure regularity in reporting. The first reports were prepared in 2003; subsequent reports are expected biennially.

In its 2003 report, Nigeria was able to report on only nine of the thirteen indicators (25); the lack of systems made it impossible to produce data for the other four. Efforts have since been made to establish systems that can generate the desired data for subsequent reports. (See Table 23-3.)

The NNRIMS has incorporated these indicators into its country-response information system. The system is being piloted in just a few states, however, and may not be able to generate nationally representative data to meet all the needs for the UNGASS report (4).

Core Indicator	2003	2005 and Beyond
1. Amount national governments spend on HIV/AIDS	Information was based on interviews with key persons; no method of validation exists	Sensitivities about the release of information will make state surveys on financial resources difficult. The tracking of funds might be limited to national expenditures rather than individual state spending in multisectoral settings.
2. National Composite Policy Index	Reported on	This should still be possible using the same format as previously undertaken.
3. Percentage of schools with teachers who have been trained in life-skills-based HIV/AIDS education and who taught it during the last academic year	Reported on by only one of the 36 states because of the lack of a documentation system	This will require funds to conduct a survey in 2005, as no monitoring system has been instituted.
4. Percentage of large enterprises with HIV/AIDS workplace policies and programs	Reported on, but information was not validated	This will require funds to conduct a survey in 2005, as no monitoring system has been instituted.
5. Percentage of patients with STIs at health care facilities who are appropriately diagnosed, treated, and counseled	Not reported on; no documentation system is in place	A health facility survey had been included in the NNRIMS but the FMOH has yet to develop a study protocol.
6. Percentage of HIV-infected pregnant women receiving a complete course of antiretroviral prophylaxis to reduce the risk of mother-to-child transmission of HIV	Reported on (the numerator was based only on those receiving care in federal government settings)	The need to include the women being treated at other public and private centers will remain a challenge.
7. Percentage of people with advanced HIV infection receiving antiretroviral combination therapy	Reported on (the numerator was based only on those receiving care in federal government settings)	The need to include patients being treated at private centers will remain a challenge until the NNRIMS is fully implemented.
8. Percentage of IDUs who have adopted behaviors that reduce HIV transmission	Reported on, based on a small sample in one of the 36 states	No plans exist for reporting on this. An IDU survey has been included in the NNRIMS but no protocol for its implementation has been developed.
9. Percentage of people aged 15 to 24 years who both correctly identify ways of preventing the sexual transmission of HIV and who reject major misconceptions about HIV transmission	Reported on	Plans exist for the FMOH to conduct regular behavior surveillance surveys.
10. Percentage of people aged 15 to 24 years reporting condom use during sexual intercourse with non-regular partners	Reported on	Plans exist for the FMOH to conduct regular behavior surveillance surveys.
11. Ratio of current school attendance among orphans to that among non-orphans aged 10 to 14 years	Reported on	Plans exist for regular NDHS to be carried out, hence this should be regularly reported.
12. Percentage of people aged 15 to 24 years who are HIV infected	Reported on	This should be possible due to the regularity with which the study is conducted.
13. Percentage of infants born to HIV-positive mothers who are infected	Not reported on	This figure may be possible using estimates, projections, and information on program coverage.

Abbreviations: FMOH: Federal Ministry of Health; IDU: injection drug user; NDHS: National Demographic and Health Survey; NNRIMS: Nigerian National Response Information Management System; UNGASS: United Nations General Assembly Special Session on HIV/AIDS

Several factors account for this inability to generate data. First, sector-level M&E systems have yet to be developed. Second, other than the health sector, most sectors are new to the national HIV/AIDS response and have yet to establish systems for conducting interventions, much less monitoring and evaluating them. The health sector can provide some information, but it is limited to indicators that the population-based behavior surveys and HIV seroprevalence surveys have generated. Indicators requiring health facility surveys and program monitoring to generate do not have robust systems in place to provide valid and reliable data.

Nigeria is making many efforts to generate data. The NNRIMS places the responsibility for measuring the indicators with the ministries relevant to the activity being measured. Some are given to the Federal Ministry of Education and the Federal Ministry of Labor and Productivity, for example, though these ministries have yet to develop mechanisms to measure these indicators.

To track progress toward achieving the Millennium Development Goals, specific goals, targets, and indicators were also set. Among the indicators developed to measure the success of this initiative were:

- the HIV prevalence rate among 15- to 24-year-old pregnant women;
- the condom use rate or contraceptive prevalence rate, particularly during the last episode of high-risk sex;
- the percentage of people aged 15 to 24 who have a comprehensive and correct knowledge of HIV/AIDS; and
- the ratio of school attendance of orphans to school attendance of non-orphans aged 10 to 14.

These indicators are expected to be collected every three to five years. Most of them are already being collected through such regular surveys as the National Demographic and Health Survey and the National HIV/AIDS and Reproductive Health Survey; the former is expected to be conducted every four years and the latter biennially.

UNAIDS developed the Country Response Information System (CRIS) to ensure that information about the epidemic could be shared on a regular basis to determine the trends of member nations. The CRIS was developed to facilitate the systematic collection, storage, analysis, retrieval, and dissemination of information on countries' responses to HIV/AIDS, thereby strengthening information systems to be able to meet the increasing needs for higher quality data and analysis as well as increasing the ability to compare situations within countries and regions. At its basic level the CRIS consists of an indicator database, a project- and resource-tracking database, a research inventory database, and the capacity to store additional important information, including surveillance and AIDS case reporting.

The NNRIMS was designed to be Nigeria's CRIS. Efforts have been made to design a computer database that can allow the easy link up with the Internet-based CRIS when fully functional. The database is still being tested for suitability, however.

Nigeria has made attempts to fulfill its reporting obligations by devising appropriate methods and mechanisms. The problem lies in the tendency to be reactive rather than proactive in designing systems to track information. The fact that little use has been made of previous findings, however, may account for the reluctance to create such systems.

Reporting on international commitments has invariably meant increased financial requirements for M&E, especially when systems are lacking. In the past, donor partners provided most such funds. While the assistance has been welcomed, it raises concerns about the sustainability and ownership of systems that are built by donors to meet the needs of international obligations, with little local access and use of the information generated.

Reports written to meet international obligations are often available on the Internet but remain inaccessible within the country. The Nigerian civil service has a code of ethics that prohibits disclosure of information without authorization. This code has many times been extended to evaluation results. This decreases the usefulness of the information to the providers and further decreases the likelihood of sustainability.

M&E reports are usually shared in stakeholders' forums before the actual submission to the international organization overseeing the commitment. After such meetings the final reports are barely accessible to the general population.

Recently several international organizations collaborated on a study on coverage of selected services for HIV/AIDS prevention, care, and support in low- and middle-income countries in 2003. Nigeria responded by checking the records of organizations working in the program areas being covered. The data were insufficient to provide information on service coverage on opportunistic infections, home-based care, family life health education, outreach services for street children, care for prisoners, men who have sex with men, injection drug users, and people receiving voluntary counseling and testing. The service coverage component of the NNRIMS is meant to address those gaps (26).

Nigeria has made significant progress in its efforts to meet its reporting obligations. Unfortunately it continues to be constrained by insufficient funds and the lack of a fully functional system to provide updated information as needed. The NNRIMS is still undergoing the pilot phase and remains constrained by the limited funds available for its implementation.

ISSUES, GAPS, AND CHALLENGES

Political and Popular Support for M&E

In the past, governments, political leaders, and program managers in Nigeria neither supported nor advocated for M&E activities, as they were not generally considered part of the program. This trend has begun to change, however, and M&E activities are receiving more support. As part of its coordinating function, NACA has established a functional M&E unit with a dedicated budget line and key personnel to coordinate M&E activities of the national response. This unit is expected to be strengthened for optimal performance of its ever-increasing tasks.

As mentioned earlier, in 2003 NACA reacted positively to the identified need for M&E by developing a potentially robust and well-coordinated management information system for monitoring and evaluating HIV/AIDS activities. This system, NNRIMS, focuses on the collection, collation, analysis, dissemination, and use of information from ongoing program efforts. NNRIMS also serves as the repository for the core indicators that guide performance of the national response to be reported on by NACA. This system is still being field-tested, and the challenge remains of providing adequate human, infrastructural, and financial resources to implement and sustain this system in Nigeria.

Demand for data and M&E results is low nationally, and until recently most M&E processes were donor driven, as many program managers saw the need for reporting as important mainly to fulfill donor requirements. That perception is changing, however, now that NACA, FMOH, and project implementers have become more proactive about M&E activities.

According to a national M&E needs assessment report that NACA produced, twice as many organizations received support from international donors as from the government (27). This survey also found that only about half of the organizations surveyed had any M&E framework. Of those without such plans, a lack of funds was the most frequently cited reason.

The HIV/AIDS Policy Environment

The successful implementation of the 2003 National Policy on HIV/AIDS is expected to help curb the spread of the virus in Nigeria. Specifically, Nigeria has mandated relevant institutions to collect, on a continuous basis, information on the epidemic and factors influencing the spread of HIV. This mandate will enable NACA to monitor and report annually on progress achieved in responding to identified HEAP objectives and subsequently the National HIV/AIDS Strategic Framework (6).

Although the policy is in place, it has yet to be fully operationalized and stepped down to the lower levels. For example, while the policy stipulates that institutions engaged in HIV/AIDS activities are expected to commit a minimum of 5% of their project budgets to facilitate M&E, not many organizations are actually implementing this policy. In addition, no policy direction exists on data use, including access to such national data sets as the NDHS for secondary analysis.

The Need to Strengthen Existing M&E Systems

The health sector response has begun to organize its M&E system to enable it to respond to the needs of the NNRIMS, but the other sectoral responses have yet to be developed well enough to provide regular data for an effective M&E system. What all the sectors critically need, however, is to establish an effective system to operationalize this work. Relevant staff needed to manage an effective M&E system is gradually being engaged, though much remains to be done to ensure good quality and appropriate numbers of personnel at all levels. Relevant equipment like computers is in short supply, and databases have yet to be set up at most levels.

No harmonization of core indicators exists to date, and the operationalization of NNRIMS is expected to create that harmonization, so all stakeholders can report on comparable indicators. The national PMTCT program—with support from the U.S. Centers for Disease Control and Prevention, APIN, and UNICEF—has made appreciable progress in standardizing data collection mechanisms and tools, and other programs will need to make reasonable progress to standardize their M&E systems

(3). Funds must be provided by all stakeholders, however, particularly NACA and FMOH, since funding appears to be the only option toward ensuring sustainability and ownership of this process.

Human and Institutional Capacity

Only in the past two decades has evaluation become fully established as a way of assessing social programs. It is now being incorporated into programming at all levels of government as well as NGOs. As a result, M&E experts are scarce globally, particularly in developing countries (18). In Nigeria, not only has the demand side been affected, but the supply side as well, as NACA and NASCP have experienced a dearth of qualified professionals in their M&E units. Although many Nigerian universities and social science departments are noted for their evaluation studies, few focus on health-related evaluations.

Resource Allocations for M&E

Monitoring efforts by UNAIDS have tracked a substantial increase in resources for HIV/AIDS programs in developing countries, as well as a growing public awareness of AIDS in countries where the epidemic is now emerging as a major problem. Current resources, however, fall substantially short of the amounts needed to conduct a comprehensive campaign against HIV/AIDS (18). Until recently, M&E activities rarely received budget lines. The situation has begun to improve both in NACA and FMOH, as funds are now available from varied sources for M&E activities. Little guidance has been given, however, on how these funds should be used. A plan that specifies fund use for M&E beyond data collection is needed as part of the development of a sustainable M&E system for responding to the epidemic in Nigeria.

Quality and Use of M&E Outputs

Data quality influences M&E results, so great care must be taken to ensure high-quality data. Many factors can help guarantee the quality of data collected, including the skill of personnel, the availability of equipment and necessary logistics, and adequate motivation of M&E personnel at all levels. A quality assurance system is needed to ensure the production and dissemination of quality data.

Skills of data producers, infrastructure, logistics, and systems for collecting, collating, validating, analyzing, and disseminating quality data need to be built at all levels. These efforts require significant financial resources on a sustainable basis, preferably from different sources.

Another obvious challenge to obtaining quality data is the difficulty in reporting small research or intervention efforts as they often feed only into process indicators that do not easily lead to outcomes or even outputs. There is poor follow-up to research results, and attempts are not usually made to find scientific explanations to any unusual findings. For example, it would be revealing to find answers to some unexpected observations in the sentinel surveys (28) and NDHS. This would reduce the tendency to speculate about possible reasons for such findings.

LESSONS LEARNED

An important aspect of evaluation is that it provides opportunities for learning. M&E managers are therefore expected to always document both positive and negative lessons as important sources of information about improving program performance.

UNAID's 2003 Progress Report on the Global Response to the HIV/AIDS Epidemic (18) detailed the following lessons:

- M&E is needed at all levels and is most useful when performed in a logical sequence, from assessing data on input, process, and output; to examining behavioral and immediate outcomes; to determining disease and social effects.
- Existing indicators should measure population-based, biological, behavioral, facility-based, and program data to determine the collective effectiveness of consolidated programs. Good contextual data should supplement these measurements.
- To minimize the data collection burden and maximize limited resources, M&E activities must be well coordinated and use ongoing systems for collecting and analyzing data.
- To increase the usefulness of evaluation results, the design, planning, analysis and reporting of M&E should actively involve key stakeholders, such as district and national managers, policy makers, community members, and program participants.
- An M&E system needs at least 10% of the total program budget to function optimally.
- Gender equality and the empowerment of women are crucial in reducing the vulnerability of women and girls to HIV/AIDS. The Declaration of Commitment agreed on several targets aimed at empowering women and girls to protect themselves from HIV infection. To assess national progress toward these goals, nine indicators requested data, asking for a breakdown by gender. Unfortunately, not even one in five countries provided these disaggregated data.

CONCLUSION

Few HIV/AIDS programs have been evaluated in Nigeria, with methodologies ranging from reviews to rapid appraisal and response monitoring. Both content and methodology gaps have hampered results-driven implementation and decision-making. Although the national response is poised for more purposeful M&E—as evidenced by progress in implementing the NNRIMS and enhancing the capacities of the agencies responsible for the sentinel and behavioral surveillance surveys—the human and institutional capacity must be developed to engage in the magnitude of efforts needed to monitor and evaluate the epidemic.

By creating NNRIMS, Nigeria has largely fulfilled its international M&E obligations, especially toward the UNGASS indicators and in compliance with UNAIDS recommendations on CRIS. Still following the UNAIDS guidelines, it has begun the pilot phase of the NNRIMS and, through the assistance of Measures Evaluation, has begun to develop a software program for gathering and collating the national data set. The progress is encouraging, but the political will to follow through will prove critical to the success of the entire process.

Although vestiges of the results-based M&E tool exist in Nigeria, systems have yet to be instituted to use the tool rigorously and to maximize the advantage of measuring performance against the targets identified both in the NNRIMS and the National Policy on HIV/AIDS. The important question here is: How do we know success when we see it? The program has failed to translate lessons learned in the field into improving program management, and no evidence suggests that such strategic information is being reflected in policy development. For example, every sentinel survey has indicated that people aged 20 to 29 years old have the highest prevalence rate, yet no meaningful interventions at scale-up levels have been directed at that age group.

The National Policy on HIV/AIDS is bland and generic, lacks a cogent policy thrust apart from its multisectoral approach, and fails to set priorities. It seems to presume that each intervention will achieve the same impact on reducing the epidemic. This presumption clearly reveals the paucity of appropriate data for making decisions on policy direction or shift.

Some painstakingly implemented policies in other countries—such as the 100%-condom–use policy among sex workers in Thailand (29) and the registration and treatment of sex workers for STIs in Senegal (30)—have produced good results. With prevalence rates ranging from 1.2% to 12%, Nigeria has multiple epidemics and must therefore prioritize its interventions, address issues of equity, expand access to programs and services, and significantly scale up its response. The country can accomplish all this by ensuring a strong policy backing and translating such policies into action. Finally, findings from evaluation and research should contribute to such policy-making and ultimately influence practice.

Specific recommendations include the following:

- **Create a demand for evaluation.** Although the demand for evaluation is on the increase through donor insistence, evaluation professionals should make concerted efforts to sensitize politicians and other policy makers to their statutory oversight functions and make it clear that evaluation can deliver more objective assessments of performance. Civil society organizations also should champion the demand for accountability.

- **Ensure supply.** While creating demand for evaluation is a continuous process, by the same token there should be expansive capacity building in M&E, including identifying and developing training institutions within the country and establishing evaluation associations to promote the culture and practice of evaluation. Collaboration with external evaluation associations and agencies, particularly the UN agencies, will go a long way toward improving the current capacity.

- **Build the systems.** Results-based M&E systems should as a matter of urgency be pushed through legislation so they become the norm. Such systems can derive and benefit from existing international standards but they should also be homegrown from the local governments to the state and federal levels. The local action committees on AIDS should develop systems that can track local indicators and feed into the information-gathering structure of the state action committees on AIDS. Data collected at the state level will also supply information to NACA's national data collection system. The guiding principles should include utility, values identification, report timeliness and dissemination, political viability, cost-effectiveness, and feasibility (31).

- **Fund the systems.** For M&E systems to survive, the UN has suggested a minimum budget of 10% of the actual program or project cost at all levels of intervention. Such funds should be disbursed as needed in a timely fashion.
- **Create incentives for sustaining the systems.** Budgetary allocations for M&E are just one kind of incentive. Other incentives should include: tying fund disbursements for continuing projects and programs to successful achievement of results for every level of implementation; increasing budgetary allocation for good performance; ensuring universal application of evaluation results for decision-making in program implementation, budgeting, and donor reporting, the National Assembly, and the presidency; and rewarding evaluators and program personnel for good performance.
- **Ensure information flow and use.** Deliberate provisions should be made to disseminate M&E results to all stakeholders. Policy makers can then apply the information to pursue evidence-based decision-making. Feedback loops will encourage data providers to continue to supply information.
- **Earmark funds for dissemination activities as well as advocacy for data use as a management tool at all levels.** The key findings from M&E activities need to be shared with those providing the data to encourage a continuous supply of necessary information to track accomplishments.
- **Ensure that research findings feed into national M&E efforts and provide additional funds for operations research.** Lessons learned from ongoing research can help improve program performance.
- **Take sociocultural factors — including economic, educational, and religious aspects — into consideration.** These factors might make local translations to answer questions raised by global indicators difficult. In developing an effective M&E system, though, it is important to take these factors into consideration, not just to fulfill a commitment to the UNGASS declaration, but also to be able to compare Nigeria's progress with that in other countries.

Nigeria must scale up its HIV/AIDS interventions massively in the next five years if it will ever be able to achieve the goal that it set for itself in the 2003 national policy and meet international obligations under the UNGASS and the Millennium Development Goals. The National HIV/AIDS Strategic Framework should set priorities and share the experiences of other African countries (32). Interventions targeted to high-risk groups such as sex workers and long-distance truck drivers should be the top priority. The second priority should be prevention of HIV transmission among young people. Sentinel surveys have found high prevalence rates among young people, who constitute more than 25% of Nigeria's population; hence investment in prevention efforts in the group will yield a high dividend. Large-scale, school-based behavior change programs and modified curricula will help significantly. Other priority areas include PMTCT, care of orphans and vulnerable children, and care and support for women and children infected and affected by HIV.

And once we have given our system a good start, I pointed out, the process of growth will be cumulative.
— PLATO IN *THE REPUBLIC*

REFERENCES

1. World Bank. Quoted in UNDP (2004) Nigerian Human Development Report. *HIV and AIDS: A Challenge to Sustainable Human Development.* Washington, DC: World Bank, 2004.

2. Rist R. Designing and building a results-based monitoring and evaluation system: a tool for Public Sector Management Policies. *IPDET Training Manual,* 2003.

3. Federal Government of Nigeria. *Nigeria National Response Information Management System (NNRIMS) Guidelines and Indicators.* Abuja: Federal Government of Nigeria, 2004.

4. National Action Committee on AIDS. *National HIV/AIDS Strategic Framework: 2005–2009.* Abuja: National Action Committee on AIDS, 2005.

5. UNAIDS. *"Three Ones" Key Principles: Coordination of National Responses to HIV/AIDS.* Geneva: UNAIDS, 2004.

6. Federal Government of Nigeria. *National Policy on HIV/AIDS.* Abuja: Federal Government of Nigeria, 2003.

7. Federal Government of Nigeria. *National HIV Sero-Prevalence Sentinel Survey: Technical Report.* Abuja: Federal Government of Nigeria, 2004.

8. Barnett T, Whiteside A. *AIDS in the Twenty-First Century: Disease and Globalization.* New York: Palgrave Macmillan, 2002.

9. Asiimwe-Okifor G, Opio AA, Musinguzi J, Madraa E, Tembo G, Carael M. Change in sexual behavior and decline in HIV infection among young pregnant women in urban Uganda. *AIDS,* 1997;11:1757–63.

10. Parker RG, Easton D, Klein CH. Structural barriers and facilitators in HIV prevention: a review of international research. *AIDS,* 2000;14(Suppl 1):S22–S32.

11. National Population Commission (Nigeria) and ORC Macro. *Nigeria Demographic and Health Survey 2003.* Calverton, Maryland: National Population Commission and ORC Macro, 2004.

12. Rossi PH, Lipsey MW, Freeman HE. *Evaluation: A Systemic Approach.* 7th ed. London: Sage Publications, 2004.

13. Trivedi P. Performance agreements in US government: lessons for developing countries. *Econ Polit Wkly,* 2003;38(46):4851–4858.

14. Federal Government of Nigeria. *Report of the National Evaluation Committee on HIV/AIDS on the National Response to the Medium-Term Plan II (1993–1997).* Abuja: Federal Government of Nigeria, 2000.

15. Federal Government of Nigeria. *Situation and Response Analysis for the Health Sector Plan.* Abuja: Federal Government of Nigeria, 2004.

16. Federal Government of Nigeria/USAID. *Nigeria: Rapid Assessment of HIV/AIDS Care in the Public and Private Sectors.* Abuja: Federal Government of Nigeria/USAID, 2004.

17. Federal Government of Nigeria. *Nigeria National HIV/AIDS Response Review (NRR) 2001–2004.* Abuja: Federal Government of Nigeria, 2005.

18. UNAIDS. *Progress Report on the Global Response to HIV/AIDS Epidemic.* Geneva: UNAIDS, 2003.

19. Department for International Development. *STD/HIV Management Project, Nigeria Phase II: End of Project Review Report, March 2003.* London: Department for International Development, 2003.

20. Ankomah A, Anyanti J. *Future Dreams Radio Campaign: A Final Evaluation Report.* Abuja: Society for Family Health, 2002.

21. Anyanti J, A Ankomah A, Omoregie G, et al. The MARCs project: a qualitative evaluation of a demonstration community level HIV prevention project. *XV International Conference on AIDS and STDs,* Bangkok, Thailand, July 11–16, 2004 (abstract MoPpD2024).

22. Department for International Development. *Benue Impact Studies.* London: Department for International Development, 2004.

23. USAID/Federal Government of Nigeria/Research Triangle Institute. *Assessing Educators' Views on the Impact of HIV/AIDS on Primary Education in Nigeria: Implications for Future Programs.* USAID/Federal Government of Nigeria/Research Triangle Institute, 2004.

24. United Nations. *Declaration of Commitment on HIV/AIDS: United Nations General Assembly Special Session on HIV/AIDS, 25–27 June 2001.* Geneva: United Nations, 2001.

25. United Nations. *A Report on the UNGASS Indicators in Nigeria: A Follow-Up to the Declaration of Commitment on HIV/AIDS, Reporting Period: January–December, 2002.* Geneva: United Nations, 2004.

26. USAID, UNAIDS, WHO, UNICEF, and the POLICY Project. *Coverage of Selected Services for HIV/AIDS Prevention, Care and Support in Low and Middle Income Countries in 2003.* USAID, UNAIDS, WHO, UNICEF, and the POLICY Project, 2004.

27. National Action Committee on AIDS. HIV/AIDS Monitoring and Evaluation. Needs Assessment Survey in Nigeria. Unpublished report. Abuja: National Action Committee on AIDS, 2002.

28. Riedner G, Dehne KL. *HIV/AIDS Surveillance in Developing Countries: Experiences and Issues.* Eschborn, Germany: Gesellschaft für Technische Zusammenarbeit, 1999.

29. World Health Organization. Disease prevention. Asia sex industry hurts AIDS efforts. *AIDS Wkly,* September 3, 2001;17.

30. Menting A. HIV prevention strategies in Africa. *Harv AIDS Rev,* Winter 2000;6–11.

31. The African Evaluation guidelines. *Eval Program Plann,* 2002;25(4):481–492.

32. Patel M, Allen KB, Keatley R, Jonsson U. Introduction: UNICEF and UNAIDS evaluations of HIV/AIDS programmes in sub-Saharan Africa. *Eval Program Plann,* 2002;25(4):317–327.

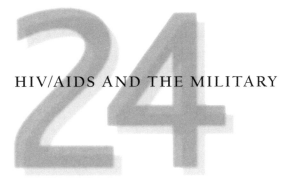

HIV/AIDS AND THE MILITARY

Ernest Ekong*

Since Nigeria's first AIDS case was reported in 1986, the health, demographic, and socioeconomic effects of the epidemic have become readily apparent. Only recently, however, has the epidemic been recognized as a national security issue. Epidemiologic evidence indicates that throughout the world men and women in the military are among the most susceptible subpopulations to sexually transmitted infections (STIs), including HIV. In peacetime, STI rates in the military are two to five times higher than in comparable civilian populations; during wartime the rates tend to climb (1). Conflict situations involving troops, vulnerable populations, and humanitarian workers further promote the transmission of HIV.

In many African countries, the uniformed services report HIV prevalence rates higher than the national averages. In Uganda, for instance, the HIV prevalence rate of 27% among the military in 1996 was more than three times the 1999 national prevalence rate of 8.3% (2). Researchers in South Africa have reported prevalence rates of 60% to 70% in the armed forces, compared with 20% in the adult population (3). In Cameroon, Nigeria's neighbor to the east, an HIV rate of 6.2% was reported in the military compared to 2% in the general population in 1993 (4). In Malawi, 25% to 50% of army officials are already HIV positive (5). Indeed, AIDS is now the leading cause of death in the military and police forces in some African countries, accounting for more than half of in-service mortality (6).

*APIN Plus/Harvard PEPFAR, Lagos, Nigeria

National leaders and military strategists must take the HIV threat seriously for several reasons. First, the capability and experience of military forces will diminish when prevalence rates are high and prevention and mitigation efforts are ineffective or insufficient. Second, some analysts speculate that when prevalence is high, soldiers increase their risk-taking behavior (7). In addition, without access to treatment, counseling, and other coping methods, soldiers with HIV face a dramatically shortened life, which reduces their drive to end conflict and work toward long-term stability. In certain cases, high prevalence has led to the extension of conflict by governments afraid to demobilize infected soldiers and to increased illegal activity among soldiers keen to earn extra money, perhaps for treatment they cannot afford (3).

HIV prevalence figures are unavailable in the public domain for Nigeria's 150,000-strong armed forces, since force-wide HIV testing has not been conducted. Nigeria is Africa's largest contributor of troops—including military observers and civilian police—to UN peacekeeping missions. Preliminary results from an ongoing study funded by the U.S. Naval Health Research Center found a 15% HIV seroprevalence rate among soldiers on active duty (5). One study of veterans of the country's peacekeeping efforts in Sierra Leone and Liberia during the 1990s suggests that 11% were infected, compared with a 5% infection rate in the general adult population (8).

This chapter examines the risk factors that favor transmission of HIV in the Nigerian military and discusses prevention and control strategies. It also highlights the special cases of demobilization, peacekeeping, and the growing proportion of women in the military, and it outlines several policy issues and recommendations that will help control the spread and limit the impact of HIV/AIDS in the military.

TRANSMISSION AND RISK FACTORS

The military community is considered a high-risk environment for HIV transmission. A number of risk factors increase the susceptibility of military personnel to HIV infection:
- Danger and risk taking are integral parts of their profession.
- They tend to be young, single, and sexually active.
- They are highly mobile and stay away from their families and home communities for extended periods.
- They are influenced by peer pressure rather than social convention.
- They are inclined to feel invincible and take risks.
- They have more ready cash than other males where they are deployed and hence are surrounded by opportunities for casual and commercial sex.

Militaries are also often closed and secretive organizations, although they are among the most likely groups to introduce successful and compulsory control measures, such as screening. A large-scale survey in the U.S. military showed that sexual activity was significantly higher in this group than in the civilian populations (9).

An important knowledge, attitudes, and practices (KAP) survey of the Nigerian Armed Forces conducted in 2001 provides an opportunity to better understand the dynamics and factors underlying the spread of HIV and other STIs in the military (4). Only 40% of respondents had good HIV transmission and prevention knowledge, while 25% of those surveyed had poor knowledge of HIV/AIDS. Four percent of those surveyed reported symptoms of STIs in the previous 12 months; more than 10% did not seek any form of orthodox medical care and treatment.

In the same KAP survey, the risk perception of HIV/AIDS was low. Forty-one percent felt they faced no risk of contracting HIV, while 22% felt they carried only a small risk despite high-risk exposures. Moreover, the respondents' condom use did not vary with the level of perceived risk. Indeed, evidence suggests that some soldiers consider the acquisition of an STI to be a symbol of sexual prowess and proof of manhood.

Only 40% of the respondents had been tested for HIV, 35% of whom had taken the test voluntarily. Eighty-nine percent indicated, however, that they would take an HIV screening test if it were provided free of charge. Military personnel scheduled for international postings undergo mandatory testing.

The survey also showed that the high-risk behavior that military personnel engaged in included multiple sexual partnering, with 15.3% of the respondents reporting having had at least two sexual partners during the previous year. Of these partners, one-third were non-regular sexual partners, including casual acquaintances, girlfriends or boyfriends, and paid sexual partners. Although less than 5% of the study population admitted having paid for sex, only slightly more than half used a condom on that occasion. The study did not ask about same-sex relationships or other potential risks.

A large proportion of respondents knew condoms could provide protection against HIV and other STIs, and 98% of the respondents knew where to obtain condoms. Only half of the respondents reported using condoms on a regular basis with their non-regular partners, however. Only one-quarter of the respondents had ever received condoms from the armed forces; of those who did, two-thirds thought the supply was inadequate.

The high mobility of the men and women in the armed forces also places them at risk of HIV infection. Two-thirds of the respondents were married, but 17% did not cohabit with their partners because they were either on peacekeeping missions or had to leave for training. Almost half of the respondents who participated in the various

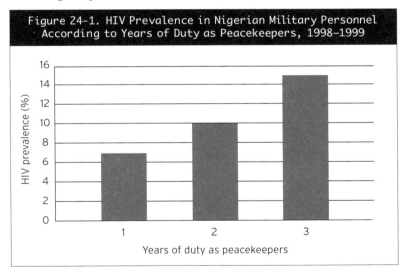

Figure 24-1. HIV Prevalence in Nigerian Military Personnel According to Years of Duty as Peacekeepers, 1998–1999

Source: Adefolalu A. AIDS in the Nigerian military. *Third All African Congress of Armed Forces and Police Medical Services*, Pretoria, South Africa, 1999.

peacekeeping operations admitted having sexual partners during their time away from home.

The longer the time spent away, the higher the chances that the soldiers had sexual partners. With these sexual partners, only half of the respondents used condoms. Deployment to unsettled areas increases their chances of acquiring HIV, as they are exposed not only to socially disrupted settings, but also to the possibility of infection through wounds and contaminated blood. Adefolalu has found that HIV prevalence in the Nigerian military increased with years of duty as peacekeepers (10) (Figure 24-1). No studies, however, have compared the proportion of HIV cases in the military that are due to sexual transmission with the proportion attributed to exposure to contaminated blood or other risk factors.

Nigerian military personnel find themselves in professional and personal situations that increase their likelihood of engaging in behavior that places them at high risk for contracting STIs, including HIV. In view of the fact that military personnel live with and interact freely with the civilian population, they could serve as a potential core transmission group to the larger population.

PREVENTION AND CONTROL

Data on HIV prevalence among the military are difficult to obtain, as governments are often unwilling to disclose high rates, for fear of seeming vulnerable to enemies and coups. For similar reasons, comprehensive HIV testing programs for military personnel in sub-Saharan Africa are rare.

While considerable attention has been paid to the role of antiretrovirals in AIDS therapy, treatment includes a range of care options, including therapies for opportunistic infections and palliative care. Furthermore, treatment itself should be seen as part of a comprehensive workplace program. Such programs are increasingly expected to include nondiscriminatory policies, education about HIV prevention, condom distribution, voluntary counseling and testing, and the provision of care, support, and treatment.

Treatment can also serve as an entry point to ensure that these other components are in place. Elements of a comprehensive workplace program response are interdependent and include sound non-discrimination and confidentiality policies that promote a secure environment for employees to receive testing as well as treatment services. Experience shows that people are more likely to take advantage of testing services when they are linked with treatment programs.

In a study to evaluate the effectiveness of a situationally based HIV risk-reduction intervention for the Nigerian uniformed services to adopt condom use with casual partners, 36% of participants in the intervention and control groups reported that they had not thought of using condoms with casual partners at baseline (11). A positive intervention effect was observed in the intervention but not the control regiment at the 6-month (40% vs. 0.9%) and 12-month (46.8% vs 4.3%) follow-up assessments ($p < 0.05$). These data confirm that a situationally based intervention with uniformed service personnel has a significant and powerful impact on reported condom use.

Prevention activities should be implemented both during and after conflicts. Such activities should be designed to be sustainable, and uniformed service personnel should offer training as peer educators. Even when soldiers are not deployed abroad they are generally posted away from their families and sexual partners. In spending months at a time in the barracks, military personnel often seek out sexual partners locally, and it is not unusual for them to have regular contact with sex workers (8).

Responsibility and respect for rank and position should be used constructively to promote the notions of safe sex and other personal protection options, as well as protection of families. All peacekeepers should have unlimited access to information about HIV/AIDS and the various ways to protect themselves. They should also have unlimited access to condoms, and the assurance of an appropriate supply of condoms should be included in logistical planning.

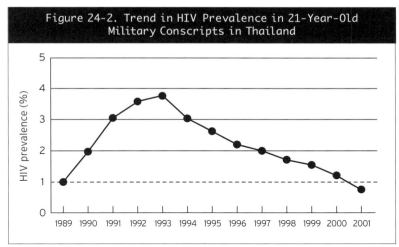

Figure 24-2. Trend in HIV Prevalence in 21-Year-Old Military Conscripts in Thailand

Source: Armed Forces Research Institute of Medical Sciences, Thailand.

The experiences of some countries suggest that HIV control programs can be effective in the military. Since the beginning of the epidemic, for example, the Royal Thai Army has realized that HIV poses a threat to individual military members as well as to national security at large. Through a strong and ongoing commitment to fight HIV in Thailand, the country has been able to control its epidemic, notably among its young soldiers, whose HIV prevalence rate dropped from nearly 4% in 1993 to under 1% in 2001 (Figure 24-2). In Uganda, HIV prevalence rates among soldiers aged 19 to 22 years decreased from 18.6% in 1991 to 4% in 2002.

SPECIAL ISSUES

A number of other issues unique to HIV/AIDS in the uniformed services include demobilized personnel, peacekeeping operations, and the growing proportion of women in the military.

Demobilized Personnel

As conflicts around the world end, military and uniformed services demobilize troops in large numbers. Demobilization—which involves reducing the number of members of uniformed personnel in national armies or disbanding and disarming irregular armies and militias—presents both a challenge and an opportunity. The challenge is to reach troops prior to demobilization with HIV/AIDS prevention and care education and information, before they function as bridge populations to the general community. Demobilization also presents a significant opportunity to create a cadre of change agents that will be reintegrated into the general civil community.

Peacekeeping Operations

Peacekeeping has become an important role for military forces the world over. National armies are increasingly requested to contribute troops and support staff to war zones and post-conflict milieu. During the past two decades, Nigerian troops have been involved in peacekeeping operations in many countries, including Congo, Côte d'Ivoire, Liberia, Sierra Leone, and Sudan. The United Nations Department of Peace Keeping Operations recommends that military personnel infected with HIV or other STIs not be deployed to peacekeeping operations and that all countries contributing peacekeepers provide their troops with standardized guidelines and training on prevention and control of HIV and other STIs (7). Once deployed, otherwise healthy HIV-positive UN peacekeepers are not repatriated on account of their HIV status; those with AIDS symptoms, however, are sent home.

Women in the Military

Although women are often in the minority in military and police forces, more and more women are enlisting in the uniformed services. In Nigeria, for instance, females constitute 6% to 10% of the military (4). These women are exposed to the same — and sometimes even greater — pressure as men to enter into casual sexual relationships. Women are also more vulnerable to HIV transmission through sex with infected partners. Efforts are needed to ensure that their needs are met through gender-sensitive AIDS control programs.

POLICY RECOMMENDATIONS

Some form of qualitative assessment should be instituted to assess the knowledge, attitudes, and practices of officers and the general military personnel about HIV and other STIs. This assessment should determine not only perceived risk and high-risk behavior, but also where they seek treatment for STIs, when they use condoms, what they do for recreation, whom they listen to for information about HIV and other STIs, and what they value. A trained counselor or health professional should conduct this assessment on a regular basis. A strategic plan based on this assessment should then integrate HIV/AIDS and other STIs programs into existing systems and structures and foster behavior change through information dissemination. A clear network of peer educators and other communication means should be developed to ensure that all soldiers have unlimited access to information and understand how to protect themselves.

Policies should be instituted to make condoms regularly available and freely distributed, with the goal of achieving a 100%-condom-use rate. This policy is particularly important when men and women are posted to foreign missions or are away from their families for more than six months.

Further studies are also needed to determine the ideal duration of time military personnel can spend away from their base yet still avoid high-risk sexual relationships.

Moreover, effective voluntary counseling and testing (VCT) and sentinel surveillance should be established in the military. Those confirmed to be HIV positive should receive assurances not only about the confidentiality of their test result, but also about their job security and the possibility of advancement in rank at least until medical discharge from the service. Such assurances will encourage people to take part in VCT without fear of stigmatization or discrimination.

Also critical is the establishment of a fully integrated and comprehensive care and support system for infected people, support groups, and their families. HIV prevention should be integrated into demobilization activities, and outreach programs should be extended to personnel who have been discharged from service. Finally, an effective monitoring and evaluation system of various strategies should be established to identify which strategies are workable and to ensure quality services at all levels.

CONCLUSION

Two decades after Nigeria's first AIDS case was reported, it is increasingly clear that the epidemic constitutes a security threat that cannot be ignored. The military is a high-risk population because of its demographic constitution, social norms, and occupational exposures. It is also clear that the walls of military bases constitute no barriers to the bidirectional transmission of HIV between military and civilian populations. With increasing funding available for HIV prevention and treatment in the country, the growing HIV epidemic in the military deserves more serious and sustained attention.

REFERENCES

1. UNAIDS. *AIDS and the Military*. Best Practice Collection. Geneva: UNAIDS, 1998.

2. U.S. Bureau of the Census, Population Division. *International Programs Center HIV/AIDS Surveillance Data*. Washington, DC: U.S. Bureau of the Census, 1998.

3. Sarin R. *A New Security Threat: HIV/AIDS in the Military*. Washington, DC: Worldwatch Institute, 2003.

4. Adebajo SB, Mafeni J, Moreland S, et al. *Knowledge, Attitudes and Sexual Behaviour Among Nigerian Military Concerning HIV/AIDS and STD: Final Technical Report*. Abuja, Nigeria: POLICY Project, 2002.

5. UNAIDS. Engaging Uniformed Services in the Fight Against HIV/AIDS. Accessed at https://uniformedservices.unaids.org on July 8, 2005.

6. Noah D, Fidas G. *The Global Infectious Disease Threat and Its Implications for the United States*. Washington, DC: National Intelligence Council, 2000.

7. United Nations. Press Release: Security Council Holds Debate on Impact of AIDS on Peace and Security in Africa. SC/6781. January 10, 2000.

8. Lovgren S. African Army hastening HIV/AIDS spread. *Jenda: A Journal of Culture and African Women Studies*, 2001;1,2.

9. Temoshok L. HIV exposure and transmission risk in military populations: uncharted prevention frontier. *XI International Conference on AIDS*, Vancouver, Canada, July 12, 1996 (abstract Mo.D.354).

10. Adefolalu A. AIDS in the military. *Third All African Congress of Armed Forces and Police Medical Services*, Pretoria, South Africa, 1999.

11. Essien J, Meshack A, Ekong E, et al. Effectiveness of a situationally-based HIV risk-reduction intervention for the Nigerian Uniformed Services on readiness to adopt condom use with casual partners. *Counselling, Psychotherapy, and Health*, 2005;1(1), 19–30.

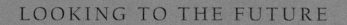

LOOKING TO THE FUTURE

Living Positively with HIV

MOHAMMED FAROUK AND HIS WIFE, MARIA, couldn't have felt happier; she was expecting twins, their first children. But then the first blow fell—she was diagnosed with HIV during routine hospital testing. Then he tested positive. Then she lost the twins. But the couple had little time to grieve. ■ Farouk, a soldier in the army, reported his diagnosis to his commandant, hoping his military benefits would allow his family additional medical

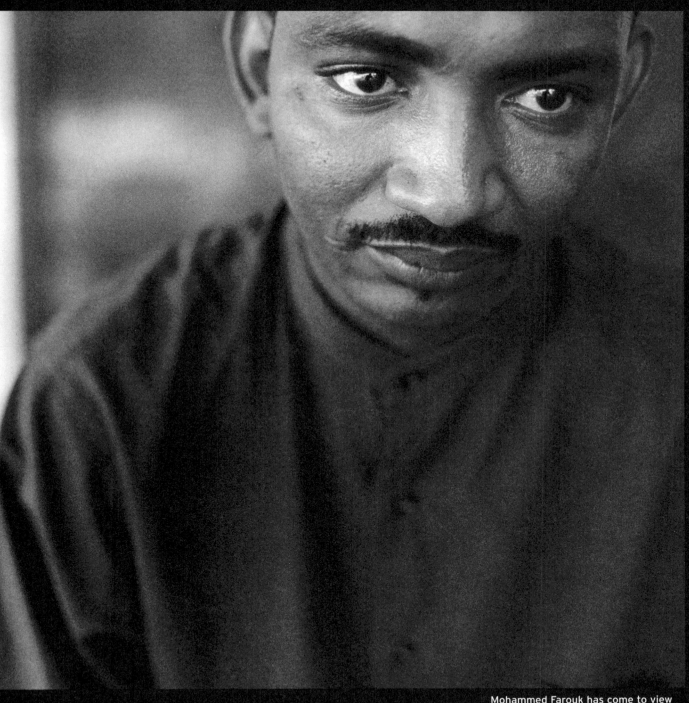

Mohammed Farouk has come to view his HIV infection as a new lease on life.

care. Instead, his superior officer ordered him locked up in the guardroom, where he remained for two weeks. Upon his release, he challenged his commandant and quit his military position, only to discover later that the army had indeed earmarked benefits for soldiers with HIV; the man responsible for the compensation fund had simply embezzled the money.

Senior officers, fearing that Farouk would expose them, referred him to a Nigerian doctor who claimed his special vaccine would cure Farouk and 30 other soldiers who were infected. The chief of army staff soon trumpeted the vaccine's success. Angered by the transparent lie, Farouk decided to take his story national.

In 1999, Farouk became one of the first Nigerians to acknowledge his HIV infection publicly. "At first," he says, "I felt stigmatized and humiliated. My colleagues, my friends, and even some of my relatives avoided me."

To gather strength, he tapped into a worldwide community of activists who were infected with HIV. In 2000, when he attended an international AIDS conference in Durban, South Africa, he met people living with HIV/AIDS who were determined to slow the spread of the virus and to give hope to other infected people. He returned home inspired to form Nigeria's first support group for people living with HIV/AIDS. Since then, as cofounder and coordinator of the AIDS Alliance in Nigeria, he has played a critical role in shaping the public response to the epidemic by involving people infected with HIV in policy and outreach efforts.

The AIDS Alliance in Nigeria now pursues three principal strategies: to convene support groups of people living with HIV; to expose and correct violations of individual rights; and to build awareness about the virus. The organization brings together people living with HIV/AIDS to meet and discuss topics central to their own lives and to the future of Nigeria. Participants also share information about health maintenance, nutrition, antiretroviral therapy, and policy developments. The groups not only function as a support network for participants, but they also offer one-on-one and group counseling by trained volunteers.

In addition, the alliance works with the government and some pharmaceutical companies to subsidize the cost of antiretrovirals for members. It also refers members to other nongovernmental organizations for help with specific issues, such as employment-related discrimination.

Since founding the alliance, Farouk has become instrumental in forming other AIDS support groups, and his work has inspired the creation of several additional ones. Farouk has also launched a newsletter, *Positive News*, which provides information about the epidemic, tracks AIDS policy developments, and tells the powerful stories of people living with HIV/AIDS.

"When I first learned I was infected, I assumed it was a death sentence," Farouk says. "I thought my life was ending. But eventually I realized the opposite had happened. My new life was just beginning. Somehow, during all the psychological trauma, stigmatization, and discrimination I suffered in the army, I found the inner strength to speak out. In life, nothing can bring you down without your permission. Even natural phenomena such as disease, war, and famine cannot stop you from living a fulfilled life. As soon as I announced my HIV status to the world, I began living more fully. Now I feel I am living positively with the virus."

CONCLUSION

When describing Nigeria, we often resort to numbers. The most populous nation in Africa, Nigeria is home to more than 130 million people. These individuals belong to more than 350 ethnic and linguistic groups, and their country is ranked among the 25 poorest in the world. And when we try to portray the country's HIV epidemic, the numbers quickly become daunting: As many as six million people already infected with the virus. HIV prevalence rates in some states as high as 12 percent. At least two million children orphaned by AIDS.

These numbers, of course, are expected to worsen as the virus continues to spread. Some experts predict that, within the decade, as many as nine million more Nigerians will become infected. But this last, tragically monolithic number is not inevitable. Despite the challenges the sheer size of its diverse population poses, Nigeria carries several distinct advantages. Its epidemic was relatively slow to develop, allowing the country time to benefit from the accumulated wisdom of other nations. Civil society organizations have shown great energy and creativity in launching interventions. Since its return to democracy in 1999, the federal government has been responsive, with the president taking a strong, personal stance. And more recently international agencies have stepped in to help.

The HIV/AIDS epidemic in Nigeria remains a formidable challenge to all sectors of society, yet it is a challenge the Nigerian people can meet. We are confident that their concerted and sustained efforts will result in a new set of figures: the number of new infections prevented, the number of HIV-infected people receiving lifesaving treatment, the number of children able to grow up with their parents.

Olusoji Adeyi, MD, MPH, DrPH
Phyllis J. Kanki, DVM, DSc
Oluwole Odutolu, MD, MBA
John A. Idoko, MD, FMCP

Lawrence Adeokun, PhD
Director, Evaluation and
Operations Research
Association for Reproductive and
Family Health
815A Army Officers Mess Road
Ikolaba GRA
P.O. Box 30259
Ibadan, Nigeria
Email: adeokun_la@yahoo.com

Isaac F. Adewole, MBBS,
FMCOG, FWACS
Provost, College of Medicine
University of Ibadan
University College Hospital
Queen Elizabeth II Road
Ibadan, Nigeria
Email: ifadewole@yahoo.co.uk

Olusoji Adeyi, MD, MPH, DrPH
Coordinator, Public Health Programs
World Bank
1818 H Street, NW
Washington, DC 20433, USA
Email: oadeyi@worldbank.org

Babatunde A. Ahonsi, PhD
Senior Program Officer
Ford Foundation (West Africa)
Akin Adesola Street V.I.
Lagos, Nigeria
Email: b.ahonsi@fordfound.org

Job Ailuogwemhe, MD
Research Associate
Department of Immunology and
Infectious Diseases
Harvard School of Public Health
651 Huntington Avenue
Boston, MA 02115
Email: jailuogw@hsph.harvard.edu

David Canning, PhD
Professor
Department of Population and
International Health
Harvard School of Public Health
665 Huntington Avenue
Boston, MA 02115, USA
Email: dcanning@hsph.harvard.edu

Ernest Ekong, MD, MPH
National Clinical Coordinator
APIN Plus/Harvard PEPFAR
c/o Nigerian Institute of Medical
Research
6 Edmond Crescent
Yaba, Lagos, Nigeria
Email: eekong@hsph.harvard.edu

Oluwole A. Fajemisin, MBBS,
MPH, MSc
National Program Officer, HIV/AIDS
World Health Organization
Block C Nalda Building
Old State Secretariat Complex
Old Airport Road
P.M.B. 208
Minna, Niger State, Nigeria
Email: woleafajemisin@yahoo.com

Adesegun O. Fatusi, MBChB, MPH,
FWACP
Senior Lecturer
Department of Community Health
College of Health Sciences
Obafemi Awolowo University
Ile-Ife, Osun State, Nigeria
Email: adesegunfatusi@yahoo.co.uk

Michael Gboun, MD, MPH
Monitoring and Evaluation Officer
UNAIDS Inter-Country Team for
East and Southern Africa

Metropark Building
351 Schoeman Street
Pretoria, South Africa
Email: mgboun@un.org.za

Tekena O. Harry, PhD
Professor of Virology
Department of Immunology and
Microbiology
University of Maiduguri Teaching
Hospital
P.M.B. 1414
Maiduguri, Nigeria
Email: tekenaharry@hotmail.com

Oni E. Idigbe, PhD
Director-General
Nigerian Institute of Medical Research
P.M.B. 2013
Yaba, Lagos, Nigeria
Email: oniidigbe@yahoo.com

Omokhudu Idogho, MD
Deputy Director/Head of Programme
Education, RSHR, HIV/AIDS and
Programme Measurement
ActionAid International Nigeria
Plot 590, Cadestral Zone
2nd Floor, NAIC Building
Central Area
Abuja, Nigeria
Email: omokhudu.idogho@actionaid.org

John A. Idoko, MD, FMCP
Professor of Medicine
Head, Infectious Diseases Program
Director, APIN and APIN Plus
Programs
Jos University Teaching Hospital
Murtala Mohammed Way
Jos, Nigeria
Email: jonidoko@yahoo.com

Akin Jimoh, MSc, MPH
Program Director
Development Communications
Network
Media Resources and Advocacy Centre
26 Adebola Street, Off Adeniran
Ogunsanya Street Surulere
Lagos, Nigeria
Email: ajimoh@devcomsnetwork.org

Oluwatoyin M. Jolayemi, MD, MPH
Program Manager
AIDS Prevention Initiative in Nigeria
990 NAL Boulevard
Central Business District
Abuja, Nigeria
Email: toyin_jolayemi@yahoo.com

Phyllis J. Kanki, DVM, DSc
Director, AIDS Prevention Initiative
in Nigeria
Principal Investigator, Harvard
PEPFAR/APIN Plus
Professor of Immunology and
Infectious Diseases
Harvard School of Public Health
651 Huntington Avenue
Boston, MA 02115, USA
Email: apin@hsph.harvard.edu

Oladapo A. Ladipo, FRCOG
Professor of Obstetrics and
Gynecology
President and CEO
Association for Reproductive and
Family Health
815A Army Officers Mess Road
Ikolaba GRA
P.O. Box 30259
Ibadan, Nigeria
Email: oladepod@yahoo.com

continued on next page

LIST OF ACRONYMS

AIDS	acquired immunodeficiency syndrome
APIN	AIDS Prevention Initiative in Nigeria
ART	antiretroviral therapy
ARV	antiretroviral
BCC	behavior change communication
CBO	community-based organization
CISCGHAN	Civil Society Consultative Group on HIV/AIDS in Nigeria
CSO	civil society organization
CSW	commercial sex worker
DFID	Department for International Development
FBO	faith-based organization
FHI	Family Health International
FMOH	Federal Ministry of Health
HAART	highly active antiretroviral therapy
HEAP	HIV/AIDS Emergency Action Plan
HIV	human immunodeficiency virus
IDU	injection drug user
IEC	information, education, and communication
JUTH	Jos University Teaching Hospital
LACA	local action committee on AIDS
LUTH	Lagos University Teaching Hospital
MARP	most-at-risk person
M&E	monitoring and evaluation
MTCT	mother-to-child transmission of HIV
MTP	Medium-Term Plan
MSM	men who have sex with men
NACA	National Action Committee on AIDS

continued on page 577

continued from previous page

Adetokunbo O. Lucas, MD
Adjunct Professor
Department of Population and
International Health
Harvard School of Public Health
665 Huntington Avenue
Boston, MA 02115, USA
Email: tokunbo@hsph.harvard.edu

Jerome O. Mafeni, MPH, MDSc, FMCDS, FWACS
Chief of Party, ENHANSE Project
The Futures Group
50 Haile Selassie Street, Asokoro
P.M.B. 533 Garki PO, FCT
Abuja, Nigeria
Email: jmafeni@futuresgroup.com

Ajay Mahal, PhD
Assistant Professor of International
Health Economics
Department of Population and
International Health
Harvard School of Public Health
665 Huntington Avenue
Boston, MA 02115, USA
Email: amahal@hsph.harvard.edu

Souleymane Mboup, PharmD, PhD
Professor of Microbiology
Laboratoire de Bacteriologie Virologie
Université Cheikh Anta Diop
CHU Le Dantec
BP 7325
Dakar, Senegal
Email: mboup@rarslbv.org

Seema Thakore Meloni, PhD, MPH
Postdoctoral Fellow
Department of Immunology and
Infectious Diseases
Harvard School of Public Health
651 Huntington Avenue
Boston, MA 02115, USA
Email: sthakore@hsph.harvard.edu

Jane Miller, MSc
Health and HIV/AIDS Adviser
Department for International
Development, Zambia
British High Commission
Plot 5210 Independence Avenue
P.O. Box 50050
Lusaka, Zambia
Email: j-miller@dfid.gov.uk

Idris Mohammed, OON, MD, FRCP, DTM&H, FAS
Professor of Medicine and Clinical
Immunology
Department of Medicine
Federal Medical Centre
Ashaka Road
Gombe, Gombe State, Nigeria
Email: iidrismohammed@netscape.net

Robert L. Murphy, MD
John Phair Professor of Medicine
Division of Infectious Diseases
Northwestern University Feinberg
School of Medicine
676 North Saint Clair Street
Suite 200
Chicago, IL 60611, USA
Email: r-murphy@northwestern.edu

Abdulsalami Nasidi, MD, PhD, OON
Director, Special Projects
Federal Ministry of Health
Federal Secretariat
Shehu Shagari Way
Maitama, Abuja, Nigeria
Email: nasidia@hotmail.com

Iyabo Obasanjo, DVM, PhD
Commissioner for Health
Ogun State Ministry of Health
Oke-Ilewo
Abeokuta, Ogun State, Nigeria
Email: iobas@hotmail.com

Georgina N. Odaibo, PhD
Lecturer I
Department of Virology
College of Medicine
University of Ibadan
University College Hospital
P.M.B. 5116
Ibadan, Nigeria
Email: foreodaibo@hotmail.com

Olakunle Odumosu, PhD
Professor
Social Development Department
Nigerian Institute of Social and
Economic Research
Oyo Road, Ojoo
Ibadan, Nigeria
Email: ofodumosu@yahoo.com

Oluwole Odutolu, MD, MBA
Senior Program Manager
AIDS Prevention Initiative in Nigeria
990 NAL Boulevard
Central Business District
Abuja, Nigeria
Email: apin@cgiar.org

**Modupe D. Oduwole, MBBS, MPH,
FWACP**
Director
Ogun State AIDS Control Program
4 Kemta Road
Idi Aba, Off Moshood Abiola Way
Abeokuta, Ogun State, Nigeria
Email: mdoduwole@yahoo.com

Irene Ogbogu, PhD
Executive Director
Women's Health, Education
and Development
Plot 288 Lagos Street, Off Samuel
Ladoke Akintola Boulevard
Garki II, Abuja, Nigeria
Email: whednigeria@yahoo.co.uk

**Folasade T. Ogunsola, MD,
FMCPath, FWACP, PhD**
Associate Professor, Medical
Microbiology
Department of Medical Microbiology
and Parasitology
College of Medicine
University of Lagos
P.M.B. 12003
Lagos, Nigeria
Email: sade.ogunsola@aoaglobal.com

continued on next page

LIST OF ACRONYMS *(continued)*

NEPWHAN	Network of People with HIV/AIDS in Nigeria
NDHS	National Demographic and Health Survey
NGO	nongovernmental organization
NIMR	Nigerian Institute of Medical Research
NISER	Nigerian Institute of Social and Economic Research
NNRIMS	Nigerian National Response Information Management System
PCR	polymerase chain reaction
PEPFAR	President's Emergency Plan for AIDS Relief
PLWHA	person living with HIV/AIDS
PMTCT	prevention of mother-to-child transmission of HIV
PSSH	Plateau State Specialist Hospital, Jos
SACA	State Action Committee on AIDS
SFH	Society for Family Health
STD	sexually transmitted disease
STI	sexually transmitted infection
SWAAN	Society for Women and AIDS in Africa, Nigeria
UCH	University College Hospital, Ibadan
UMTH	University of Maiduguri Teaching Hospital
UNAIDS	Joint United Nations Program on HIV/AIDS
UNFPA	United Nations Population Fund
VCT	voluntary counseling and testing
WHED	Women's Health, Education and Development

continued from previous page

Akinyemi Ojesina, MD
APIN Fellow
AIDS Prevention Initiative in Nigeria
Harvard School of Public Health
651 Huntington Avenue
Boston, MA 02115, USA
Email: aojesina@hsph.harvard.edu

Prosper Okonkwo, MD, FMCPH
Program Manager
AIDS Prevention Initiative in Nigeria
c/o IITA HQ
ELO Building 35/38
P.M.B. 5320, Oyo Road
Ibadan, Nigeria
Email: p.okonkwo@cgiar.org

David O. Olaleye, DVM, PhD
Professor of Virology
Head, Department of Virology
College of Medicine
University of Ibadan
University College Hospital
P.M.B. 5116
Ibadan, Nigeria
Email: ibvirology@yahoo.com

Viola Adaku Onwuliri, PhD
Associate Professor
Department of Biochemistry
Faculty of Medical Sciences
University of Jos
P.M.B. 2084
Jos, Nigeria
Email: vonwuliri@yahoo.com

Atiene Solomon Sagay, MBBS, FWACS, MRCOG
Associate Professor
Department of Obstetrics and
Gynaecology
Faculty of Medical Sciences
University of Jos
P.M.B. 2084
Jos, Nigeria
Email: atsagay58@yahoo.com

Lateef Salako, MBBS, PhD, DSc, FRCP
Chief Executive
Federal Vaccine Production
Laboratory
Yaba, Lagos, Nigeria
Email: lateefsalako@yahoo.com

Jean-Louis Sankalé, PharmD, DSc
Senior Research Scientist
AIDS Prevention Initiative in Nigeria
Department of Immunology and
Infectious Diseases
Harvard School of Public Health
651 Huntington Avenue
Boston, MA 02115, USA
Email: jsankale@hsph.harvard.edu

Abdoulaye Dieng Sarr, PharmD, DSc
Senior Research Scientist
Department of Immunology and
Infectious Diseases
Harvard School of Public Health
651 Huntington Avenue
Boston, MA 02115, USA
Email: adsarr@hsph.harvard.edu

Adedoyin Soyibo, PhD
Director, Health Policy Training and
Research Programme
Department of Economics
University of Ibadan
Ibadan, Nigeria
Email: adedoyin.soyibo@mail.ui.edu.ng

Babafemi Taiwo, MD
Fellow in Infectious Diseases
Division of Infectious Diseases
Northwestern University Feinberg
School of Medicine
676 North Saint Clair Street
Suite 200
Chicago, IL 60611, USA
Email: b-taiwo@northwestern.edu